Surgical Oncology Manual

Frances C. Wright • Jaime M. Escallon
Moises Cukier • Melanie E. Tsang
Usmaan Hameed
Editors

Surgical Oncology Manual

Third Edition

Springer

Editors
Frances C. Wright
Department of Surgery
University of Toronto
Toronto, ON
Canada

Jaime M. Escallon
Department of Surgery
University of Toronto
Toronto, ON
Canada

Moises Cukier
Department of Surgery
University of Toronto
Toronto, ON
Canada

Melanie E. Tsang
Department of Surgery
University of Toronto
Toronto, ON
Canada

Usmaan Hameed
Department of Surgery
University of Toronto
Toronto, ON
Canada

Originally published by the Department of Surgery, University of Toronto, Canada (March 25, 2013)
ISBN 978-3-030-48362-3 ISBN 978-3-030-48363-0 (eBook)
https://doi.org/10.1007/978-3-030-48363-0

This Springer imprint is published by the registered company Springer Nature Switzerland AG
The registered company address is: Gewerbestrasse 11, 6330 Cham, Switzerland

Preface

Dear Colleagues,

I am delighted to present the third edition of *The University of Toronto Surgical Oncology Manual*. This is a collaborative work between the breast, general surgical oncology, hepatopancreatobiliary- transplant and minimally invasive fellowship programmes at the University of Toronto as well as our colleagues in medical oncology, radiation oncology, plastic surgery, thoracic surgery, interventional radiology, dermatology, geriatrics and pathology.

The manual represents a concise, usable and practical manual for the busy resident, fellow and staff looking for the latest information on cancers that are treated surgically. Although the focus of this manual is surgical treatment of cancers, we have also included discussion of systemic and radiation treatments and how these treatments interact with surgery as well as non-surgical loco-regional therapies administered by surgeons as it reflects our current practice.

For this particular edition, we have introduced three new chapters: geriatric surgical oncology, which will be an increasingly large focus of our practice, oesophageal cancer and malignancy of unknown primary.

I am truly grateful for the many hours of work all present and past authors and editors have put into both this current edition as well as previous editions. Thank you to all for all your efforts.

With Thanks,

Toronto, ON, Canada Frances C. Wright, MD, Med, FRCSC MD, Med, FRCSC

Acknowledgement

To all fellows and staff for their invaluable contribution.

To the General Surgery Oncology Fellowship Program for their financial support.

The Editors would also like to acknowledge with thanks the following individuals who have kindly granted us permission for the use of material in this publication:

Previous Fellows
Dan Charlton
Juan Camilo Correa
Gareth Eeson
Mai Kim Gervais
Trevor Hamilton
Usmaan Hameed
Jessica Maxwell
Andrea MacNeill
Vanessa Palter
Jennifer Racz
Amanda Roberts
Koji Tomiyama
Amelie Tremblay

Previous Authors
Martin Blackstein
Zane Cohen
Bernard Cummings
Paul Karanicolas
Peter Kim
Robin McLeod
Paul Ridgway
Corwyn Rowsell

Contents

Contributors

Wadid W. K. Abadir Department of Dermatology, University of Toronto, Toronto, ON, Canada

Albiruni R. Abdul Razak Department of Medicine, University of Toronto, Toronto, ON, Canada

Shabbir M. H. Alibhai Division of Geriatric Medicine, Department of Medicine, University of Toronto, Toronto, ON, Canada

Institute of Health Policy, Management, and Evaluation, University of Toronto, Toronto, ON, Canada

Department of Medicine, University Health Network, Toronto, ON, Canada

Naser AlQurini Division of Geriatric Medicine, Department of Medicine, University of Toronto, Toronto, ON, Canada

Department of Medicine, University of Toronto, Toronto, ON, Canada

Shady Ashamalla Department of Surgery, University of Toronto, Toronto, ON, Canada

Angela Assal Department of Medicine, University of Toronto, Toronto, ON, Canada

Nancy N. Baxter Department of Surgery, University of Toronto, Toronto, ON, Canada

Melbourne School of Population and Global Health, University of Melbourne, Melbourne, Victoria, Australia

Danielle Bischof Department of Surgery, Sinai Health System, Toronto, ON, Canada

Jessica Bogach General Surgical Oncology, University of Toronto, Toronto, ON, Canada

Jean-Francois Boileau Department of Surgery, Sir Mortimer B. Davis Jewish General Hospital, McGill University, Montreal, QC, Canada

Savtaj S. Brar Department of Surgery, University of Toronto, Toronto, ON, Canada

James Brierley Department of Radiation Oncology, University of Toronto, Toronto, ON, Canada

Marcus J. Burnstein Department of Surgery, University of Toronto, Toronto, ON, Canada

Marcus O. Butler Department of Medical Oncology and Hematology, University of Toronto, Toronto, ON, Canada

Department of Medicine, University of Toronto, Toronto, ON, Canada

Dario Callegaro MD General Surgical Oncology, University of Toronto, Toronto, ON, Canada

Charles Catton MD, FRCPC Department of Radiation Oncology, University of Toronto, Toronto, ON, Canada

Tyler R. Chesney Department of Surgery, University of Toronto, Toronto, ON, Canada

General Surgical Oncology, University of Toronto, Toronto, ON, Canada

William Chu Department of Radiation Oncology, University of Toronto, Toronto, ON, Canada

Tulin Cil Department of Surgery, University of Toronto, Toronto, ON, Canada

Sean Cleary Department of Surgery, Mayo Clinic, Rochester, MN, USA

Natalie G. Coburn Department of Surgery, Sunnybrook Health Sciences Centre, University of Toronto, Toronto, ON, Canada

Department of Surgery, University of Toronto, Toronto, ON, Canada

Mark Corrigan Department of Surgery, Cork University Hospital, Cork, Ireland

Andrea M. Covelli General Surgical Oncology, University of Toronto, Toronto, ON, Canada

Moises Cukier Department of Surgical Oncology, National Cancer Institute, Panama City, Panama

Gail Darling Department of Surgery, University of Toronto, Toronto, ON, Canada

Nicolas Devaud Complex General Surgical Oncology, University of Toronto, Toronto, ON, Canada

Karen Devon Department of Surgery, University of Toronto, Toronto, ON, Canada

Brendan C. Dickson MD, MSc, FCAP, FRCPC Department of Laboratory Medicine and Pathobiology, University of Toronto, Toronto, ON, Canada

Alexandra M. Easson Department of Surgery, University of Toronto, Toronto, ON, Canada

Hyeyoun (Elise) Min Division of Plastic & Reconstructive Surgery, Sunnybrook University of Toronto, Toronto, ON, Canada

Christine Elser Department of Medical Oncology, Princess Margaret Cancer Centre, Toronto, ON, Canada

Department of Medical Oncology, University of Toronto, Toronto, ON, Canada

Jaime M. Escallon Department of Surgery, University of Toronto, Toronto, ON, Canada

Samir Fasih Medical Oncology, University of Toronto, Toronto, ON, Canada

Peter C. Ferguson MD, FRCSC, FAOA Department of Surgery, University of Toronto, Toronto, ON, Canada

Steven Gallinger Department of Surgery, University of Toronto, Toronto, ON, Canada

Ralph George Department of Surgery, University of Toronto, Toronto, ON, Canada

Rebecca A. Gladdy MD, PhD, FRCSC, FACS Department of Surgery, University of Toronto, Toronto, ON, Canada

Anand Govindarajan Department of Surgery, University of Toronto, Toronto, ON, Canada

Paul D. Greig Abdominal Organ Transplant and Hepatopancreatobiliary Surgery, Department of Surgery, University of Toronto, Toronto, ON, Canada

Robert Gryfe Department of Surgery, University of Toronto, Toronto, ON, Canada

Abha A. Gupta MD, MSc, FRCPC Division of Medical Oncology, University of Toronto, Toronto, ON, Canada

Vaibhav Gupta General Surgery Resident, University of Toronto, Toronto, ON, Canada

Julie Hallet Department of Surgery, University of Toronto, Toronto, ON, Canada

Usmaan Hameed Department of Surgery, University of Toronto, Toronto, ON, Canada

Moska Hamidi Department of Surgery, University of Toronto, Toronto, ON, Canada

General Surgical Oncology, University of Toronto, Toronto, ON, Canada

Lucy K. Helyer Department of Surgery, Dalhousie University, Halifax, NS, Canada

Naama Hermann Sunnybrook & University Health Network, University of Toronto, Toronto, ON, Canada

Claire Holloway Department of Surgery, University of Toronto, Toronto, ON, Canada

Ali Hosni Department of Radiation Oncology, University of Toronto, Toronto, ON, Canada

Eugene Hsieh Department of Pathology, University of Toronto, Toronto, ON, Canada

Shiva Jayaraman Department of Surgery, University of Toronto, Toronto, ON, Canada

Anthony M. Joshua Kinghorn Cancer Centre, St Vincents Hospital, Sydney, NSW, Australia

Ricky Jrearz General Surgical Oncology, University of Toronto, Toronto, ON, Canada

Paul J. Karanicolas Department of Surgery, University of Toronto, Toronto, ON, Canada

Erin Kennedy Department of Surgery, University of Toronto, Toronto, ON, Canada

Mohammadali Khorasani General Surgical Oncology, University of Toronto, Toronto, ON, Canada

Sepehr Khorasani Colorectal Surgery, University of Toronto, Toronto, ON, Canada

Richard Kirsch Department of Pathology, University of Toronto, Toronto, ON, Canada

Michael Ko Department of Surgery, University of Toronto, Toronto, ON, Canada

Monika K. Krzyzanowska Department of Medicine, University of Toronto, Toronto, ON, Canada

Girish S. Kulkarni Department of Surgery, University of Toronto, Toronto, ON, Canada

Nicholas Latchana Department of Surgery, University of Toronto, Toronto, ON, Canada

Lawrence Lau Department of Surgery, University of Toronto, Toronto, ON, Canada

Calvin H. L. Law Department of Surgery, University of Toronto, Toronto, ON, Canada

David W. Lim Breast Surgical Oncology, University of Toronto, Toronto, ON, Canada

Breast Surgical Oncology, Sunnybrook & University Health Network, University of Toronto, Toronto, ON, Canada

Sunnybrook & University Health Network, University of Toronto, Toronto, ON, Canada

Joan E. Lipa Department of Surgery, Division of Plastics and Reconstructive Surgery, University of Toronto, Toronto, ON, Canada

Department of Medical Oncology and Hematology, University of Toronto, Toronto, ON, Canada

Nicole J. Look Hong Department of Surgery, Division of Surgical Oncology, University of Toronto, Toronto, ON, Canada

Michail N. Mavros Complex General Surgical Oncology & HPB Surgery, University of Toronto, Toronto, ON, Canada

Andrea McCart Department of Surgery, University of Toronto, Toronto, ON, Canada

David R. McCready Department of Surgery, Division of Surgical Oncology, University of Toronto, Toronto, ON, Canada

Carol-anne E. Moulton Department of Surgery, University of Toronto, Toronto, ON, Canada

Janice R. Mulcahy St. Michael's Hospital, University of Toronto, Toronto, ON, Canada

Sten Myrehaug Department of Radiation Oncology, University of Toronto, Toronto, ON, Canada

Grainne M. O'Kane Department of Medical Oncology, University of Toronto, Toronto, ON, Canada

Jesse D. Pasternak Department of Surgery, University of Toronto, Toronto, ON, Canada

Teresa M. Petrella Department of Medical Oncology, University of Toronto, Toronto, ON, Canada

Aman Pooni Colorectal Surgery, University of Toronto, Toronto, ON, Canada

Fayez A. Quereshy Department of Surgery, University of Toronto, Toronto, ON, Canada

Jennifer M. Racz Department of Surgery, Mayo Clinic, Rochester, MN, USA

Lorne Rotstein Department of Surgery, University of Toronto, Toronto, ON, Canada

Erin M. Sadler General Surgery, University of Toronto, Toronto, ON, Canada

Department of Surgery, University of Toronto, Toronto, ON, Canada

Gonzalo Sapisochin Abdominal Organ Transplant and Hepatopancreatobiliary Surgery, Department of Surgery, University of Toronto, Toronto, ON, Canada

Blayne Amir Sayed Abdominal Organ Transplant and Hepatopancreatobiliary Surgery, Department of Surgery, University of Toronto, Toronto, ON, Canada

Eran Shlomovitz Department of Surgery, University of Toronto, Toronto, ON, Canada

Christopher R. Shubert Hepatopancreatobiliary Surgery, University of Toronto, Toronto, ON, Canada

Simron Singh Department of Medicine, University of Toronto, Toronto, ON, Canada

Laura Snell Department of Surgery, University of Toronto, Toronto, ON, Canada

Peter K. Stotland Department of Surgery, University of Toronto, Toronto, ON, Canada

Alexander Sun Department of Radiation Oncology, University of Toronto, Toronto, ON, Canada

Carol J. Swallow Department of Surgery, University of Toronto, Toronto, ON, Canada

Melanie E. Tsang Department of Surgery, University of Toronto, Toronto, ON, Canada

David R. Urbach Department of Surgery, University of Toronto, Toronto, ON, Canada

Alice C. Wei Department of Surgery, Memorial Sloan Kettering Cancer Center, New York, NY, USA

Edward Weiss Department of Medicine, University of Toronto, Toronto, ON, Canada

Frances C. Wright Department of Surgery, University of Toronto, Toronto, ON, Canada

Jonathan C. Yeung Department of Surgery, University of Toronto, Toronto, ON, Canada

Lu Yin Breast Surgical Oncology, Sunnybrook & University Health Network, University of Toronto, Toronto, ON, Canada

Tumors of the Adrenal Gland

1

Moska Hamidi, Michail N. Mavros, Karen Devon, Girish S. Kulkarni, Calvin H. L. Law, David R. Urbach, Julie Hallet, and Jesse D. Pasternak

Adrenal Incidentaloma

Background

An adrenal mass identified on an imaging study performed for reasons other than cancer staging or adrenal disease is considered an incidentaloma. Typically, this refers to lesions that are 1 cm or greater. According to autopsy series, clinically inapparent adrenal masses have a 2.1% prevalence, increasing up to 7% among those 70 years of age or older. However, literature reviews report an incidentalomas rate of 1–5% [1–3]. These lesions can be classified as functional or nonfunctional benign masses, and malignant tumors. More than 80% of incidentalomas are nonfunctional tumors, with cortical adenomas dominating as the most commonly identified incidentaloma. Of the remainder, approximately 5% cause subclinical or clinical Cushing syndrome (SCS), 5% are pheochromocytomas, 1% are aldosteronoma, while <5% make up adrenocortical carcinoma (ACC), and 2.5% are a metastatic lesion [4] (See Box 1.1).

Moska Hamidi and Michail N. Mavros contributed equally with all other contributors.

M. Hamidi · K. Devon · G. S. Kulkarni · C. H. L. Law · D. R. Urbach · J. Hallet
J. D. Pasternak (✉)
Department of Surgery, University of Toronto, Toronto, ON, Canada
e-mail: moh350@mail.harvard.edu; karen.devon@wchospital.ca; Girish.kulkarni@uhn.ca; Calvin.Law@sunnybrook.ca; david.urbach@wchospital.ca; julie.hallet@sunnybrook.ca; Jesse.Pasternak@uhn.ca

M. N. Mavros
Complex General Surgical Oncology & HPB Surgery, University of Toronto, Toronto, ON, Canada
e-mail: michail.mavros@mail.utoronto.ca

F. C. Wright et al. (eds.), *Surgical Oncology Manual*,
https://doi.org/10.1007/978-3-030-48363-0_1

Box 1.1 Differential diagnosis for adrenal incidentaloma

Functional Tumours	Pheochromocytoma	Cortisol Producing Adenoma	Aldosteronoma	Primary Adrenal Hyperplasia
Nonfunctional Tumours	Adenoma	Myelolipoma	Cyst	Ganglioneuroma
Malignant Tumours	Adrenocortical Carcinoma	Metastases		

Workup [4]

- When an adrenal mass is identified on imaging, the patient should be evaluated further to determine these key features that will help direct future management:
  - Determine if the tumor is functionally active (i.e., hypersecreting adrenal hormones)
  - Determine the risk of malignancy
- This should start with a detailed history and physical examination of the patient. The exam should focus on signs or symptoms of hormone excess, a personal history of cancer.
- To determine if the lesion is functional, a biochemical evaluation is required (see *algorithm 1*). Finally, a detailed review of the imaging which identified the lesion is required, followed with any further imaging, if necessary (Fig. 1.1).

Imaging

- Imaging is used to help distinguish between the different types of adrenal lesions in Box 1.1. Most adrenal lesions are described with CT scan or MRI [2].
- Adrenal CT protocol, which includes an unenhanced, early contrast-enhanced and delayed contrast-enhanced phase can help identify adenomas and differentiate lipid-poor adenomas from other lesions [2].
- While a formal adrenal protocol can help differentiate between adrenal adenoma, pheochromocytoma, metastatic lesions, and possibly adrenal cortical carcinoma, it does not take the place of formal biochemical testing [4].
- To differentiate the diagnosis of an adrenal lesion, radiologists rely on several imaging characteristics, including contrast enhancement, washout, and the Hounsfield units of different tumor types (see Table 1.1).
  - Size can be helpful to determine risk of malignancy as larger lesions have a much higher rate of cancer than smaller masses.
  - Specific criteria which increase the risk of a lesion include size greater than 4–6 cm on CT, tumors with $\geq$10 HU, a delayed washout of contrast (<40% at 15 min), calcification, irregular margins, or invasion into surrounding structures are all concerning features for malignancy [4, 5].
  - Malignant lesions typically have rapid initial enhancement with slow washout, in contrast to adenomas where contrast washout is rapid [5].

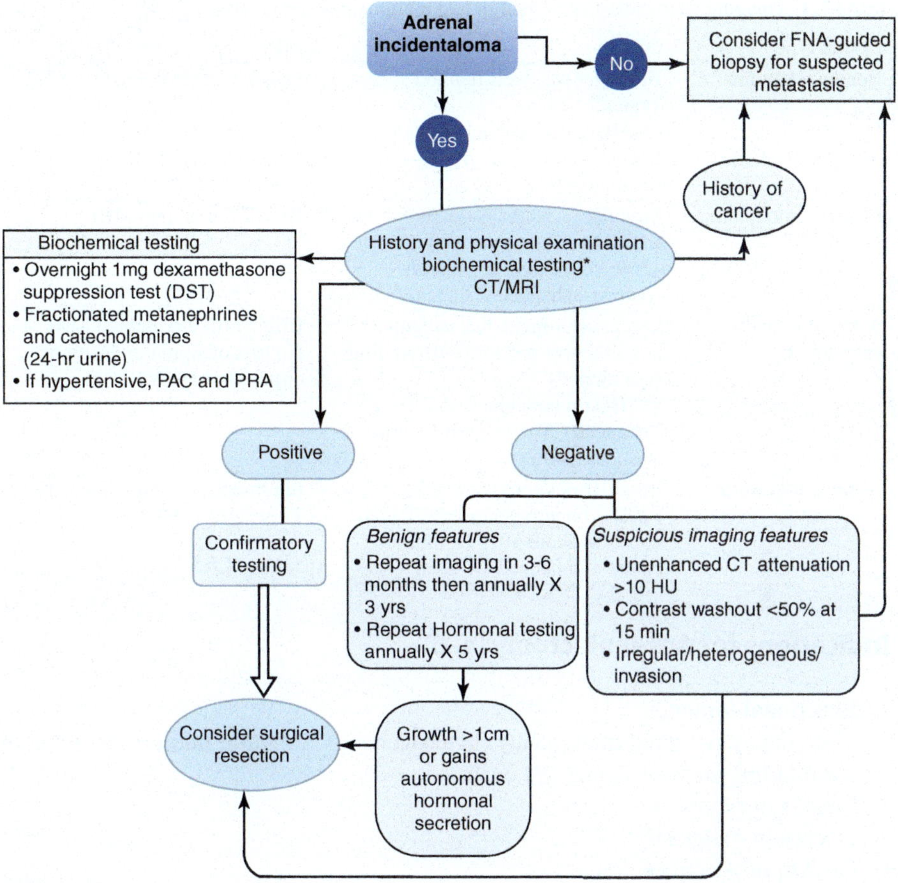

Fig. 1.1 Algorithm for workup and management of adrenal incidentaloma [23, 24]

Management and Follow-Up [4]

- There is a risk of mass enlargement or becoming functionally active.
  - One-, 2-, and 5-year risk of growth is 6%, 14%, and 29%, respectively.
  - One-, 2- and 5-year risk of hypersecreting hormones is 17%, 29%, and 47%, respectively.
- Therefore, lesions that do not meet criteria for surgical resection should be followed.
  - Repeat imaging at 6 months, then annually for 1–2 years.
  - Repeat functional testing can be considered.

Table 1.1 Imaging characteristics of benign and malignant adrenal masses [2, 4]

Lesion type	CT	MRI
Benign adenoma	Homogenous, well-defined Typically <4 cm <10HU on nonenhanced scan Enhanced CT scan with 15-min washout ≥40%	Low T2 signal intensity on MRI Loss of signal intensity on opposed-phase chemical shift sequences on MRI
Pheochromocytoma	Vascular >20HU on nonenhanced CT scan <50% washout at 15 min on contrast-enhanced CT scan	High T2 signal on MRI
Adrenocortical carcinoma	Large, heterogeneous, irregular, possible invasion into surrounding structures >18HU on nonenhanced CT scan Enhanced CT scan with 15-min washout ≤40%	Bright on T2-weighted MRI No loss of signal intensity on opposed-phase MRI images
Adrenal metastases	Irregular nonhomogeneous >20HU on nonenhanced CT scan <50% washout after 15 min on contrast-enhanced CT scan	Intermediate to high intensity on T2-weighted MRI

Indications for Adrenalectomy [4–6]

- Functional tumor
- Malignancy/potential malignancy (heterogeneous, irregular borders, invasion of surrounding structures, size ≥4 cm)
- Local symptoms
- Uncertain diagnosis
- Growth of >1 cm

Functional Adrenal Tumors

Pheochromocytoma

Overview

Workup

- All incidentalomas suspected of pheochromocytoma should be evaluated through history and physical examination.
  - Episodic headache.
  - Sweating.
  - Tachycardia.
  - Palpitations.
  - Tremor.
  - Hypertension.

Table 1.2 Workup and management of pheochromocytoma [4, 25]

Workup	Perioperative management	Surgical management	Adjunctive therapy (malignant disease)	Follow-up
History and physical *Laboratory investigations* Consider confirmatory test (i.e., clonidine suppression test) *Imaging* Thin-cut spiral CT or MRI MIBG scan (to assess for multiple tumors or malignancy) If MRI/CT negative and diagnosis still suspected >10 cm adrenal mass or paraganglionoma	*Preoperative* Alpha adrenergic blockade Fluid and electrolyte repletion Beta-blockade after alpha-blockade, as needed	*Benign disease* Laparoscopic adrenalectomy Minimal tumor handling to decrease excess catecholamine surge Early division of adrenal vein in laparoscopic anterior approach Close communication with anesthesia *Malignant disease* Resect primary and metastatic lesions if possible to reduce symptoms of hormone excess May improve efficacy of subsequent treatment	*Chemotherapy* [7] Consider in unresectable or rapidly growing tumors Combination of vincristine, cyclophosphamide, dacarbazine, doxorubicin ~50% will respond *Radiation* For bulky symptomatic primaries Bony metastases *I-131 MIBG* [8] If tumor takes up MIBG (60% of tumors) Response rate of 30% *Consider 68-Ga DOTATE or PRRT*	*Completely resected disease* Q6–12 months H&P BP check Plasma metane-phrines Annually Consider imaging *Incompletely resected disease* Q3–4 months H&P BP check Plasma metane-phrines Imaging

- Investigation for biochemical evidence of pheochromocytoma using measurement of plasma fractionated metanephrines and normetanephrines (more sensitive) OR 24-hour urinary metanephrines and fractionated catecholamines (more specific) [9] (see Table 1.2).
- If metastatic pheochromocytoma is suspected, further imaging may be indicated [9].
  - MIBG scan.
  - Somatostatin receptor-based imaging (i.e., ^{68}Ga-dotate PET/CT scintigraphy)[a].
  - FDG-PET/CT[b]

[a]^{68}Ga-dotatate PET/CT is more sensitive than somatostatin receptor scintigraphy for determining somatostatin receptor status [9]

[b]Both FDG-PET/CT and ^{68}Ga-dotatate PET/CT scintigraphy have >90% sensitivity, but signal intensity was significantly greater in the latter, with lower background activity [10]

Perioperative Considerations

- All patients should have α-adrenergic blockade for 1–3 weeks preoperatively [4].
  - Always start with α-blockers (e.g., phenoxybenzamine 10 mg BID or doxazosin).
  - Titrate dose until patient is normotensive or intolerable side effects develop (i.e., orthostatic hypotension).
  - May need to add β-blockade if they have persistent tachycardia or arrhythmias. Propranolol 10–40 mg q6–8 h most commonly used.
    Must not use β-blocker if alpha-blockade not optimized.
- Encourage liberal fluid and salt intake to counteract the intravascular volume depletion caused by pheochromocytoma.
- Intraoperative hypertension should be controlled with nitroprusside, nicardipine, nitroglycerine, or phentolamine. If tachyarrhythmia develops, treat with esmolol/ lidocaine.
- Monitor for hypotension and hypoglycemia in immediate postoperative period
- Hold all antihypertensive agents postoperatively; add back agents as needed as some patients have underlying essential hypertension.
- Do not abruptly stop β-blockers in patients treated chronically, especially older patients with ischemic heart disease [4].

Genetic Testing

- 25% of patients with pheochromocytoma have an associated genetic syndrome [4, 11].
  - These patients tend to present at a younger age and some with bilateral disease.
- Autosomal dominant familial disorders associated with adrenal pheochromocytoma.

Von-Hippel-Lindau (VHL) [12]
Pheochromocytoma (20%); paraganglioma; hemangioblastoma; retinal angioma; renal cell carcinoma; pancreatic neuroendocrine tumors; cystadenomas of pancreas, broad ligament and epididymis.
Multiple endocrine neoplasia type 2 (MEN-2) [12]
Pheochromocytoma (50%); medullary thyroid cancer (100%); primary hyperparathyroidism (20%); primary lichen amyloidosis (5%).
Only 3–5% of pheochromocytoma in MEN-2 are malignant. Highest risk seen in RET codon mutations 918, 634, 883).
Neurofibromatosis type 1 [12]
Pheochromocytoma (2%); café au lait patches; CNS gliomas; cognitive deficits; bony abnormalities.
Familial pheochromocytoma [12]
Germ-line mutations of genes encoding succinate dehydrogenase subunits B, C, and D.
Individuals with succinate dehydrogenase B mutations are more likely to develop malignant disease [13].

- Due to a high association of pheochromocytoma with genetic disease, all patients should be considered for screening.
- Testing includes mutations for RET, VHL genes, and subunits of succinate dehydrogenase genes [4].

Cushing Syndrome

Overview

Workup [4]

- Patients should also be evaluated for cardiovascular and metabolic comorbidities (diabetes, hypertension, osteoporosis) along with signs of hypercortisolism:
  - Weight gain.
  - Proximal muscle weakness.
  - Easy bruising, striae, skin atrophy.
  - Central obesity, dorsal cervical fat pad, "moon face."
- Severe hypercortisolism suppresses immunity and predisposes to severe infections [16].
- Patients with an adenoma without physical signs of hypercortisolism may have subclinical Cushing syndrome (SCS) and require further testing (see Table 1.3).
  - A diagnosis of SCS is still controversial, and many consider it a continuum between no functional excess and Cushing Syndrome; however, many con-

Table 1.3 Workup and management of cortisol-producing adenoma

Workup	Perioperative management	Surgical management	Medical Management
History and physical *Laboratory investigations* Screen with one of the following [14, 15]: 1 mg overnight dexamethasone suppression test Midnight salivary cortisol (≥2) 24-h UFC ≥ 2 Confirmatory testing if +ve If hypercortisolemic, perform serum ACTH (8 am cortisol) *Imaging* Thin-cut adrenal CT ± MRI	*Preoperative* VTE prophylaxis (>10-fold greater risk of VTE) Manage hyperglycemia Manage HTN Postoperative Maintain glucocorticoid therapy—may need stress dosing Manage hyperglycemia	Adrenalectomy[b] Unilateral for confirmed cortisol-producing tumor Bilateral for AIMAH or PPNAD	If surgical treatment not possible or to control cortisol secretion while waiting for surgery Agents include metyrapone, ketoconazole

UFC urine free cortisol, *AIMAH* ACTH-independent macronodular adrenal hyperplasia, *PPNAD* primary pigmented nodular adrenocortical disease

sider the diagnosis established if the serum cortisol is >5.0 ng/dL after a 1-mg DST [4], while excluded if ≤50 nmol/L (≤1.8 μg/dL) [6].
  - May need a 2-day low-dose DST to confirm the diagnosis—consider referral to endocrinologist.
- The overnight 1 mg DST should be administered at 11 pm and fasting plasma cortisol and ACTH level measured between 8 and 9 AM the following day [4].
  - Cortisol suppression <1.8 ng/dL has the best negative predictive value for Cushing syndrome.

Perioperative Considerations

- Patients with SCS should have individualized treatment plan.
  - No consensus on long-term benefits of adrenalectomy (see Table 1.4)
  - Adrenalectomy typically reserved for younger patients with recent onset or worsening HTN, diabetes, dyslipidemia, or osteoporosis [4].
- Patients with long-standing hypercortisolism should be considered immunosuppressed and given antibiotic and peptic ulcer prophylaxis.
- Increased thromboembolic risk precludes preoperative VTE prophylaxis.
- Those with cortisol-producing adenomas have a suppressed HPA axis should receive glucocorticoids postoperatively until recovery (which may take 6–18 months), there has been some evidence to check ACTH stimulated cortisol in the immediate postoperative period which if not suppressed can guide steroid replacement [4].

Autonomous Cortisol Secretion (Subclinical Cushing Syndrome (SCS))

- Patients have an elevated cortisol without overt signs or symptoms of Cushing syndrome.

Table 1.4 Metabolic outcomes after adrenalectomy for SCS [18–20]

Study	Author (year)	Methods	Results
Biochemical and clinical benefits of unilateral adrenalectomy in patients with subclinical hypercortisolism and bilateral adrenal incidentalomas	Perogamvros et al. (2015) [18]	33 pts with bilateral AI 14 pts underwent unilateral adrenalectomy 19 pts f/u only Measured 0800 h plasma ACTH, 12 AM serum cortisol (MSF), 24-h urinary-free cortisol (UFC) and serum cortisol after a 2-day low-dose-dexamethasone-suppression test Assessed arterial HTN, impaired glucose tolerance or diabetes mellitus, dyslipidemia, and osteoporosis	Surgical group had a statistically significant reduction in all biochemical markers ($p < 0.05$) Comorbidities only improved in the surgical group as measured by objective tests and medication use (OGGT, BP readings, DEXA)

Table 1.4 (continued)

Study	Author (year)	Methods	Results
Adrenalectomy may improve cardiovascular and metabolic impairment and ameliorate quality of life in patients with adrenal incidentalomas and subclinical Cushing syndrome	Iacobone et al. (2012) [19]	20 pts with AI underwent laparoscopic adrenalectomy 15 managed nonoperatively Measured corticosteroid secretion, arterial blood pressure (BP), glycometabolic profile (lipid profile, hemoglobin A1C, fasting serum glucose, BMI), and quality of life (by the SF-36 questionnaire) at baseline and the end of follow-up Follow-up was median 36 months	Compared to conservatively managed group (which had no improvements): Lab corticosteroid parameters normalized in all surgical pts ($P < 0.001$) A decrease in BP occurred in 53%, glycometabolic control improved in 50%, and BMI decreased ($P < 0.01$) SF-36 evaluation improved ($P < 0.05$)
Outcome of adrenalectomy for subclinical hypercortisolism and Cushing syndrome	Raffaelli et al. (2017) [20]	Retrospective review of 29 pts with SCS and 50 pts with CS who underwent unilateral laparoscopic adrenalectomy Assessed baseline and follow-up comorbidities (BMI, HTN, diabetes) Measured ACTH, AM cortisol, 1 mg DST, UFC, blood glucose Outcomes: OR time, intraoperative/postoperative complications, need for postoperative glucocorticoid replacement, clinical and hormonal outcomes Mean F/U 51 months	Hypercortisolism resolved in all patients At long-term f/u HTN and diabetes improved significantly for all patients (no differences seen between SCS and CS groups)

Pts patients, *AI* adrenal incidentaloma, *F/U* follow-up, *HTN* hypertension, *OGGT* oral glucose tolerance test, *DEXA* dual energy X-ray absorptiometry, *SCS* subclinical Cushing syndrome, *CS* Cushing syndrome

  – However, many observational studies have reported complications typical of hypercortisolism such as obesity, diabetes, hypertension, dyslipidemia, and osteoporosis [16].
- Data is lacking for which localization studies may be effective in diagnosing SCS in patients with bilateral adrenal nodules.
- SCS is reported in 5–48% of incidentalomas making it the most frequent hormonal abnormality among these patients [17].

- The clinical relevance and optimal management of SCS are still in question [16].
- Several retrospective studies have evaluated the outcomes after adrenalectomy on patients with SCS (see Table 1.4).
- Both American and European practice guidelines recommend an individualized approach to management of these patients, accounting for age, onset, and duration of any comorbidities and how well they are controlled by medical management in addition to the extent of end-organ damage (European practice guidelines/AAES) [4, 6].
- The AACE/AAES Adrenal Incidentaloma guidelines specify those <40 years with recent onset or worsening of diabetes, hypertension, or osteoporosis should be considered for surgery, while older patients should have a more individualized approach [4].

Primary Aldosteronism

Overview

Workup [4, 6, 26]

- While only 1% of adrenal incidentalomas are aldosterone-producing adenomas, a screening workup to rule this out should still be performed specifically for those with hypertension (see Table 1.5).
- History and physical may reveal hypertension, headaches, fatigue, polydipsia, polyuria, nocturia.
- It should be emphasized that many patients with aldosteronomas *do not* have hypokalemia.

Table 1.5 Workup and management of aldosterone-producing adenoma [4]

Workup	Perioperative management	Surgical management	Medical management
History and physical *Laboratory Investigations* Electrolytes, creatinine PAC:PRA >20 Confirmatory testing if positive *Imaging* Thin-cut adrenal CT ± MRI Adrenal vein sampling (AVS) if indicated (see below)	*Preoperative* Control of HTN Manage hypokalemia (spironolactone, KCl)	Adrenalectomy Unilateral for confirmed lateralization on AVS	If no lateralization or bilateral involvement (cortical adrenal hyperplasia): K+-sparing diuretics and restriction of sodium intake (<100 mEq/day)

- A plasma aldosterone concentration (PAC) (ng/dL) to plasma renin activity (PRA) (ng/mL) (aldosterone-to-renin ratio [ARR]) should be measured when patient is off any mineralocorticoid receptor blockers.
  - A ratio >20 should prompt confirmatory testing.
  - One study reported a sensitivity and specificity of 90% and 91%, respectively, with a PAC:PRA >30 combined with a PAC >20 ng/dL.
  - This is most sensitive when measured in the morning after being seated for 5–15 min.
  - Spironolactone/eplerenone should be held for 4–6 weeks.
  - ACE inhibitors and ARBs can improve the diagnostic power of the PAC:PRA.
  - β-blockers and clonidine suppress the PRA➔ increased false positive rate.
- Confirmatory testing is positive if aldosterone or ARR suppression occurs with:
  - Oral Na + load (with >200 mEq/day of Na × 3 days) and 24-hr urine aldosterone.
  - IV Na + load (2–3 L of NaCl 0.9% over 4–6 h) with plasma aldosterone measurement.
  - Fludrocortisone suppression and ARR measurement.
  - Captopril challenge.

Adrenal Vein Sampling

- Primary hyperaldosteronism can be due to an aldosteronoma, primary (unilateral) adrenal hyperplasia (PAH).
- Adrenal vein sampling (AVS) can be performed to delineate between these lesions.
- Those with unilateral microadenomas (<1 cm) or bilateral abnormal appearing glands should be considered for AVS [27].
- It is important to have AVS done by a high volume center who is comfortable with ACTH stimulation.
- Spironolactone should be held for 6 weeks and eplerenone for 4 weeks prior to AVS [4].
- A "lateralization index" or corrected aldosterone to cortisol ratio > 4:1 is indicative of unilateral source of aldosterone excess.
  - These patients are more likely responsive to adrenalectomy [4].
- Factors associated with lateralization on AVS include an adrenal mass ≥ 3 cm on CT scan, a low renin value and high plasma ARR [28].

Perioperative Considerations

- All patients with unilateral primary hyperaldosteronism should be considered for surgical resection.

  - Untreated hyperaldosteronism can lead to myocardial fibrosis, increased clotting and ischemic events, left ventricular hypertrophy, and increased mortality from CHF [4].
  - These changes occur despite medical management of hypertension and hypokalemia.
- Preoperative medications for most patients include mineralocorticoid receptor antagonist, antihypertensive agents, potassium chloride to maintain normokalemia.
- These agents are stopped postoperatively; if blood pressure remains elevated, add back antihypertensive medications [5].
  - Normotension (without medication) may take several weeks.
  - 90% of patients will have significant reductions in blood pressure, with reduction in dosing and number of antihypertensive medication.
  - 30–60% will discontinue all medications.
  - 100% will achieve normokalemia.

Prediction of Cure (Aldosterone Resolution Score)

- There are numerous factors associated with hypertension resolution after adrenalectomy.
- Zarnegar et al. developed an aldosterone resolution score (ARS) to predict resolution of hypertension based on 4 clinical variables [21].
  - ≤2 antihypertensive medications.
  - BMI ≤25 kg/m^2.
  - Duration of HTN ≤6 years.
  - Female sex.
- Taking two or fewer antihypertensive medications has the strongest independent predictor of resolution [21].
- Other factors that have been implicated include ≤1 first-degree relative with hypertension, higher preoperative ARR, higher urinary aldosterone secretion, and strong positive response to spironolactone [22].

Adrenocortical Carcinoma

- Adrenocortical carcinomas (ACCs) are rare tumors occurring with an incidence of 0.5–2 per million patients per year. ACC has a bimodal age distribution with increased incidence in children <6 years and in adults in their 40s and 50s [29]. ACCs may be either nonfunctional or associated with symptoms of hormonal excess. An overview of the workup and management of ACC is presented in Table 1.6.
- ACC appears to be mostly sporadic; however, in ~10% of cases it is associated with a hereditary cancer syndrome including [30]:
  - Li-Fraumeni syndrome (4–8% of adult-onset ACC) or SBLA syndrome (sarcoma, breast cancer, lung cancer, and ACC) [31]

Table 1.6 The ENSAT staging system for ACC

Presentation	5-year overall survival
Tumor ≤5 cm confined to the adrenal gland without local invasion [Stage I, T1N0M0]	82%
Tumor >5 cm confined to the adrenal gland without local invasion [Stage II, T2N0M0]	61%
Any size with local invasion, ± invasion to adjacent organs/great vessels (T3–4) or regional lymph nodes (N1) [Stage III, T3-4N0-1M0]	50%
Distant metastasis [Stage IV, TxNxM1]	13%

  - Lynch syndrome (MLH1, MSH2, MSH6, PMS2 mutations) in ~3% of ACC cases (all ACCs should be screened for microsatellite instability).
  - Multiple endocrine neoplasia (MEN) type 1 [parathyroid, pituitary and pancreatic neuroendocrine tumors and adrenal tumors (ACC << adrenal adenomas)] in 1–2% of ACC cases [32].
- 60% of ACCs present with symptoms of hormone excess [29].
  - 40% Cushing syndrome alone.
  - 25% mixed virilization and Cushing.
  - <10% virilization alone.
  - <10% feminizing (all feminizing tumours in men are malignant).
  - <10% hyperaldosteronism—this is usually to cross reactivity of the aldosterone receptor from cortisol at high concentrations.

Preoperative Workup [33]

- Biochemical evaluation (as per incidentaloma)
- Imaging:
  - CT chest (evaluate for pulmonary metastases)
  - CT abdomen (adrenal protocol: precontrast, portal, and delayed venous phase) and/or MRI
  - Bone scan (if clinical suspicion)
  - FDG-PET/CT reserved for indeterminate sites of potential metastases
  - CT characteristics: Irregular, heterogeneous (due to tumor necrosis), unilateral, >20HU (Hounsfield units), heterogeneous enhancement with IV contrast, delayed washout, possible tumor calcification.
- Biopsy:
  - Generally not advisable due to low sensitivity and risk for tract seeding. Indications for biopsy include unresectable cases (where tissue is needed for initiation of systemic therapy) or high suspicion for adrenal metastasis. It is important to consider that adrenalectomy is a good diagnostic procedure as well for atypical lesions and may take the place of biopsies. Pheochromocytoma must be ruled out prior to consideration for biopsy.

Prognostic Factors

1. Stage (as per the European Network for The Study of Adrenal Tumors [ENSAT], see Table 1.6) [34]
2. GRAS parameters (Grade, R status, Age, Secretion)

- Grade: Weiss' histological scoring system includes 9 features (nuclear grade, mitotic rate, atypical mitoses, clear cell component, diffuse architecture, tumor necrosis, invasion of venous or sinus structures, or tumor capsule) [35] Weiss score <3 usually indicates benign tumor [35], while score >6 has been associated with decreased overall survival ($p = 0.03$) [36]. Markers of proliferation (KI-67 and mitotic rate) also indicate poorer prognosis [36–38].
  - R status: R0 (margin-negative) resection was the sole independent predictor of overall survival in a recent multi-institutional study (5-year OS 64.8% for R0 vs 33.8% for R1 resection, $p < 0.001$) [39]. R0 resection is also a significant predictor of recurrence (5-year RFS 30% for R0 vs 14% for R1 resection, $p = 0.03$) [39–41].
  - Age: Older age has been associated with worse survival [36, 41].
  - Secretion: Hormone secretion, especially cortisol, is associated with worse survival [36, 39, 41].

Operative Considerations

- The operation of choice is radical surgical excision with wide margins and en bloc resection of adjacent involved organs (if needed) [33].
- The role of regional lymphadenectomy is still debated, but recent retrospective studies suggest it may offer a survival benefit [42–44]. Both indications and extent need to be clarified.
- An open approach is currently recommended for ACC resection due to its friable thin capsule and potential for seeding [33]. The use of laparoscopy for ACC is being explored in Europe where retrospective series reported similar oncologic outcomes for laparoscopically resected Stage I–II tumors in highly selected patients [45, 46].
- For patients presenting with oligometastatic disease at time of initial diagnosis, surgical resection of all disease may be beneficial (in addition to systemic therapy) in selected patients specifically patients with functional disease [30, 47].

Adjuvant and Systemic Therapy

- Traditionally mitotane has been offered in the adjuvant setting, especially for high-risk tumors (Stage III, R1 resection, or Ki-67 > 10%) based on earlier retrospective studies from Europe [48, 49], but recent studies failed to demonstrate any benefit [50, 51]. The ADIUVO trial (open-label RCT comparing adjuvant

Table 1.7 Overview of the workup and management of adrenocortical carcinoma

Workup	Management		Follow-up
	Localized disease	Metastatic disease	
History and physical exam Labs: As per incidentaloma [33] Imaging: CT abdomen +/− MRI CT chest Bone scan (if clinically suspicious) PET (for indeterminate remote metastases) Biopsy: Should be avoided (risk of seeding and limited usefulness in differentiating benign vs malignant). May perform if unresectable and needed to initiate systemic therapy or if suspicious for adrenal metastasis	Surgical excision with en bloc resection of adjacent involved organs if needed Consider adjuvant mitotane and/or radiation therapy, especially in high-risk cases	Complete resection of limited oligometastatic resectable disease may be beneficial in highly selected patients Radiation for bony metastases if symptomatic RFA or embolization for hepatic metastases Mitotane monotherapy Mitotane plus chemotherapy (etoposide, doxorubicin, cisplatin)	Clinically: Cushing syndrome Virilization syndrome Labs and imaging (q 6 months): Urinary cortisol CT scan chest/abdo/pelvis for 5 years

RFA radiofrequency ablation

mitotane vs observation in Stage I–III ACC, R0 resection, and Ki-67 < 10%) completed accrual and is expect to shed further light [52].

- Adjuvant external beam radiation has been offered in the adjuvant setting for high-risk tumors and was shown to decrease local recurrence in small retrospective series [53]. Further research is needed to identify the patients in whom radiation may offer a survival advantage.
- For advanced unresectable and metastatic ACC, EDP (etoposide, doxorubicin, cisplatin)-mitotane is considered first-line therapy based on one RCT comparing it with streptozocin-mitotane [54]. Single-agent therapy with mitotane is an alternative (less toxicity). Local therapeutic measures (radiation, ablation, chemoembolization) may also be of value [55].
- Molecular targeted agents and immune checkpoint inhibitors are currently being investigated for ACC (Table 1.7).

Special Notes:

There may be role for repeat surgery for recurrent disease in patients with recurrence-free interval >12 months and completely resectable disease [56].

Metastases to the Adrenal Gland

- In patients with no history of malignancy, <1% of adrenal tumors represent metastatic disease. In patients with a history of malignancy, however, 70% of adrenal tumors represent metastases from other sites.

- The adrenal gland is the fourth most common site of metastasis after the lungs, liver, and bone.
- In Western countries, lung, breast, melanoma, kidney, thyroid, and colon cancer primaries are most common. In a large retrospective series (including autopsies) from Hong Kong, most common primaries included lung (35%), gastric (14%), esophageal (12%), hepatobiliary (11%), or pancreatic (7%) cancer [57].

Workup

- Imaging characteristics: Irregular, heterogeneous, frequently bilateral, >20 HU, enhancement with IV contrast, delayed washout.
- Workup as by the primary malignancy
- Role of FNA
  - Main utility of FNA is for diagnostic uncertainty in the setting an indeterminate adrenal lesion which may represent a metastasis and excision by adrenalectomy is not first choice by treatment team [58].
  - *Must* rule out pheochromocytoma prior to biopsy [59].
  - Laparoscopic adrenalectomy is performed for diagnostic and therapeutic purposes in adrenal incidentaloma or metastatic disease.

Indications for Resection of Adrenal Metastasis

- Potential benefit in survival for selected patients.
- Non-small-cell lung cancer: median survival 26 months [60], 5-year overall survival 34% vs 0% [61, 62].
- Colorectal cancer: median survival 29 months [60].
  - Laparoscopic approach is becoming standard for resection of metastatic disease due to lower perioperative morbidity and faster recovery and return to chemotherapy [63, 64].

References

1. Taffel M, Haji-Momenian S, Nikolaidis P, Miller F. Adrenal imaging: a comprehensive review. Radiol Clin North Am. 2012;50:219–43.
2. Kim Y, Park BK, Kim CK, Park SY. Adenoma characterization: adrenal protocol with dual-energy CT. Radiology. 2013;266(2):514–20.
3. Davenport C, Liew A, Doherty B, et al. The prevalence of adrenal incidentaloma in routine clinical practice. Endocrine. 2011;40:80–3.
4. Zeiger M, Thompson G, Duh Q, Hamrahian A, et al. AACE/AAES adrenal incidentaloma guidelines. Endocr Pract. 2009;15:1–20.
5. Lee JM, Kim MK, Ko SH, Koh JM, Kim BY, Kim SW, et al. Clinical guidelines for the management of adrenal incidentaloma. Endocrinol Metab. 2017;32(2):200–18.
6. Fassnacht M, Arlt W, Bancos I, et al. Management of adrenal incidentalomas: European Society of Endocrinology Clinical Practice Guideline in collaboration with the European Network for the Study of Adrenal Tumors. Eur J Endocrinol. 2016;175:G1–G34.

7. Averbuch SD, Steakley CS, Young RC, et al. Malignant pheochromocytoma: effective treatment with a combination of cyclophosphamide, vincristine, and dacarbazine. Ann Intern Med. 1988;109(4):267–73.
8. Rose B, Matthay KK, Price D, et al. High-dose 131I-metaiodobenzylguanidine therapy for 12 patients with malignant pheochromocytoma. Cancer. 2003;98(2):239–48.
9. National Comprehensive Cancer Network. Neuroendocrine and adrenal tumors (version 3.2018). https://www.nccn.org/professionals/physician_gls/pdf/neuroendocrine.pdf. Accessed 2 Jan 2018.
10. Chang CA, Pattison DA, Tothill RW, et al. (68)Ga-DOTATATE and (18)F-FDG PET/CT in Paraganglioma and Pheochromocytoma: utility, patterns and heterogeneity. Cancer Imaging. 2016;16(1):22. https://doi.org/10.1186/s40644-016-0084-2.
11. Neumann HP, Bausch B, McWhinney SR, et al. Germ-line mutations in nonsyndromic pheochromocytoma. N Engl J Med. 2002;346(19):1459–66.
12. Chen H, Sippel RS, O'Dorisio MS, et al. The North American Neuroendocrine Tumor Society consensus guideline for the diagnosis and management of neuroendocrine tumors: pheochromocytoma, paraganglioma, and medullary thyroid cancer. Pancreas. 2010;39(6):775–83.
13. Gimenez-Roqueplo AP, Favier J, Rustin P, et al. Mutations in the SDHB gene are associated with extra-adrenal and/or malignant pheochromocytomas. Cancer Res. 2003;63(17):5615–21.
14. Nieman LK, Biller BM, Findling JW, et al. Treatment of Cushing's syndrome: an endocrine society clinical practice guideline. J Clin Endocrinol Metab. 2015;100(8):2807–31.
15. Nieman LK, Biller BM, Findling JW, et al. The diagnosis of Cushing's syndrome: an Endocrine Society Clinical Practice Guideline. J Clin Endocrinol Metab. 2008;93(5):1526–40.
16. Chiodini I, Morelli V, Salcuni A, et al. Beneficial metabolic effects of prompt surgical treatment in patients with an adrenal incidentaloma causing biochemical hypercortisolism. J Clin Endocrinol Metab. 2010;95(6):2736–45.
17. Young W, Kebebew E. The adrenal incidentaloma. In: Lacroix A, editor, UpToDate; 2018 [updated 2018 Feb 20]. Available from: https://www.uptodate.com/contents/the-adrenal-incidentaloma?
18. Perogamvros D, Vassiladi D, Karapanou O, et al. Biochemical and clinical benefits of unilateral adrenalectomy in patients with subclinical hypercortisolism and bilateral adrenal incidentalomas. Eur J Endocrinol. 2015;173:719–25.
19. Iacobone M, Citton M, Viel M, et al. Adrenalectomy may improve cardiovascular and metabolic impairment and ameliorate quality of life in patients with adrenal incidentalomas and subclinical Cushing's syndrome. Surgery. 2012;152(6):991–7.
20. Raffaelli M, De Crea C, D'Amato G, et al. Outcome of adrenalectomy for subclinical hypercortisolism and Cushing syndrome. Surgery. 2017;161(1):264–71.
21. Cho E. Update on the aldosterone resolution score and lateralization in patients with primary aldosteronism. Endocrinol Metab (Seoul). 2018;33(3):352–4.
22. Funder JW, Carey RM, Fardella C, et al. Case detection, diagnosis, and treatment of patients with primary aldosteronism: an endocrine society clinical practice guideline. J Clin Endocrinol Metab. 2008;93(9):3266–81.
23. Grumbach MM, Biller BM, Braunstein GD, et al. Management of the clinically inapparent adrenal mass ("incidentaloma"). Ann Intern Med. 2003;138(5):424–9.
24. Mansmann G, Lau J, Balk E, et al. The clinically inapparent adrenal mass: update in diagnosis and management. Endocr Rev. 2004;25(2):309–40.
25. Harari A, Inabnet WB 3rd. Malignant pheochromocytoma: a review. Am J Surg. 2011;201(5):700–8.
26. Mattsson C, Young WF Jr. Primary aldosteronism: diagnostic and treatment strategies. Nat Clin Pract Nephrol. 2006;2(4):198–208. quiz, 1 p following 230.
27. Young WF, Stanson AW, Thompson GB, et al. Role for adrenal venous sampling in primary aldosteronism. Surgery. 2004;136(6):1227–35.
28. Mathur A, Kemp CD, Dutta U, et al. Consequences of adrenal venous sampling in primary hyperaldosteronism and predictors of unilateral adrenal disease. J Am Coll Surg. 2010;211(3):384–90.

29. Ng L, Libertino JM. Adrenocortical carcinoma: diagnosis, evaluation and treatment. J Urol. 2003;16929:5–11.
30. Dickson PV, Kim L, Yen TWF, Yang A, Grubbs EG, Patel D, et al. Adjuvant and neoadjuvant therapy, treatment for advanced disease, and genetic considerations for adrenocortical carcinoma: an update from the SSO Endocrine and Head and Neck Disease Site Working Group. Ann Surg Oncol. 2018;2540:3453–9.
31. Hisada M, Garber JE, Fung CY, Fraumeni JF, Li FP. Multiple primary cancers in families with Li-Fraumeni syndrome. J Natl Cancer Inst. 1998;9036:606–11.
32. Brandi ML, Gagel RF, Angeli A, Bilezikian JP, Beck-Peccoz P, Bordi C, et al. Guidelines for diagnosis and therapy of MEN type 1 and type 2. J Clin Endocrinol Metab. 2001;8640:5658–71.
33. Dickson PV, Kim L, Yen TWF, Yang A, Grubbs EG, Patel D, et al. Evaluation, staging, and surgical management for adrenocortical carcinoma: an update from the SSO Endocrine and Head and Neck Disease Site Working Group. Ann Surg Oncol. 2018;2540:3460–8.
34. Fassnacht M, Johanssen S, Quinkler M, Bucsky P, Willenberg HS, Beuschlein F, et al. Limited prognostic value of the 2004 International Union Against Cancer staging classification for adrenocortical carcinoma: proposal for a Revised TNM Classification. Cancer. 2009;11530:243–50.
35. Weiss LM, Medeiros LJ, Vickery AL. Pathologic features of prognostic significance in adrenocortical carcinoma. Am J Surg Pathol. 1989;1331:202–6.
36. Libé R, Borget I, Ronchi CL, Zaggia B, Kroiss M, Kerkhofs T, et al. Prognostic factors in stage III-IV adrenocortical carcinomas (ACC): an European Network for the Study of Adrenal Tumor (ENSAT) study. Ann Oncol. 2015;2638:2119–25.
37. Stojadinovic A, Ghossein RA, Hoos A, Nissan A, Marshall D, Dudas M, et al. Adrenocortical carcinoma: clinical, morphologic, and molecular characterization. J Clin Oncol. 2002;2032:941–50.
38. Morimoto R, Satoh F, Murakami O, Suzuki T, Abe T, Tanemoto M, et al. Immunohistochemistry of a proliferation marker Ki67/MIB1 in adrenocortical carcinomas: Ki67/MIB1 labeling index is a predictor for recurrence of adrenocortical carcinomas. Endocr J. 2008;5529:49–55.
39. Margonis GA, Kim Y, Prescott JD, Tran TB, Postlewait LM, Maithel SK, et al. Adrenocortical carcinoma: impact of surgical margin status on long-term outcomes. Ann Surg Oncol. 2016;2329:134–41.
40. Ip JC, Pang TC, Glover AR, Soon P, Clarke S, Richardson A, et al. Improving outcomes in adrenocortical cancer: an Australian perspective. Ann Surg Oncol. 2015;2235:2309–16.
41. Ayala-Ramirez M, Jasim S, Feng L, Ejaz S, Deniz F, Busaidy N, et al. Adrenocortical carcinoma: clinical outcomes and prognosis of 330 patients at a tertiary care center. Eur J Endocrinol. 2013;16934:891–9.
42. Reibetanz J, Jurowich C, Erdogan I, Nies C, Rayes N, Dralle H, et al. Impact of lymphadenectomy on the oncologic outcome of patients with adrenocortical carcinoma. Ann Surg. 2012;25530:363–9.
43. Miller BS, Doherty GM. Regional lymphadenectomy for adrenocortical carcinoma. Ann Surg. 2013;25732:e13–4.
44. Gerry JM, Tran TB, Postlewait LM, Maithel SK, Prescott JD, Wang TS, et al. Lymphadenectomy for adrenocortical carcinoma: is there a therapeutic benefit? Ann Surg Oncol. 2016;23(Suppl 5):708–13.
45. Lombardi CP, Raffaelli M, De Crea C, Boniardi M, De Toma G, Marzano LA, et al. Open versus endoscopic adrenalectomy in the treatment of localized (stage I/II) adrenocortical carcinoma: results of a multiinstitutional Italian survey. Surgery. 2012;15234:1158–64.
46. Autorino R, Bove P, De Sio M, Miano R, Micali S, Cindolo L, et al. Open versus laparoscopic adrenalectomy for adrenocortical carcinoma: a meta-analysis of surgical and oncological outcomes. Ann Surg Oncol. 2016;2332:1195–202.
47. Wängberg B, Khorram-Manesh A, Jansson S, Nilsson B, Nilsson O, Jakobsson CE, et al. The long-term survival in adrenocortical carcinoma with active surgical management and use of monitored mitotane. Endocr Relat Cancer. 2010;1729:265–72.

48. Berruti A, Grisanti S, Pulzer A, Claps M, Daffara F, Loli P, et al. Long-term outcomes of adjuvant mitotane therapy in patients with radically resected adrenocortical carcinoma. J Clin Endocrinol Metab. 2017;10232:1358–65.
49. Else T, Williams AR, Sabolch A, Jolly S, Miller BS, Hammer GD. Adjuvant therapies and patient and tumor characteristics associated with survival of adult patients with adrenocortical carcinoma. J Clin Endocrinol Metab. 2014;9930:455–61.
50. Grubbs EG, Callender GG, Xing Y, Perrier ND, Evans DB, Phan AT, et al. Recurrence of adrenal cortical carcinoma following resection: surgery alone can achieve results equal to surgery plus mitotane. Ann Surg Oncol. 2010;1729:263–70.
51. Postlewait LM, Ethun CG, Tran TB, Prescott JD, Pawlik TM, Wang TS, et al. Outcomes of adjuvant mitotane after resection of adrenocortical carcinoma: a 13-institution study by the US Adrenocortical Carcinoma Group. J Am Coll Surg. 2016;22232:480–90.
52. http://clinicaltrials.gov/ct2/show/NCT00777244. Accessed 22 Apr 2019.
53. Polat B, Fassnacht M, Pfreundner L, Guckenberger M, Bratengeier K, Johanssen S, et al. Radiotherapy in adrenocortical carcinoma. Cancer. 2009;11541:2816–23.
54. Fassnacht M, Terzolo M, Allolio B, Baudin E, Haak H, Berruti A, et al. Combination chemotherapy in advanced adrenocortical carcinoma. N Engl J Med. 2012;36651:2189–97.
55. Fassnacht M, Dekkers O, Else T, Baudin E, Berruti A, de Krijger RR, et al. European Society of Endocrinology Clinical Practice Guidelines on the management of adrenocortical carcinoma in adults, in collaboration with the European Network for the Study of Adrenal Tumors. Eur J Endocrinol. 2018;179:G1–G46.
56. Erdogan I, Deutschbein T, Jurowich C, Kroiss M, Ronchi C, Quinkler M, et al. The role of surgery in the management of recurrent adrenocortical carcinoma. J Clin Endocrinol Metab. 2013;9829:181–91.
57. Lam KY, Lo CY. Metastatic tumours of the adrenal glands: a 30-year experience in a teaching hospital. Clin Endocrinol (Oxf). 2002;5629:95–101.
58. Mazzaglia PJ, Monchik JM. Limited value of adrenal biopsy in the evaluation of adrenal neoplasm: a decade of experience. Arch Surg. 2009;14433:465–70.
59. Vanderveen KA, Thompson SM, Callstrom MR, Young WF, Grant CS, Farley DR, et al. Biopsy of pheochromocytomas and paragangliomas: potential for disaster. Surgery. 2009;14634:1158–66.
60. Moreno P, de la Quintana Basarrate A, Musholt TJ, Paunovic I, Puccini M, Vidal O, et al. Adrenalectomy for solid tumor metastases: results of a multicenter European study. Surgery. 2013;15434:1215–22; discussion 22–3.
61. Tanvetyanon T, Robinson LA, Schell MJ, Strong VE, Kapoor R, Coit DG, et al. Outcomes of adrenalectomy for isolated synchronous versus metachronous adrenal metastases in non-small-cell lung cancer: a systematic review and pooled analysis. J Clin Oncol. 2008;2635:1142–7.
62. Raz DJ, Lanuti M, Gaissert HC, Wright CD, Mathisen DJ, Wain JC. Outcomes of patients with isolated adrenal metastasis from non-small cell lung carcinoma. Ann Thorac Surg. 2011;9233:1788–92; discussion 93.
63. Strong VE, D'Angelica M, Tang L, Prete F, Gönen M, Coit D, et al. Laparoscopic adrenalectomy for isolated adrenal metastasis. Ann Surg Oncol. 2007;1440:3392–400.
64. Duh QY. Laparoscopic adrenalectomy for isolated adrenal metastasis: the right thing to do and the right way to do it. Ann Surg Oncol. 2007;1440:3288–9.

Ampullary Cancer

2

Lawrence Lau, Nicholas Latchana, Shiva Jayaraman, Sean Cleary, and Carol-anne E. Moulton

Introduction

Periampullary neoplasms arise in proximity of the ampulla of Vater (within 2 cm) and can originate from the duodenum, pancreatic head, distal common bile duct, or the ampullary complex. Ampullary tumors are those arising directly from the structures of the ampullary complex distal to the confluence of the bile duct and pancreatic duct and represent roughly 7% of periampullary neoplasms. These rare tumors represent 0.5% of all GI cancers, though a subtle increase of 0.9% per year has been observed in recent decades [1].

Ampullary carcinoma carries a notably more favorable prognosis than other pancreaticobiliary malignancies. This is likely attributed to presentation with early clinical jaundice, and potentially, a more favorable disease biology. Curative-intent resection is possible in 50% of patients presenting with ampullary cancer compared with 10% for patients with pancreatic cancer [2]. Specific risk factors for ampullary cancer have not been identified, but duodenal adenomas and periampullary malignancies are a well-described feature of the familial adenomatous polyposis syndrome.

The large majority of ampullary cancers are adenocarcinoma and are broadly categorized into pancreaticobiliary and intestinal histologic subtypes based on their morphological appearance, immunohistochemical staining pattern, and molecular features. Intestinal-type tumors (CDX2 positive, MUC1 negative) have a more favorable prognosis compared with pancreaticobiliary type (CDX2

L. Lau · N. Latchana · S. Jayaraman · C.-a. E. Moulton (✉)
Department of Surgery, University of Toronto, Toronto, ON, Canada
e-mail: Nicholas.Latchana@mail.utoronto.ca; Shiva.Jayaraman@unityhealth.to; Carol-anne.Moulton@uhn.ca

S. Cleary
Department of Surgery, Mayo Clinic, Rochester, MN, USA
e-mail: Cleary.Sean@mayo.edu

F. C. Wright et al. (eds.), *Surgical Oncology Manual*,
https://doi.org/10.1007/978-3-030-48363-0_2

Table 2.1 Prognosis based on tumor extent at presentation [1, 6, 7]

Presentation	Prognosis 5-year overall survival (OS)
Local	45–67%
Regional	31–55%
Distant	4–14%

negative, MUC1 positive) (~60% vs. ~20% at 5 years; median OS 116 vs. 22 months) [3, 4]. Prognosis is determined by the stage at presentation (Table 2.1). Lymph node positivity is among the strongest prognostic factors and is closely correlated with the size of the primary tumor: <1 cm = 9%, 1–1.5 cm = 25%, and >1.5 cm 40–50% [4]. The recommended staging system is the International Union Against Cancer and American Joint Committee on Cancer (UICC/AJCC) 8th edition [5].

Several factors conspire against the formulation of large prospective randomized studies for ampullary carcinoma: the rarity of the disease, histologic heterogeneity, differentiating from other periampullary tumors preoperatively, and the amalgamation with other pancreaticobiliary cancers. As such, no prospective studies exclusively evaluating ampullary carcinoma have been published, and management recommendations are based largely on extrapolation from the management of pancreatic adenocarcinoma and consensus guidelines (Table 2.2).

Special Notes

- In Ontario, all patients with known or suspected ampullary adenocarcinoma should be referred for management at a high-volume hepatopancreaticobiliary surgical oncology center.
- *Endoscopic resection* of ampullary adenomas is associated with lower morbidity than surgical resection, but has a fivefold increased rate of recurrence [9]. Endoscopic biopsy has a false negative rate of 16–24% for invasive adenocarcinoma [10–12]. The likelihood of coexistent adenocarcinoma increases with adenoma size (>2–3 cm), the presence of high-grade dysplasia, pancreatic duct involvement with dilation >7 mm, and endoscopic signs of malignancy (friability, ulceration, spontaneous bleeding, and firm consistency) [9, 11–13].
- *Role of Frozen Section*: Frozen section is used to confirm metastatic/unresectable disease. In cases where a lesion is not endoscopically resectable, but is amenable to local resection (transduodenal ampullectomy), frozen section is used to determine margin status and to determine the need to proceed to pancreaticoduodenectomy.
- *Laparoscopic Staging*: It has limited use in upstaging ampullary carcinoma since the advent of high-quality multidetector CT. Appropriate in selected patients at increased risk of metastatic disease in the absence of unresectability on preoperative imaging (e.g., elevated CA 19-9, larger tumors [14]).

Table 2.2 Management of resectable periampullary tumors

Clinical scenario	Work-up	Surgical management	Adjuvant therapy	Follow-up (F/U)
Benign adenoma	History and physical exam Labs: Ca 19–9, CEA Staging: CT chest, biphasic CT abdo/pelvis	*Local resection* recommended: endoscopic resection, duodenotomy with polypectomy and/or ampullectomy[a] [8]	No adjuvant therapy indicated	Following local resection surveillance is required with a side-viewing endoscope
In situ disease	MRI/MRCP +/− EUS to evaluate the extent of local invasion or for biopsy +/− Staging laparo-scopy[a]	*Pancreaticoduodenectomy* should be considered for high-grade dysplasia/in situ disease in young patients and good performance status; otherwise local excision is recommended		CT chest/abdo/pelvis every 3–6 months for the first 2 years, then every 6 months to 1 year thereafter
Invasive disease	Consider biliary decompression if jaundice present (ERCP or PTC) and immediate resection not available	*Pancreaticoduodenectomy* recommended [8] Local resection for cT1 disease is associated with R1 resection rate of 25–60% and higher local recurrence. Not recommended for good operative candidates Lymphadenectomy: Routine LN dissection includes peripancreatic, CBD and pyloric nodes Extended LN dissection not indicated as no demonstrated improvement in outcomes	No consensus of optimal therapy Consider: Chemotherapy alone[a] Chemoradiotherapy[a] Observation	

MRCP magnetic resonance cholangiopancreatography, *ERCP* endoscopic retrograde cholangiopancreatography, *PTC* percutaneous transhepatic cholangiography, *EUS* endoscopic ultrasound, *LN* lymph node

[a]See Special Notes

- *Medical Oncology*: No consensus exists regarding optimal systemic therapy for ampullary carcinoma [6]. The largest RCT evaluating adjuvant chemotherapy for resected periampullary cancers (ESPAC-3 trial, n = 297 ampullary) showed a statistically nonsignificant improvement in overall survival with gemcitabine or 5-FU over observation alone [15]. The role of molecular targeted agents remains to be evaluated in ampullary cancer. Treatment approaches follow guidelines established for pancreatic cancer regardless of subtype [16]. Patients should be referred for discussion of adjuvant therapy.

Table 2.3 Management strategy for duodenal polyps in patients with familial adenomatous polyposis [22]

Stage	Size (mm)	Histology	Management
1	0	Normal	EGD q 5 years
2	1–2	Adenoma	EGD q 3 years
3	2.1–10	Adenoma	EGD q6 months
4	2.1–10 >10	HGD Adenoma	Endoscopic or surgical resection
5	Any	Adenocarcinoma	Radical surgery (e.g., pancreaticoduodenectomy)

EGD esophagoduodenoscopy (with side-viewing scope), *HGD* high-grade dysplasia

- *Radiotherapy*: The role of adjuvant radiation is controversial. Several observational studies suggest improved survival with chemoradiation (CRT) for tumors with adverse features (node positive, poorly differentiated, T3/T4) [17–20]. The only prospective RCT evaluating CRT for resected pancreatic and periampullary cancers failed to demonstrate a survival benefit for the subgroup of mixed periampullary tumors (n = 104) [21].

Special Case: Familial Adenomatous Polyposis (FAP)

- 50–90% of patients diagnosed with FAP have duodenal adenomas.
- Overall lifetime risk of duodenal cancer is ~5%.
- Duodenal cancer in FAP has a later onset than colorectal cancer (median age 52).
- FAP patients require regular side-viewing duodenoscopy and biopsy of suspicious lesions, starting at 25 years.
- A practical and effective surveillance strategy for upper GI malignancies in FAP patients has been developed at the University of Toronto (Table 2.3).

Landmark Trials

Prospective RCTs regarding the management of ampullary carcinoma are few, due to the relative rarity of the disease and inclusion in pancreatic adenocarcinoma trials. As such, treatment protocols have largely been extrapolated from trials evaluating periampullary malignancies that included subsets of ampullary carcinoma [15, 21]. Surgical management is largely dictated by consensus statements [8].

Referring to Multidisciplinary Cancer Conference (MCC)

1. High-risk features (R1 resection, poorly differentiated, T3/T4, node positive, pancreaticobiliary histology).
2. Locally advanced disease.
3. Unresectable disease (Table 2.4).

Table 2.4 Management of unresectable/metastatic ampullary adenocarcinoma

Criteria of unresectability	Management
Metastatic disease: Liver, lung, peritoneum, and distant lymph nodes (celiac, SMA nodes, tail of pancreas) Patient factors: Prohibitive comorbidities or functional status Anatomical factors: Criteria similar to those applied to pancreatic head cancers, e.g., arterial encasement, portal vein involvement which precludes reconstruction	Radical resection not indicated Consider nonoperative palliation interventions (e.g., stent/PTC placement) Consider surgery for palliation only Improved PFS and median survival have been demonstrated with platinum + anti-metabolite regimens [23, 24] Consider radiotherapy

SMA superior mesenteric artery, *PTC* percutaneous transhepatic cholangiography/catheter, *PFS* progression-free survival

Toronto Pearls

- Biliary obstruction associated with ampullary lesions can be intermittent (ball-valve effect).
- Lesions with high-grade dysplasia or carcinoma in situ on endoscopic biopsies have high rate of invasive cancer on final pathology. Formal resection (pancreaticoduodenectomy) or intraoperative frozen section at ampullectomy should be considered in these patients.
- Formal pancreaticoduodenal resection should be considered for malignant ampullary lesions.
- Pylorus-preserving pancreaticoduodenectomy is generally not advised for ampullary lesions.
- Luminal obstruction by ampullary lesions can be palliated by endoscopic resection and/or endoluminal stent placement.

References

1. Albores-Saavedra J, et al. Cancers of the ampulla of vater: demographics, morphology, and survival based on 5,625 cases from the SEER program. J Surg Oncol. 2009;100(7):598–605.
2. O'Connell JB, et al. Survival after resection of ampullary carcinoma: a national population-based study. Ann Surg Oncol. 2008;15(7):1820–7.
3. Chang DK, et al. Histomolecular phenotypes and outcome in adenocarcinoma of the ampulla of vater. J Clin Oncol. 2013;31(10):1348–56.
4. Heinrich S, Clavien PA. Ampullary cancer. Curr Opin Gastroenterol. 2010;26(3):280–5.
5. Herman JM, et al. Ampulla of Vater. In: Amin MB, et al., editors. AJCC cancer staging manual. 8th ed. New York: Springer; 2017. p. 327–35.
6. Stiles ZE, et al. Ampullary adenocarcinoma: defining predictors of survival and the impact of adjuvant therapy following surgical resection for stage I disease. J Surg Oncol. 2018;117:1500–8.
7. Jiang ZQ, et al. A retrospective study of ampullary adenocarcinomas: overall survival and responsiveness to fluoropyrimidine-based chemotherapy. Ann Oncol. 2013;24(9):2349–53.

8. Kondo S, et al. Guidelines for the management of biliary tract and ampullary carcinomas: surgical treatment. J Hepato-Biliary-Pancreat Surg. 2008;15(1):41–54.
9. Onkendi EO, et al. Adenomas of the ampulla of vater: a comparison of outcomes of operative and endoscopic resections. J Gastrointest Surg. 2014;18:1588–96.
10. Roggin KK, et al. Limitations of ampullectomy in the treatment of nonfamilial ampullary neoplasms. Ann Surg Oncol. 2005;12(12):971–80.
11. Lee HS, et al. Diagnostic accuracy of the initial endoscopy for ampullary tumors. Clin Endosc. 2015;48(3):239–46.
12. Kang SH, et al. Therapeutic outcomes of endoscopic papillectomy for ampullary neoplasms: retrospective analysis of a multicenter study. BMC Gastroenterol. 2017;17(1):69.
13. Kim HN, et al. Prediction of carcinoma after resection in subjects with ampullary adenomas on endoscopic biopsy. J Clin Gastroenterol. 2013;47:346–51.
14. Alexakis N, et al. High serum CA 19-9 but not tumor size should select patients for staging laparoscopy in radiological resectable pancreas head and peri-ampullary cancer. Eur J Surg Oncol. 2015;41(2):265–9.
15. Neoptolemos JP, et al. Effect of adjuvant chemotherapy with fluorouracil plus folinic acid or gemcitabine vs observation on survival in patients with resected periampullary adenocarcinoma: the ESPAC-3 periampullary cancer randomized trial. JAMA. 2012;308(2):147–56.
16. Ghosn M, et al. Where does chemotherapy stand in the treatment of ampullary canrcinoma? A review of literature. World J Gastrointest Oncol. 2016;8(10):745–50.
17. Bhatia S, et al. Adjuvant therapy for ampullary carcinomas: the Mayo Clinic experience. Int J Radiat Oncol Biol Phys. 2006;66(2):514–9.
18. Narang AK, et al. Evaluation of adjuvant chemoradiation therapy for ampullary adenocarcinoma: the Johns Hopkins Hospital-Mayo Clinic collaborative study. Radiat Oncol. 2011;6:126.
19. Kim K, et al. Role of adjuvant chemoradiotherapy for ampulla of Vater cancer. Int J Radiat Oncol Biol Phys. 2009;75(2):436–41.
20. Krishnan S, et al. Role of adjuvant chemoradiation therapy in adenocarcinomas of the ampulla of vater. Int J Radiat Oncol Biol Phys. 2008;70(3):735–43.
21. Klinkenbijl JH, et al. Adjuvant radiotherapy and 5-fluorouracil after curative resection of cancer of the pancreas and periampullary region: phase III trial of the EORTC gastrointestinal tract cancer cooperative group. Ann Surg. 1999;230(6):776–82. discussion 782–4.
22. Serrano PE, et al. Progression and management of duodenal neoplasia in familial adenomatous polyposis: a cohort study. Ann Surg. 2015;261(6):1138–44.
23. Valle J, et al. Cisplatin plus gemcitabine versus gemcitabine for biliary tract cancer. N Engl J Med. 2010;362(14):1273–81.
24. Overman MJ, et al. Phase II study of capecitabine and oxaliplatin for advanced adenocarcinoma of the small bowel and ampulla of Vater. J Clin Oncol. 2009;27(16):2598–603.

Anal Cancer

3

Tyler R. Chesney, Edward Weiss, Monika K. Krzyzanowska, Ali Hosni, James Brierley, and Alexandra M. Easson

Introduction

Anal cancer is uncommon, representing 2.5% of all gastrointestinal tract malignancies, with an annual incidence rate of 1.8 per 100,000 in the USA and approximately 500 incident cases yearly in Canada [1–3]. Nearly two-thirds of incident cases are in women [2, 3]. Over the past decade, incidence has risen by 2% per year [2, 4]. Squamous cell carcinomas account for most anal cancers and are the focus of this chapter, but other histologic types including adenocarcinoma (mostly from anal glands), melanoma, neuroendocrine, and sarcoma occur in the anus rarely [5]. Annual incidence is higher in those with immunodeficiency: 6–12 per 100,000 after solid organ transplantation, and 50 to 145 per 100,000 in those with HIV infection [6–9].

T. R. Chesney (✉)
General Surgical Oncology, University of Toronto, Toronto, ON, Canada

E. Weiss · M. K. Krzyzanowska
Department of Medicine, University of Toronto, Toronto, ON, Canada
e-mail: edward.weiss@uhn.ca; monika.krzyzanowska@uhn.ca

A. Hosni · J. Brierley
Department of Radiation Oncology, University of Toronto, Toronto, ON, Canada
e-mail: Ali.Hosni@rmp.uhn.on.ca; james.brierley@rmp.uhn.ca

A. M. Easson
Department of Surgery, University of Toronto, Toronto, ON, Canada
e-mail: alexandra.easson@uhn.ca

F. C. Wright et al. (eds.), *Surgical Oncology Manual*,
https://doi.org/10.1007/978-3-030-48363-0_3

Terminology

- *Anal canal* The anal canal extends from the anorectal ring (the palpable upper border of the anal sphincter at the puborectalis muscles) to the lowermost edge of the sphincter complex corresponding to the anal verge or introitus of the anal orifice (Fig. 3.1) [10]. Anal cancer is classified as anal canal cancer if the lesion cannot be fully visualized with gentle traction of the buttocks [11, 12]. Proximal to distal, the anal canal contains several types of mucosa: glandular/columnar, transitional (anal transition zone), nonkeratinizing squamous (anoderm), keratinizing squamous (the dentate line divides keratinizing and nonkeratinizing), and merges with the hair-bearing perianal skin (true epidermis with epidermal appendages) at the mucocutaneous junction (anal verge). The treatment of anal canal

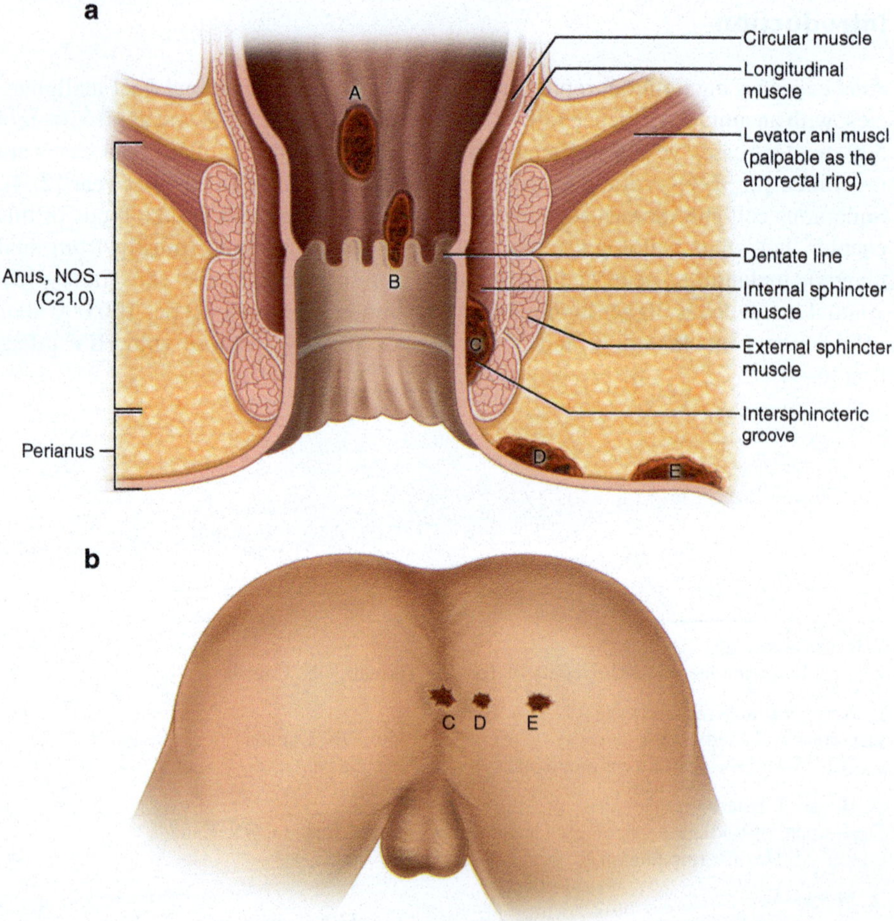

Fig. 3.1 Anal cancer (A–C), perianal cancer (D), and skin cancer (E). (**a**) coronal cross-section (**b**) perineal view

tumors has been standardized for all squamous cell carcinomas irrespective of histological subtype (keratinizing or non-keratinizing, epidermoid, transitional, basaloid, or cloacogenic) due to similar prognosis and response to treatment [13].

- *Perianal* The perianal skin (previously anal margin) begins at the anal verge and extends over a 5 cm radius (Fig. 3.1). It is further defined by the presence of epidermal appendages, and contains the pigmented skin. Perianal cancers are those that can be fully visualized with gentle traction of the buttocks [11, 12]. Those further than 5 cm from the anal orifice are classified as skin cancers.
- *Regional lymph nodes* The proximal anal canal (above the dentate line) has lymphatic drainage to the mesorectal, superior rectal, and internal iliac nodes. Distal to the dentate line, drainage is to the inguinal nodes and external iliac nodes.
- *Precursor lesions (anal squamous intraepithelial lesions)* The Lower Anogenital Squamous Terminology (LAST) should be used [14, 15]. HPV-related squamous anogenital precursor lesions are divided into low-grade squamous intraepithelial lesions (LSILs) and high-grade squamous intraepithelial lesions (HSILs) based on mitotic activity, depth of dermal involvement, and abnormalities in squamous cell differentiation. LSIL can then be subclassified into condyloma (raised papillary proliferation with low-grade viral cytopathologic changes), and flat lesions labelled anal intraepithelial neoplasia 1 (AIN1). HSIL can be subclassified into AIN2 and AIN3 based on depth of abnormal cells. Generally, LSIL is observed, and HSIL is treated. Older terms such as high-grade anal intraepithelial neoplasia (HGAIN) and low-grade anal intraepithelial neoplasia (LGAIN), Bowen disease, and carcinoma in situ should not be used. Similarly, these squamous lesions are differentiated from extramammary Paget disease which is an apocrine neoplasm from sweat glands; pagetoid spread, known as secondary extramammary Paget disease, can occur from adjacent colorectal adenocarcinoma, urothelial carcinoma, or melanoma [15].
- *Superficially invasive squamous cell carcinoma (SISCCA)* Invasive squamous carcinoma that invades ≤3 mm from the basement membrane has a horizontal spread ≤7 mm, and must have been completely excised to confirm limited extent of the tumor [14]. These are classified as T1 anal carcinomas by AJCC [11]. SISCCA are typically identified by high-resolution anoscopy (HRA) and ongoing studies are investigating the role of excision alone as treatment for these lesions [16].

Risk Factors and Precursor Lesions

Anal cancer is an human papillomavirus (HPV)-associated cancer, like cervical, vaginal, penile, and oropharyngeal cancers, with 80–90% attributable to HPV [4, 17–19]. High-risk HPV types include HPV 16 and HPV 18 in 80–90% of cases, as well as HPV 31, 33, 45, 52, and 58 in a lesser proportion [17, 18, 20]. Oncogenesis is associated with persistent infection with high-risk HPV producing oncoproteins E6 and E7 which bind cellular proteins, including p53 and pRb from the tumor suppressor genes TP53 and retinoblastoma, deregulating DNA repair and apoptosis, and stimulating cell-cycle progression [21].

Table 3.1 Risk factors for anal cancer

HPV exposure [26–29]	Immunodeficiency	Other
Lifetime number of sexual partners Prior sexually transmitted infection Prior anogenital warts (condyloma) Anoreceptive intercourse Prior HPV-associated squamous anogenital cancers (cervical, vulvar, vaginal, penile)	HIV infection [6, 9, 30] Autoimmune disorder [31] Solid organ transplantation [6, 7] Immunosuppressive medications [32]	Female sex [33] Smoking [34] Age

Risk factors for anal cancer largely relate to HPV exposure and immunodeficiency enabling persistence of HPV infection (Table 3.1) [22, 23]. Benign anal conditions such as hemorrhoids and fissures, and inflammatory bowel diseases, are not associated with an increased risk of anal cancer [24, 25].

HPV-related precursor lesions can be (1) clinically apparent raised condylomata, (2) incidentally found in anorectal surgical specimens, or (3) subclinical flat lesions seen on HRA or as subtle plaques, erythema, pigmentation, or pruritis. Histologically they are classified as LSIL or HSIL. LSIL represents morphologic features of HPV infection, while HSIL is a non-obligate precancerous lesion [14]. Typically, condylomata are LSIL, and flat lesions can be LSIL or HSIL.

Anal condyloma acuminata (anal warts) are the most common HPV-related anogenital lesions, and present as exophytic, soft, cauliflower-like masses [15]. Typically associated with low-risk HPV types 6 and 11, condylomata are low-risk lesions that may recur but have little, if any, risk of progression to carcinoma [12]. A small proportion of condylomata, more so anal canal lesions, may be associated with high-risk HPV and may progress to HSIL and invasive carcinoma, but this association is not fully clear [15]. A condyloma is distinguished from skin stags and hemorrhoids clinically. Flat LSIL (AIN1) are typically within the anal canal. They should be differentiated from seborrheic keratosis and psoriasiform dermatitis, and can be histologically similar to reactive changes [14, 15]. HSIL can arise in a condyloma, but typically are a flat lesion. Because the morphologic features of AIN2 fall between HPV infection (LSIL) and precancer (HSIL), immunohistochemical staining for p16, a biomarker for HPV-related cell proliferation is used to confirm HSIL when morphological features of AIN2 are present [14]. AIN2 that is p16 negative is classified as LSIL. Use of the LAST criteria limits inter-rater discordance in pathology interpretation [14, 15].

LSIL may spontaneously regress or progress to HSIL. HSIL is less likely to regress, and may progress to anal cancer. Population-based estimates of the rate of progression from HSIL to anal cancer may be as high as 2% per year (10% at 5 years), and may be higher in those with HIV [16, 35–40]. Spontaneous regression of HSIL may occur in some [36, 41]. There is no conclusive evidence that treatment of HSIL effectively prevents incident anal cancer; retrospective studies show variable results comparing treatment of HSIL to watchful waiting [16, 42–45]. Two ongoing randomized clinical trials (ANCHOR and HPV-SAVE) aim to investigate this question [46, 47]. The management of anal squamous intraepithelial lesions is detailed in Table 3.2

Table 3.2 Management of anal squamous intraepithelial lesions (precursor lesions)

		Treatment		
	Work-up	Primary	Recurrence	Follow-up
LSIL (condyloma, AIN 1)	Comprehensive history Digital anorectal examination. High-resolution anoscopy (HRA) with acetic acid 3% and Lugol's iodine [48] Gynecological examination in female patients, with cervical cancer screening as appropriate Genital examination in male patients to exclude HPV-related disease HIV testing Consider pathology review to confirm diagnosis by LAST criteria [14].	Biopsy to rule out HSIL Watchful waiting recommended, may regress and low risk of progression Condylomata may regress, or can be treated with the same modalities as HSIL or other treatments (cryotherapy, sinecatechins [49], podophyllotoxin [50])	Same as primary	No clear evidence to guide method or frequency. History, DRE, conventional anoscopy or HRA, and/or anal cytology, are all available options [43, 51]
HSIL (AIN 2, AIN 3)		Watchful waiting with history, DRE, conventional anoscopy or HRA every 4–6 months Patient-applied topical/intra-anal treatment 5% imiquimod cream 3/week for 16 weeks [52–54] 5% fluorouracil for 9–16 weeks [53, 55] Cidofovir 1% gel for 6 weeks [56, 57] Local/ablative treatments with HRA Trichloroacetic acid (TCA) [58, 59] Electrocautery ablation [53, 60–62] Radiofrequency ablation provides circumferential treatment [63] Infrared coagulation [64, 65] Cryotherapy	High rate of recurrence with all treatment options available Retreatment and surveillance possible	If watchful waiting, history, DRE, simple anoscopy or HRA every 4–6 months After complete treatment, no clear evidence to guide method or frequency. History, DRE, conventional anoscopy or HRA, and/or anal cytology, are all available options. At least yearly, and some recommend every 6 months particularly in those with HIV [43, 51]

Thorough clinical assessment should be done to exclude concomitant anal cancer.

Treatment choice based on location (canal or perianal), extent (>30–50% circumference in canal), availability, preference (patient- or physician-applied). A topical/intra-anal can be used for greater extent or patient preference for self-application; local/ablative treatment for smaller or remaining lesions [16, 43, 51].

Ablation requires destructive ablation of only the epidermal layer; margins are not required. for ablative techniques within the anal canal, avoid potential stenosis by ablating <30–50% of circumference at one treatment.

If access to HRA is not available, clinical assessment, ablative treatments, and follow-up can be done with conventional anoscopy with or without acetic acid 3%, but recurrence may be increased due to decreased sensitivity [51]

Recurrence of HSIL is common (20–50% at 1 year), but can be retreated; recurrence may decrease with HRA-directed therapy allowing adequate lesion recognition and eradication [16, 60, 61, 66]

With improved topical and ablative techniques as well as HRA, mapping procedures and wide local excision are no longer needed even for diffuse disease. Wide excision causes extensive tissue destruction, wound complications, and does not have lower recurrence risk [67]. If HRA is not available, can consider mapping procedure under general anesthesia in high-risk patients to determine extent of HSIL and assist with surveillance intensity. If considering wide local excision (>1 cm margins), this should be done only if the lesion is <30% of the anal circumference with no sphincter involvement. With wide local excision, recurrence rates are up to 63% in 1 year

AIN anal intraepithelial lesion, *HRA* high-resolution anoscopy, *HSIL* high-grade squamous intraepithelial lesion, *LSIL* low-grade squamous intraepithelial lesion

Anal Cancer

Almost half of patients present with bleeding; a third with mass sensation; some may have pain, irritation, or pruritis; and a fifth are asymptomatic [51, 68]. Diagnostic delay may occur if nonspecific anorectal symptoms are attributed to benign anorectal pathology such as hemorrhoids [51]. Pain and itching should be treated seriously even if invasion cannot be confirmed on biopsy. The onset of pain and symptoms is a key indicator of possible recurrence.

The Union for International Cancer Control's (UICC)/American Joint Committee on Cancer (AJCC) eighth edition is the recommended anal cancer staging system [11]. This is based on tumor size, invasion of adjacent structures, regional nodal involvement, and distant metastases. Notable changes from UICC/AJCC seventh edition include staging perianal cancers such as anal canal cancers rather than squamous cell skin cancers as previously done; removal of N2 and N3 categories and defining N1a, N1b, and N1c; and revision of stage groupings including subclassification of stage II into IIA and IIB with differing prognosis [69]. Tumor size determines T-category: ≤2 cm (T1), >2 to ≤5 cm (T2), >5 cm (T3), and T4 can be any size but invades adjacent organ (e.g., vagina, urethra, bladder) [11]. Any regional nodal involvement is staged N1; this is subclassified into N1a (mesorectal, internal iliac, or inguinal), N1b (external iliac only), N1c (any N1a with external iliac) [11]. Regarding stage classifications, any distant metastasis is stage IV, any regional nodal metastasis or T4 category are stage III, larger tumors (>2 cm) without nodal involvement is stage II, and small tumors without nodal involvement (≤2 cm) are stage I.

At presentation, 50% are localized, 30% regional, and 15% distant, with population-based overall survival at 5 years of 82%, 64%, and 30%, respectively [2]. Tumor size >5 cm, regional nodal and extrapelvic metastases are the most important prognostic features influencing overall survival [69, 70]. Tumor >5 cm and tumor invasion to other organs are frequently identified as risk factors for colostomy [70–72]. Currently, there are no other prognostic or predictive biomarkers established for routine clinical use [73].

Historically, anal cancers were treated with radical surgery by abdominoperineal resection; however, in a few centers radical radiation without chemotherapy was used to facilitate sphincter preservation. In 1974, Nigro et al. first described preoperative combined chemoradiotherapy in an attempt to reduce recurrence rates after abdominoperineal resection and observed complete clinical response in the first three patients and complete pathological response in the two that underwent surgery [74]. This led to the investigation of what has now become the standard treatment – concurrent radiation and chemotherapy without surgery as primary treatment, reserving surgery for treatment salvage of persistent or recurrent disease. Concurrent radiation and chemotherapy results in sphincter preservation in the majority of cases and allows prophylactic treatment to uninvolved nodes reducing of nodal recurrence [75, 76]. The management of anal cancer is detailed in Tables 3.3, and 3.4. Table 3.5 summarizes landmark studies in anal cancer treatment.

Table 3.3 Management of anal cancer: local/regional disease (any T, any N, M0)

		Treatment		
	Work-up	Primary	Recurrence	Follow-up

Anal canal cancer, any local or regional (T1–T4, N0, or N+)
Perianal cancer, 2 cm or more or regional disease (T2–T4, N0, or any T, N+)
	• Comprehensive history
	• Digital anorectal examination
	• Clinical assessment of inguinal lymph nodes (FNAB if suspicious)
	• Conventional anoscopy, biopsy primary tumor for histologic confirmation
	• Gynecological examination in female patients, with cervical cancer screening as appropriate
	• Genital examination in male patients to exclude HPV-related disease
	• HIV testing
	• Fertility preservation considerations
	• Imaging
	  • CT thorax
	  • CT abdomen and pelvis
	  • Pelvic MRI for locoregional staging and assessing sphincter involvement.
	  • PET for tumors >T1N0, may alter radiation planning [13, 51, 77, 78]
		• Primary curative-intent treatment is concurrent radiation and chemotherapy (CRT) with 5FU + MMC to the primary lesion and regional nodal basins (for N+ disease or elective node irradiation if N-) [13, 51, 78–83]
		• CRT with 5FU + MMC better DFS and OS than CRT with 5FU + Cis [84, 85]
		• Induction chemotherapy prior to CRT or maintenance chemotherapy after CRT has no added benefit [80, 85, 86]
		• CRT with 5FU + MMC better local recurrence, colostomy-free, and DFS than CRT with 5FU alone [82]
		• Primary surgical management should be reserved for select cases based on patient factors such as prior pelvic radiation, incontinence, fistula, and should follow a discussion at a MCC
		• Surgery for defunctioning stoma if fistula or fecal incontinence that will lead to greater skin toxicity during CRT
			Local persistence (>6 months or progression) or recurrence after cCR
			  • Salvage surgery with abdominoperineal resection and multivisceral resection of adherent structures
			  • 20–30% will have persistent or recurrent disease [51]
			  • R0 resection achieved in 60–90% [87–94]
			  • Locoregional recurrence after salvage surgery 30–75% [87–94]
			  • 5-year OS 25–85% [87–94]
			Regional recurrence
			  • Recurrence rates <5% in those who receive elective radiation to inguinal regions
			  • Formal groin dissection and/or consideration of inguinal irradiation (if the inguinal region has not received prior radiation therapy) +/– chemotherapy; limited data to guide this treatment choice [75, 95–97]
				Assess for cCR after CRT starting 8–12 weeks after CRT [13, 51, 78, 85]
				  • History, DRE, inguinal lymph nodes, anoscopy as indicated
				  • Persistent disease after CRT, reassess every 4 weeks up to 6 months. 30% may take 6 months for cCR [85, 98]
				  • Progression or persistence after 6 months, biopsy to confirm, restage, discussion for salvage surgery
				  • No biopsy to confirm cCR
				  • Radiation proctitis is meaningful long-term toxicity
				Surveillance after cCR or curative surgery [13, 51, 78]
				  • History, physical examination including DRE, anoscopy if indicated every 3 months for 2 years, then every 6 months for 1 year, then annually until 5 years
				  • CT chest, abdomen, pelvis if T3–4 or N+ (MRI if recommended by radiologist), every 6 months for 3 years, starting 3 months after treatment

Table 3.3 (continued)

	Work-up	Treatment		Follow-up
		Primary	Recurrence	
Perianal cancer, <2 cm, well-differentiated (T1, N0)		• Wide local excision provided that sphincter function is not compromised [13, 51, 99] • There is no agreement on what margin of resection constitutes an "adequate" margin, particularly with respect to the deep margin. In surgical planning, 1 cm radial margins are recommended [23, 47]		Perianal cancer treated with wide local excision • For residual HSIL, observation or 5% imiquimod cream 3/week for 16 weeks [52–54] • Consider referral for HRA surveillance of recurrence or incident HSIL • Consider anal cytology or HPV-DNA testing in surveillance

- Ensure that the lesion is biopsy-proven squamous cell carcinoma prior to proceeding with comprehensive staging investigations.
- Patients presenting with clinical or radiographic evidence of inguinal lymph node metastases should undergo pretreatment FNA biopsy to confirm the diagnosis if the result may alter radiation treatment planning.
- Consider HIV testing if the patient has a known risk factor. Patients with HIV should receive concomitant management of HIV infection by their primary care physician or infectious disease specialist. otherwise, patients with HIV should be treated similarly to those without HIV [13, 51, 78].
- If invasive SCC found incidentally on surgical specimen, discuss at MCC regarding re-excision vs CRT
- Superficially invasive squamous cell carcinoma (SISCCA), which invades ≤3 mm and is ≤7 mm wide, usually seen on HRA, if completely excised with margins ≥1 mm, some consider omission of CRT even if within the anal canal [16]
- Due to the need for wide lateral margins and prior pelvic RT, patients undergoing salvage surgery experience a high rate of postoperative complications (35–75%) particularly perineal infections and delayed wound healing [87–91]. Use of a myocutaneous flap for perineal reconstruction should be part of surgical planning [87–91, 100].
- Monitor for, counsel, and treat anorectal, urinary, and sexual function, fertility, and lymphedema [13, 68, 78]

5FU 5-fluorouracil, *cCR* complete clinical response, *Cis* cisplatin, *CRT* chemoradiotherapy, *DRE* digital rectal examination, *FNAB* fine-needle aspiration biopsy, *MCC* multidisciplinary cancer conference, *MMC* mitomycin C, *OS* overall survival

Table 3.4 Management of anal canal and perianal cancer: metastatic (any T, any N, M+)

Work-up	Treatment
Comprehensive history Digital anorectal examination Clinical assessment of inguinal lymph nodes (FNAB if suspicious) Conventional anoscopy, biopsy primary tumor for histologic confirmation Gynecological examination in female patients, with cervical cancer screening as appropriate Genital examination in male patients to exclude HPV-related disease HIV testing Hepatitis serology in preparation for systemic therapy Fertility preservation considerations Imaging CT thorax CT abdomen and pelvis Pelvic MRI	Most common sites are liver, lung, and extrapelvic lymph nodes; 10–20% of patients [85, 101, 102] Limited data to guide treatment choices [78] Systemic treatments are the main treatment options. 5FU + Cis has been most published and supported by guidelines as first-line albeit results are modest and treatment is associated with substantial toxicity [13, 78] Other combinations are being actively studied including docetaxel+5FU + Cis and immunotherapy [78, 103–105] There are very little data to support local treatments of metastatic disease including surgery or radiotherapy [106] If the primary cancer and/or symptomatic regional node metastases are present, consider the addition of chemoradiation or surgical excision for local control (as described for M0 disease)

5FU 5-fluorouracil, *Cis* cisplatin, *DRE* digital rectal examination, *FNAB* fine-needle aspiration biopsy

Prevention and Screening

Vaccination should be routinely administered to everyone between ages 9–13 to prevent initial HPV infection, and later if not previously immunized including MSM and those with immunodeficiency [13, 20, 114, 115]. HPV-9 nonvalent vaccine targets high-risk HPV types 16, 18, 31, 33, 45, 52, and 58, as well as low-risk HPV 6 and 11, accounting for nearly all causes of HPV-associated cancers and condyloma [20, 116]. Efficacy for preventing persistent infection is over 90% [117–119]. The prior quadrivalent vaccine targeted HPV 16, 18, 6, 11 [117]. Safer sex practices including routine condom use, as well as smoking cessation should also be advocated [8].

Screening is proposed for well-established high-risk groups including persons living with HIV, men who have sex with men (MSM), and MSM with HIV infection who have even greater risk [9, 28, 30, 40, 51, 120, 121]. Screening may allow early detection of HPV-related precursor lesions which can be treated to prevent anal cancer. However, evidence is not yet available to demonstrate reduced anal cancer incidence, mortality benefit, cost-effectiveness, or optimal screening approach and follow-up [43, 120, 122]. Ongoing studies will inform screening strategies [46, 47, 123]. At least, for those in high-risk populations, discussion of the risk of anal cancer and symptoms that should prompt clinical assessment and routine digital anorectal examination is appropriate [124]. Screening methods include anal cytology, HPV testing, high-resolution anoscopy, and directed biopsies [120–122, 125, 126]. A strategy analogous to cervical cancer screening includes anal cytology or HPV testing to triage use of HRA and directed biopsy. Anal cytology is categorized using

Table 3.5 Landmark studies

Topic	Study	Methods	Results
First use of CRT (preoperative)	Nigro et al. (1974) [74]	Case reports, $n = 3$ Concurrent 30 Gy RT + 5FU + MMC APR after 6 weeks	CRT can induce CR Two patients had a complete pathologic response at time of APR One patient declined surgery, but had a complete clinical response which was sustained at 1-year follow-up
Radical CRT (surgery only if persistent or recurrent disease)	Cummings et al. (1980) [107]	Single-arm cohort, $n = 6$ Concurrent 45 Gy RT + 5FU + MMC	CRT without surgery is a possible treatment option All patients had cCR with retained continence No local recurrence with 6–20-month-follow-up
CRT protocols (surgery only if persistent or recurrent disease)	UKCCCR ACT I (1996) [79] 13-year update (2010) [102]	RCT, $n = 585$ RT alone vs. CRT (RT + 5FU + MMC)	CRT is superior to RT alone (reporting at 12 years) cCR (30% vs. 39%) Locoregional recurrence (59% vs. 34%; HR 0.46, 95% CI 0.35–0.60, $p < 0.001$) Colostomy-free survival (20% vs 30%; HR 0.76, 95% CI 0.63–0.91, $p = 0.004$) Anal cancer-specific survival (51% vs. 64%; HR 0.67, 95% CI 0.51–0.88, $p = 0.004$) OS not statistically different (at 12 years, 28% vs. 33%; HR 0.86, 95% CI 0.70–1.04), $p = 0.12$)
	EORTC 22861 (1997) [81]	Multicenter RCT, $n = 110$ RT alone vs. CRT (RT + MMC-5FU)	CRT is superior to RT alone (reporting at 5 years) cCR (54% RT vs. 80% CRT) Locoregional recurrence (18% higher, $p = 0.02$) Colostomy-free rate (32% higher, $p = 0.002$) Event-free survival (absolute difference not reported, $p = 0.03$) OS not statistically different (54% vs. 58%, $p = 0.17$)
	RTOG 87–04 (1996) [82]	RCT, $n = 310$ RT + 5FU vs. RT + MMC-5FU.	CRT with MMC + 5FU is superior to CRT with 5FU alone, but increased toxicity (at 4 years) Locoregional recurrence (16% vs. 34%, $p < 0.001$) Colostomy-free rate (78% vs. 91%; $p = 0.002$ DFS (51% vs. 73%; $p < 0.001$) Toxicity in MMC group higher (7% vs. 23% grade 4 and 5 toxicity, $p < 0.001$) OS not different at 4 years

Table 3.5 (continued)

Topic	Study	Methods	Results
CRT intensification (surgery only if persistent or recurrent disease)	RTOG 98–11 (2008) [80] 5-year update (2012) [84]	RCT, $n = 682$ RT + 5FU+MMC vs. induction Cis-5FU then RT + Cis-5FU	CRT with MMC-5FU is superior to induction chemotherapy (Cis-5FU) followed by CRT with Cis-5FU (reporting at 5 years) DFS (68% vs. 58%; HR 1.39, 95% CI, 1.10–1.76, $p = 0.006$) OS (78% vs. 70%; HR 1.37, 95% CI 1.04–1.81, $p = 0.026$) Colostomy-free survival (72% vs 65%, HR 1.29, 95% CI, 0.99–1.67, $p = 0.05$). MMC arm higher acute toxicity (62% vs 42% grade 3–4 toxicity, $p < 0.001$)
	ACCORD 03 (2012) [86]	RCT, $n = 307$ 2x2 factorial trial (4 arms) Induction Cis-5FU then RT + Cis-5FU then standard dose RT boost. Induction Cis-5FU then RT+ Cis-5FU then high- dose RT boost RT + Cis-5FU then standard dose RT boost RT + Cis-5FU then high- dose RT boost	The addition of induction chemotherapy or high-dose RT boost did not demonstrate improved colostomy-free survival Induction Cis-5FU vs. no induction; 68% vs 58%, $p = 0.37$. Standard-dose RT boost vs. high-dose RT boost; 73.7% vs. 77.8%, $p = 0.067$.
	ACT II (2013) [85]	RCT, $n = 940$ 2x2 factorial trial (4 arms) RT + 5FU + MMC + maintenance 5FU + Cis (2 doses) RT + 5FU + MMC + no maintenance RT + 5FU + Cis + maintenance 5FU + Cis (2 doses) RT + 5FU + Cis + no maintenance	CRT with MMC- 5FU vs Cis-5FU is similar (reporting at 5 years) cCR similar (90% vs 90%; absolute difference – 0.9%, 95% CI -4.9–3.1, 30% without cCR at 11 weeks had cCR by 26 weeks Colostomy-free survival (68% vs 67%) DFS similar (69% vs. 69%; HR 0.95, 95% CI 0.75–1.19) OS similar (79% vs. 77%; HR 1.05, 95% CI 0.80–1.38) Maintenance chemotherapy did not offer improvement over CRT alone Colostomy-free survival (69% vs 66%) DFS (70% vs. 69%; HR 0.95, 95% CI 0.75–1.21). OS (76% vs. 79%, HR 1.07 CI 0.81–1.41).

(continued)

Table 3.5 (continued)

Topic	Study	Methods	Results
Intensity modulated radiation therapy (IMRT) to reduce toxicity	RTOG 0529 (2013) [108]	Phase 2 trial, $n = 63$ IMRT+MMC-5FU	Outcomes in this prospective single-arm study were compared to conventional RT + MMC-5FU in RTOG98–11 Grade 2+ gastrointestinal/genitourinary adverse events similar (77% in both trials) IMRT had improved acute grade 2+ hematologic, 73% (98–11 85%, $p = 0.032$), grade 3+ gastrointestinal, 21% (98–11 36%, $p = 0.008$), and grade 3+ dermatologic adverse events 23% (98–11 49%, $P < 0.0001$)
	Hosni et al. 2018 [109]	Prospective single-arm cohort, $n = 101$ IMRT+MMC-5FU	Most common acute grade ≥ 3 toxicities were skin (42%) and hematological (31%). 5-year OS 83% 5-year DFS 76% 5-year CFS 75%
Surgery	Correa et al. 2013 [110]	Retrospective single-arm cohort, $n = 111$ Salvage surgery for persistence or recurrence after CRT	83% required APR with en bloc resection of local structures (mostly vagina and uterus) 77% R0 resection margin 5-year OS 25% (95% CI 16–17%)
	Lefèvre et al. 2012 [111]	Retrospective single-arm cohort, $n = 105$ Salvage surgery for persistence or recurrence after CRT (7% primary surgery for contraindication to radiation)	All received APR (no report of en bloc resection) 82% R0 resection margin 5-year OS 61%
	Eeson et al. 2011 [96]	Retrospective single-arm cohort, $n = 51$ Salvage surgery for persistence or recurrence after CRT	All APR 63% Ro resection margin 5-year OS 29%
	ACT II 2016 (abstract) [112]	RCT, $n = 940$ Reporting on 291 patients with persistent or recurrent disease	107 (31%) underwent attempted salvage surgery with abdominoperineal resection 2-year OS 54% (95%CI 43–63%)
	Penderson et al. 2018 [113]	Retrospective single-arm cohort, $n = 47$ Salvage surgery for persistence or recurrence after CRT	33% required APR with en bloc resection (almost all hysterectomy) 85% R0 resection margin 5-year OS 50%

Table 3.5 (continued)

Topic	Study	Methods	Results
Systemic treatment for metastatic or unresectable disease	KEYNOTE-028 [105]	Phase Ib trial, *n* = 25 Pembrolizumab (anti-PD-1 immunotherapy)	Overall response rate 17% (95%CI 5–37%). Disease control rate 58% Adverse events 64%, most common diarrhea, fatigue, and nausea
	NCI9673 [104]	Phase 2 trial, *n* = 37 Nivolumab (anti-PD-1 immunotherapy)	Overall response rate 24% (95% CI 15–33%); 5% complete response. Grade 3 adverse event 14% (anemia, fatigue, rash, and hypothyroidism)
	Epitopes-HPV02 [103]	Phase 2 trial, *n* = 69 Docetaxel+5FU + Cis	Progression-free survival at 1 year 48%. Grade 3–4 adverse event 70%, most common neutropenia, diarrhea

5FU 5-fluorouracil, *APR* abdominoperineal resection, *cCR* complete clinical response, *Cis* cisplatin, *CRT* chemoradiotherapy, *DFS* disease-free survival, *MMC* mitomycin C, *OS* overall survival

the Bethesda system into negative, atypical squamous cells of undetermined significance (ASC-US), low-grade squamous intraepithelial lesion (LSIL); atypical squamous cells, cannot exclude HSIL (ASC-H); or HSIL [127]. Those with any abnormal cytology (ACS-US or more) are then screened with HRA and directed biopsies [51, 120, 128]. Anal cytology testing and interpretation, HRA, and follow-up strategies require expertise, and use of screening strategies should not be done without local expertise [48, 51, 129–131].

Referring to Medical Oncology

1. All patients with a biopsy-proven diagnosis of anal canal carcinoma should be referred to a medical oncologist for consideration of primary combined-modality chemoradiotherapy.
2. All patients with a biopsy-proven diagnosis of perianal carcinoma not suitable for local excision should be referred to a medical oncologist for consideration of primary combined-modality chemoradiotherapy.

Referring to Radiation Oncology

1. All patients with a biopsy-proven diagnosis of anal canal carcinoma should be referred to a radiation oncologist for consideration of primary combined-modality chemoradiotherapy.
2. All patients with a biopsy-proven diagnosis of perianal carcinoma not suitable for local excision should be referred to radiation oncologist for consideration of primary combined-modality chemoradiotherapy.

Referring to Multidisciplinary Cancer Conference

1. All patients with clinically suspected or biopsy-proven persistent or recurrent anal carcinoma following primary combined-modality or surgical treatment should be discussed at a Multidisciplinary Cancer Conference (MCC).
2. Patients not suitable for combined-modality chemoradiotherapy as the primary treatment of an anal carcinoma (due to patient comorbidities or tumor-related factors such as prior pelvic radiation, incontinence, fistula) should be discussed at an MCC, and considered for radical radiation alone or radical surgery (possibly with adjuvant preoperative or postoperative radiation with/without chemotherapy).
3. Patients presenting with metastatic disease should be discussed at MCC.
4. All patients with a biopsy-proven diagnosis of *adenocarcinoma* of the anal canal or perianal area should be discussed at MCC. Standard of care remains multimodality treatment including surgery as well as chemotherapy and radiation, like that in rectal adenocarcinoma. Several small series (including the Toronto experience) have found that local control can be achieved in about 50% of cases with adenocarcinomas, less than about 3 cm in size using combination chemoradiation alone. Treatment plans should be individualized on a case-by-case basis.

Toronto Pearls

- For patients undergoing chemoradiotherapy, the use of intensity modulated radiation therapy is associated with less treatment toxicity and better quality of life [132, 133].
- For patients undergoing radical salvage surgery, the use of a myocutaneous flap for perineal reconstruction is recommended.
- In order to achieve an R0 resection in locally advanced or recurrent disease, a multidisciplinary surgical team (including uro-oncology, plastic surgery, and/or orthopedic surgery) should be used in the context of multivisceral pelvic resections.
- HIV-positive patients should be managed similarly to non-HIV-infected patients. The risk of excessive reaction to radiation and/or chemotherapy is low. Treatment should be adjusted on an individual basis based on toxicity and side-effect profile.
- Previous pelvic radiation is a relative, but not an absolute, contraindication to radiation and chemotherapy for anal cancer. Such patients should be referred to a radiation oncologist for assessment and discussed at an MCC.

References

1. Canadian Cancer Statistics Advisory Committee. Anal Cancer statistics. In: Can. Cancer Soc. 2013. http://www.cancer.ca/en/cancer-information/cancer-type/anal/statistics/?region=on. Accessed 11 Dec 2018.
2. SEER Cancer Stat Facts: Anal Cancer. Natl Cancer Inst. 2018. https://seer.cancer.gov/statfacts/html/anus.html. Accessed 11 Dec 2018.

3. Siegel RL, Miller KD, Jemal A. Cancer statistics, 2018 CA: a cancer. J Clin. 2017;68:7–30.
4. Van Dyne EA, Henley SJ, Saraiya M, Thomas CC, Markowitz LE, Benard VB. Trends in human papillomavirus–associated cancers—United States, 1999–2015. Morb Mortal Wkly Rep. 2018;67:918.
5. Klas JV, Rothenberger DA, Wong WD, Madoff RD. Malignant tumors of the anal canal: the spectrum of disease, treatment, and outcomes. Cancer Interdiscip Int J Am Cancer Soc. 1999;85:1686–93.
6. Grulich AE, Van Leeuwen MT, Falster MO, Vajdic CM. Incidence of cancers in people with HIV/AIDS compared with immunosuppressed transplant recipients: a meta-analysis. Lancet. 2007;370:59–67.
7. Madeleine MM, Finch JL, Lynch CF, Goodman MT, Engels EA. HPV-related cancers after solid organ transplantation in the United States. Am J Transplant. 2013;13:3202–9.
8. Medford RJ, Salit IE. Anal cancer and intraepithelial neoplasia: epidemiology, screening and prevention of a sexually transmitted disease. Can Med Assoc J. 2015;187:111–5.
9. Silverberg MJ, Lau B, Justice AC, Engels E, Gill MJ, Goedert JJ, Kirk GD, D'souza G, Bosch RJ, Brooks JT. Risk of anal cancer in HIV-infected and HIV-uninfected individuals in North America. Clin Infect Dis. 2012;54:1026–34.
10. Goligher JC, Leacock AG, Brossy J. The surgical anatomy of the anal canal. Br J Surg. 1955;43:51–61.
11. Amin MB, Edge S, Greene F, et al, editors. AJCC cancer staging manual. 8th ed. Switzerland: Springer International Publishing.
12. Longacre TA, Kong CS, Welton ML. Diagnostic problems in anal pathology. Adv Anat Pathol. 2008;15:263–78.
13. Glynne-Jones R, Nilsson PJ, Aschele C, Goh V, Peiffert D, Cervantes A, Arnold D. Anal cancer: ESMO-ESSO-ESTRO clinical practice guidelines for diagnosis, treatment and follow-up. Ann Oncol. 2014;25:iii10–20.
14. Darragh TM, Colgan TJ, Cox JT, Heller DS, Henry MR, Luff RD, McCalmont T, Nayar R, Palefsky JM, Stoler MH. The lower anogenital squamous terminology standardization project for HPV-associated lesions: background and consensus recommendations from the College of American Pathologists and the American Society for Colposcopy and Cervical Pathology. Arch Pathol Lab Med. 2012;136:1266–97.
15. Yang EJ, Kong CS, Longacre TA. Vulvar and anal intraepithelial neoplasia: terminology, diagnosis, and ancillary studies. Adv Anat Pathol. 2017;24:136–50.
16. Berry-Lawhorn JM, Palefsky JM. Progression of anal high-grade squamous intraepithelial lesions to anal squamous cell carcinoma and clinical management of anal superficially invasive squamous cell carcinoma. In: Semin. Colon Rectal Surg. Elsevier; 2017. p. 91–6.
17. De Vuyst H, Clifford GM, Nascimento MC, Madeleine MM, Franceschi S. Prevalence and type distribution of human papillomavirus in carcinoma and intraepithelial neoplasia of the vulva, vagina and anus: a meta-analysis. Int J Cancer. 2009;124:1626–36.
18. Saraiya M, Unger ER, Thompson TD, Lynch CF, Hernandez BY, Lyu CW, Steinau M, Watson M, Wilkinson EJ, Hopenhayn C. US assessment of HPV types in cancers: implications for current and 9-valent HPV vaccines. JNCI J Natl Cancer Inst. 2015;107(6):djv086.
19. Plummer M, de Martel C, Vignat J, Ferlay J, Bray F, Franceschi S. Global burden of cancers attributable to infections in 2012: a synthetic analysis. Lancet Glob Heal. 2016;4:e609–16.
20. Salvadori MI. Human papillomavirus vaccine for children and adolescents. 2018.
21. Viarisio D, Gissmann L, Tommasino M. Human papillomaviruses and carcinogenesis: well-established and novel models. Curr Opin Virol. 2017;26:56–62.
22. Conley LJ, Ellerbrock TV, Bush TJ, Chiasson MA, Sawo D, Wright TC. HIV-1 infection and risk of vulvovaginal and perianal condylomata acuminata and intraepithelial neoplasia: a prospective cohort study. Lancet. 2002;359:108–13.
23. Rodríguez AC, Schiffman M, Herrero R, Wacholder S, Hildesheim A, Castle PE, Solomon D, Burk R, Group PEG. Rapid clearance of human papillomavirus and implications for clinical focus on persistent infections. J Natl Cancer Inst. 2008;100:513–7.
24. Frisch M, Olsen JH, Bautz A, Melbye M. Benign anal lesions and the risk of anal cancer. N Engl J Med. 1994;331:300–2.

25. Frisch M, Johansen C. Anal carcinoma in inflammatory bowel disease. Br J Cancer. 2000;83:89.
26. Tseng H-F, Morgenstern H, Mack TM, Peters RK. Risk factors for anal cancer: results of a population-based case–control study. Cancer Causes Control. 2003;14:837–46.
27. Frisch M, Glimelius B, van den Brule AJC, Wohlfahrt J, Meijer CJLM, Walboomers JMM, Goldman S, Svensson C, Adami H-O, Melbye M. Sexually transmitted infection as a cause of anal cancer. N Engl J Med. 1997;337:1350–8.
28. Schwartz LM, Castle PE, Follansbee S, Borgonovo S, Fetterman B, Tokugawa D, Lorey TS, Sahasrabuddhe VV, Luhn P, Gage JC. Risk factors for anal HPV infection and anal precancer in HIV-infected men who have sex with men. J Infect Dis. 2013;208:1768–75.
29. Edgren G, Sparén P. Risk of anogenital cancer after diagnosis of cervical intraepithelial neoplasia: a prospective population-based study. Lancet Oncol. 2007;8:311–6.
30. Tong WWY, Hillman RJ, Kelleher AD, Grulich AE, Carr A. Anal intraepithelial neoplasia and squamous cell carcinoma in HIV-infected adults. HIV Med. 2014;15:65–76.
31. Sunesen KG, Nørgaard M, Thorlacius-Ussing O, Laurberg S. Immunosuppressive disorders and risk of anal squamous cell carcinoma: a nationwide cohort study in Denmark, 1978–2005. Int J Cancer. 2010;127:675–84.
32. Albuquerque A, Cappello C, Cuming T, De Masi A, Bowring J, Rosenthal AN, Nathan M. Anal high-grade squamous intraepithelial lesions in pharmacologically immunocompromised patients followed in a referral center. Dis Colon Rectum. 2018;61:1267–72.
33. Joseph DA, Miller JW, Wu X, Chen VW, Morris CR, Goodman MT, Villalon-Gomez JM, Williams MA, Cress RD. Understanding the burden of human papillomavirus-associated anal cancers in the US. Cancer. 2008;113:2892–900.
34. Daling JR, Madeleine MM, Johnson LG, Schwartz SM, Shera KA, Wurscher MA, Carter JJ, Porter PL, Galloway DA, McDougall JK. Human papillomavirus, smoking, and sexual practices in the etiology of anal cancer. Cancer. 2004;101:270–80.
35. Lee GC, Kunitake H, Milch H, Savitt LR, Stafford CE, Bordeianou LG, Francone TD, Ricciardi R. What is the risk of anal carcinoma in patients with anal intraepithelial neoplasia III? Dis Colon Rectum. 2018;61:1350–6.
36. Tong WWY, Jin F, McHugh LC, Maher T, Sinclair B, Grulich AE, Hillman RJ, Carr A. Progression to and spontaneous regression of high-grade anal squamous intraepithelial lesions in HIV-infected and uninfected men. AIDS. 2013;27:2233–43.
37. Tinmouth J, Peeva V, Amare H, Blitz S, Raboud J, Sano M, Steele L, Salit IE. Progression from perianal high-grade anal intraepithelial neoplasia to anal cancer in HIV-positive men who have sex with men. Dis Colon Rectum. 2016;59:836–42.
38. Fazendin EA, Crean AJ, Fazendin JM, Kucejko RJ, Gill HS, Poggio JL, Stein DE. Condyloma acuminatum, anal intraepithelial neoplasia, and anal cancer in the setting of HIV: do we really understand the risk? Dis Colon Rectum. 2017;60:1078–82.
39. Cajas-Monson LC, Ramamoorthy SL, Cosman BC. Expectant management of high-grade anal Dysplasia in people with HIV: long-term data. Dis Colon Rectum. 2018;61:1357–63.
40. Machalek DA, Poynten M, Jin F, Fairley CK, Farnsworth A, Garland SM, Hillman RJ, Petoumenos K, Roberts J, Tabrizi SN. Anal human papillomavirus infection and associated neoplastic lesions in men who have sex with men: a systematic review and meta-analysis. Lancet Oncol. 2012;13:487–500.
41. Tong WWY, Shepherd K, Garland S, Meagher A, Templeton DJ, Fairley CK, Jin F, Poynten IM, Zaunders J, Hillman RJ. Human papillomavirus 16–specific T-cell responses and spontaneous regression of anal high-grade squamous intraepithelial lesions. J Infect Dis. 2014;211:405–15.
42. Factor SH, Cooperstein A, Pereira GA, Goldstone SE. Are colon and rectal surgeons ready to screen for anal dysplasia? Results of a survey on attitudes and practice. Sex Transm Dis. 2014;41:246–53.
43. Alam NN, White DA, Narang SK, Daniels IR, Smart NJ. Systematic review of guidelines for the assessment and management of high-grade anal intraepithelial neoplasia (AIN II/III). Color Dis. 2016;18:135–46.

44. Crawshaw BP, Russ AJ, Stein SL, Reynolds HL, Marderstein EL, Delaney CP, Champagne BJ. High-resolution anoscopy or expectant management for anal intraepithelial neoplasia for the prevention of anal cancer: is there really a difference? Dis Colon Rectum. 2015;58:53–9.
45. Goldstone SE. One step forward, two steps. Dis Colon Rectum. 2018;61:1339–41.
46. Topical or ablative treatment in preventing anal cancer in patients with HIV and anal high-grade squamous intraepithelial lesions (ANCHOR). In: (Identification No. NCT02135419). 2014. https://clinicaltrials.gov/ct2/show/NCT02135419. Accessed 14 Dec 2018.
47. The HPV-SAVE Study Team: HPV screening and vaccine evaluation in men who have sex with men (HPV-SAVE). In: (Identification No. NCT02503111). 2015. https://clinicaltrials.gov/ct2/show/NCT02503111. Accessed 14 Dec 2018.
48. Hillman RJ, Cuming T, Darragh T, Nathan M, Berry-Lawthorn M, Goldstone S, Law C, Palefsky J, Barroso LF, Stier EA. 2016 IANS international guidelines for practice standards in the detection of anal cancer precursors. J Low Genit Tract Dis. 2016;20:283–91.
49. Stockfleth E, Beti H, Orasan R, Grigorian F, Mescheder A, Tawfik H, Thielert C. Topical Polyphenon® E in the treatment of external genital and perianal warts: a randomized controlled trial. Br J Dermatol. 2008;158:1329–38.
50. Tyring S, Edwards L, Cherry LK, Ramsdell WM, Kotner S, Greenberg MD, Vance JC, Barnum G, Dromgoole SH, Killey FP. Safety and efficacy of 0.5% podofilox gel in the treatment of anogenital warts. Arch Dermatol. 1998;134:33–8.
51. Stewart DB, Gaertner WB, Glasgow SC, Herzig DO, Feingold D, Steele SR. The American society of colon and rectal surgeons clinical practice guidelines for anal squamous cell cancers (revised 2018). Dis Colon Rectum. 2018;61:755–74.
52. Fox PA, Nathan M, Francis N, Singh N, Weir J, Dixon G, Barton SE, Bower M. A double-blind, randomized controlled trial of the use of imiquimod cream for the treatment of anal canal high-grade anal intraepithelial neoplasia in HIV-positive MSM on HAART, with long-term follow-up data including the use of open-label imiquimod. AIDS. 2010;24:2331–5.
53. Richel O, de Vries HJC, van Noesel CJM, Dijkgraaf MGW, Prins JM. Comparison of imiquimod, topical fluorouracil, and electrocautery for the treatment of anal intraepithelial neoplasia in HIV-positive men who have sex with men: an open-label, randomised controlled trial. Lancet Oncol. 2013;14:346–53.
54. van der Snoek EM, den Hollander JC, van der Ende ME. Imiquimod 5% cream for five consecutive days a week in an HIV-infected observational cohort up to 32 weeks in the treatment of high-grade squamous intraepithelial lesions. Sex Transm Infect. 2015;91(4):245–7.
55. Richel O, Wieland U, De Vries HJC, Brockmeyer NH, Van Noesel C, Potthoff A, Prins JM, Kreuter A. Topical 5-fluorouracil treatment of anal intraepithelial neoplasia in human immunodeficiency virus-positive men. Br J Dermatol. 2010;163:1301–7.
56. Stier EA, Goldstone SE, Einstein MH, Jay N, Berry JM, Wilkin T, Lee JY, Darragh TM, Da Costa M, Panther L. Safety and efficacy of topical cidofovir to treat high-grade perianal and vulvar intraepithelial neoplasia in HIV-positive men and women. AIDS. 2013;27:545.
57. Sendagorta E, Bernardino JI, Álvarez-Gallego M, Feíto M, Feltes R, Beato MJ, Pérez-Molina JA, Yllescas M, Díaz-Almirón M, Arribas JR. Topical cidofovir to treat high-grade anal intraepithelial neoplasia in HIV-infected patients: a pilot clinical trial. AIDS. 2016;30:75–82.
58. Singh JC, Kuohung V, Palefsky JM. Efficacy of trichloroacetic acid in the treatment of anal intraepithelial neoplasia in HIV-positive and HIV-negative men who have sex with men. J Acquir Immune Defic Syndr. 2009;52:474.
59. Cranston RD, Baker JR, Liu Y, Wang L, Elishaev E, Ho KS. Topical application of trichloroacetic acid is efficacious for the treatment of internal anal high-grade squamous intraepithelial lesions in HIV-positive men. Sex Transm Dis. 2014;41:420–6.
60. Marks DK, Goldstone SE. Electrocautery ablation of high-grade anal squamous intraepithelial lesions in HIV-negative and HIV-positive men who have sex with men. JAIDS J Acquir Immune Defic Syndr. 2012;59:259–65.
61. Pineda CE, Berry JM, Jay N, Palefsky JM, Welton ML. High-resolution anoscopy targeted surgical destruction of anal high-grade squamous intraepithelial lesions: a ten-year experience. Dis Colon Rectum. 2008;51:829–37.

62. Burgos J, Curran A, Landolfi S, Navarro J, Tallada N, Guelar A, Crespo M, Ocaña I, Ribera E, Falcó V. The effectiveness of electrocautery ablation for the treatment of high-grade anal intraepithelial neoplasia in HIV-infected men who have sex with men. HIV Med. 2016;17:524–31.
63. Goldstone RN, Hasan SR, Goldstone SE. Brief report: radiofrequency ablation therapy for anal intraepithelial neoplasia results from a single-center prospective pilot study in HIV+ participants. JAIDS J Acquir Immune Defic Syndr. 2017;76:e93–7.
64. Weis SE, Vecino I, Pogoda JM, Susa JS. Treatment of high-grade anal intraepithelial neoplasia with infrared coagulation in a primary care population of HIV-infected men and women. Dis Colon Rectum. 2012;55:1236–43.
65. Sirera G, Videla S, Piñol M, Coll J, García-Cuyás F, Vela S, Cañadas M, Darwich L, Pérez N, Gel S. Long-term effectiveness of infrared coagulation for the treatment of anal intraepithelial neoplasia grades 2 and 3 in HIV-infected men and women. AIDS. 2013;27:951–9.
66. Goldstone SE, Johnstone AA, Moshier EL. Long-term outcome of ablation of anal high-grade squamous intraepithelial lesions: recurrence and incidence of cancer. Dis Colon Rectum. 2014;57:316–23.
67. Steele SR, Varma MG, Melton GB, Ross HM, Rafferty JF, Buie WD. Practice parameters for anal squamous neoplasms. Dis Colon Rectum. 2012;55:735–49.
68. Shridhar R, Shibata D, Chan E, Thomas CR. Anal cancer: current standards in care and recent changes in practice. CA Cancer J Clin. 2015;65:139–62.
69. Goffredo P, Garancini M, Robinson TJ, Frakes J, Hoshi H, Hassan I. A national-level validation of the new American joint committee on cancer 8th edition subclassification of stage IIA and B anal squamous cell cancer. Ann Surg Oncol. 2018;25(6):1–7.
70. Gunderson LL, Moughan J, Ajani JA, Pedersen JE, Winter KA, Benson AB III, Thomas CR Jr, Mayer RJ, Haddock MG, Rich TA. Anal carcinoma: impact of TN category of disease on survival, disease relapse, and colostomy failure in US gastrointestinal intergroup RTOG 98-11 phase 3 trial. Int J Radiat Oncol Biol Phys. 2013;87:638–45.
71. Glynne-Jones R, Kadalayil L, Meadows HM, Cunningham D, Samuel L, Geh JI, Lowdell C, James R, Beare S, Begum R. Tumour-and treatment-related colostomy rates following mitomycin C or cisplatin chemoradiation with or without maintenance chemotherapy in squamous cell carcinoma of the anus in the ACT II trial. Ann Oncol. 2014;25:1616–22.
72. Bilimoria KY, Bentrem DJ, Rock CE, Stewart AK, Ko CY, Halverson A. Outcomes and prognostic factors for squamous-cell carcinoma of the anal canal: analysis of patients from the National Cancer Data Base. Dis Colon Rectum. 2009;52:624–31.
73. Jones CM, Goh V, Sebag-Montefiore D, Gilbert DC. Biomarkers in anal cancer: from biological understanding to stratified treatment. Br J Cancer. 2017;116:156.
74. Nigro ND, Vaitkevicius VK, Considine B. Combined therapy for cancer of the anal canal: a preliminary report. Dis Colon Rectum. 1974;17:354–6.
75. Gerard J, Chapet O, Samiei F, Morignat E, Isaac S, Paulin C, Romestaing P, Favrel V, Mornex F, Bobin J. Management of inguinal lymph node metastases in patients with carcinoma of the anal canal: experience in a series of 270 patients treated in Lyon and review of the literature. Cancer. 2001;92:77–84.
76. Ortholan C, Resbeut M, Hannoun-Levi J-M, Teissier E, Gerard J-P, Ronchin P, Zaccariotto A, Minsat M, Benezery K, François E. Anal canal cancer: management of inguinal nodes and benefit of prophylactic inguinal irradiation (CORS-03 Study). Int J Radiat Oncol Biol Phys. 2012;82:1988–95.
77. Mahmud A, Poon R, Jonker D. PET imaging in anal canal cancer. 2017. Toronto: Cancer Care Ontario. Program in evidence- based care recommendation report no.: PET-17, available on the CCO website https://www.cancercareontario.ca/sites/ccocancercare/files/guidelines/full/pebcpet-17f_0.pdf.
78. Benson AB, Venook A, Al-Hawary M, et al. Anal Carcinoma, Version 2.2018. J Natl Compr Cancer Netw. 2018;16:852–71.
79. Party UACTW. Epidermoid anal cancer: results from the UKCCCR randomised trial of radiotherapy alone versus radiotherapy, 5-fluorouracil, and mitomycin. Lancet. 1996;348:1049–54.

80. Ajani JA, Winter KA, Gunderson LL, Pedersen J, Benson AB, Thomas CR, Mayer RJ, Haddock MG, Rich TA, Willett C. Fluorouracil, mitomycin, and radiotherapy vs fluorouracil, cisplatin, and radiotherapy for carcinoma of the anal canal: a randomized controlled trial. JAMA. 2008;299:1914–21.
81. Bartelink H, Roelofsen F, Eschwege F, Rougier P, Bosset JF, Gonzalez DG, Peiffert D, Van Glabbeke M, Pierart M. Concomitant radiotherapy and chemotherapy is superior to radiotherapy alone in the treatment of locally advanced anal cancer: results of a phase III randomized trial of the European Organization for Research and Treatment of Cancer Radiotherapy and Gastro. J Clin Oncol. 1997;15:2040–9.
82. Flam M, John M, Pajak TF, Petrelli N, Myerson R, Doggett S, Quivey J, Rotman M, Kerman H, Coia L. Role of mitomycin in combination with fluorouracil and radiotherapy, and of salvage chemoradiation in the definitive nonsurgical treatment of epidermoid carcinoma of the anal canal: results of a phase III randomized intergroup study. J Clin Oncol. 1996;14:2527–39.
83. Spithoff K, Cummings B, Jonker D, Biagi J, Gastrointestinal Cancer Disease Site Group. Management of squamous cell cancer of the anal canal. Toronto: Cancer Care Ontario. Program in Evidence-based Care Evidence-Based Series No.: 2–8 Version 2 2013.
84. Gunderson LL, Winter KA, Ajani JA, Pedersen JE, Moughan J, Benson AB III, Thomas CR Jr, Mayer RJ, Haddock MG, Rich TA. Long-term update of US GI intergroup RTOG 98-11 phase III trial for anal carcinoma: survival, relapse, and colostomy failure with concurrent chemoradiation involving fluorouracil/mitomycin versus fluorouracil/cisplatin. J Clin Oncol. 2012;30:4344.
85. James RD, Glynne-Jones R, Meadows HM, Cunningham D, Myint AS, Saunders MP, Maughan T, McDonald A, Essapen S, Leslie M. Mitomycin or cisplatin chemoradiation with or without maintenance chemotherapy for treatment of squamous-cell carcinoma of the anus (ACT II): a randomised, phase 3, open-label, 2× 2 factorial trial. Lancet Oncol. 2013;14:516–24.
86. Peiffert D, Tournier-Rangeard L, Gérard J-P, Lemanski C, François E, Giovannini M, Cvitkovic F, Mirabel X, Bouché O, Luporsi E. Induction chemotherapy and dose intensification of the radiation boost in locally advanced anal canal carcinoma: final analysis of the randomized UNICANCER ACCORD 03 trial. J Clin Oncol. 2012;30:1941–8.
87. Tan KK, Pal S, Lee PJ, Rodwell L, Solomon MJ. Pelvic exenteration for recurrent squamous cell carcinoma of the pelvic organs arising from the cloaca–a single institution's experience over 16 years. Color Dis. 2013;15:1227–31.
88. Schiller DE, Cummings BJ, Rai S, Le LW, Last L, Davey P, Easson A, Smith AJ, Swallow CJ. Outcomes of salvage surgery for squamous cell carcinoma of the anal canal. Ann Surg Oncol. 2007;14:2780–9.
89. Harris DA, Williamson J, Davies M, Evans MD, Drew P, Beynon J, Group SPO. Outcome of salvage surgery for anal squamous cell carcinoma. Color Dis. 2013;15:968–73.
90. Nilsson PJ, Svensson C, Goldman S, Glimelius B. Salvage abdominoperineal resection in anal epidermoid cancer. Br J Surg. 2002;89:1425–9.
91. Sunesen KG, Buntzen S, Tei T, Lindegaard JC, Nørgaard M, Laurberg S. Perineal healing and survival after anal cancer salvage surgery: 10-year experience with primary perineal reconstruction using the vertical rectus abdominis myocutaneous (VRAM) flap. Ann Surg Oncol. 2009;16:68–77.
92. Hallemeier CL, You YN, Larson DW, Dozois EJ, Nelson H, Klein KA, Miller RC, Haddock MG. Multimodality therapy including salvage surgical resection and intraoperative radiotherapy for patients with squamous-cell carcinoma of the anus with residual or recurrent disease after primary chemoradiotherapy. Dis Colon Rectum. 2014;57:442–8.
93. Hannes S, Reinisch A, Bechstein WO, Habbe N. Salvage abdominoperineal excisions in recurrent anal cancer—impact of different reconstruction techniques on outcome, morbidity, and complication rates. Int J Color Dis. 2016;31:653–9.
94. Bignell M, Chave H, Branagan G. Outcome of surgery for recurrent anal cancer–results from a tertiary referral centre. Colorectal Dis. 2018;20(9):771–7.

95. Akbari RP, Paty PB, Guillem JG, Weiser MR, Temple LK, Minsky BD, Saltz L, Wong WD. Oncologic outcomes of salvage surgery for epidermoid carcinoma of the anus initially managed with combined modality therapy. Dis Colon Rectum. 2004;47:1136–44.
96. Eeson G, Foo M, Harrow S, McGregor G, Hay J. Outcomes of salvage surgery for epidermoid carcinoma of the anus following failed combined modality treatment. Am J Surg. 2011;201:628–33.
97. Blinde SE, Schasfoort R, Mens JW, Verhoef C, Olofsen M, Nuyttens JJ. Inguinal lymph node recurrence in the untreated groin of patients with anal carcinoma. Dis Colon Rectum. 2014;57:578–84.
98. Glynne-Jones R, Sebag-Montefiore D, Meadows HM, Cunningham D, Begum R, Adab F, Benstead K, Harte RJ, Stewart J, Beare S. Best time to assess complete clinical response after chemoradiotherapy in squamous cell carcinoma of the anus (ACT II): a post-hoc analysis of randomised controlled phase 3 trial. Lancet Oncol. 2017;18:347–56.
99. Chai CY, Cao HT, Awad S, Massarweh NN. Management of stage I squamous cell carcinoma of the anal canal. JAMA Surg. 2018;153:209–15.
100. Renehan AG, Saunders MP, Schofield PF, O'Dwyer ST. Patterns of local disease failure and outcome after salvage surgery in patients with anal cancer. Br J Surg Inc Eur J Surg Swiss Surg. 2005;92:605–14.
101. Cummings BJ. Metastatic anal cancer: the search for cure. Oncol Res Treat. 2006;29:5–6.
102. Northover J, Glynne-Jones R, Sebag-Montefiore D, James R, Meadows H, Wan S, Jitlal M, Ledermann J. Chemoradiation for the treatment of epidermoid anal cancer: 13-year follow-up of the first randomised UKCCCR Anal Cancer Trial (ACT I). Br J Cancer. 2010;102:1123.
103. Kim S, François E, André T, Samalin E, Jary M, El Hajbi F, Baba-Hamed N, Pernot S, Kaminsky M-C, Bouché O. Docetaxel, cisplatin, and fluorouracil chemotherapy for metastatic or unresectable locally recurrent anal squamous cell carcinoma (Epitopes-HPV02): a multicentre, single-arm, phase 2 study. Lancet Oncol. 2018;19:1094–106.
104. Morris VK, Salem ME, Nimeiri H, Iqbal S, Singh P, Ciombor K, Polite B, Deming D, Chan E, Wade JL. Nivolumab for previously treated unresectable metastatic anal cancer (NCI9673): a multicentre, single-arm, phase 2 study. Lancet Oncol. 2017;18:446–53.
105. Ott PA, Piha-Paul SA, Munster P, Pishvaian MJ, Van Brummelen EMJ, Cohen RB, Gomez-Roca C, Ejadi S, Stein M, Chan E. Safety and antitumor activity of the anti-PD-1 antibody pembrolizumab in patients with recurrent carcinoma of the anal canal. Ann Oncol. 2017;28:1036–41.
106. Pawlik TM, Gleisner AL, Bauer TW, Adams RB, Reddy SK, Clary BM, Martin RC, Scoggins CR, Tanabe KK, Michaelson JS. Liver-directed surgery for metastatic squamous cell carcinoma to the liver: results of a multi-center analysis. Ann Surg Oncol. 2007;14:2807–16.
107. Cummings BJ, Harwood AR, Keane TJ, Thomas GM, Rider WD. Combined treatment of squamous cell carcinoma of the anal canal: radical radiation therapy with 5-fluorouracil and mitomycin-C, a preliminary report. Dis Colon Rectum. 1980;23:389–91.
108. Kachnic LA, Winter K, Myerson RJ, Goodyear MD, Willins J, Esthappan J, Haddock MG, Rotman M, Parikh PJ, Safran H. RTOG 0529: a phase 2 evaluation of dose-painted intensity modulated radiation therapy in combination with 5-fluorouracil and mitomycin-C for the reduction of acute morbidity in carcinoma of the anal canal. Int J Radiat Oncol Biol Phys. 2013;86:27–33.
109. Hosni A, Han K, Le LW, Ringash J, Brierley J, Wong R, Dinniwell R, Brade A, Dawson LA, Cummings BJ. The ongoing challenge of large anal cancers: prospective long term outcomes of intensity-modulated radiation therapy with concurrent chemotherapy. Oncotarget. 2018;9:20439.
110. Correa JHS, Castro LS, Kesley R, Dias JA, Jesus JP, Olivatto LO, Martins IO, Lopasso FP. Salvage abdominoperineal resection for anal cancer following chemoradiation: a proposed scoring system for predicting postoperative survival. J Surg Oncol. 2013;107:486–92.
111. Lefèvre JH, Corte H, Tiret E, Boccara D, Chaouat M, Touboul E, Svrcek M, Lefrancois M, Shields C, Parc Y. Abdominoperineal resection for squamous cell anal carcinoma: survival and risk factors for recurrence. Ann Surg Oncol. 2012;19:4186–92.

112. Glynne-Jones R, Meadows HM, Lopes A, Adams RA, Samuel LM, Hill J, Renehan A, Hawkins MA, Sebag-Montefiore D, Study ACTII. Salvage surgery with abdominoperineal excision of the rectum (APER) following loco-regional failure after chemoradiation (CRT) using mitomycin (MMC) or cisplatin (CisP), with or without maintenance 5FU/CisP chemotherapy (CT) in squamous cell carcinoma of the anus (SCCA) and the impact on long-term outcomes: results of ACT II. 2016.
113. Pedersen TB, Gocht-Jensen P, Klein MF. 30-day and long-term outcome following salvage surgery for squamous cell carcinoma of the anus. Eur J Surg Oncol. 2018;44:1518–21.
114. Petrosky E, Bocchini JJA, Hariri S, Chesson H, Curtis CR, Saraiya M, Unger ER, Markowitz LE. Use of 9-valent human papillomavirus (HPV) vaccine: updated HPV vaccination recommendations of the advisory committee on immunization practices. MMWR Morb Mortal Wkly Rep. 2015;64:300–4.
115. National Advisory Committee on Immunization. Update on the recommended human papillomavirus (HPV) vaccine immunization schedule. Public Heal. Agency Canada. 2015.
116. Patel C, Brotherton JML, Pillsbury A, Jayasinghe S, Donovan B, Macartney K, Marshall H. The impact of 10 years of human papillomavirus (HPV) vaccination in Australia: what additional disease burden will a nonavalent vaccine prevent? Eurosurveillance. 2018;23(41):1700737.
117. Palefsky JM, Giuliano AR, Goldstone S, Moreira ED Jr, Aranda C, Jessen H, Hillman R, Ferris D, Coutlee F, Stoler MH. HPV vaccine against anal HPV infection and anal intraepithelial neoplasia. N Engl J Med. 2011;365:1576–85.
118. Arbyn M, Xu L. Efficacy and safety of prophylactic HPV vaccines. A Cochrane review of randomized trials. Expert Rev Vaccines. 2018;17(12):1–7.
119. Signorelli C, Odone A, Ciorba V, Cella P, Audisio RA, Lombardi A, Mariani L, Mennini FS, Pecorelli S, Rezza G. Human papillomavirus 9-valent vaccine for cancer prevention: a systematic review of the available evidence. Epidemiol Infect. 2017;145:1962–82.
120. Palefsky JM. Screening to prevent anal cancer: current thinking and future directions. Cancer Cytopathol. 2015;123:509–10.
121. Leeds IL, Fang SH. Anal cancer and intraepithelial neoplasia screening: a review. World J Gastrointest Surg. 2016;8:41.
122. Clarke MA, Wentzensen N. Strategies for screening and early detection of anal cancers: a narrative and systematic review and meta-analysis of cytology, HPV testing, and other biomarkers. Cancer Cytopathol. 2018;126(7):447–60.
123. Machalek DA, Grulich AE, Hillman RJ, Jin F, Templeton DJ, Tabrizi SN, Garland SM, Prestage G, McCaffery K, Howard K. The Study of the Prevention of Anal Cancer (SPANC): design and methods of a three-year prospective cohort study. BMC Public Health. 2013;13:946.
124. Berry JM, Jay N, Cranston RD, Darragh TM, Holly EA, Welton ML, Palefsky JM. Progression of anal high-grade squamous intraepithelial lesions to invasive anal cancer among HIV-infected men who have sex with men. Int J Cancer. 2014;134:1147–55.
125. Sambursky JA, Terlizzi JP, Goldstone SE. Testing for human papillomavirus strains 16 and 18 helps predict the presence of anal high-grade squamous intraepithelial lesions. Dis Colon Rectum. 2018;61:1364–71.
126. Schofield AM, Sadler L, Nelson L, Gittins M, Desai M, Sargent A, McMahon RFT, Hill J, Crosbie EJ, Patnick J. A prospective study of anal cancer screening in HIV-positive and negative MSM. AIDS. 2016;30:1375–83.
127. Nayar R, Wilbur DC The Bethesda system for reporting cervical cytology: definitions, criteria, and explanatory notes. Switzerland: Springer; 2015.
128. Jin F, Grulich AE, Poynten IM, Hillman RJ, Templeton DJ, Law CLH, Farnsworth A, Garland SM, Fairley CK, Roberts JM. The performance of anal cytology as a screening test for anal HSILs in homosexual men. Cancer Cytopathol. 2016;124:415–24.
129. Templeton DJ, Roberts JM, Poynten IM, Law C, Hillman RJ, Farnsworth A, Fairley CK, Tabrizi SN, Garland SM, Grulich AE. Prevalence and predictors of unsatisfactory anal cytol-

ogy tests in a cohort of gay and bisexual men in Sydney, Australia: baseline findings from the Study of the Prevention of Anal Cancer (SPANC). Eur J Cancer Prev. 2017;26:212–6.
130. Darragh TM, Tokugawa D, Castle PE, Follansbee S, Borgonovo S, LaMere BJ, Schwartz L, Gage JC, Fetterman B, Lorey T. Interrater agreement of anal cytology. Cancer Cytopathol. 2013;121:72–8.
131. Darragh TM, Winkler B, Souers RJ, Laucirica R, Zhao C, Moriarty AT. Room for improvement: initial experience with anal cytology: observations from the College of American Pathologists interlaboratory comparison program in nongynecologic cytology. Arch Pathol Lab Med. 2013;137:1550–4.
132. Han K, Cummings BJ, Lindsay P, Skliarenko J, Craig T, Le LW, Brierley J, Wong R, Dinniwell R, Bayley AJ. Prospective evaluation of acute toxicity and quality of life after IMRT and concurrent chemotherapy for anal canal and perianal cancer. Int J Radiat Oncol Biol Phys. 2014;90:587–94.
133. Glynne-Jones R, Tan D, Hughes R, Hoskin P. Squamous-cell carcinoma of the anus: progress in radiotherapy treatment. Nat Rev Clin Oncol. 2016;13:447.

Breast Cancer

4

David W. Lim, Lu Yin, Janice R. Mulcahy, Naama Hermann, Hyeyoun (Elise) Min, Jean-Francois Boileau, Mark Corrigan, Tulin Cil, Alexandra M. Easson, Jaime M. Escallon, Ralph George, Claire Holloway, Joan E. Lipa, and David R. McCready

Hyeyoun (Elise) Min contributed equally with all other contributors.

D. W. Lim · L. Yin
Breast Surgical Oncology, Sunnybrook & University Health Network, University of Toronto, Toronto, ON, Canada
e-mail: David.Lim@wchospital.ca

J. R. Mulcahy
St. Michael's Hospital, University of Toronto, Toronto, ON, Canada

N. Hermann
Sunnybrook & University Health Network, University of Toronto, Toronto, ON, Canada

H. (Elise) Min
Division of Plastic & Reconstructive Surgery – Sunnybrook, University of Toronto, Toronto, ON, Canada

J.-F. Boileau
Department of Surgery, Sir Mortimer B. Davis Jewish General Hospital, McGill University, Montreal, QC, Canada

M. Corrigan
Department of Surgery, Cork University Hospital, Cork, Ireland
e-mail: mark.corrigan@ucc.ie

T. Cil · A. M. Easson · J. M. Escallon · R. George · C. Holloway
Department of Surgery, University of Toronto, Toronto, ON, Canada
e-mail: Tulin.Cil@uhn.ca; Alexandra.Easson@uhn.ca; Jaime.Escallon@sinaihealth.ca; GeorgeR@smh.ca

J. E. Lipa
Department of Surgery, Division of Plastics and Reconstructive Surgery, University of Toronto, Toronto, ON, Canada
e-mail: Joan.Lipa@sunnybrook.ca

D. R. McCready (✉)
Department of Surgery, Division of Surgical Oncology, University of Toronto, Toronto, ON, Canada
e-mail: David.McCready@uhn.ca

F. C. Wright et al. (eds.), *Surgical Oncology Manual*,
https://doi.org/10.1007/978-3-030-48363-0_4

Introduction

Breast cancer is the most common cancer among Canadian women with the exception of non-melanoma skin cancer. An estimated 26, 300 new cases occurred in Canada in 2017. Breast cancer is responsible for 26% of all new cancers in women and 13% of all cancer-related deaths in women. One in every 8 women is expected to develop breast cancer during her lifetime, and 1 in 31 women will die of breast cancer [1].

Presentation	Prognosis 5-Year overall survival (OS)
Early breast cancer[a] (75–80%)	90–100%
Locally advanced breast cancer[a] (10–20%)	36–67%
Distant metastasis (5%)	22%

[a]See definitions in this chapter

The recommended staging system is the eighth edition of American Joint Committee on Cancer (AJCC) [2].

The surgical management of breast cancer requires an understanding of the complete spectrum of breast pathology, both malignant and premalignant. As a result, an overview of this continuum is presented: from high-risk pathologies, through preinvasive disease, to invasive disease and the management of some of its various subtypes.

Benign, but Worrisome

There exist pathological entities affecting the breast which bridge the divide between benign and malignant. They can present difficulty to the clinician, in terms of their appropriate management and—like many aspects of breast treatment—they are under constant review. Below we have summarized the clinical and pathological features as well as management of several of the more commonly encountered entities:

Entity	Definition and diagnosis	Treatment [3, 4]	Comments
Atypical ductal hyperplasia (ADH) [3]	A proliferation of uniform epithelial cells with monomorphic round nuclei filling part, but not all, of the involved duct Same cytology and architecture as low-grade DCIS but extent is <2 mm or less than 2 involved ducts Diagnosis: asymptomatic, incidental, often calcifications on mammography	If found on CNB, the area should be removed to ensure that no adjacent carcinoma is present If found at the margins of an excised lesion, re-excision is not generally considered necessary unless bordering on the diagnosis of DCIS, or concern that target lesion was not completely excised	Upgrade rate to DCIS or invasive carcinoma often 10–20% [3] Atypical hyperplasia confers a substantial increase in the risk of subsequent breast cancer (RR 3.7–5.3) [5] Follow with clinical exam every 6–12 months and annual screening mammogram (not before age 30); NCCN recommends consideration of tomosynthesis and annual MRI [6], but Cancer Care Ontario currently does not endorse annual MRI [7]
Atypical lobular hyperplasia (ALH) [3]	Often an incidental finding on breast biopsies done for other reasons Proliferation of monomorphic, evenly spaced, dyscohesive cells filling part, but not all, of the involved lobule ALH can also involve ducts (DIAL: duct involvement by atypical lobular cells) Same cytology and architecture of LCIS but quantitatively lesser in extent Diagnosis: asymptomatic, incidental, loss of E-cadherin [8]	If found on CNB, the area should be removed if there is imaging-pathologic discordance If found at the margins of an excised lesion, re-excision is not generally considered necessary	Upgrade rate to DCIS or invasive cancer after diagnosis of incidental ALH on CNB is <3% (usually very small, low-grade invasive carcinomas) Routine excision is not advocated if there is radiologic-pathologic concordance and no other lesions requiring excision are present [4] Similar risk of subsequent breast cancer as ADH (RR 3.7–5.3) [3] ALH is associated with an increased risk of both ipsilateral and contralateral breast cancer, with the Nurses' Health Study demonstrating that only 56% of cancers developing in women with ALH occurred in the ipsilateral breast. The cumulative incidence of breast cancer over 30 years in patients with ALH approached 35% [9] Follow with clinical exam every 6–12 months and annual screening mammogram (not before age 30); NCCN recommends consideration of tomosynthesis and annual MRI [6], but Cancer Care Ontario currently does not endorse annual MRI [7]

(continued)

Entity	Definition and diagnosis	Treatment [3, 4]	Comments
Lobular carcinoma in situ (LCIS) [3]	Abnormal cell growth in the lobules of the breast that represents an increased risk of cancer rather than being a premalignant condition per se Distinguish between classical (cLCIS) and pleomorphic (pLCIS) to plan treatment Diagnosis: asymptomatic, incidental, lacks clinical and mammographic signs, loss of E-cadherin [8]	If found on CNB, the area should be removed if there is imaging-pathologic discordance Excise any nonclassical LCIS (e.g., pleomorphic LCIS, LCIS with necrosis) If found at the margins of an excised lesion (including invasive cancer), re-excision is not generally considered necessary (unless nonclassical LCIS is found at the margin) Multifocal/extensive LCIS involving >4 terminal ductal lobular units on CNB may be associated with an increased risk of invasive cancer on excision [6]	Relative risk of developing invasive cancer is 7–11-fold; absolute risk is 1%/year and is lifelong [3] If there is radiologic-pathologic concordance and no other lesions with risk of concomitant malignancy (i.e., ADH, papilloma, radial scar) are present, upgrade rate is <5% [4] and can observe with close clinical and imaging follow-up [3] or excision [6] Follow-up with clinical exam every 6–12 months and annual screening mammogram (not before age 30); NCCN recommends consideration of tomosynthesis and annual MRI [6], but Cancer Care Ontario currently does not endorse annual MRI [7] Pleomorphic LCIS is an aggressive variant of LCIS often sharing pathologic features with DCIS (central necrosis and calcifications), and is often treated with excision to clear margins, similar to DCIS [10]
Papillary lesions, including intraductal papilloma [11]	Intraluminal epithelial fronds that may exhibit a variety of alterations from atypia or DCIS to carcinoma Diagnosis: breast lump, nipple discharge (often bloody), or nodule on ultrasound or by ductoscopy	Generally, the advice is for excision given the risk of malignancy, especially if palpable or atypia present. If the absence of atypia can be proven, however, there might be a role for observation, but the literature on papillary lesions without atypia is mixed with little consensus	Without atypia, the chance of malignancy is very small (<10%), but with atypia, some authors have reported the associated rate of coexistent cancer to be as high as 67% [12]. One of the largest multicenter series (n = 238) reported an upgrade rate of 14.4%, with only 3.7% upgraded to invasive cancer. Older age and presence of atypia on core biopsy were associated with risk of malignancy [13] Incidental, benign papillary lesions can be followed [3]
Sclerosing adenosis [11]	A benign lobular lesion with increased fibrous tissue and interspersed glandular cells Diagnosis: occasional lump/nodules or pain, and occasional microcalcifications. Perform CNB	No treatment is needed [11] After CNB, excision is only recommended in the following situations: Limited sampling Presence of atypia Radiological discordance	Risk of subsequent cancer is small [11]

Microglandular adenosis	A rare type of adenosis, resembling tubular carcinoma, where irregular clusters of small tubules are present in adipose or fibrous tissues Diagnosis: may present as mass Perform CNB	Given risk of carcinoma, perform excision	Microglandular adenosis is poorly studied, but is associated with a carcinoma rate of approximately 23% [14, 15]
Radial scars and complex sclerosing lesions [11]	Benign, spiculated masses characterized by a sclerotic-appearing (scar-like) center with peripheral entrapped normal breast ducts and lobules Diagnosis: asymptomatic. Perform imaging and CNB	The standard management is to excise if detected as a mammographic lesion However, if the radial scar is an incidental finding on a CNB performed to investigate a suspected different lesion and atypia is not identified, there may be a role for observation	Risk of subsequent breast cancer is twofold [16]
Pseudoangiomatous stromal hyperplasia (PASH) [11]	Benign, stromal (myofibroblast) proliferation that simulates a vascular lesion More common in premenopausal women, possible hormonal etiology Presents as painless mass or imaging abnormality Most common appearance on mammogram/US is a solid, well-defined, noncalcified mass	If diagnosed conclusively on CNB, PASH can be managed expectantly Excise if discordance with imaging or increase in size of lesion	Although PASH is benign, recurrence after excision is reported in 15–22% of cases Excise if suspicious imaging findings, interval growth, and symptomatic lesions No increased risk of subsequent breast cancer

(continued)

Entity	Definition and diagnosis	Treatment [3, 4]	Comments
Columnar cell lesions (CCLs) without or with atypia (CCL-A, the latter also being known as flat epithelial atypia, FEA) [3]	Often seen on CNB performed for mammographic calcifications Enlarged terminal ductal lobular units with replacement of native epithelial cells by 1 or more layers of columnar epithelial cells with or without atypia Diagnosis: asymptomatic. Perform imaging and CNB	CCLs with associated ADH should be excised FEA without associated ADH has historically been excised but it can now be reasonably observed if there are no other indications for excision or concerning residual microcalcifications	Similar risk of subsequent breast cancer as proliferative disease without atypia (RR 1.47) [3] Systematic review of 24 studies showed that the upgrade rate to DCIS on excision was 1.5% for pure CCLs, 9% for CCL-A (FEA), and 20% for CCLs with ADH [4] Women with pure FEA on excisional biopsy can be followed with routine surveillance (no need for high-risk screening) [3]
Fibroepithelial lesions, including fibroadenoma and phyllodes tumors [3, 11]	Present as mass on physical examination or nodule on mammogram or ultrasound [11] Simple fibroadenomas are benign tumors containing glandular and fibrous tissue Complex fibroadenomas contain other proliferative changes (i.e., duct epithelial hyperplasia, sclerosing adenosis, calcification, apocrine change) Phyllodes tumors on histology show leaf-like architecture with elongated cleft-like spaces containing papillary projections of epithelial-lined stroma with degrees of hyperplasia and atypia	If found at the margins of an excised lesion, re-excision is not generally considered necessary [3] Fibroadenomas do not require excision unless rapid growth, symptomatic, or patient preference. Excise giant fibroadenomas (>10 cm in size) Management of complex fibroadenomas is controversial, with some advocating for excision and others recommending expectant management [11] Excise phyllodes tumors with negative margins (aim for >1 cm margin during surgery); SLNB is not necessary [11] Excise fibroepithelial lesions "not further defined" for diagnosis (including "cellular fibroadenoma," "cellular fibroepithelial lesion," or "fibroepithelial lesion with cellular stroma")	CNB findings associated with phyllodes tumor on excision include increased stromal cellularity, stromal mitoses, stromal overgrowth, fragmentation, nuclear pleomorphism, and infiltration of adipose tissue, but this is not consistent [4] There may be a role for close imaging follow-up for indeterminate fibroepithelial lesions [4] Phyllodes tumors are further classified as benign, borderline, or malignant, based on pathologic features (e.g., degree of stromal cellular atypia, mitoses, infiltrative vs. circumscribed margins, and presence of stromal overgrowth) [11] Core biopsy has a 25–30% false-negative rate when used to diagnose phyllodes tumors so excise solid masses that grow rapidly or become symptomatic after an initial benign CNB Consider adjuvant radiotherapy for borderline or malignant, but not benign, phyllodes tumors. Chemotherapy is reserved for large, high-risk (>10 cm) or recurrent malignant phyllodes tumors Pathologic margins >1 mm is acceptable for borderline/malignant phyllodes, while a negative margin is acceptable for benign phyllodes [17]
Mucocele-like lesions (MLLs) [4]	Rare lesion of dilated ducts filled with mucin; epithelial lining of the duct can have a range of abnormal pathology (atypia, DCIS, or cancer) May or may not be a precursor lesion to mucinous DCIS or mucinous carcinoma	Excise all MLLs with associated atypia Consider excision of benign MLLs if a finding of atypia would change patient management, but there may be a role for close observation [4]	Rate of upgrade from benign MLL on CNB to malignancy on excision is low (<5%), with the upgrade usually to just atypia [4]

ALND axillary lymph node dissection, *CLL* columnar cell-like lesion, *CLL-A* columnar cell-like lesion with atypia, *CNB* core needle biopsy, *DCIS* ductal carcinoma in situ, *FEA* flat epithelial atypia, *MLL* mucocele-like lesion, *MRI* magnetic resonance imaging, *RR* relative risk, *US* ultrasound

Ductal Carcinoma In Situ

Ductal carcinoma in situ (DCIS) is a preinvasive epithelial breast cancer that does not penetrate the basement membrane. With the advent of organized screening, the incidence of DCIS markedly increased from 5.8 per 100,000 women in the 1970s to 32.5 per 100,000 women in 2004 and then reached a plateau [18]. Approximately 90% are asymptomatic and not palpable, with the remainder presenting as a lump, discharge, or Paget's disease of the nipple. When DCIS is observed in the breast lobule, the process is referred to as "cancerization of the lobule."

Although evidence suggests that a significant proportion of DCIS lesions do not progress to invasive cancer, it is currently not possible to accurately distinguish which will progress and which will not. Furthermore, DCIS frequently coexists with invasive disease, and up to 15% of surgical specimens excised for a preoperative diagnosis of DCIS on core biopsy will be upgraded to invasive breast cancer [18]. These factors have led to an aggressive approach to all DCIS [19, 20].

The indications for breast-conserving surgery (e.g., lumpectomy) versus mastectomy are similar in DCIS as with invasive disease, with mastectomy indicated where:

1. Area of DCIS is large, relative to breast size.
2. Disease is multicentric.
3. Radiotherapy is contraindicated.
4. Clear margins cannot be obtained with breast conservation.

The lack of true randomized data regarding breast-conserving surgery (BCS) and mastectomy for DCIS should be noted. The first indication that BCS—in conjunction with adjuvant radiotherapy—was acceptable treatment for DCIS came from a subset analysis of 78 patients in the NSABP B-06 study [21]. Originally enrolled because of presumed invasive breast cancer, these women were downgraded to DCIS on pathologic reanalysis. The local recurrence rate was 9% in those that underwent radiotherapy versus 43% in those that did not. Retrospective studies have since confirmed that BCS provides survival rates similar to mastectomy; however, local recurrence is higher, even with radiotherapy [22, 23]. The recommended surgical margin of 2 mm for DCIS is discussed further below. In patients with DCIS and microinvasion (no invasive focus >1 mm), the DCIS margin guideline should be used, as systemic treatment decisions in these patients are driven by their DCIS. This is in contrast to patients with invasive breast cancer with a DCIS component, where the margin for invasive breast cancer (no ink on tumor) should be used [24].

As mentioned, similar to invasive disease, there is good evidence for radiotherapy following a breast-conserving approach:

Study	Methods	Results
NSABP-B17 Fisher et al. [25]	*N* = 818 RCT Patients assigned to lumpectomy alone vs. lumpectomy and RT	At 7.5 years, RT reduced the incidence of ipsilateral invasive disease (13.4% to 3.9%) as well as ipsilateral DCIS (13.4% to 8.2%) A subset analysis from this study also demonstrated that comedonecrosis was a risk factor for recurrence At 17.25 years, RT reduced ipsilateral breast tumor recurrence by 52% (HR 0.48) [26]
EORTC 10853 Julien et al. [27]	*N* = 1010 RCT Patients with DCIS and BCS randomized to receive no further treatment or RT	RT reduced overall noninvasive recurrence at 10.5 years by 48% and invasive recurrence by 42% At 15.8 years, RT reduced the risk of any local recurrence by 48% (HR 0.52) [28]
UK/ANZ DCIS Cuzick et al. [29] SweDCIS Wärnberg et al. [30]	*N* = 1701 RCT Patients with excised DCIS randomized to receive RT, tamoxifen, both or none *N* = 1046 RCT Patients randomized to RT or not after BCS for DCIS	RT reduced ipsilateral invasive recurrence at 12.7 years by 68% and DCIS by 62%, but with no effect on contralateral breast cancer Relative risk reduction of 37.5% of ipsilateral breast event after 20 years of follow-up

BCS breast-conserving surgery, *HR* hazard ratio, *NSABP* National Surgical Adjuvant Breast and Bowel Project, *RT* radiotherapy, *RCT* randomized controlled trial

These studies, such as NSABP B-17 [25] and EORTC 10853 [27], are marked by limitations relating to the pathological assessment of tumors (such as tumor size measurement and free margin definition), and lack of routine specimen imaging and postoperative mammography [31], thereby questioning the completeness of excision in both studies. As a result, many believe that these data strengthen the argument for complete surgical resection rather than an approach that relies on radiotherapy as a means of dealing with residual disease.

There is some evidence, however, that radiotherapy may be safely omitted in some cases of DCIS. The University of Southern California/Van Nuys prognostic index for DCIS uses four prognostic factors (tumor size, margin width, patient age, and pathologic classification as determined by both nuclear grade and presence or absence of comedonecrosis) to stratify patients by their risk of recurrence at 12 years of follow-up. Patients with low scores (4, 5, or 6) had a combination of being over the age of 60 with tumors less than 1.5 cm in size that were non-high grade (nuclear grade 1 or 2) and without necrosis, and a margin size greater than 10 mm. These patients with low scores, and patients who score 7 but have margins ≥3 mm, were found to gain no additional benefit from adjuvant radiotherapy following BCS in their 12-year local recurrence-free survival [32].

More recently, a prospective study of 670 patients [33] demonstrated a 5-year recurrence of 15% for high-grade DCIS, but only 6% for low- or intermediate-grade DCIS, when excised with a minimum of 3 mm margins. However, the authors note an increase in recurrences beyond 5 years for all grades of DCIS and urge caution in applying these results to clinical practice. Another prospective trial of wide excision alone (over 1 cm margin) for low-to-intermediate grade DCIS found an unacceptably high local recurrence rate of 12% at 5 years and 15.6% at 10 years [34]. A recent prospective trial found that the local recurrence rate continues to rise after 12 years of follow-up, even in patients with favorable DCIS features [35]. While some studies using contemporary cohorts report that postoperative radiation after BCS for DCIS is associated with a reduced risk for ipsilateral recurrence with no survival benefit compared to observation alone [33], others report that the benefit in survival offered by radiation after BCS is dependent on patient factors and tumor biology [36, 37].

Given the difficulty in determining which patients with DCIS may be safely treated with wide excision alone [38], it remains the standard of practice at the University of Toronto to offer radiation to all patients having undergone breast-conserving surgery (BCS) for DCIS. Whole-breast radiation following lumpectomy decreases DCIS recurrence rates by 50% [39]. The standard dose of adjuvant radiotherapy following BCS for completely excised DCIS is 4000 cGy in 15 fractions or 4250 cGy in 16 fractions, with consideration for a boost of 1000 cGy (in 4 or 5 additional fractions) to the tumor bed for any of the following criteria: age ≤ 50 years, high grade, or close (<2 mm) or positive margins [40].

The Oncotype DX® DCIS score is a multigene assay that provides additional molecular information from the tumor that may help guide treatment recommendations for adjuvant radiotherapy [41]. The DUCHESS (Evaluation of the DCIS Score for Decisions on Radiotherapy in Patients with Low/Intermediate Risk DCIS) trial is a Canadian multicenter prospective cohort study currently recruiting women with low- to moderate-risk DCIS to evaluate the utility of the Oncotype DX® DCIS score in guiding radiation treatment decisions following BCS, the results of which are eagerly awaited [42]. Recently, the updated NCCN guidelines have added that select patients may be considered for accelerated partial breast irradiation if they meet the definition of low-risk DCIS as defined by the RTOG 9804 trial: screen-detected DCIS, low to intermediate grade, tumor size ≤2.5 cm, and surgical excision with margins over 3 mm [39].

Adjuvant radiotherapy is generally not recommended for patients with DCIS who are adequately treated with mastectomy. Close or positive DCIS margins following mastectomy may lead to the consideration of postmastectomy radiation. However, the rates of chest wall recurrence following mastectomy for DCIS are low, even with positive or close margins [43, 44].

The NSABP B-24 study demonstrated that adjuvant tamoxifen following BCS and radiation for DCIS reduces a second breast event [45, 46], and subsequent randomized trials showed no difference between tamoxifen and aromatase inhibitors in their efficacy [47]. The benefit gained from endocrine therapy has to be weighed against their known adverse effects (i.e., menopausal symptoms, mood and sleep disturbances, arthralgias, cataracts/deep vein thrombosis/pulmonary embolism/uterine cancer for tamoxifen, and decreased bone mineral density for aromatase inhibitors). Adjuvant endocrine therapy is not routinely offered at the University of Toronto because the additional benefit gained from endocrine therapy for DCIS is felt to be small following both surgical excision with clear margins and radiotherapy relative to the risks of adverse events. Patients with DCIS may be considered for adjuvant endocrine therapy on a case-by-case basis in discussion with a medical oncologist, in patients with a strong personal preference for avoiding radiation following BCS, or who decline additional surgery in the setting of a positive margin, but this is not standard of care [39, 48–49].

DCIS Recurrence

Approximately 50% of recurrences are invasive disease [39, 50]. Factors associated with an increased risk of recurrence include palpable mass, larger size, higher grade, close or involved margins, presence of comedonecrosis, and age at diagnosis <50 years [39].

Margin status is an important predictor of DCIS local recurrence [22]. The NSABP-B17 [25], NSABP-B24 [45], and EORTC clinical trials [27] have all revealed that clear margins significantly decrease recurrence. No trials, however, have rigorously examined the optimum excision width. An analysis of pooled data from both randomized and nonrandomized studies in 2005 concluded that a margin of 2 mm when excising DCIS was as safe as a larger margin when followed by radiotherapy [51]. In 2016, the Society of Surgical Oncology, American Society of Clinical Oncology, and American Society for Radiation Oncology jointly released a consensus statement recommending a 2 mm margin for BCS with whole-breast radiation for treatment of DCIS [50, 52–53]. In their meta-analysis of studies examining varying margin widths (>0–1 mm, 2 mm, 3 mm, and 10 mm), there was no difference in recurrence when comparing 2 mm to 10 mm margins, while narrower margins (>0 or 1 mm) had a statistically significant increase in recurrence compared to 2 mm margins [54]. The consensus panel did recommend clinical judgment when deciding upon the need for re-excision when DCIS margins are less than 2 mm [50, 52–53], as there is no difference in locoregional recurrence for patients with margins <2 mm or ≥ 2 mm if adjuvant radiotherapy is given [24, 55–56]. Patients with DCIS that do require additional excision following BCS include those with margins <2 mm and do not plan to receive radiotherapy have multiple very close margins or evidence of residual malignant-appearing calcifications on mammography [24].

Although a high-grade lesion was originally thought to be a risk factor for recurrence [27], a 2006 review of the EORTC data [57] with a 10-year follow-up suggested that this might not be the case. That study did confirm that comedonecrosis is an independent risk factor for recurrence, with 3 of 10 patients recurring by 10 years [57]. A 2013 study found that larger DCIS size, margins <1 mm, and presence of lobular neoplasia, but not grade, were associated with increased risk of local DCIS recurrence [58]. Several studies with longer follow-up have since corroborated that high nuclear grade is not associated with DCIS recurrence [59, 60]. High nuclear grade, however, may be associated with invasive recurrence [61]. It may be that nuclear grade becomes less of a risk factor for recurrence in the modern era when DCIS is appropriately treated with surgical excision (with clear margins) and adjuvant radiotherapy (with or without endocrine therapy).

Age is also a significant factor in DCIS recurrence. The EORTC trial demonstrated a higher recurrence rate in young women under 40, quoting a hazard ratio (HR) of 2.54 [27]. Similarly, the NSABP B-24 trial found that the rate of ipsilateral (invasive and in situ) disease in women under 49 years old was 33/1000 women per year as opposed to 13/1000 for those over 49 years of age [45, 62]. A 2014 study of 5752 DCIS cases in Ontario from 1994 to 2003 found that young age < 45 was significantly associated with both DCIS (HR 2.6) and invasive (HR 3.0) recurrence [63]. Interestingly, one study found that women <40 years of age with DCIS were at higher risk for invasive recurrence than DCIS recurrence (15.8% vs. 11.5% 10-year recurrence risk), although mortality remained low, while the risks appeared equivalent in women ≥40 years of age [64].

The management of recurrence is largely dependent on the type of recurrence, the surgical treatment of prior DCIS, and whether radiotherapy has been administered. For DCIS recurrence, if radiotherapy has not been previously received, then a local resection may be possible followed by adjuvant radiotherapy; otherwise, a mastectomy should be offered [65]. There is increasing interest in the consideration of repeat resection and irradiation for local recurrence, with studies showing that this approach is safe and feasible in the setting of recurrence. However, the data remains limited by short follow-up and is largely confined to the setting of invasive disease rather than DCIS [66–68] and this approach is, therefore, not universally accepted. Invasive recurrences should be treated according to principles outlined in the subsequent section "Invasive Breast Cancer" and will be dependent on previous DCIS treatment and whether radiotherapy has been previously administered.

DCIS and the Axilla

The incidence of axillary metastases in DCIS is <1%, and these are likely to represent missed invasive disease, rather than true DCIS metastases. For DCIS diagnosed preoperatively on core biopsy, 15% will subsequently be found to have invasive cancer on final postoperative pathology [18]. It should be borne in mind that the majority of reported sentinel lymph node (SLN) involvement in DCIS is revealed by immunohistochemical (IHC) techniques as isolated tumor cells or micrometastases, and the clinical significance of these is uncertain even in true invasive disease [52, 53].

The American Society of Clinical Oncology has recommended that axillary staging in patients with DCIS treated by BCS be reserved for those with invasive disease. For those undergoing mastectomy or immediate reconstruction for DCIS, sentinel lymph node biopsy (SLNB) is recommended, with a view to avoid axillary lymph node dissection in the event of an upgrade from DCIS to invasive carcinoma on final pathology of the mastectomy specimen, as SLNB is not possible after mastectomy [69]. The current NCCN guidelines also offer similar recommendations, reserving SLNB for DCIS treated with mastectomy or excised in an anatomic location that may compromise the performance of a future SLNB (e.g., extreme upper outer quadrant lesions near the axilla and central lesions involving the nipple-areolar complex, both likely disrupting lymphatic drainage of the breast) [39].

Invasive Breast Cancer

In this section, the management of invasive breast cancer is discussed, focusing on tumors less than 5 cm with no evidence of matted or fixed axillary lymph nodes, corresponding to T0, T1, T2 and N0, N1 (stages 0, I, IIA, and IIB).

Work-up	Surgical management	Follow-up (F/U)
History and physical exam Imaging: Review bilateral mammogram and ultrasound (assess for multifocal/multicentric disease, as well as contralateral disease) Axillary US Breast MRI if indicated (see below) Core needle biopsy to confirm the diagnosis Apply clip if neoadjuvant therapy is considered CCO staging recommendations [70]: Routine bone scanning, liver ultrasonography, and chest radiography are not indicated before surgery Postoperatively: In women with stage I tumors, routine bone scanning, liver ultrasonography, and chest radiography are not indicated as part of baseline staging In women who have pathological stage II tumors, a postoperative bone scan is recommended as part of baseline staging In women who have pathological stage III tumors, bone scan, chest radiography, and liver ultrasound are recommended postoperatively	Breast (local): Breast-conservative surgery plus breast irradiation or mastectomy +/− postmastectomy radiation therapy [71] Axilla (regional): Sentinel lymph node biopsy for clinical N0 patients Axillary lymph node dissection for clinical N1 Consider and discuss neoadjuvant chemotherapy in the following cases: Triple-negative Young patients (<40) Her2/neu + Reducing the size of tumor to facilitate BCS Node-positive patients	Regular clinical breast exam Mammogram every 12 months

BCS breast-conserving surgery, *MRI* magnetic resonance imaging, *CCO* Cancer Care Ontario, *US* ultrasound

Special Notes

- It is standard of care to obtain the diagnosis of invasive breast cancer with core needle biopsy. While the primary use of core needle biopsy is to establish a diagnosis, it is also useful in providing receptor status if neoadjuvant chemotherapy is considered. Furthermore, positive margin rates and the need for reoperation are reduced in women who have been assessed with core needle biopsy preoperatively [72].

- In breast cancer of a more advanced stage, Cancer Care Ontario has recommended that in women with pathological stage III tumors, bone scanning, liver ultrasonography, or CT abdomen and chest radiography are recommended postoperatively as part of baseline staging. However, in women for whom treatment options are restricted to tamoxifen or hormone therapy, or for whom no further treatment is indicated because of age or other factors, routine bone scanning, liver ultrasonography, and chest radiography are not indicated as part of baseline staging [70].
- Mammography remains the mainstay of breast imaging. MRI of the breast is considered an adjunct to mammography. Preoperative diagnostic MRI detects additional ipsilateral lesions in up to 32% of patients and contralateral lesions in 7% of patients. Sensitivity ranges from 75 to 100% and specificity from 80 to 100% [73]. However, several studies have failed to show a decreased rate of positive margins in BCS for patients undergoing MRI [74, 75] while also showing an increased likelihood of mastectomy in such patients [75].
- According to the American College of Radiology, current indications for diagnostic MRI are as follows:
  - Axillary adenocarcinoma with unknown primary.
  - Evaluation of response to neoadjuvant chemotherapy.
  - Assessment of extent of DCIS and IDC.
  - Assessment of invasion of deep fascia.
  - Evaluation of possible recurrence.
- Diagnostic MRI can also be considered in patients with invasive lobular carcinoma, as there is some evidence that MRI reduces the need for re-excision surgery in this subset of patients, but at the cost of an increased likelihood of upfront mastectomy [74].
- Be aware that mucinous carcinomas often lack suspicious features on imaging and can be mistaken for fibroadenomas. Consider serial imaging or repeat core biopsies of breast lesions suggestive of fibroadenomas in older patients [76].
- The eighth edition of the AJCC introduced changes to breast cancer staging such that in addition to anatomic features, the biology of breast cancers are considered in determining prognosis [2]. In addition to TNM status, biologic markers of tumor grade and receptor status (estrogen receptor, progesterone receptor, and HER2/neu receptor) and results of genomic assays (including Oncotype DX® and EndoPredict) were included.

Breast-Conserving Surgery

The aim of breast conservation is to achieve a balance between complete resection of the tumor with negative margins and preservation of as much normal breast tissue as possible. Volume loss is the major determinant of cosmesis after BCS. A good cosmetic outcome maximizes the psychosocial benefits of breast preservation [77].

In patients with no contraindication to BCS, there are several points to be discussed with the patient	BCS includes the lumpectomy to a negative margin, margin revision being necessary in about 20% of cases If the margin is positive after appropriate attempts at therapeutic breast-conserving surgery, the patient should be considered for mastectomy
	BCS for DCIS and invasive breast cancer includes administration of radiotherapy
	When compared with mastectomy, BCS may have a slightly higher risk of local recurrence. Both approaches, however, have equivalent survival outcomes

Absolute Contraindications to BCS

1. Early pregnancy, if radiation deemed necessary to be performed during pregnancy.
2. Multicentric IDC—diffuse-appearing suspicious microcalcifications or inability to resect the evident disease with acceptable cosmetic results.
3. Any contraindication to radiation therapy (e.g., active collagen vascular disease with severe vasculitis, ataxia telangiectasia).

Relative Contraindications to BCS

1. A history of collagen vascular disease, in remission.
2. Large tumor size in relation to the breast size.
3. A history of prior therapeutic irradiation to the breast region.

For invasive cancer, another consideration in the choice of surgical treatment of the primary tumor is the management of the axilla after positive SLNB. The ACOSOG Z0011 trial—detailed in sect. IV of this chapter—supports omission of axillary lymph node dissection (ALND) after positive SLNB in many patients treated with BCS. However, patients treated with mastectomy were excluded and the current standard remains completion of ALND in those cases. This may factor into the decision-making process for the patient and surgeon.

Trials for BCS Versus Mastectomy

Study	Methods	Results
NSABP-B06 Fisher et al. [62]	$N = 1851$ RCT Patients in stages I and II were assigned total mastectomy/ALND, lumpectomy/ALND alone or lumpectomy/ALND + breast irradiation Margins—no cancer cell at the surgical margin	Follow-up—20 years No significant differences in disease-free survival and overall survival Recurrence rate in the ipsilateral breast was 14.3% in the lumpectomy/ALND plus breast irradiation group and 39.2% in the lumpectomy/ALND-alone group

Study	Methods	Results
Milan Group Veronesi et al. [23]	$N = 701$ RCT Patients with tumor <2 cm were assigned radical mastectomy vs. quadrantectomy/ALND + radiotherapy Margins—1.5–2.0 cm, with the overlying skin and deep fascia	Follow-up—20 years No statistical difference in overall survival Recurrence rate higher in the BCS group (8.8% vs. 2.3%)

RCT randomized controlled trial

Meta-analysis to Assess Surgical Margins in BCS for Early Breast Cancer

Study	Methods	Results
Houssami et al. [77]	33 studies $N = 28{,}162$ patients (1506 with LR) Impact of surgical margins on LR Model 1—effect of margin status in relation to LR Model 2—effect of margin distance to LR (1 mm vs. 2 mm vs. 5 mm)	Higher probability of LR associated with positive/close margins vs. negative margins (OR 1.97) No difference in LR with 1 mm vs. 2 mm vs. 5 mm margin distance Wider margins unlikely to increase long-term local control

LR local recurrence, *OR* odds ratio

This work by Houssami et al. formed the basis of the Society of Surgical Oncology-American Society for Radiation Oncology (SSO-ASTRO) consensus guidelines for breast-conserving surgery for early-stage breast cancer. Using this data, a multidisciplinary panel concluded that "no ink on tumor" should be adopted as the standard for an adequate margin for invasive breast cancer [78]. This guideline has since been endorsed by the American Society of Clinical Oncology (ASCO) and the American Society of Breast Surgeons (ASBrS) [79].

Genetic Testing

In Ontario, patients who qualify for government-funded genetic testing include the following [80]:

1. Male breast cancer patients.
2. Female breast cancer under age 35.
3. Ashkenazi Jewish patients with breast cancer < age 50 and/or ovarian cancer at any age.
4. Affected breast cancer patients with 2 cases of breast and/or ovarian cancer on the same side of the family.
5. Unaffected patient but has relative with known BRCA1 or BRCA2 mutation.

6. Unaffected Ashkenazi Jewish patient with first- or second-degree relative with breast or ovarian cancer.
7. Unaffected individual with a strong pedigree of breast or ovarian cancer (>10% chance of carrying a pathogenic mutation).

Note that NCCN offers similar guidelines on genetic testing, which includes individuals with triple-negative breast cancer diagnosed ≤60 years old [81]. The ASBrS has also recently published a consensus guideline recommending that genetic testing be considered and discussed for all patients with a new diagnosis of breast cancer [82].

The Axilla

Management of the axilla is arguably the most controversial aspect of the breast cancer treatment paradigm. Many changes have occurred in the past 20 years. From considering axillary lymph node dissection (ALND) as the standard of care for all breast cancer patients, to now omitting selected patients with proven axillary metastases from further surgery, it is a complex facet of the management of invasive breast cancer.

Authors such as Steele et al. [83] in the 1980s challenged the belief that all breast cancer patients should have an ALND. They endorsed a system of axillary node sampling, whereby four nodes were "cherry picked" from level one of the axilla, and if negative for disease, no further surgery was performed. This limited axillary node sampling may be seen as the grandfather of SLNB, a technique which has supplanted ALND as the standard of care in staging the clinically negative axilla.

Several key trials have demonstrated the efficacy of SLNB

Study	Methods	Results
Multicenter Validation Study Krag et al. [84] 1998	*N* = 443 All patients underwent both SLNB and then ALND	It demonstrated that this technique could be used by surgeons At least 1 SLN was identified in 98% of cases and the predictive value of a negative SLN was 96%, with a false-negative rate of 11%
ASCO Review Lyman et al. [85] 2005	*N* = 8059 Systematic review of 69 SLNB trials	SLN identification was successful in 95% of patients The false-negative rate was 7.3% (range 0–29%). Using both radiocolloid and blue dye was more successful than blue dye alone
ALMANAC Mansel et al. [86] 2006	*N* = 1031 RCT Patients randomly assigned to ALND vs. SLNB with delayed ALND if SLN positive	SLNB group had less arm morbidity SLNB group had better quality of life and arm functioning scores

Study	Methods	Results
NSABP B-32 Technical results Krag et al. [87] 2007 NSABP B-32 OS results Krag et al. [88] 2010	$N = 5611$ RCT Comparing SLNB, followed by ALND (group 1) vs. SLNB, followed by ALND for positive SLN (group 2)	Lymphatic mapping was successful in 97.2% when using both radioactive and blue dye The FNR was 9.8% in group 1. The FNR was inversely associated with the number of SLNs removed, such that the FNR was 17.7% when only one SLN was removed, 10% when 2 SLNs were removed, and so forth No significant differences were observed in regional control or OS between groups at follow-up of 8 years No significant differences in nodal recurrence as first event between the two groups

ALND axillary lymph node dissection, *ASCO* American Society of Clinical Oncology, *FNR* false-negative rate, *NSABP* National Surgical Adjuvant Breast and Bowel Project, *OS* overall survival, *SLN* sentinel lymph node, *SLNB* sentinel lymph node biopsy, *RCT* randomized controlled trial

Approach to the Axilla in Early-Stage Breast Cancer

The contribution of ALND to survival in women with breast cancer has been questioned since the publication of the NSABP B-04 [89] trial. It has often been the basis of argument against mandatory ALND. In this study, clinically node-negative patients were randomized to radical mastectomy (RM), total mastectomy (TM), plus postoperative axillary irradiation or TM alone. Forty percent of the RM group had subclinical lymph node involvement. One can assume that the TM plus irradiation and the TM alone groups also had 40% of subclinical axillary lymph involvement because of randomization. Despite not having any treatment to the axilla, the axillary recurrence rate, as a first failure, was only 19% in the TM alone group. Moreover, the three groups had a similar overall survival [90].

In the era of SLNB, the contribution of axillary dissection to survival was revisited in the ACOSOG Z0011 trial [91]. In this prospective randomized noninferiority trial, women with T1-T2 breast cancers who were clinically node negative (T1-T2cN0), receiving breast-conserving therapy with only one or two positive SLNs and with no gross extracapsular extension, were randomized to SNLB-alone versus ALND groups. All patients received adjuvant systemic therapy and opposing tangential field whole-breast irradiation. One criticism of this study was the relatively short follow-up (median: 6.3 years) period when it was first published in 2006. However, subsequent results published in 2017 still showed no difference in 10-year overall survival (86.3% in the SLND alone group vs. 83.6% in the ALND group with a noninferiority $p = 0.02$) [92]. Ten-year disease-free survival was also similar between groups, with 78.2% in the ALND group versus 80.2% in the SLNB-alone group. This study demonstrated the noninferiority of SLNB to ALND for patients with T1-T2 tumors, and 1 or 2 positive SLNs who are treated with lumpectomy, adjuvant radiation and systemic therapy, with a noninferiority hazard ratio of 1.3.

Studies in support of ALND *after positive SLNB*

Study	Methods	Results
SEER Database Analysis Joslyn. [93] 2002	Retrospective review *N* = 257,157 Women diagnosed with breast cancer in the SEER database between 1988 and 2000	Women undergoing ALND had an increased survival With an increasing ratio of positive nodes to total number removed, there was a consistent trend towards reduced survival
Truong et al. [94] 2002	Retrospective population-based cohort *N* = 8038 Patients treated for T1–2 breast cancer in British Columbia between 1989 and 1998	Overall and cancer-specific 5-year survival rates were significantly worse in those who had not undergone ALND (68% vs. 85% and 86% vs. 91%, respectively). Note that the much larger difference in overall survival suggests large heterogeneity between groups
Early Breast Cancer Trialists' Collaborative Group Analysis Clarke et al. [95] 2005	78 RCTs *N* = 42,000 Comparing the effect of different types of local treatment on recurrence and survival	While not directly examining ALND, the study showed that local control affects overall survival, a fact which is often used in support of ALND Local recurrence positively impacted on the 15-year survival

RCT randomized controlled trials, *ALND* axillary lymph node dissection, *SEER* surveillance epidemiology and end results (US National Cancer Institute)

Studies suggesting ALND does not affect overall survival

Study	Methods	Results
NSABP B-04 Fisher et al. [96] 1985	*N* = 1843 RCT Women were assigned to radical mastectomy vs. simple mastectomy plus local nodal irradiation, or simple mastectomy with delayed ALND if needed	There was no effect on survival of prophylactic ALND vs. nodal radiotherapy vs. no initial axillary treatment This study is criticized for being underpowered and also for including many women with simple mastectomy who had some nodes removed with the breast specimen
The Breast Carcinoma Collaborative Group of the Institut Curie Cabanes et al. [97] 1992	*N* = 658 RCT Patients assigned to lumpectomy alone or lumpectomy plus ALND All received RT, and women with positive LNs received chemotherapy	ALND was initially associated with significantly better 5-year survival (97% vs. 93%) However, after 10–15 years of follow-up, survival rates were similar (~75%). Regional recurrence was lower in women who had ALND. However, this needs to take into consideration the fact that the only women who received chemotherapy were in the ALND group

NSABP National Surgical Adjuvant Breast and Bowel Project, *RCT* randomized controlled trials, *ALND* axillary lymph node dissection, *RT* radiotherapy, *LN* lymph node

Studies in support of ALND omission *after limited positive SLNB*

Study	Methods	Results
Z0011 Guiliano et al. [91, 92] 2010, 2017	*N* = 891 RCT T1-T2cN0 invasive breast cancer ALND vs. no ALND for women with 1 or 2 positive SLNB Exclusion: 3 or more positive SLNs, matted nodes, gross extranodal extension, neoadjuvant treatment Planned adjuvant systemic therapy and opposing tangential field whole-breast irradiation to all patients	At median follow-up of 9.3 years, the 10-year overall survival was 83.6% in ALND and 86.3% in those with SLNB. Importantly, 10-year disease-free survival was also similar, with 78.2% in ALND and 80.2% with SLNB It is criticized for its low numbers and an approximately 20% lost to follow-up rate (unlike NSABP-B32 < 1%) Inconsistent field of adjuvant radiation therapy (from the radiation reports available for 605 patients, 89% received whole-breast radiation and 15% also received radiation to the supraclavicular region) [98] Powered for 1900 patients but closed earlier due to lower than expected mortality rate
AMAROS Donker et al. [99] 2014 IBCSG 23–01 Galimberti et al. [100] 2018	*N* = 4806 → 1425 (29.7%) found to have positive SLNB RCT, noninferiority trial From 2001 to 2010, patients with cT1–2 N0 invasive breast cancer were enrolled in the EORTC phase III noninferiority AMAROS trial. Patients with neoadjuvant systemic treatment were excluded from the study Protocol was amended in 2006 to include cT3 and multifocal disease Patients were randomized to ALND or ART prior to SLNB and breast-conserving surgery or mastectomy. Patients with positive SLNs were then included in analysis. ART included radiation to level I, II, III, and supraclavicular lymph nodes Primary endpoint was 5-year axillary recurrence rate RandomisedRandomized noninferiority phase 3 trial Primary endpoint: disease-free survival in T1-T2 tumors with only micrometastasis randomized to ALND or no ALND	5-year axillary recurrence was 0.43% after axillary lymph node dissection and 1.19% after axillary radiotherapy. Due to the accrual and low number of events, the noninferiority test was underpowered and the study was statistically inconclusive Clinical signs of lymphedema were noted more often following ALND than ART, 23% vs. 11% at 5 years ($p < 0.0001$). Rates of subjectively measured lymphedema were not different between groups. Range of motion and quality of life measurements were not significantly different between the two groups No significant difference in 10-year disease-free survival (74.9% in the ALND group vs. 76.8% in the no ALND group) with a hazard ratio of 0.85 (95% CI 0.65–1.11). This study showed noninferiority as a hazard ratio of less than 1.25 Higher rate of sensory neuropathy, motor neuropathy, and lymphedema in the ALND group

RCT randomized controlled trial, *ALND* axillary lymph node dissection, *LN* lymph node, *SLNB* sentinel lymph node biopsy, *RT* radiotherapy, *EORTC* European Organisation for Research and Treatment of Cancer, *AMAROS* the after-mapping of the axilla: radiotherapy or surgery?, *ART* axillary radiation therapy, *NSABP* National Surgical Adjuvant Breast and Bowel Project, T1 or T2 and clinically N0

Special Notes

- Although by no means an exhaustive examination of the literature, the above studies do help demonstrate the controversy surrounding ALND. It should be always remembered that with the rapid changes in adjuvant therapy for breast cancer, one must examine the older literature with a certain degree of care. Certainly, it seems that the benefit of extensive axillary surgery is questionable in this era of effective adjuvant therapy. Given the limitations of the Z0011 study, however, it is difficult at the present time to completely advocate a definitive move away from the procedure. Both NCCN guidelines and the American Society of Breast Surgeons endorse that if all Z0011 criteria are met, ALND is not required after SLNB.
- At the University of Toronto, we also forego axillary dissection in patients meeting the Z0011 inclusion criteria.

Isolated Tumor Cells and Micrometastases

Isolated tumor cells (ITCs)	Micrometastases
Defined by the eighth edition of AJCC as "small clusters of cells not greater than 0.2 mm, or nonconfluent or nearly confluent clusters of cells not exceeding 200 cells in a single histologic lymph node cross section are classified as isolated tumour cells" [2] (pN0(i+)) No further surgery, radiotherapy, or chemotherapy is indicated by their presence. However, in the neoadjuvant setting, their significance is less clear [101].	Defined by a separate designation of pN1mi (>0.2 mm and no greater than 2.0 mm) to indicate micrometastases alone [2] NSABP B-32 showed a 1.2% lower 5-year survival ($p = 0.03$) in patients with occult micrometastases, compared to those that were pathologically node-negative [88]. Thus, although larger than ITCs, micrometastasis are of limited clinical significance

Special Notes

- The literature is populated by much discussion regarding the significance of isolated tumor cells (ITCs) and micrometastases. This debate has been largely superseded by the publication of Z0011 and its findings relating to the significance of macrometastases [91], along with Weaver et al. who demonstrated statistical but no clinical significance to their presence [102].

Extranodal Extension

Extranodal extension (ENE) is defined as tumor breach outside of the lymph node capsule. In the literature, it has been associated with worse prognosis and involvement of further non-sentinel lymph nodes with disease [103, 104]. The ACOSOG Z0011 trial excluded patients with gross ENE but did not further analyze the presence of microscopic ENE [91]. In a study by Gooch et al., in 331 patients with ENE out of 11,730 patients meeting ACOSOG Z0011 criteria, ENE was associated with increased axillary burden [105]. ENE > 2 mm was the strongest predictor of greater than 4 positive lymph nodes at completion ALND on multivariate analysis (33% of patients with ENE >2 mm vs 9% of patients with ENE ≤2 mm vs 3% of patients with no ENE had more than 4 positive LNs at completion ALND, $p < 0.0001$). Another smaller study demonstrated similar recurrence and mortality in patients with no ENE compared to patients with ENE ≤2 mm [106]. Therefore, one could consider avoiding ALND if only microscopic or focal ENE (≤ 2 mm) is identified on SLNB.

SLNB Following Neoadjuvant Systemic Therapy

- For patients undergoing neoadjuvant chemotherapy, studies such as SENTINA, ACOSOG Z1071, and SN FNAC have demonstrated the feasibility and accuracy of SLNB following neoadjuvant systemic therapy if dual-agent lymphatic mapping is used and more than 2 SLNs are retrieved. These studies are described in more detail in the *Locally Advanced Breast Cancer* section.

Summary: Management of the Clinically Node-Negative Axilla in Patients Who Have Not Received Neoadjuvant Chemotherapy

- SLNs are pathologically negative or contain only ITCs:
  - SLNB is the standard for staging and axillary surgery [107].
- SLNs contain micrometastatic disease on pathologic examination:
  - SLNB alone can safely manage burden of disease. However, case should be discussed at Multidisciplinary Cancer Conference (MCC) to determine if identification of macrometastases would alter adjuvant therapy recommendations. If so, completion ALND may be considered if the patient does not meet inclusion criteria for Z0011 [107].
- SLNs contain macrometastatic disease on pathologic examination:
  - If meets all inclusion criteria for Z0011 (T1 or T2 tumor, clinical N0, 1, or 2 positive SLNs, no gross extranodal extension, breast-conserving therapy, whole-breast radiotherapy planned, no neoadjuvant chemotherapy), no further ALND is required [107].

    If three or more positive SLNs and/or gross extranodal disease, consider completion ALND [107].
  - If patient has undergone mastectomy, has multicentric tumor, or is pregnant, a discussion at MCC is warranted to review the benefits/risks of completion ALND versus axillary radiotherapy.

Considerations of Adjuvant Treatment for Invasive Breast Cancer

Genomic Assays

In addition to providing prognostic information regarding breast cancers and the risk of recurrence, genomic assays are also being used to guide the recommendation for adjuvant therapies. Studies are ongoing to include node-positive patients.

TAILORx Study—Sparano et al. [108]

Methods	Results	Implications for clinical practice
N = 10, 273 RCT Patients aged 18–75 with hormone receptor-positive, HER2-negative, axillary node-negative breast cancers with mid-range Oncotype DX® recurrence scores (11–25) were randomly assigned to either chemoendocrine or endocrine therapy alone Noninferiority study to determine if chemotherapy can be safely omitted in patients with mid-range (intermediate) recurrence scores	Endocrine therapy was not inferior to chemotherapy in these patients with regard to: Invasive disease-free survival Freedom from recurrence of breast cancer at a distant or local-regional site Overall survival Chemotherapy was associated with some benefit in women 50 years old and younger with Oncotype DX® recurrence scores in the 16–25 range 9-year rate of distant recurrence: ~5% for women with recurrence scores of 11–25 ~3% for women with recurrence scores of 10 or less	Adjuvant chemotherapy can be omitted in patients with HR-positive, HER2-negative, node-negative breast cancers who have Oncotype DX® recurrence scores <25 if over the age of 50 Adjuvant chemotherapy should be discussed and offered to women under the age of 50 with HR-positive, HER2-negative, node-negative breast cancers who have Oncotype DX® recurrence scores in the 16–25 range

HR hormone receptor, *RCT* randomized controlled trial

Ovarian Function Suppression

Ovarian function suppression with LHRH (luteinizing hormone-releasing hormone) analogs (e.g., goserelin (Zoladex), leuprolide (Lupron)) should be considered in high-risk hormone receptor-positive premenopausal women requiring chemotherapy [109, 110]. Ovarian function suppression may also be considered to protect ovarian function in premenopausal women during chemotherapy [111, 112].

Locally Advanced Breast Cancer

Locally advanced breast cancer (LABC) is a heterogeneous entity. The term includes T3: tumors greater than 5 cm in maximum diameter, T4: tumors that directly invade skin or chest wall, as well as inflammatory breast cancer, and tumors that have extensive regional lymph node involvement (matted ipsilateral lymph nodes N2–N3) without evidence of distant metastatic disease at initial presentation. These tumors fall into the category of stage IIB (T3 N0) and III disease as per AJCC eighth edition staging. It is clinically useful to separate LABC into operable and inoperable (situations in which surgery is unlikely to remove all disease). This decision is made clinically based on physical examination and review of breast imaging. Approximately 25–30% of LABC are inoperable on presentation [113]. Up to 20% of patients with stage III disease are metastatic after staging [39]. Signs of questionable operable benefit or inoperability include the following [114]:

1. Extensive skin edema.
2. Satellite nodule in the skin.
3. Inflammatory breast cancer.
4. Involvement of supraclavicular or internal mammary lymph nodes.
5. Preoperative upper limb edema.
6. Skin ulceration.
7. Fixation to the chest wall.
8. Fixed, matted ALN.

Optimal management of LABC requires multimodality treatment [39]. The usual order of treatment varies according to the patient and the tumor clinical stage and characteristics:

Work-up	Inoperable LABC	Operable LABC	Follow-up (F/U)
Obtain the ER, PR, and HER2/neu status Imaging: Breast MRI CT scan chest, abdomen, and pelvis Bone scan PET/CT (optional) Apply a radiologic marker to breast cancer and biopsy-proven involved node preinitiation of chemotherapy Precise tumor measurement and documentation of skin changes Consider discussion in MCC Refer to Fertility, if premenopausal	Neoadjuvant systemic therapy and reassess response after each cycle If response—continue until completion of planned treatment or maximal response—then surgical management If no response—discuss again in MCC. Options: Alternate systemic therapy regimen If operable: Ssurgical management If nonoperable: radiotherapy +/− planned surgical treatment	Consider neoadjuvant chemotherapy in: Any patient who will need adjuvant chemotherapy [115] and in whom surgical pathology information is not required to determine regimen High-grade tumors [115, 116] HER2+ [116] Triple negative (ER/PR/HER2−) [117] Luminal B [115] – Young patients <35 years [118] Patient has large tumor and seeks breast conservation Patients with node-positive disease Surgical management of the breast (usually mastectomy unless downstaging with optional reconstruction) and axilla (see below: SLNB vs. axillary dissection)	Regular clinical breast exam 1–4 times a year for 5 years, then annual Mammogram every 12 months

ER estrogen receptor, *PR* progesterone receptor, *HER2* human epidermal growth factor receptor 2, *MCC* Multidisciplinary Cancer Conference, *SLNB* sentinel lymph node biopsy

Special Notes

- Radiation therapy will be recommended postmastectomy or post-BCS to patients with LABC.
- Advantages of neoadjuvant chemotherapy:
  - Evaluation of in vivo response to chemotherapy.
  - Downstaging to facilitate breast conservation and omission of ALND in some cases.

    Conversion from mastectomy to BCS occurs in approximately 23% of patients [119]. The extent of conversion depends on the criteria for performing BCS set by the individual trial.
  - Local recurrence rates in this conversion group were slightly higher than in the mastectomy group (15.9% vs. 9.9%, not significant) in the NSABP B-18 study [120] and in a 2018 Early Breast Cancer Trialists' Collaborative Group (EBCTCG) meta-analysis of ten randomized trials from 1983 to 2002 [121]. A 2012 combined analysis of NSABP B-18 and B-27 found that the 10-year cumulative incidence of locoregional recurrence after NACT was 12.3% for

mastectomy (without radiation) versus 10.3% for BCS (with radiation) [122]. A more recent 2016 meta-analysis of eight trials from 2000 to 2015 with a total of 3215 patients found that following neoadjuvant chemotherapy, the prevalence of local recurrence was 9.2% in the BCS group versus 8.3% in the mastectomy group (not significant) [123].
  - Early introduction of chemotherapy to treat occult potential systemic metastases.

Neoadjuvant chemotherapy studies

Study	Methods	Results
NSABP B18 Wolmark et al. [120]	*N* = 1493 RCT Operable T1–3 N0–1 M0 patients assigned to preoperative chemo (4 cycles of AC) vs. postoperative chemo (4 cycles of AC)	Follow-up—9 years No differences in OS (70% and 69%) or DFS (53% and 55%) Marginally statistically significant treatment by age interactions appears to be emerging for survival and DFS, suggesting that younger patients may benefit from preoperative therapy, whereas the reverse may be true for older patients
EORTC Trial 10,902 van der Hage et al. [119]	*N* = 698 RCT Patients with T1c, T2, T3, T4b, N0 to 1, and M0 breast cancer were assigned to preoperative vs. postoperative chemotherapy (4 cycles—FEC)	Median follow-up—56 months No differences in terms of PFS, OS, and LRR Preoperative chemotherapy enabled more patients to be treated with breast-conserving surgery (rate of downstaging was 23%)
Fisher et al. 2011 [124]	*N* = 385 Retrospective chart review Patients with stage I, II, or III and triple-negative breast cancer treated with neoadjuvant or adjuvant chemotherapy	There is a trend towards survival benefit in patients with pCR following neoadjuvant chemotherapy However, patients undergoing neoadjuvant chemotherapy with residual disease had significantly worse survival compared to patients receiving adjuvant therapy, with a trend towards worse survival compared to patients receiving neoadjuvant chemotherapy with pCR

AC doxorubicin/adriamycin + cyclophosphamide, *RCT* randomized controlled trial, *DFS* disease-free survival, *FEC* fluorouracil, epirubicin, and cyclophosphamide, *OS* overall survival, *PFS* progression-free survival, *LRR* locoregional recurrence, *pCR* complete pathologic response

- Potential candidates for BCS after neoadjuvant chemotherapy:
  - Ideally unifocal disease (However, multifocal and even multicentric disease can now be removed using oncoplastic techniques, thus allowing for BCS. This is discussed further in the "Oncoplastics" section.)
  - No inflammatory skin involvement.
  - Radiographic abnormalities (e.g., suspicious calcifications) resectable with lumpectomy.
  - No contraindication to adjuvant radiotherapy.
- Neoadjuvant endocrine therapy may be considered for patients who are not candidates for systemic chemotherapy and have markers for endocrine responsive-

ness or chemotherapy unresponsiveness such as ER and PR positivity, low grade, invasive lobular histology, and low Ki67 [115].

- SLNB has been investigated both before and after the completion of neoadjuvant chemotherapy [125]. When performed before neoadjuvant chemotherapy, it is both accurate (identification rate between 93 and 100%) and safe, with a low rate of regional recurrence reported. However, it potentially delays the initiation of chemotherapy in an era where lymph node status does not influence the choice of chemotherapy. Conversely, SLN biopsy after neoadjuvant chemotherapy has the advantage of reducing the number of operative procedures needed, as well as being both accurate and safe [125]. A 2016 meta-analysis examining the accuracy rate of SLNB after neoadjuvant chemotherapy found that in 1456 patients with initially clinically node-negative breast cancer from 16 studies, the SLNB detection rate was 96% (95% CI: 95–97%), with a false-negative rate of 6% [126]. Furthermore, in comparison to performing SLNB prior to chemotherapy, SLNB performed after neoadjuvant chemotherapy has similar SLN identification and false-negative rates, has lower nodal positivity rates (with fewer subsequent axillary dissections for T2 and T3 disease), and does not lead to higher locoregional failure rates [127]. Thus, in patients whose initial ipsilateral axillary evaluation is negative (cN0), sentinel lymph node biopsy is preferably performed after neoadjuvant systemic therapy [39].
- Three clinical trials examined the accuracy and false-negative rates of SLNB performed after neoadjuvant chemotherapy in patients with cN1 disease. The ACOSOG Z1071 (Alliance) Trial had a SLNB identification rate of 92.7% (which was higher when using dual tracer vs. single tracer, 93.8% vs. 88.9%) with a false-negative rate of 12.6% when 2 or more sentinel lymph nodes were examined [128]. The Canadian SN FNAC study showed a SLN identification rate of 87.6% after chemotherapy (less than the predefined optimal SLN identification rate of 90%), but has shown an acceptable false-negative rate of 8.4% when immunohistochemistry (IHC) is used and sentinel node metastases of any size (thus including isolated tumor cells) are considered positive. After neoadjuvant therapy, accuracy of SLNB is further increased by the use of both blue dye and radiolabeled tracer, as well as harvesting more than one sentinel node if possible [101]. In the SENTINA study C arm (patients who converted from cN+ to clinically node negative after neoadjuvant chemotherapy), the SLN detection rate was 80.1% with an overall FNR of 14.2% (24.3% when one node removed vs. 18.5% when two sentinel nodes removed vs. consistently <10% when three or more sentinel nodes removed) [129]. A recent updated meta-analysis of 19 studies from 2016 demonstrated a pooled SLN identification rate of 91% for patients with clinically node-positive breast cancer treated with neoadjuvant chemotherapy, with a pooled FNR of 13% [130].
- Residual nodal disease in the axilla following neoadjuvant treatment is felt to represent chemoresistant disease, and chemoresistant disease is also felt to be

resistant to radiotherapy [131]. As a result, in patients who are node positive on presentation, axillary lymph node dissection should be performed if the axilla remains clinically positive following neoadjuvant systemic therapy. If the axilla becomes clinically negative after neoadjuvant systemic therapy, SLNB may be performed; otherwise, axillary lymph node dissection should be pursued. SLNB has a > 10% false-negative rate in this setting but this rate can be improved by: (1) targeted removal of clipped nodes that were biopsy-proven positive prior to neoadjuvant systemic therapy [132, 133], (2) use of dual tracer localization, (3) removal of two (as per SN FNAC) or more (as per ACOSOG Z1071) sentinel nodes [39], and (4) use of IHC and planned ALND for any persistent disease in sentinel nodes (including isolated tumor cells). Alternatively, intraoperative frozen section may be undertaken at the time of SLNB, with planned completion axillary lymph node dissection if any residual nodal disease is identified on frozen section. Axillary lymph node dissection should be pursued for any residual nodal disease following neoadjuvant systemic therapy on final pathology, including isolated tumor cells.

- Axillary imaging after neoadjuvant chemotherapy has not been found to be a reliable predictor of axillary pathology after neoadjuvant chemotherapy. In the SN FNAC study, the accuracy of axillary ultrasound post-NAC was 62%, with an 81% positive-predictive value and a 48% negative-predictive value [101]. In the ACOSOG Z1071 study, 57% of 430 patients with normal axillary ultrasounds had nodal positivity [128]. Radiologic response by MRI has also not been found to predict axillary response following neoadjuvant chemotherapy [134].
- Future Directions: Two ongoing randomized controlled trials are investigating the potential de-escalation of therapy for patients with initial clinical N1 disease who receive neoadjuvant chemotherapy. (1) In breast cancer patients with cT1-3 N1 disease who have positive sentinel lymph nodes after receiving neoadjuvant chemotherapy, the Alliance A11202 trial is a prospective randomized phase III trial that is randomizing them to either no further axillary surgery (with radiation to breast (if BCS)/chest wall (if mastectomy) and nodal basins including levels 1–3 of the axilla and supraclavicular fossa) or completion level 1–2 axillary lymph node dissection (with radiation to breast (if BCS)/chest wall (if mastectomy) and nodal basins including level 3 axillary nodes and supraclavicular fossa). The primary endpoint is invasive breast cancer recurrence-free survival. As of May 2019, the study has enrolled 2918 participants [135]. (2) In breast cancer patients with cT1-3 N1 disease who have negative axillary nodes following neoadjuvant chemotherapy (determined histologically negative either by ALND or SLNB +/− ALND), the B-51/RTOG 1304 (NRG 9353) trial is randomizing patients to receive either regional nodal radiotherapy (with radiation to breast (if BCS)/chest wall (if mastectomy)) or no regional nodal radiotherapy (with whole-breast radiotherapy if BCS but no chest wall radiotherapy if mastectomy). The primary endpoint is to determine if the addition of comprehensive regional nodal

radiotherapy significantly reduces breast cancer recurrence in this population, with secondary outcomes examining overall survival, locoregional recurrence, and distant recurrence. As of May 2019, this study has accrued 1231 patients (75.2% of anticipated sample size) with an estimated completion date of April 2020 [136].

- Following standard neoadjuvant chemotherapy for triple-negative breast cancer, adjuvant capecitabine is now offered for patients with residual disease at surgery (Create-X trial) [137]. For HER-2 positive patients with no residual disease after neoadjuvant chemotherapy, patients will complete up to 1 year of HER2-targeted therapy with trastuzumab (Herceptin) with or without pertuzumab [39]. For HER2-positive patients with residual invasive disease at surgery, 14 cycles of ado-trastuzumab emtansine (TDM-1) is now recommended (Katherine trial) [138].

Inflammatory Breast Cancer

Inflammatory breast cancer (IBC) is a rare clinicopathological entity (1–6% of all breast cancer) characterized by rapid progression and aggressive behavior, with higher metastatic potential. IBC presents with erythema and edema with exaggerated hair-follicle pits, causing a peau d'orange appearance of the skin [139]. Diffuse erythema of more than one-third of the skin overlying the breast distinguishes IBC (T4d) from neglected noninflammatory LABC with skin involvement (T4a-c) [139, 140]. Diagnostic criteria include rapid onset of erythema, edema and/or peau d'orange with or without a palpable mass occupying at least one-third of the breast, duration not greater than 6 months, and pathological confirmation of invasive cancer [141]. Skin biopsy can aid in diagnosis and was recommended by an international consensus [141]. Most IBC are ductal carcinoma of high nuclear grade; 17–30% are triple negative and 18–44% are HER2-positive [140]. Dermal lymphatic emboli are present in 75% of cases; their absence does not exclude the diagnosis [139, 140]. All women with IBC should undergo staging investigation with at least bone scan and CT scans of the chest, abdomen, and pelvis [141].

After ruling out metastasis, patients are treated with preoperative chemotherapy followed by modified radical mastectomy and radiation in those who clinically respond to chemotherapy [39, 139–143]. Nonresponders may be considered for palliative radiotherapy, as surgery does not appear to benefit this subgroup; mastectomy may be considered for symptom palliation [39, 139]. The trimodality approach of chemotherapy, surgery, and radiation improves the outcome of patients with IBC, as Li et al. in 2008 reported a 5-year survival rate of 40–50% [139].

Special Considerations

Pregnancy and Breast Cancer

Pregnancy-associated breast cancer (PABC) is defined as breast cancer diagnosed during pregnancy or within 1 year of delivery. It is one of the most common malignancies diagnosed during pregnancy. Incidence is estimated to be 1 in 3000–10,000 pregnancies, and 0.2–3.8% of all breast cancers are pregnancy-related [144].

PABC has been demonstrated to have worse prognosis in terms of recurrence and death when compared with non-pregnancy-related breast cancer. Suggested causes include the following:

1. Aggressive disease caused by hormonal and immune changes, and breast involution [145].
2. Diagnosis at an advanced stage, possibly due to a lack of awareness and difficulty in assessing the pregnant breast [145].
3. Use of suboptimal treatments [146].

Management of PABC requires multidisciplinary approach, ensuring best care both for the mother and the fetus. Of note, there is no evidence showing that termination of the pregnancy affects prognosis. However, termination during the first trimester should be discussed with the patient, as it can help avoid delays in treatments that are contraindicated during organogenesis [39].

Treatment of PABC depends on the stage of the cancer, and is similar to that of the non-pregnant patient, with modifications dependent on the gestational age of the pregnancy at diagnosis of PABC [147].

Work-up	Surgical management	Adjuvant therapy
Physical exam Breast and axillary ultrasound Mammogram (with fetal protection) Biopsy	BCT vs. mastectomy: same as for the non-pregnant patient Exception is a patient in the first trimester where chemotherapy is not indicated. Since radiation will be delayed to the postpartum period, mastectomy may offer maximal oncological safety SLNB vs. ALND: same as for the non-pregnant patient SLNB: technetium-99 lymphoscintigraphy is considered safe, but blue dye is contraindicated Reconstruction is usually delayed until after delivery, as achieving symmetry is difficult due to pregnancy-associated breast engorgement	Radiation: Wwhen indicated, should be delayed to the postpartum period Chemotherapy: can be administered, as adjuvant or neoadjuvant treatment, beginning after the first trimester and up to week 35 or 3 weeks before the planned delivery

ALND axillary lymph node dissection, *BCT* breast-conserving therapy, *SLNB* sentinel lymph node biopsy

Special Notes

- Breast MRI should not be performed during pregnancy due to inability to administer gadolinium.
- Fluorouracil, doxorubicin, and cyclophosphamide can be used during the second and third trimesters of pregnancy; paclitaxel may be acceptable if clinically indicated [39].
- The use of trastuzumab is contraindicated in all trimesters due to renal and pulmonary complications [39].
- Tamoxifen is associated with a 20% birth defect risk and, if indicated, should be initiated postpartum [147].

Breast Cancer in the Elderly

With improving life expectancy, the geriatric population is expected to become a significant proportion of the Canadian population. Cancer care decisions in the elderly is complicated by competing medical comorbidities.

Regarding screening, the Canadian Task Force on Preventative Health Breast Cancer Update in 2018 offered no recommendations on screening for patients age 75 and older [148]. A 2009 update from the United States Preventative Services Task Force on screening for breast cancer also acknowledged the lack of studies on the effectiveness of mammography screening in decreasing breast cancer mortality in women aged 70 years and older [149]. The lag time to benefit from screening for breast cancer with mammography is estimated to be 10 years, which should also factor into the consideration for screening the geriatric population [150]. In women over the age of 75, the American Geriatric Society has recommended that medical comorbidities, individual life expectancy and the risks of screening, overdiagnosis, and overtreatment should be considered when making the decision to screen for breast cancer [151].

Special Notes

- Breast cancers in the elderly are more likely to be hormone receptor-positive and less frequently HER2-positive.
- A Cochrane Review comparing surgery (with and without adjuvant endocrine therapy) versus endocrine therapy alone as primary treatment for hormone receptor-positive breast cancer in the elderly showed no difference in survival but increased local control with surgery [152]. Individual life expectancy, medical comorbidities, and the risks of overtreatment should be considered in treatment decisions for breast cancer in the elderly.
- A 2017 systematic review and meta-analysis found that elimination of axillary staging in the elderly affected regional control but did not impact survival [153]. The Society of Surgical Oncology Choosing Wisely campaign also recommends not routinely using axillary staging in clinically node-negative women over the age of 70 years old with hormone receptor-positive breast cancer [154].

- The CALGB 9343 randomized controlled trial showed that in women over 70 years of age with stage 1 (T1N0M0) estrogen receptor-positive breast cancer and clinically negative axilla treated with lumpectomy and endocrine therapy, the addition of adjuvant radiotherapy resulted in an 8% improvement in local-regional control but no additional benefit on survival after 12 years of median follow-up [155].
- Tools such as ePrognosis (eprognosis.ucsf.edu) or a comprehensive geriatric assessment [156] can help predict morbidity and mortality in older patients with cancer. These tools may help evaluate elderly patients in the consideration for surgical treatment of breast cancer.

Dense Breasts

Increased breast density is recognized as an independent risk factor for breast cancer [157]. Mammographic screening is less effective in detecting lesions in women with dense breast tissue. To avoid missing breast cancers on mammograms, supplemental screening modalities including ultrasonography and MRI have been used to increase breast cancer detection rates [158]. This is an area requiring further research. Additional breast imaging modalities increase false-positive rates [158, 159] and their effects on breast cancer outcomes remain unclear [159].

Paget's Disease of the Nipple

Paget's disease of the nipple is an uncommon presentation of breast cancer (1–3%). It presents as a scaly, raw, eczematous, or ulcerated lesion that begins on the nipple and then spreads to the areola. Bloody discharge is occasionally present and bilaterality has been described. An underlying breast cancer (DCIS or invasive disease) is present in 85–88% of cases, often without an associated mass on exam or mammographic finding [160].

Paget's disease is often mistaken in its initial assessment for eczema or dermatitis and treated with a short course of topical steroids. Lesions suspected of Paget's disease of the nipple and persistent nipple abnormalities following treatment with topical steroids should undergo skin punch biopsy. The histologic hallmark of Paget's disease of the nipple are Paget cells, which are malignant intraepithelial adenocarcinoma cells within the epidermis of the nipple. Following the diagnosis of Paget's disease of the nipple, bilateral mammography and ultrasound should be performed to identify an underlying cancer (with bilateral breast MRI if both mammogram and ultrasound are negative).

If an underlying cancer is identified preoperatively, both the cancer and the nipple-areolar complex require excision, either as BCS or mastectomy. In clinically node-negative patients, axillary SLNB should be performed if invasive disease is confirmed preoperatively or if undertaking mastectomy for DCIS. Patients with a clinically positive or suspicious axilla should undergo ultrasound-guided fine needle aspiration or core needle biopsy of the palpable nodes. If FNA or core biopsy is positive, axillary lymph node dissection at the time of surgery is recommended. If FNA or core biopsy is negative, proceed to SLNB. For patients treated with neoadjuvant chemotherapy, SLNB may be considered for select patients with initial cN1 disease that convert to cN0.

For women with Paget's disease of the nipple without a palpable mass or mammographic abnormality, and where cancer is not identified preoperatively, central lumpectomy (removing the nipple-areolar complex) followed by whole-breast radiotherapy is appropriate. SLNB as a second operation may be pursued if invasive breast cancer is identified postoperatively [160].

Male Breast Cancer

Male breast cancer is a rare condition, with less than 1% of all breast cancers occurring in men [161]. The peak age of incidence is 71 for sporadic cancer and in the 50s for BRCA2-associated male breast [162]. Men tend to be 5–10 years older than women at diagnosis. The most frequent type is invasive ductal carcinoma, accounting for 90% of the cases [163]. The vast majority of male breast cancer is hormone receptor-positive.

The main risk factors for male breast cancer are a strong family history of breast cancer and BRCA mutation (men with BRCA2 mutation have a greater risk of breast cancer (6% absolute lifetime risk) than men with BRCA1 mutation, and an 80-fold increased risk over the general population) [164, 165]. Other conditions associated with increased levels of estrogen and/or decreased levels of androgen, such as Klinefelter syndrome, cirrhosis, gynecomastia, obesity, alcoholism, exogenous treatment with testosterone or estrogen-containing compounds, and testicular diseases (e.g., orchitis, cryptorchidism, testicular injury), are also risk factors.

The presentation (usually a subareolar painless, firm mass), diagnostic work-up (with mammography, ultrasound and biopsy), and staging of male breast cancer mirror that of breast cancer seen in women. One should keep in mind that a new diagnosis of male breast cancer should prompt genetic testing and counseling, as well as screening for prostate cancer.

The management of male breast cancer is similar to breast cancer seen in women. Treatment principles, including the indications for neoadjuvant and adjuvant systemic therapy and management of the axilla, are extrapolated from treatment principles in women, although most studies do not include men. Thus, male breast cancer cases should be discussed in the setting of a multidisciplinary conference.

Surgical management of male breast cancer is simple mastectomy and SLNB or ALND for invasive cancer. Adjuvant radiotherapy is recommended if there is involvement of the chest wall or lymph nodes. There is emerging data that BCS may be attempted for patient preference if there is sufficient breast tissue to obtain a clear margin. In this setting, adjuvant radiotherapy is also recommended, similar to women with breast cancer undergoing BCS [166].

For hormone-sensitive tumors, adjuvant endocrine therapy is recommended. In this setting, tamoxifen has been more studied and is recommended, given the insufficient evidence to support aromatase inhibitor therapy in men [167]. For men who cannot tolerate tamoxifen (e.g., hypercoagulable state), an aromatase inhibitor may be given in combination with an LHRH agonist (e.g., goserelin, leuprolide, buserelin). Later-line hormonal treatments include anti-androgen drugs (e.g., flutamide, bicalutamide). Bilateral orchiectomy can be used to lower estrogen/androgen levels but given its psychological and physical impact, medical options are preferred over this last resort [161, 166].

Following a personal history of breast cancer, men should be surveyed with annual mammography [165]. Screening recommendations for men with a strong family history or genetic predisposition for breast cancer include semiannual clinical exam starting at age 35 and baseline mammography at age 40, with further annual mammography if increased breast density is observed on baseline mammogram [165].

Until recently, it was thought that male breast cancer was associated with a worse prognosis than women. This may be related to male breast cancer being typically diagnosed at a later stage than female breast cancer, owing to a lack of awareness of male breast cancer and a lack of screening in this population [166]. A 2012 study reported a 5-year survival rate of 74% in men compared to 83% in women [168]. However, more contemporary studies of both male and female breast cancer with careful matching for age at diagnosis, grade, and stage are revealing an improvement in survival with time, such that survival is no longer significantly worse in men than women [166].

Metastatic Breast Cancer

Approximately 4.1% of newly diagnosed breast cancer patients will have metastases at presentation. Improved systemic therapy has seen an increase in the 5-year survival of such patients in the past 5 years [169].

Until recently, surgery had a limited role in the management of patients with metastasis [170, 171]. However, there is an emerging body of evidence to support the concept that removing the primary may provide a survival advantage for such patients [169–171]. A 2002 retrospective review of 16,023 patients from the National Cancer Data Base found that overall survival was improved in women with de novo stage IV breast cancer who underwent surgical resection, with 3-year survival rates of 17% for the no-surgery group, 26% for the partial mastectomy group, and 35% for the mastectomy group [170]. Multiple other retrospective studies have reported survival benefits following surgical resection of the breast primary in patients with metastases [172–180]. However, Cady et al. [181] in 2008 challenged this view through a case-matched retrospective analysis of 808 patients with metastatic breast cancer. They found that case matching either diminishes or eliminates the survival advantage obtained with surgery. This finding was further supported by a 2011 study by Dominici et al. [182]. These retrospective studies highlighted the need for randomized controlled trials to examine the benefit of surgery in the de novo metastatic population.

In a 2015 open-label randomized controlled trial of patients with de novo metastatic breast cancer who responded to frontline chemotherapy, Badwe et al. found that locoregional treatment of the primary tumor and axillary nodes in 173 women had no impact on overall survival, as compared to the 177 women who did not receive locoregional treatment [183]. In a 2018 multicenter, phase III RCT randomizing 138 patients to upfront surgery (following chemotherapy) and 136 patients to systemic therapy only, Soran et al. found that median survival was not different at 36 months but was improved at 40 months with upfront surgery (HR 0.66, 95% CI: 0.49–0.88). Subgroup analyses found that this benefit was seen for estrogen- or progesterone-receptor positivity, HER2 negativity, patients younger than 55 years of age, and patients with bone oligometastasis [184]. Additional trials are ongoing [185]. We believe that these cases constitute special situations that need a multidisciplinary approach. Each decision needs to be tailored according to patient symptoms (e.g., pain, bleeding, nonhealing wound), comorbidities, and life expectancy.

Locoregional Recurrence of Breast Cancer

Breast cancer recurrence can be divided into breast recurrence after breast-conserving therapy, recurrence after mastectomy, and axillary recurrences [186].

Breast recurrence after BCT	Recurrence after mastectomy	Axillary recurrence

Rate of LR after BCT—0.5–1% per year [187]
Risk factors:
  Age < 45 years
  High grade
  Extensive DCIS
  Node positive
  HER2/neu overexpression
  Positive margins
  Lack of radiotherapy [188]
Most recurrences occur in the same quadrant as the primary tumor
Usually detected by physical examination and/or mammography
Metastatic work-up is required to rule out systemic disease
Due to previous radiotherapy, mastectomy is the standard of care, although data is beginning to emerge examining possible repeat excision and radiotherapy [67–68, 188].
Repeat SLNB may be attempted if ALND was not previously performed [39]
	Rate of chest wall recurrence: 5–7%
	The main predicting factor of chest wall recurrence is tumor size >4 cm and 4 or more positive nodes [188]
	Usually the recurrence after mastectomy carries a worse outcome than that after BCT
	Metastatic work-up is indicated
	If systemic disease is ruled out, the local treatment involves wide local excision with or without radiotherapy (depending if previously received); repeat SLNB attempt is discouraged [39]
		Rule out distant metastases and then patients treated with surgical excision of gross disease (i.e., completion axillary node dissection) have better regional control than those treated by radiation therapy [188, 189]. If not technically resectable, consider systemic therapy to gauge response, then resect if becomes feasible [39]
		Isolated axillary recurrence has a 5-year survival of 50% [190]
		There is limited data on repeat irradiation of a previously irradiated axilla, and it should be discussed in the setting of a multidisciplinary meeting [68]
		For supraclavicular and internal mammary node recurrence, NCCN recommends radiation therapy [39], while UpToDate recommends initial systemic therapy, with consideration for either surgery (if previous irradiation) or radiation or both if restaging does not show metastatic progression [191]

BCT breast-conserving therapy, *LR* local recurrence

Referral to Medical Oncology

1. All invasive breast cancers need to be evaluated by medical oncology or discussed in MCC for consideration of systemic therapy.

Referral to Radiation Oncology

1. In situ or invasive carcinoma treated with breast-conserving therapy.
2. Positive or very close margins after mastectomy.
3. Any tumor more than 5 cm irrespective of the surgical treatment offered.
4. Locally advanced and inflammatory breast cancer.
5. Node-positive breast cancer.
6. Paget's disease of the nipple treated with central lumpectomy.

Referring to Multidisciplinary Cancer Conference

Ideally all patients where time allows; however, the following should be discussed:

1. Any case in which a deviation from the standard of care is considered.
2. Axillary lymph node metastases.
3. To review imaging and assess the extent of the disease for the purpose of planning surgical therapy.
4. Disease progression on neoadjuvant chemotherapy with borderline resectability.
5. Patient with metastasis to contralateral axilla.
6. Patient with axillary metastasis and unknown primary cancer.
7. Locoregional recurrence.
8. Metastatic breast cancer in which surgery is being considered.

Technical Aspects of Breast Surgery

Oncoplastic Breast Surgery

Oncoplastic breast surgery (OPBS) is defined as breast reshaping and breast volume displacement and replacement techniques that extend breast-conserving surgery (BCS) options in order to avoid mastectomy [192]. It aims to preserve aesthetic outcome as well as quality of life for breast cancer patients without compromising disease control. Longer term follow-up data confirms not only the oncologic safety of these techniques, but also a lower rate of positive margins when OPBS is utilized, given the wider area of resection [193, 194]. To date, OPBS has been widely accepted and utilized in Europe and the United Kingdom. In a recent MD Anderson Cancer Center analysis of 9861 patients with operable breast cancer, the addition of OPBS permitted a nearly fourfold increase in the percentage of all BCS performed (from 4% to 15%) between 2007 and 2014 [195].

There are two levels of oncoplastic breast surgery [192]:

- Level I: Basic glandular reshaping with local glandular flaps. There is no skin excision and the nipple-areolar complex may be recentralized.
- Level II: Therapeutic mammoplasties, mastopexies and contralateral balancing procedures. The resulting breast is usually smaller, rounder, and higher.

Whenever there is an anticipated poor cosmetic outcome with standard BCS, OPBS should be considered. Excision volume, tumor location, and glandular density are three important elements that should be considered for the choice of the appropriate OPBS technique [196]. Up to 50% of the breast volume can be excised using OPBS. As a general rule, when resection of less than 20% of the breast is planned, Level I parenchymal reshaping can be used. Tumors located in the upper outer quadrant are in the most favorable location for larger volume resections, whereas the upper inner and lower quadrants are the least favorable and can result in significant deformity without OPBS. Regarding the breast glandular density, fatty and scattered fibroglandular breasts are at more risk of fat necrosis after extensive undermining. On the other hand, heterogeneously dense and extremely dense breasts are ideally suited for mobilizing during Level I OPBS.

Comparing Level I and Level II OPBS [196]

Level	Indications	Technique	Pitfalls/comments
I Parenchymal reshaping	Anticipated poor cosmetic outcome with standard BCS Resection of less than 20% of the breast volume is planned	Subcutaneous undermining following mastectomy plane up to ¼ to 2/3 of the breast envelope Excision of the tumor and mobilization from the pectoralis fascia NAC can be recentralized away from the lumpectomy area	Fat necrosis if extensive undermining in fatty breasts
II	Resection of 20–50% of the breast volume is planned		
Round-block	Upper pole and upper inner quadrant tumors (but virtually any location) 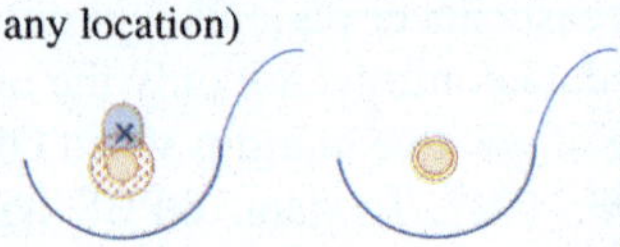	Two concentric periareolar incisions followed by deepithelialization of the skin between the 2 incisions Skin undermining circumferentially starting from outer edge of incision and lumpectomy NAC recentralization	NAC is supplied by posterior glandular base This is a versatile technique and can be applied to tumors in any location

Level	Indications	Technique	Pitfalls/comments
Superior pedicle mammoplasty with inverted T scar	Lower pole tumors 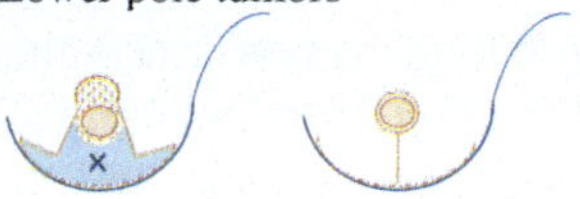	Periareolar and inferior quadrant incisions Deepithelialization and elevation of superior pedicle Lumpectomy and re-approximation of medial and lateral parenchymal flaps NAC recentralization	Foregoing deepithelialization of the area around the NAC and elevation of the NAC would result in "bird beak" deformity
Batwing	Upper inner quadrant tumors 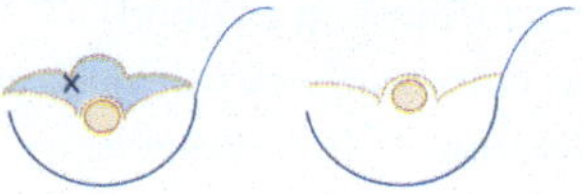	Batwing (or hemi-batwing) incision Lumpectomy with removal of skin between upper incision and NAC Re-approximation of batwing incision	The lateral drawing lines should be greater than the round central diameter in length for optimal results [197]
Racquet mammoplasty	Upper outer quadrant tumors 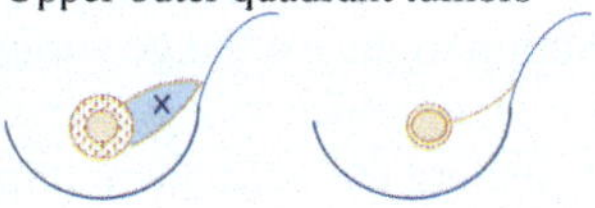	Racquet incision periareolar and upper outer quadrant Periareolar deepithelialization, quadrant undermining, and lumpectomy Complete detachment of retroareolar gland to allow volume redistribution in lateral space NAC recentralization	An incomplete detachment of the retroareolar gland will not permit maximal mobility to fill the defect

BCS breast-conserving surgery, *NAC* nipple-areolar complex

This table illustrates some examples of level 2 oncoplastic techniques but is not exhaustive.

Technical Aspects of Breast Reconstruction aAfter Mastectomy

Breast reconstruction after mastectomy seeks to restore breast appearance and feel, and patient-reported outcome measures demonstrate its benefit in psychosocial and physical well-being [199]. Ultimately, the decision to pursue reconstruction is up to the patient's preference, but it is our goal to enable our patients to make an informed decision in a timely fashion. The possibility of breast reconstruction should be discussed with the patient who is undergoing mastectomy, and if immediate reconstruction is desired and appropriate, a timely referral to a plastic surgeon is encouraged.

Types of Reconstruction

After a skin-sparing or nipple-sparing mastectomy is performed, there are two main types of reconstruction: prosthetic (use of implants) versus autologous (use of one's own body tissue). The choice between these two options and the timing of the reconstruction (delayed vs. immediate) require a discussion based on the need for adjuvant chemotherapy or radiation, donor tissue availability, medical comorbidities, patient's preference, and lifestyle [200].

Implant-Based Reconstruction

Implant-based reconstruction can be performed two-staged (using a temporary tissue expander) or single-staged (via a direct-to-implant method).

The two-staged reconstruction is more commonly performed, and this process involves a tissue expander placement at the time of the mastectomy. In the immediate few weeks after the operation, the mastectomy skin envelope undergoes expansion as saline fluid is injected into the tissue expander via a syringe needle every 1–2 weeks in the office setting until the expander reaches the desired volume. The subsequent operation involves the tissue expander exchange for a permanent implant. The time between the initial operation to the exchange varies per individual but is generally around 6 months.

The direct-to-implant method involves placing the permanent implant at the time of the mastectomy. This single-staged reconstruction is more successful when there is good mastectomy flap vascularity and no significant stretch or tension in the mastectomy flaps after the implant placement. This method would be ideal for patients with native breasts that are non-ptotic and small with the desired volume that is similar or smaller than the native volume.

In implant-based reconstruction, acellular dermal matrix (ADM)—a processed cadaveric dermis—is commonly used to provide extra coverage of the device in the lower breast pole as an extension of the pectoralis major muscle [201, 202], improve definition of the inferior pole [203], and potentially reduce capsular contracture [204]. However, ADM is costly with a potentially added risk [205] and its selective use is encouraged. In a preoperative setting, ADM use is anticipated in patients with larger breast volumes, nipple-sparing procedures, and direct-to-implant reconstruction, and when postoperative radiation treatment is anticipated. In an intraoperative setting, ADM use is considered in patients with compromised pectoralis major muscle integrity, a high pectoralis insertion, relative skin excess in the setting of a well-perfused mastectomy skin flap, and positive sentinel lymph node status (increases the possibility of receiving adjuvant radiation therapy). Poor flap vascularity is a contraindication for acellular dermal matrix use because it will not incorporate and may lead to persistent seroma, infection, and ultimate loss of the reconstruction [206].

In the past two decades, a subpectoral (dual plane) placement of the implant has been commonly used [207] and remains widely used. In recent years, a prepectoral placement of the implants has also become an acceptable option as it allows the benefits of no animation deformity or absence of pectoralis major muscle spasm and less discomfort [208]. However, for a prepectoral reconstruction to be successful, a reasonable thickness of the mastectomy flap ensuring the flap vascularity is critical [208]. Other considerations include BMI < 30, mild to moderate breast volume, nonsmokers, minimal ptosis, and prophylactic mastectomy patients in order to decrease the risk of delayed wound healing, mastectomy flap necrosis, infection, seroma, and reconstructive failure [209, 210].

Implant-based reconstruction requires a detailed discussion regarding the safety concerns of the implants. Both silicone and saline implants that are currently available in practice are deemed safe. However, it is important to discuss implant-related risks that include implant infection, rupture, extrusion, capsular contracture, the possible need for additional implant exchanges in the future, and the risk for breast implant-associated anaplastic large cell lymphoma (BIA-ALCL).

BIA-ALCL is a rare peripheral T cell lymphoma which recent evidence suggests an increased incidence with textured implants [211]. Patients may present with periprosthetic fluid collection years after the initial implant operation in these cases, or with a periprosthetic mass. The work-up would involve a cytological analysis of at least 50 cc of a periprosthetic aspirate for lymphoma protocol with flow cytometry, and immunohistochemistry checking for malignant cells that are CD30+ and ALK-negative. Confirmed cases of BIA-ALCL require total capsulectomy and implant removal, with the need for possible adjuvant therapy if there is lymph node or extracapsular involvement or systemic disease. At this time, there is no confirmed case of BIA-ALCL in a patient with a smooth implant-only history where the full implant history of the patient is known.

Autologous Reconstruction

Autologous reconstruction involves using one's own tissue. There are two types—pedicled and free flaps.

Pedicled flaps involve transposing regional tissue while keeping the blood supply intact, such as the pedicled latissimus dorsi (LD) flap or a pedicled transverse rectus abdominis myocutaneous (TRAM) flap that gets transposed to the chest. The pedicled LD flap is a faster operation than a free flap but likely requires additional volume using a prosthetic device (tissue expander changed to implant). This is an option for patients who have previously received radiation to the chest or those who are not candidates for a free flap due to inadequate tissue availability or medical comorbidities. The pedicled TRAM flap is less frequently used today as it increases the risk of abdominal bulge/hernia from having the entire rectus muscle taken but it remains an option in certain situations.

Free flaps involve a distant transfer of tissue that requires a reestablishment of the blood supply via the use of microsurgical techniques. The most commonly used flaps are the deep inferior epigastric perforator (DIEP) flap or muscle-sparing transverse rectus abdominus (MS-TRAM) free flap from the abdomen. Alternative free flaps use tissues from the buttocks and thighs in cases where there is insufficient abdominal tissue or the patient has already undergone abdominoplasty. Free flaps are generally longer operations (8–10 hours) that require a 3-day stay in the hospital to monitor the flap perfusion in the first few days. Patients with an autologous reconstruction have been found to have a higher long-term satisfaction than those who underwent an implant-based reconstruction on patient-reported outcome measures [199].

Timing of Reconstruction

Reconstruction is offered in an immediate, delayed, or delayed-immediate time frame. An immediate reconstruction is performed at the time of the mastectomy and can include both autologous and implant-based reconstruction options. In an immediate reconstruction, adequate perfusion of the mastectomy flap is critical to obtain a successful reconstruction. Delayed reconstruction is often recommended in patients who are anticipated to undergo adjuvant radiation as the reconstruction failure and complication rate is increased in this population [212]. Delayed autologous reconstruction would allow breast reconstruction using healthy tissue and decrease reconstruction failure rates [200]. Delayed-immediate reconstruction is for patients who are at an increased risk for needing postmastectomy radiation therapy and who wish to have a breast form in place while waiting for final pathology and/or during the period of postmastectomy radiation therapy. A tissue expander is placed at the time of skin-sparing mastectomy and those who do not require postmastectomy radiation therapy, based on final pathology, can undergo a definitive breast reconstruction soon after the initial operation with an implant or a flap [213]. If radiation therapy is required, the expander can be radiated, and following a post-recovery period the expander can be replaced with autologous tissue. In this manner, more skin is preserved (but still not as much as with an immediate reconstruction), and radiation of the final reconstruction can be avoided. However, there may still be complications related to radiation of the expander so that it may require premature removal and place the patient back into the realm of delayed reconstruction.

Surveillance [214, 215]

Surveillance for breast cancer recurrence in the reconstructed breast is completed clinically. There is no evidence to support radiographic screening of the reconstructed breast unless the patient has palpable findings suggestive of recurrence. Suspicious masses or symptoms should be imaged and completely worked up. Fat necrosis is relatively common and benign following breast reconstruction.

Toronto Pearls

- When localizing a lesion for breast conservation, some radiologists will mark the site of the lesion on the skin, but this is not always true. It is helpful to remember that the point of entry and the nipple are the only fixed points. The cranial-caudal (CC) view of a preoperative mammogram defines medial versus lateral and lesion along the nipples line will be either 12′ or 6 o'clock. The medial-lateral

(ML) view defines upper versus lower half and lesions located at the nipple line will be located at either 3′ or 9 o'clock.

- Z0011 results are integrated into our surgical practice: clinically node-negative patients who have undergone lumpectomy and SLNB with positive nodes and who meet Z0011 criteria are not routinely offered completion axillary dissection.
- In cases of locally advanced breast cancer, we perform the SLNB after neoadjuvant chemotherapy if nodes were clinically and radiologically negative prior to treatment. FNA of any suspicious axillary nodes is attempted pretreatment. If nodes were positive and the axilla becomes clinically negative after neoadjuvant systemic therapy, SLNB may be performed; otherwise, axillary lymph node dissection should be pursued.
- Oncoplastic procedures in breast conservation are considered on a case-by-case basis, as are contralateral balancing procedures such as reduction mammoplasty (in conjunction with plastic surgery).
- Contralateral prophylactic mastectomy (CPM) is not routinely recommended in the absence of a genetic mutation resulting in increased lifetime risk of developing a new breast cancer. In discussing CPM for patients without a gene mutation, the following must be considered: CPM does not offer an overall survival benefit in comparison to clinical and radiographic surveillance [198]. It does decrease the risk of developing a contralateral breast cancer. CPM has no effect on local recurrence of the ipsilateral cancer. CPM may be considered in non-gene mutation carriers who are unable/unwilling to undergo continued surveillance and in those who wish to have immediate autologous flap-based reconstruction for optimal symmetry.

References

1. Canadian Cancer Society's Advisory Committee on Cancer Statistics. Canadian cancer statistics 2017. Toronto: Canadian Cancer Society; 2017.
2. Hortobagyi GN, Connolly JL, Edge SB, et al. American Joint Committee on Cancer cancer staging manual. 8th ed. New York: Springer International Publishing; 2017.
3. Sabel M, Collins L. Atypical and lobular carcinoma in situ: high-risk lesions of the breast. In: Chagpar AB, editor. UptoDate; 2017. Retrieved March 23, 2019 from https://www.uptodate.com/contents/atypia-and-lobular-carcinoma-in-situ-high-risk-lesions-of-the-breast.
4. American Society of Breast Surgeons. Consensus guideline on concordance assessment of image-guided breast biopsies and management of borderline or high-risk lesions. 2016. Retrieved from https://www.breastsurgeons.org/about/statements/PDF_Statements/Concordance_and_High%20RiskLesions.pdf.
5. Hartmann LC, Sellers TA, Frost MH, et al. Benign breast disease and the risk of breast cancer. N Engl J Med. 2005;353:229–37.
6. National Comprehensive Cancer Network. Breast cancer screening and diagnosis (Version 3.2018). http://www.nccn.org/professionals/physician_gls/pdf/breast-screening.pdf.
7. Warner E, Messersmith H, Causer P, Eisen A, Shumak R, Plewes D. Mangetic resonance imaging screening of women at high risk for breast cancer. Warner E, Agbassi C, reviewers. Toronto (ON): Cancer Care Ontario; 2012 Aug 31 [Endorsed 2018 Jan]. Program in Evidence-based Care Evidence-based Guideline No.: 15–11 Version 3 ENDORSED. Accessed March 30, 2019 from https://www.cancercareontario.ca/en/guidelines-advice/types-of-cancer/2051.

8. Mastracci TL, Tjan S, Bane AL, et al. E-cadherin alterations in atypical lobular hyperplasia and lobular carcinoma in situ of the breast. Mod Pathol. 2015;18(6):741–51.
9. Collins LC, Baer HJ, Tamimi RM, et al. Magnitude and laterality of breast cancer risk according to histologic type of atypical hyperplasia: results from the Nurses' Health Study. Cancer. 2007;109:180–7.
10. Masannat YA, Bains SK, Pinder SE, et al. Challenges in the management of pleomorphic lobular carcinoma in situ of the breast. Breast. 2013;22(2):194–6.
11. Sabel M. Overview of benign breast disease. In: Chagpar AB, editor. UptoDate. 2018. Retrieved March 23, 2019 from https://www.uptodate.com/contents/overview-of-benign-breast-disease.
12. Sydnor MK, Wilson JD, Hijaz TA, et al. Underestimation of the presence of breast carcinoma in papillary lesions initially diagnosed at core-needle biopsy. Radiology. 2007;242:58–62.
13. Foley NM, Racz JM, Al-Hilli A, et al. An international multicenter review of the malignancy rate of excised papillomatous breast lesions. Ann Surg Oncol. 2015;22(Suppl 3):S385–90.
14. James BA, Cranor ML, Rosen PP. Carcinoma of the breast arising in microglandular adenosis. Am J Clin Pathol. 1993;100:507–13.
15. Koenig C, Dadmanesh F, Bratthauer GL, et al. Carcinoma arising in microglandular adenosis: an immunohistochemical analysis of 20 intraepithelial and invasive neoplasms. Int J Surg Pathol. 2000;8:303–15.
16. Racz JM, Carter JM, Degnim AC. Challenging atypical breast lesions including flat epithelial atypia, radial scar, and intraductal papilloma. Ann Surg Oncol. 2017;24(10):2842–7.
17. Spanheimer PM, Murray MP, Zabor EC, et al. Long-term outcomes after surgical treatment of malignant/borderline phyllodes tumors of the breast. Ann Surg Oncol. 2019;26(7):2136–43.
18. Virnig BA, Tuttle TM, Shamliyan T, et al. Ductal carcinoma in situ of the breast: a systematic review of incidence, treatment, and outcomes. J Natl Cancer Inst. 2010;102(3):170.
19. Collins LC, Tamimi RM, Baer HJ, et al. Outcome of patients with ductal carcinoma in situ untreated after diagnostic biopsy: results from the Nurses' Health Study. Cancer. 2005;103:1778–84.
20. Sanders ME, Schuyler PA, Dupont WD, et al. The natural history of low-grade ductal carcinoma in situ of the breast in women treated by biopsy only revealed over 30 years of long-term follow-up. Cancer. 2005;103:2481–4.
21. Fisher ER, Anderson S, Redmond C, et al. Pathologic findings from the national surgical adjuvant breast project protocol B-06. 10-year pathologic and clinical prognostic discriminants. Cancer. 1993;71:2507–14.
22. Boland GP, Chan KC, Knox WF, et al. Value of the Van Nuys prognostic index in prediction of recurrence of ductal carcinoma in situ after breast-conserving surgery. Br J Surg. 2003;90:426–32.
23. Veronesi U, Cascinelli N, Mariani L, et al. Twenty-year follow-up of a randomized study comparing breast-conserving surgery with radical mastectomy for early breast cancer. N Engl J Med. 2002;347(16):1227–32.
24. Kuerer HM, Smith BD, Chavez-MacGregor M, et al. DCIS margins and breast cancer: MD Anderson Cancer Center multidisciplinary practice guidelines and outcomes. J Cancer. 2017;8(14):2653–62.
25. Fisher B, Dignam J, Wolmark N, et al. Lumpectomy and radiation therapy for the treatment of intraductal breast cancer: findings from National Surgical Adjuvant Breast and Bowel Project B-17. J Clin Oncol. 1998;16(2):441–52.
26. Wapnir IL, Dignam JJ, Fisher B, et al. Long-term outcomes of invasive ipsilateral breast tumor recurrences after lumpectomy in NSABP B-17 and B-24 randomized clinical trials for DCIS. J Natl Cancer Inst. 2011;103(6):478–88.
27. Julien JP, Bijker N, Fentiman IS, et al. Radiotherapy in breast-conserving treatment for ductal carcinoma in situ: first results of the EORTC randomised phase III trial 10853. Lancet. 2000;355(9203):528–33.
28. Donker M, Litière S, Werutsky G, et al. Breast-conserving treatment with or without radiotherapy in ductal carcinoma in situ: 15-year recurrence rates and outcome after a recurrence, from the EORTC 10853 randomized phase III trial. J Clin Oncol. 2013;31(32):4054–9.

29. Cuzick J, Sestak I, Pinder SE, et al. Effect of tamoxifen and radiotherapy in women with locally excised ductal carcinoma in situ: long-term results from the UK/ANZ DCIS trial. Lancet Oncol. 2011;12:21–9.
30. Wärnberg F, Garmo H, Emdin S, et al. Effect of radiotherapy after breast-conserving surgery for ductal carcinoma in situ: 20 years follow-up in the randomized SweDCIS Trial. J Clin Oncol. 2014;32(32):3613–8.
31. Cutuli B, Bernier J, Poortmans P. Radiotherapy in DCIS, an underestimated benefit? Radiother Oncol. 2014;112(1):1–8.
32. Silverstein MJ, Lagios MD. Treatment selection for patients with ductal carcinoma in situ (DCIS) of the breast using the University of Southern California/Van Nuys (USC/VNPI) prognostic index. Breast J. 2015;21(2):127–32.
33. Hughes LL, Wang M, Page DL, et al. Local excision alone without irradiation for ductal carcinoma in situ of the breast: a trial of the Eastern Cooperative Oncology Group. J Clin Oncol. 2009;27(32):5319–24.
34. Wong JS, Chen YH, Gadd MA, et al. Eight-year update of a prospective study of wide excision alone for small low- or intermediate-grade ductal carcinoma in situ (DCIS). Breast Cancer Res Treat. 2014;143(2):343–50.
35. Solin LJ, Gray R, Hughes LL, et al. Surgical excision without radiation for ductal carcinoma in situ of the breast: 12-year results from the ECOG-ACRIN E5194 study. J Clin Oncol. 2015;33(33):3938–44.
36. Sagara Y, Freedman RA, Vaz-Luis I, et al. Patient prognostic score and associations with survival improvement offered by radiotherapy after breast-conserving surgery for ductal carcinoma in situ: a population-based longitudinal cohort study. J Clin Oncol. 2016;34(11):1190–6.
37. McCormick B, Winter K, Hudis C, et al. RTOG 9804: a prospective randomized trial for good-risk ductal carcinoma in situ comparing radiotherapy with observation. J Clin Oncol. 2015;33(7):709–15.
38. Shah C, Vicini FA, Berry S, et al. Ductal carcinoma in situ of the breast: evaluating the role of radiation therapy in the management and attempts to identify low-risk patients. Am J Clin Oncol. 2015;38(5):526–33.
39. NCCN Clinical Practice Guidelines in Oncology: Breast Cancer. Version 1.2019. 14/03/2019. Available at: http://www.nccn.org/professionals/physician_gls/pdf/breast.pdf. Accessed 16 Mar 2019.
40. Smith BD, Bellon JR, Blitzblau R, et al. Radiation therapy for the whole breast: executive summary of an American Society for Radiation Oncology (ASTRO) evidence-based guideline. Pract Radiat Oncol. 2018;8(3):145–52.
41. Lalani N, Rakovitch E. Improving therapeutic ratios with the Oncotype DX® ductal carcinoma in situ (DCIS) score. Cureus. 2017;9(4):e1185. https://doi.org/10.7759/cureus.1185.
42. Evaluation of the DCIS score for decisions on radiotherapy in patients with low/intermediate risk DCIS (DUCHESS). ClinicalTrials.gov [Internet]. Bethesda: National Library of Medicine (US). 2016. Identifier NCT02766881. Cited 2018 Jan 27. Available from: http://clinicaltrials.gov/ct2/show/NCT02766881.
43. Klein J, Kong I, Paszat L, et al. Close or positive resection margins are not associated with an increased risk of chest wall recurrence in women with DCIS treated by mastectomy: a population-based analysis. Springerplus. 2015;4:335. https://doi.org/10.1186/s40064-015-1032-5.
44. Childs SK, Chen YH, Duggan MM, et al. Impact of margin status on local recurrence after mastectomy for ductal carcinoma in situ. Int J Radiat Oncol Biol Phys. 2013;85(4):948–52.
45. Fisher B, Dignam J, Wolmark N, et al. Tamoxifen in treatment of intraductal breast cancer: national surgical adjuvant breast and bowel project B-24 randomised controlled trial. Lancet. 1999;353:1993–2000.
46. Allred DC, Anderson SJ, Palk S, et al. Adjuvant tamoxifen reduces subsequent breast cancer in women with estrogen receptor-positive ductal carcinoma in situ: a study based on NSABP protocol B-24. J Clin Oncol. 2012;30(12):1268–73.

47. Forbes JF, Sestak I, Howell A, et al. Anastrozole versus tamoxifen for the prevention of locoregional and contralateral breast cancer in postmenopausal women with locally excised ductal carcinoma in situ (IBIS-II DCIS): a double-blind, randomized controlled trial. Lancet. 2016;387(10021):866–73.
48. Anderson C, Meyer AM, Wheeler SB, et al. Endocrine therapy initiation and medical oncologist utilization among women diagnosed with ductal carcinoma in situ. Oncologist. 2017;22(5):535–41.
49. Anderson C, Winn AN, Dusetzina SB, Nichols HB. Endocrine therapy initiation among older women with ductal carcinoma in situ. J Cancer Epidemiol. 2017;2017:6091709. https://doi.org/10.1155/2017/6091709.
50. Morrow M, Van Zee KJ, Solin LJ, et al. Society of Surgical Oncology-American Society for Radiation Oncology-American Society of Clinical Oncology consensus guideline on margins for breast-conserving surgery with whole-breast irradiation in ductal carcinoma in situ. J Clin Oncol. 2016;34(33):4040–6.
51. Kell MR, Morrow M. An adequate margin of excision in ductal carcinoma in situ. BMJ. 2005;331:789–90.
52. Morrow M, Van Zee KJ, Solin LJ, et al. Society of Surgical Oncology-American Society for Radiation Oncology-American Society of Clinical Oncology consensus guideline on margins for breast-conserving surgery with whole-breast irradiation in ductal carcinoma in situ. Pract Radiat Oncol. 2016;6(5):287–95.
53. Morrow M, Van Zee KJ, Solin LJ, et al. Society of Surgical Oncology-American Society for Radiation Oncology-American Society of Clinical Oncology consensus guideline on margins for breast-conserving surgery with whole-breast irradiation in ductal carcinoma in situ. Ann Surg Oncol. 2016;23(12):3801–10.
54. Marinovich ML, Azizi L, Macaskill P, et al. The association of surgical margins and local recurrence in women with ductal carcinoma in situ treated with breast-conserving therapy: a meta-analysis. Ann Surg Oncol. 2016;23(12):3811–21.
55. Van Zee KJ, Subhedar P, Olcese C, et al. Relationship between margin width and recurrence of ductal carcinoma in situ: analysis of 2996 women treated with breast-conserving surgery for 30 years. Ann Surg. 2015;262(4):623–31.
56. Tadros AB, Smith BD, Shen Y, et al. Ductal carcinoma in situ and margins <2 mm: contemporary outcomes with breast conservation. Ann Surg. 2019;269(1):150–7.
57. Bijker N, Meijnen P, Peterse JL, et al. Breast-conserving treatment with or without radiotherapy in ductal carcinoma-in-situ: ten-year results of European Organisation for Research and Treatment of Cancer randomized phase III trial 10853 – a study by the EORTC Breast Cancer Cooperative Group and EORTC Radiotherapy Group. J Clin Oncol. 2006;24(21):3381–7. Epub 2006 Jun 26.
58. Collins LC, Achacoso N, Haque R, et al. Risk factors for non-invasive and invasive local recurrence in patients with ductal carcinoma in situ. Breast Cancer Res Treat. 2013;139(2):453–60.
59. Subhedar P, Olcese C, Patil S, et al. Decreasing recurrence rates for ductal carcinoma in situ: analysis of 2996 women treated with breast-conserving surgery over 30 years. Ann Surg Oncol. 2015;22(10):3273–81.
60. Rakovitch E, Gray R, Baehner FL, et al. Refined estimates of local recurrence risks by DCIS score adjusting for clinicopathological features: a combined analysis of ECOG-ACRIN E5194 and Ontario DCIS cohort studies. Breast Cancer Res Treat. 2018;169(2):359–69.
61. Wallis MG, Clements K, Kearins O, et al. The effect of DCIS grade on rate, type and time to recurrence after 15 years of follow-up of screen-detected DCIS. Br J Cancer. 2012;106(10):1611–7.
62. Fisher B, Land S, Mamounas E, et al. Prevention of invasive breast cancer in women with ductal carcinoma in situ: an update of the national surgical adjuvant breast and bowel project experience. Semin Oncol. 2001;28:400–18.
63. Kong I, Narod SA, Taylor C, et al. Age at diagnosis predicts local recurrence in women treated with breast-conserving surgery and postoperative radiation therapy

for ductal carcinoma in situ: a population-based outcomes analysis. Curr Oncol. 2014;21(1):e96–e104.

64. Cronin PA, Olcese C, Patil S, et al. Impact of age on risk of recurrence of DCIS: outcomes of 2996 women treated with breast-conserving surgery over 30 years. Ann Surg Oncol. 2016;23(9):2816–24.
65. Solin LJ, Fourquet A, Vicini FA, et al. Salvage treatment for local recurrence after breast-conserving surgery and radiation as initial treatment for mammographically detected ductal carcinoma in situ of the breast. Cancer. 2001;91(6):1090–7.
66. Resch A, Fellner C, Mock U, et al. Locally recurrent breast cancer: pulse dose rate brachytherapy for repeat irradiation following lumpectomy- a second chance to preserve the breast. Radiology. 2002;225:713–8.
67. Arthur DW, Winter KA, Kuerer HM, et al. NRG Oncology-Radiation Therapy Oncology Group Study 1014: 1-year toxicity report from a phase 2 study of repeat breast-preserving surgery and 3-dimensional conformal partial-breast reirradiation for in-breast recurrence. Int J Radiat Oncol Biol Phys. 2017;98(5):1028–35.
68. Harms W, Budach W, Dunst J, et al. DEGRO practical guidelines for radiotherapy of breast cancer VI: therapy of locoregional breast cancer recurrences. Strahlenther Onkol. 2016;192(4):199–208.
69. Lyman GH, Temin S, Edge SB, et al. Sentinel lymph node biopsy for patients with early-stage breast cancer: American Society of Clinical Oncology clinical practice guideline update. J Clin Oncol. 2014;32:1365–83.
70. Hamm C, Tey R, reviewers. Baseline staging tests in primary breast cancer. Toronto: Cancer Care Ontario; 2011. Available at: https://www.cancercare.on.ca/common/pages/UserFile.aspx?fi leId=13868.
71. Meric F, Mirza NQ, Vlastos G, et al. Positive surgical margins and ipsilateral breast tumor recurrence predict disease-specific survival after breast-conserving therapy. Cancer. 2003;97:926–33.
72. Hanley C, Kessaram R. Quality of diagnosis and surgical management of breast lesions in a community hospital: room for improvement? Can J Surg. 2006;49:185–92.
73. Warner E. Systematic review: using magnetic resonance imaging to screen for women at high risk for breast cancer. Ann Intern Med. 2008;148(9):671–9.
74. Sardanelli F, Boetes C, Borish B. Magnetic resonance imaging of the breast: recommendations from the EUSOMA working group. Eur J Cancer. 2010;46:1296–316.
75. Houssami N, Turner R, Morrow M. Preoperative magnetic resonance imaging in breast cancer: meta-analysis of surgical outcomes. Ann Surg. 2013;257(2):249–55.
76. Tan JZY, Waugh J, Kumar B, et al. Mucinous carcinomas of the breast: imaging features and potential for misdiagnosis. J Med Imaging Radiat Oncol. 2013;57(1):25–31.
77. Houssami N, Macaskill P, Marinovich ML. The association of surgical margins and local recurrence in women with early-stage invasive breast cancer treated with breast-conserving therapy: a meta-analysis. Ann Surg Oncol. 2014;21(3):717–30.
78. Moran MS, Schnitt SJ, Giuliano AE, et al. Society of surgical oncology-american society for radiation oncology consensus guideline on margins for breast-conserving surgery with whole-breast irradiation in stages I and II invasive breast cancer. Ann Surg Oncol. 2014;21(3):704–16.
79. Buchholz TA, Somerfield MR, Griggs JJ, et al. Margins for breast-conserving surgery with whole-breast irradiation in stage I and II invasive breast cancer: American Society of Clinical Oncology endorsement of the Society of Surgical Oncology/American Society for Radiation Oncology consensus guideline. J Clin Oncol. 2014;32(14):1502–6.
80. Ontario Ministry of Health and Long Term Care guidelines on breast cancer genetic counseling and testing. Available at: http://www.health.gov.on.ca/en/pro/programs/ohip/bulletins/4381/bul4381a.aspx.
81. NCCN clinical practice guidelines in oncology: genetic/familial high-risk assessment: breast and ovarian. Version 3.2019. 18/01/2019. Available at: http://www.nccn.org/professionals/physician_gls/pdf/genetics_screening.pdf. Accessed 12 May 2019.

82. American Society of Breast Surgeons. Consensus guideline on genetic testing for hereditary breast cancer. 2019. Retrieved from https://www.breastsurgeons.org/docs/statements/Consensus-Guideline-on-Genetic-Testing-for-Hereditary-Breast-Cancer.pdf. Accessed 12 May 2019.
83. Steele RJ, Forrest AP, Gibson T, et al. The efficacy of lower axillary sampling in obtaining lymph node status in breast cancer: a controlled randomized trial. Br J Surg. 1985;72:368–9.
84. Krag D, Weaver D, Ashikaga T, et al. The sentinel node in breast cancer—a multicenter validation study. N Engl J Med. 1998;339:941–6.
85. Lyman GH, Giuliano AE, Somerfield MR, et al. American society of clinical oncology guideline recommendations for sentinel lymph node biopsy in early-stage breast cancer. J Clin Oncol. 2005;23:7703–20.
86. Mansel RE, Fallowfield L, Kissin M, et al. Randomized multicenter trial of sentinel node biopsy versus standard axillary treatment in operable breast cancer: the ALMANAC trial. J Natl Cancer Inst. 2006;98:599–609.
87. Krag DN, Anderson SJ, Julian TB, et al. Technical outcomes of sentinel-lymph-node resection and conventional axillary-lymph-node dissection in patients with clinically node-negative breast cancer: results from the NSABP B-32 randomised phase III trial. Lancet Oncol. 2007 Oct;8(10):881–8.
88. Krag DN, Anderson SJ, Julian TB, et al. Sentinel-lymph-node resection compared with conventional axillary-lymph-node dissection in clinically node-negative patients with breast cancer: overall survival findings from the NSABP B-32 randomised phase 3 trial. Lancet Oncol. 2010;11(10):927–33.
89. Fisher B, Montague E, Redmond C, et al. Findings from NSABP protocol no. B-04-comparison of radical mastectomy with alternative treatments for primary breast cancer. I. Radiation compliance and its relation to treatment outcome. Cancer. 1980;46:1–13.
90. Newman LA, Mamounas EP. Review of breast cancer clinical trials conducted by the National Surgical Adjuvant Breast Project. Surg Clin North Am. 2007;87:279–305. Vii.
91. Giuliano AE, McCall L, Beitsch P, et al. Locoregional recurrence after sentinel lymph node dissection with or without axillary dissection in patients with sentinel lymph node metastases: the American College of Surgeons Oncology Group Z0011 randomized trial. Ann Surg. 2010;252:426–32.
92. Giuliano AE, Ballman KV, McCall L, et al. Effect of axillary dissection vs no axillary dissection on 10-year overall survival among women with invasive breast cancer and sentinel node metastasis: the ACOSOG Z0011 (Alliance) Randomized Clinical Trial. JAMA. 2017;318(10):918–26. https://doi.org/10.1001/jama.2017.11470.
93. Joslyn SA. Hormone receptors in breast cancer: racial differences in distribution and survival. Breast Cancer Res Treat. 2002;73:45–59.
94. Truong PT, Bernstein V, Wai E, et al. Age-related variations in the use of axillary dissection: a survival analysis of 8038 women with T1-ST2 breast cancer. Int J Radiat Oncol Biol Phys. 2002;54:794–803.
95. Clarke M, Collins R, Darby S, et al. Effects of radiotherapy and of differences in the extent of surgery for early breast cancer on local recurrence and 15-year survival: an overview of the randomised trials. Lancet. 2005;366:2087–106.
96. Fisher B, Bauer M, Margolese R, et al. Five-year results of a randomized clinical trial comparing total mastectomy and segmental mastectomy with or without radiation in the treatment of breast cancer. N Engl J Med. 1985;312:665–73.
97. Cabanes PA, Salmon RJ, Vilcoq JR, et al. Value of axillary dissection in addition to lumpectomy and radiotherapy in early breast cancer. The Breast Carcinoma Collaborative Group of the Institut Curie. Lancet. 1992;339:1245–8.
98. Jagsi R, Chadha M, Moni J, et al. Radiation field design in the ACOSOG Z0011 (Alliance) trial. J Clin Oncol. 2014 Nov 10;32(32):3600–6.
99. Donker M, van Tienhoven G, Straver ME, et al. Radiotherapy or surgery of the axilla after a positive sentinel node in breast cancer (EORTC 10981–22023 AMAROS): a randomised, multicentre, open-label, phase 3 non-inferiority trial. Lancet Oncol. 2014;15:1303–10.

100. Galimberti V, Cole BF, Viale G, et al. International breast Cancer Study Group Trial 23-01. Axillary dissection versus no axillary dissection in patients with breast cancer and sentinel-node micrometastases (IBCSG 23-01):10-year follow-up of a randomised, controlled phase 3 trial. Lancet Oncol. 2018;19(10):1385–93.
101. Boileau JF, Poirier B, Basik M, Holloway C, et al. Sentinel node biopsy following neoadjuvant chemotherapy in biopsy proven node positive breast cancer: the SN FNAC study. J Clin Oncol. 2015;33(3):258–64.
102. Weaver DL, Ashikaga T, Krag DN, et al. Effect of occult metastases on survival in node-negative breast cancer. N Engl J Med. 2011;364:412–21.
103. Altinyollar H, Berberoglu U, Gulben K, et al. The correlation of extranodal invasion with other prognostic parameters in lymph node positive breast cancer. J Surg Oncol. 2007;95(7):567–71.
104. Joseph KA, El-Tamer M, Komenaka I, et al. Predictors of nonsentinel node metastasis in patients with breast cancer after sentinel node metastasis. Arch Surg. 2004;139(6):648–51.
105. Gooch J, King TA, Eaton A, et al. The extent of extracapsular extension may influence the need for axillary lymph node dissection in patients with T1-T2 breast cancer. Ann Surg Oncol. 2014;21(9):2897–903.
106. Choi AH, Blount S, Perez MN, et al. Size of extranodal extension on sentinel lymph node dissection in the American College of Surgeons Oncology Group Z0011 Trial Era. JAMA Surg. 2015;150(12):1141–8.
107. Pilewskie ML, Morrow M. Management of the clinically node-negative axilla: what have we learned from the clinical trials? Oncology (Williston Park). 2014;28(5):371–8.
108. Sparano JA, Gray RJ, Makower DF, et al. Adjuvant chemotherapy guided by a 21-gene expression assay in breast cancer. N Engl J Med. 2018;379:111–21.
109. Francis PA, Regan MM, Fleming GF, et al. Adjuvant ovarian suppression in premenopausal breast cancer. N Engl J Med. 2015;372:436–66.
110. Pagani O, Regan MM, Waley MD, et al. Adjuvant exemestane with ovarian suppression in premenopausal breast cancer. N Engl J Med. 2014;371:107–18.
111. Moore HC, Unger JM, Phillips KA, et al. Goserelin for ovarian protection during breast-cancer adjuvant chemotherapy. N Engl J Med. 2015;372:923–32.
112. Park WC. Role of ovarian function suppression in premenopausal women with early breast cancer. J Breast Cancer. 2016;19(4):341–8.
113. Kwon DS, Kelly CM, Ching CD. Chapter 2 Invasive breast cancer. In: Feig BW, Ching CD, editors. The MD Anderson surgical oncology handbook. 5th ed. Philadelphia: Lippincott Williams & Wilkins; 2012. p. 20–65. Print.
114. Chia S, Swain SM, Byrd DR, et al. Locally advanced and inflammatory breast cancer. J Clin Oncol. 2008;26:786–90.
115. Kaufmann M, von Minckwitz MG, Bear HD, et al. Recommendations from an international expert panel on the use of neoadjuvant (primary) systemic treatment of operable breast cancer: new perspectives 2006. Ann Oncol. 2007;18:1927–34.
116. Colleoni M, Viale G, Zahrieh D, et al. Expression of ER, PgR, HER1, HER2, and response: a study of preoperative chemotherapy. Ann Oncol. 2008;19:465–72.
117. Rody A, Karn T, Solbach C, et al. The erbB2+ cluster of the intrinsic gene set predicts tumor response of breast cancer patients receiving neoadjuvant chemotherapy with docetaxel, doxorubicin and cyclophosphamide within the GEPARTRIO trial. Breast. 2007;16:235–40.
118. Spring L, Greenup R, Niemierko A, et al. Pathologic complete response after neoadjuvant chemotherapy and long-term outcomes among young women with breast cancer. J Natl Compr Cancer Netw. 2017;15(10):1216–23.
119. van der Hage JA, van de Velde CJ, Julien JP, et al. Preoperative chemotherapy in primary operable breast cancer: results from the European Organization for Research and Treatment of Cancer trial 10902. J Clin Oncol. 2001;19:4224–37.
120. Wolmark N, Wang J, Mamounas E, et al. Preoperative chemotherapy in patients with operable breast cancer: nine-year results from National Surgical Adjuvant Breast and Bowel Project B-18. J Natl Cancer Inst Monogr. 2001:96–102.

121. Early Breast Cancer Trialists' Collaborative Group (EBCTCG). Long-term outcomes for neoadjuvant versus adjuvant chemotherapy in early breast cancer: meta-analysis of individual patient data from ten randomized trials. Lancet Oncol. 2018;19(1):27–39.
122. Mamounas EP, Anderson SJ, Dignam JJ, et al. Predictors of locoregional recurrence after neoadjuvant chemotherapy: results from combined analysis of National Surgical Adjuvant Breast and Bowel Project B-18 and B-27. J Clin Oncol. 2012;30(32):3960–6.
123. Zhou X, Li Y. Local recurrence after breast-conserving surgery and mastectomy following neoadjuvant chemotherapy for locally advanced breast cancer – a meta-analysis. Breast Care (Basel). 2016;11(5):345–51.
124. Fisher CS, Ma CX, Gillanders WE, et al. Neoadjuvant chemotherapy is associated with improved survival compared with adjuvant chemotherapy in patients with triple-negative breast cancer only after complete pathologic response. Ann Surg Oncol. 2012;19:253–8.
125. Sabel MS. Sentinel lymph node biopsy before or after neoadjuvant chemotherapy: pros and cons. Surg Oncol Clin N Am. 2010;19:519–38.
126. Geng C, Chen X, Pan X, et al. The feasibility and accuracy of sentinel lymph node biopsy in initially clinically node-negative breast cancer after neoadjuvant chemotherapy: a systematic review and meta-analysis. PLoS One. 2016;11(9):e0162605.
127. Hunt KK, Yi M, Mittendorf EA, et al. Sentinel lymph node surgery after neoadjuvant chemotherapy is accurate and reduces the need for axillary dissection in breast cancer patients. Ann Surg. 2009;250(4):558–66.
128. Boughey JC, Suman VJ, Mittendorf EA, Ahrendt GM, et al. Sentinel lymph node surgery after neoadjuvant chemotherapy in patients with node-positive breast cancer. The ACOSOG Z1071 (Alliance) clinical trial. JAMA. 2013;310(14):1455–61.
129. Kuehn T, Bauerfeind I, Fehm T, et al. Sentinel-lymph-node biopsy in patients with breast cancer before and after neoadjuvant chemotherapy (SENTINA): a prospective, multicenter cohort study. Lancet Oncol. 2013;14(7):609–18.
130. El Hage CH, Headon H, El Tokhy O, et al. Is sentinel lymph node biopsy a viable alternative to complete axillary dissection following neoadjuvant chemotherapy in women with node-positive breast caner at diagnosis? An updated meta-analysis involving 3,398 patients. Am J Surg. 2016;212(5):969–81.
131. Rycaj K, Tang DG. Cancer stem cells and radioresistance. Int J Radiat Biol. 2014;90(8):615–21.
132. Boughey JC, Ballman KV, Le-Petross HT, et al. Identification and resection of clipped node decreases the false-negative rate of sentinel lymph node surgery in patients presenting with node-positive breast cancer (T0-T4, N1-N2) who receive neoadjuvant chemotherapy: results from ACOSOG Z1071 (Alliance). Ann Surg. 2016;263(4):802–7.
133. Caudle AS, Yang WT, Krishnamurthy S, et al. Improved axillary evaluation following neoadjuvant therapy for patients with node-positive breast cancer using selective evaluation of clipped nodes: implementation of targeted axillary dissection. J Clin Oncol. 2016;34(10):1072–8.
134. Weber JJ, Jochelson MS, Eaton A, et al. MRI and prediction of pathologic complete response in the breast and axilla after neoadjuvant chemotherapy for breast cancer. J Am Coll Surg. 2017;225(6):740–6.
135. ClinicalTrials.gov [Internet]. Comparison of axillary lymph node dissection with axillary radiation for patients with node-positive breast cancer treated with chemotherapy. Bethesda: National Library of Medicine (US); 2013. Identifier NCT01901094. 2019 Feb 20 [cited 2019 March 10]. Available from: http://clinicaltrials.gov/ct2/show/NCT01901094.
136. ClinicalTrials.gov [Internet]. Standard or comprehensive radiation therapy in treating patients with early-stage breast cancer previously treated with chemotherapy and surgery. Bethesda: National Library of Medicine (US); 2013. Identifier NCT01872975. 2017 May 16 [cited 2019 March 21]. Available from: http://clinicaltrials.gov/ct2/show/NCT01872975.
137. Masuda N, Lee SJ, Ohtani S, et al. Adjuvant capecitabine for breast cancer after preoperative chemotherapy. N Engl J Med. 2017;376:2147–59.
138. von Minckwitz G, Huang CS, Mano MS, et al. Trastuzumab emtansine for residual invasive HER2-positive breast cancer. N Engl J Med. 2019;380:617–28.

139. Li BD, Sicard MA, Ampil F, et al. Trimodal therapy for inflammatory breast cancer: a surgeon's perspective. Oncology. 2010;79:3–12.
140. Mamouch F, Berrada N, Aoullay Z, et al. Inflammatory breast cancer: a review. World J Oncol. 2018;9(5–6):129–35.
141. Dawood S, Merajver SD, Viens P, et al. International expert panel on inflammatory breast cancer: consensus statement for standardized diagnosis and treatment. Ann Oncol. 2011;22(3):515–23.
142. Robertson FM, Bondy M, Yang W, et al. Inflammatory breast cancer: the disease, the biology, the treatment. CA Cancer J Clin. 2010;60:351–75.
143. Ueno NT, Espinosa Fernandez JR, Cristofanilli M, et al. International consensus on the clinical management of inflammatory breast cancer from the Morgan Welch Inflammatory Breast Cancer Research Program 10th Anniversary Conference. J Cancer. 2018;9(8):1437–47.
144. Hartman EK, Eslick GD. The prognosis of women diagnosed with breast cancer before, during and after pregnancy: a meta-analysis. Breast Cancer Res Treat. 2016;160:347–60.
145. Ruiz R, Herrero C, Strasser-Weippl K, et al. Epidemiology and pathophysiology of pregnancy-associated breast cancer: a review. Breast. 2017;35:136–41.
146. Peccatori FA, Lambertini M, Scarfone G, et al. Biology, staging, and treatment of breast cancer during pregnancy: reassessing the evidences. Cancer Biol Med. 2018;15:6–13.
147. Cordeiro CN, Gemignani ML. Breast cancer in pregnancy: avoiding fetal harm when maternal treatment is necessary. Breast J. 2017;23(2):200–5.
148. Klarenbach S, Sims-Jones N, Lewin G, et al. Recommendations on screening for breast cancer in women aged 40-74 years who are not at increased risk for breast cancer. CMAJ. 2018;190(49):E1441–51.
149. Nelson HD, Tyne K, et al.; U.S. Preventive Services Task Force. Screening for breast cancer: an update for the U.S. Preventive Services Task Force. Ann Intern Med. 2009;151(10):727–37, W237–42.
150. Lee SJ, Boscardin WJ, Stijacic-Cenzer I, et al. Time lag to benefit after screening for breast and colorectal cancer: meta-analysis of survival data from the United States, Sweden, United Kingdom, and Denmark. BMJ. 2013;346:e8441.
151. American Geriatrics Society. Ten things clinicians and patients should question. 2014 [updated 2015 Apr 23]. Choosing Wisely. Accessed May 25, 2019 from https://www.choosingwisely.org/societies/american-geriatrics-society/.
152. Hind D, Wyld L, Reed MW. Surgery, with or without tamoxifen, vs tamoxifen alone for older women with operable breast cancer: cochrane review. Br J Cancer. 2007;96(7):1025–9.
153. Liang S, Hallet J, Simpson JS, et al. Omission of axillary staging in elderly patients with early stage breast cancer impacts regional control but not survival: a systematic review and meta-analysis. J Geriatr Oncol. 2017;8(2):140–7.
154. Choosing Wisely. The Socieyt of Surgical Oncology Encourages Doctors, Patients to question specific commonly-used tests and treatments as part of choosing wisely campaign. 2016. Accessed May 25, 2019 from http://www.choosingwisely.org/the-society-of-surgical-oncology-joins-choosing-wisely-campaign/.
155. Hughes KS, Schnaper LA, Bellon JR, et al. Lumpectomy plus tamoxifen with or without irradiation in women age 70 years or older with early breast cancer: long-term follow-up of CALGB 9343. J Clin Oncol. 2013;31(19):2382–7.
156. Extermann M, Hurria A. Comprehensive geriatric assessment for older patients with cancer. J Clin Oncol. 2007;25(14):1824–31.
157. Nazari SS, Mukherjee P. An overview of mammographic density and its association with breast cancer. Breast Cancer. 2018;25(3):259–67.
158. Melnikow J, Fenton JJ, Whitlock EP, et al. Supplemental screening for breast cancer in women with dense breasts: a systematic review for the U.S. Preventive Services Task Force. Ann Intern Med. 2016;164(4):268–78.
159. Lee JM, Arao RF, Sprague BL, et al. Performance of screening ultrasonography as an adjunct to screening mammography in women across the spectrum of breast cancer risk. JAMA Intern Med. 2019; https://doi.org/10.1001/jamainternmed.2018.8372. [Epub ahead of print].

160. Sabel, M., & Weaver, D. L. (2018) Paget disease of the breast. In: Chagpar AB, Hayes DF, Pierce LJ, editors. UptoDate. Retrieved May 12, 2019 from https://www.uptodate.com/contents/paget-disease-of-the-breast.
161. Canadian Cancer Society. Breast cancer in men. Accessed March 29, 2019 from http://www.cancer.ca/en/cancer-information/cancer-type/breast/breast-cancer/breast-cancer-in-men/.
162. FentimanIS,FourquetA,HortobagyiGN.Malebreastcancer.Lancet.2006;367(9510):595–604.
163. Serdy KM, Leone JP, Dabbs DJ, et al. Male breast Cancer. Am J Clin Pathol. 2017;147(1):110–9.
164. Pritzlaff M, Summerour P, McFarland R, et al. Male breast cancer in a multi-gene panel testing cohort: insights and unexpected results. Breast Cancer Res Treat. 2017;161(3):575–86.
165. Block WD, Muradali D. Breast cancer in men. CMAJ. 2013;185(14):1247. https://doi.org/10.1503/cmaj.122056.
166. Gradishar WJ, Ruddy KJ. Breast cancer in men. In: Chagpar AB, Hayes DF, editors. UpToDate. 2019. Retrieved April 20, 2019, from https://www.uptodate.com/contents/breast-cancer-in-men.
167. Zagouri F, Sergentanis TN, Azim HA Jr, et al. Aromatase inhibitors in male breast cancer: a pooled analysis. Breast Cancer Res Treat. 2015;151(1):141–7.
168. Greif JM, Pezzi CM, Klimberg VS, et al. Gender differences in breast cancer: analysis of 13,000 breast cancers in men from the National Cancer Data Base. Ann Surg Oncol. 2012;19(10):3199–204.
169. Pockaj BA, Wasif N, Dueck AC, et al. Metastasectomy and surgical resection of the primary tumor in patients with stage IV breast cancer: time for a second look? Ann Surg Oncol. 2010;17:2419–26.
170. Khan SA, Stewart AK, Morrow M. Does aggressive local therapy improve survival in metastatic breast cancer? Surgery. 2002;132:620–6.
171. Beslija S, Bonneterre J, Burstein HJ, et al. Third consensus on medical treatment of metastatic breast cancer. Ann Oncol. 2009;20:1771–85.
172. Fields RC, Jeffe DB, Trinkaus K, et al. Surgical resection of the primary tumor is associated with increased long-term survival in patients with stage IV breast cancer after controlling for site of metastasis. Ann Surg Oncol. 2007;14:3345–51.
173. Babiera GV, Rao R, Feng L, et al. Effect of primary tumor extirpation in breast cancer patients who present with stage IV disease and an intact primary tumor. Ann Surg Oncol. 2006;13:776–82.
174. Blanchard DK, Shetty PB, Hilsenbeck SG, et al. Association of surgery with improved survival in stage IV breast cancer patients. Ann Surg. 2008;247:732–8.
175. Neuman HB, Morrogh M, Gonen M, et al. Stage IV breast cancer in the era of targeted therapy: does surgery of the primary tumor matter? Cancer. 2010;116:1226–33.
176. Bafford AC, Burstein HJ, Barkley CR, et al. Breast surgery in stage IV breast cancer: impact of staging and patient selection on overall survival. Breast Cancer Res Treat. 2009;115:7–12.
177. Hazard HW, Gorla SR, Scholtens D, et al. Surgical resection of the primary tumor, chest wall control, and survival in women with metastatic breast cancer. Cancer. 2008;113:2011–9.
178. Ly BH, Vlastos G, Rapiti E, et al. Local-regional radiotherapy and surgery is associated with a significant survival advantage in metastatic breast cancer patients. Tumori. 2010;96:947–54.
179. Gnerlich J, Jeffe DB, Deshpande AD, et al. Surgical removal of the primary tumor increases overall survival in patients with metastatic breast cancer: analysis of the 1988-2003 SEER data. Ann Surg Oncol. 2007;14:2187–94.
180. Rao R, Feng L, Kuerer HM, et al. Timing of surgical intervention for the intact primary in stage IV breast cancer patients. Ann Surg Oncol. 2008;15:1696–702.
181. Cady B, Nathan NR, Michaelson JS, et al. Matched pair analyses of stage IV breast cancer with or without resection of primary breast site. Ann Surg Oncol. 2008;15:3384–95.
182. Dominici L, Najita J, Hughes M, et al. Surgery of the primary tumor does not improve survival in stage IV breast cancer. Breast Cancer Res Treat. 2011;129(2):459–65.

183. Badwe R, Hawaldar R, Nair N, et al. Locoregional treatment versus no treatment of the primary tumor in metastatic breast cancer: an open-label randomized controlled trial. Lancet Oncol. 2015;16(13):1380–8.
184. Soran A, Ozmen V, Ozbas S, et al. Randomized trial comparing resection of primary tumor with no surgery in stage IV breast cancer at presentation: protocol MF07-01. Ann Surg Oncol. 2018;25(11):3141–9.
185. Khan SA. Early surgery or standard palliative therapy in treating patients with stage IV breast cancer. Available from: http://clinicaltrials.gov/show/NCT01242800. Updated 01 January 2019. Accessed 16 Mar 2019.
186. Easson AM, McCready DR. Management of local recurrence of breast cancer. Expert Rev Anticancer Ther. 2004;4:219–26.
187. Cabioglu N, Hunt KK, Buchholz TA, et al. Improving local control with breast-conserving therapy: a 27-year single-institution experience. Cancer. 2005;104:20–9.
188. Mahvi DA, Liu R, Grinstaff MW, et al. Local cancer recurrence: the realities, challenges, and opportunities for new therapies. CA Cancer J Clin. 2018;68(6):488–505.
189. Recht A, Pierce SM, Abner A, et al. Regional nodal failure after conservative surgery and radiotherapy for early-stage breast carcinoma. J Clin Oncol. 1991;9:988–96.
190. Willner J, Kiricuta IC, Kolbl O. Locoregional recurrence of breast cancer following mastectomy: always a fatal event? Results of univariate and multivariate analysis. Int J Radiat Oncol Biol Phys. 1997;37:853–63.
191. Hirsch A, Sabel MS, Hayes DF. Management of locoregional recurrence of breast cancer after mastectomy. In: Burstein HJ, editor. UpToDate. 2018. Retrieved March 16, 2019, from https://www.uptodate.com/contents/management-of-locoregional-recurrence-of-breast-cancer-after-mastectomy.
192. Campbell EJ, Romics L. Oncological safety and cosmetic outcomes in oncoplastic breast conservation surgery: a review of the best level of evidence literature. Breast Cancer (Dove Med Press). 2017;9:521–30.
193. Kaur N, Petit JY, Rietjens M, et al. Comparative study of surgical margins in oncoplastic surgery and quadrantectomy in breast cancer. Ann Surg Oncol. 2005;12(7):539–45.
194. Spear SL, Pelletiere CV, Wolfe AJ, et al. Experience with reduction mammaplasty combined with breast conservation therapy in the treatment of breast cancer. Plast Reconstr Surg. 2003;111(3):1102–9.
195. Carter SA, Lyons GR, Kuerer HM, et al. Operative and oncologic outcomes in 9861 patients with operable breast cancer: single-institution analysis of breast conservation with oncoplastic reconstruction. Ann Surg Oncol. 2016;23(10):3190–8.
196. Clough KB, Kaufman GJ, Nos C, et al. Improving breast cancer surgery: a classification and quadrant per quadrant atlas for oncoplastic surgery. Ann Surg Oncol. 2010;17(5):1375–91.
197. Sanidas EE, Schrenk P. Part II: breast conserving oncoplastic techniques: Batwing technique. In: Fitzal F, Schrenk P, editors. Oncoplastic breast surgery, a guide to clinical practice. 2nd ed. Vienna: Springer; 2015. p. 21–5. Print.
198. Wong SM, Freedman RA, Sagara Y, et al. Growing use of contralateral prophylactic mastectomy despite no improvement in long-term survival for invasive breast cancer. Ann Surg. 2017;265(3):581–9.
199. Santosa KB, Qi J, Kim HM, et al. Long-term patient-reported outcomes in postmastectomy breast reconstruction. JAMA Surg. 2018;153(10):891–9.
200. Lee CN-H, Deal AM, Huh R, et al. Quality of patient decisions about breast reconstruction after mastectomy. JAMA Surg. 2017;152(8):741–8.
201. Rawlani V, Buck DW II, Johnson SA, et al. Tissue expander breast reconstruction using prehydrated human acellular dermis. Ann Plast Surg. 2011;66:593–7.
202. Kim JY, Connor CM. Focus on technique: two-stage implant-based breast reconstruction. Plast Reconstr Surg. 2012;130(Suppl 2):104S–15S.
203. Spear SL, Sher SR, Al-Attar A. Focus on technique: supporting the soft-tissue envelope in breast reconstruction. Plast Reconstr Surg. 2012;130(Suppl 2):89S–94S.

204. Salzberg CA, Dunavant C, Nocera N. Immediate breast reconstruction using porcine acellular dermal matrix (Strattice) long-term outcomes and complications. J Plast Reconstr Aesthet Surg. 2013;66:323–8.
205. Ho G, Nguyen TJ, Shahabi A, et al. A systematic review and meta-analysis of complications associated with acellular dermal matrix-assisted breast reconstruction. Ann Plast Surg. 2012;68:346–56.
206. Jordan SW, Khavanin N, Fine NA, et al. An algorithmic approach for selective acellular dermal matrix use in immediate two-stage breast reconstruction: indications and outcomes. Plast Reconstr Surg. 2014;134:178–88.
207. Corderiro PG, Jazayeri L. Two-stage implant-based breast reconstruction: an evolution of the conceptual and technical approach over a two-decade period. Plast Reconstr Surg. 2016;138:1–11.
208. Nahabedian MY. Current approaches to prepectoral breast reconstruction. Plast Reconstr Surg. 2018;142:871–80.
209. Sigalove S, Maxwell GP, Sigalove NM, et al. Prepectoral implant-based breast reconstruction: rationale, indications, and preliminary results. Plast Reconstr Surg. 2017;139:287–94.
210. Sbitany H, Piper M, Lentz R. Prepectoral breast reconstruction: a safe alternative to submuscular prosthetic reconstruction following nipple-sparing mastectomy. Plast Reconstr Surg. 2017;140:432–43.
211. Leberfinger AN, Behar BJ, Williams NC, et al. Breast implant-associated anaplastic large cell lymphoma: a systematic review. JAMA Surg. 2017;152(12):1161–8.
212. Nelson JA, Disa JJ. Breast reconstruction and radiation therapy: an update. Plast Reconstr Surg. 2017;140(5S):60S–8S.
213. Kronowitz SJ. Delayed-immediate breast reconstruction: technical and timing considerations. Plast Reconstr Surg. 2010;125(2):463–74.
214. Shea-Budgell M, Quan ML, Mehling B, et al. Breast reconstruction following prophylactic or therapeutic mastectomy for breast cancer: recommendations from an evidence-based provincial guideline. Plast Surg. 2014;22(2):103–11.
215. Zakireh J, Fowble B, Esserman LJ. Application of screening principles to the reconstructed breast. J Clin Oncol. 2010;28:173–80.

Cholangiocarcinoma

5

Nicholas Latchana, Sean Cleary,
and Carol-anne E. Moulton

Introduction

Cholangiocarcinoma is an uncommon cancer that occurs within the intrahepatic and extrahepatic portions of the bile duct system. In North America, the incidence of extrahepatic cholangiocarcinoma is 0.5–2 per 100,000 and 0.95 per 100,000 for intrahepatic cholangiocarcinoma [1]. Up to 50% of patients will be lymph node (LN) positive at presentation, 5% are multifocal tumors, and 10–20% will have peritoneal involvement at presentation (see Table 5.1). Risk factors for cholangiocarcinoma are primary sclerosing cholangitis (PSC) with a lifetime risk 10–40% [2, 3], parasitic infection [1], previous sphincteroplasty [4], congenital anomalies of the biliary tree (choledochal cyst, Caroli's disease, anomalous pancreaticobiliary duct junction) [5], and chronic biliary inflammatory disease (hepatitis B/C, liver cirrhosis [6], recurrent pyogenic cholangitis) (see Table 5.2). The most common presentation is painless jaundice and weight loss in the setting of extrahepatic duct involvement. In Western countries, 80% are extrahepatic (20% distal and 60% hilar) and 20% are intrahepatic (see Tables 5.3 and 5.4).

The recommended staging system is the Union for International Cancer Control and American Joint Committee on Cancer (UICC/AJCC) 8th edition. ICC and ECC are staged differently.

N. Latchana (✉) · C.-a. E. Moulton
Department of Surgery, University of Toronto, Toronto, ON, Canada
e-mail: Nicholas.Latchana@mail.utoronto.ca; Carol-anne.Moulton@uhn.ca

S. Cleary
Department of Surgery, Mayo Clinic, Rochester, MN, USA
e-mail: Cleary.Sean@mayo.edu

F. C. Wright et al. (eds.), *Surgical Oncology Manual*,
https://doi.org/10.1007/978-3-030-48363-0_5

Table 5.1 Clinical outcome

Presentation	Prognosis 5-year overall survival (OS)
Distal extrahepatic localized, LN negative Hilar extrahepatic localized, LN negative Intrahepatic localized, LN negative	37–54% (fully resected disease) 20–50% (fully resected disease) 20–43% (fully resected disease)
LN positive—resectable	20–25% [7] (median survival 22 months with positive margins, 60 months with negative margins) [8]
Metastatic or unresectable disease	<5%

LN lymph node

Table 5.2 Special cases

Primary sclerosing cholangitis	Congenital cysts
6.8% of patients develop cholangiocarcinoma over 10 years (10–40% lifetime risk) Incidence: 0.6% per year Usually presents within the first 2 years after diagnosis of PSC [10] Screening recommendations: q6 month biliary imaging (CT or MRI/MRCP), Ca 19–9 for 2 years. However, no validated surveillance program in this population [1, 5] There is some emerging evidence to support the use of EUS with biopsy/brushings in this scenario	Incidence of cholangiocarcinoma <1% per year Overall lifetime incidence of 28%, if left untreated [11] Upon identification, ductal imaging is necessary with MRCP; ERCP if needed Recommend cyst excision with hepaticojejunostomy reconstruction Cyst enterostomy is not recommended [12]

PSC primary sclerosing cholangitis, ERCP endoscopic retrograde cholangiopancreatography

Table 5.3 Intrahepatic cholangiocarcinoma

Work-up	Management	Follow-up
History and physical exam Lab work: Ca 19–9, AFP, CEA Imaging: CT chest, multiphasic CT A/P MRI/MRCP Search for primary adenocarcinoma of other site: Endoscopy, chest CT, mammography [13]	Surgical resection is the only potential cure Removal of involved liver segments There is emerging evidence that recommends a routine hilar LN dissection for its prognostic value [14] M1 disease includes involvement of celiac, periaortic, caval LN	CT C/A/P q3–6 months × 2 years However, there is no data to support that aggressive postoperative surveillance as it has not been shown to alter outcome in this disease

LN lymph nodes, *CT C/A/P* computed tomography of chest, abdomen, and pelvis

Table 5.4 Extrahepatic cholangiocarcinoma

Site	Work-up	Management	Follow-up
Distal bile duct (below the cystic duct)	History and physical exam Labs: Ca 19–9 Imaging: CT chest, multiphasic CT A/P MRI/MRCP Consider biliary decompression if: Jaundice present with ERCP/PTC Consider EUS for biopsy of lesion and lymph nodes (biopsy should be avoided in surgically resectable patients) [13] Specificity of brush cytology is almost 100%, but sensitivity only 18–40% [16] Consider serum IgG4 to rule out IgG4 related sclerosing cholangitis	Surgical resection is the only potential cure Pancreaticoduodenectomy including en bloc resection of extrahepatic bile duct and gallbladder Regional nodes include: Hilar (CBD, common hepatic, portal, cystic) Posterior and anterior pancreaticoduodenal Nodes along SMV Nodes along right lateral wall of SMA	CT C/A/P q3–6 months for 2 years There is no data to support that aggressive surveillance alters outcome in this disease
Hilar (above the cystic duct)		En bloc resection of extrahepatic bile duct and gallbladder, including right and left hepatectomy, or extended right/left hepatectomy [7] Caudate lobe should be removed [13] Regional nodes include: Hilar (CBD, hepatic, portal, cystic) Pericholedochal nodes in hepatoduodenal ligament	

ERCP endoscopic retrograde cholangiopancreatography, *PTC* percutaneous transhepatic cholangiography, *EUS* endoscopic ultrasound, *CBD* common bile duct, *SMV* superior mesenteric vein, *SMA* superior mesenteric artery

Definitions/Terminology

- *Extrahepatic Cholangiocarcinoma* (Bismuth/Corlett Classification system) [9].
  - Type 1: Distal to hepatic duct bifurcation *(distal).*
  - Type 2: Involving the bifurcation *(hilar).*
  - Type 3a/3b: Occlusion of common and either right (a) or left hepatic duct (b).
  - Type 4: Multicentric or involve bifurcation and both right and left hepatic ducts.

Special Notes

- Ca 19–9 can be elevated in up to 85% of patients with cholangiocarcinoma, but is not specific; elevation can also occur in the setting of obstructive jaundice without malignancy. If it remains elevated after biliary decompression, it could indicate the presence of malignancy. Elevated pre- and postoperative Ca 19–9 predict poor survival [15].
- For perihilar tumors, decisions regarding which side of the liver to resect depend on right- or left-sided dominance, volume of future liver remnant, and the extent of vascular and ductal involvement.
- Some centers report that 30–50% of tumors will be deemed unresectable at the time of surgery, despite accurate preoperative imaging (see Table 5.5) [11].
- Quality Indicators: Pathologic Analysis—R0 margin, regional lymphadenectomy includes three or more LN.

Special Notes

- In Ontario, all patients with known or suspected cholangiocarcinoma should be referred for management at a high-volume hepatopancreaticobiliary surgical oncology center.
- *Radiologic assessment* should include the following: level of involvement of the biliary tree, extent of vascular involvement, identification of hepatic lobar atrophy, and identification of metastatic disease [17].
- *Role of Frozen Section*: Although frozen section is frequently employed intraoperatively, it has differing uses depending on the type of cholangiocarcinoma.

Table 5.5 Unresectable/metastatic disease

Criteria of unresectability	Management
Metastatic disease: Liver, lung, peritoneum, distant lymph nodes (N2 disease: celiac, SMA nodes) Patient factors: Comorbidities rendering patient unable to tolerate potentially curative surgery Anatomical factors: (adapted from Jarnagin et al. [20], JHPB surgery guidelines [23]) Encasement of bilateral hepatic arteries or proper hepatic artery Extension into secondary biliary radicals bilaterally with no chance for an R0 resection Extension into biliary radicals unilaterally, with contralateral hepatic artery encasement/occlusion or contralateral atrophy of one hepatic lobe Relative contraindication: Atrophy of one hepatic lobe with contralateral portal vein encasement/occlusion—dependent upon the extent of portal vein involvement, this can be resected and reconstructed	Consider transplant candidacy (Mayo protocol) if unresectable for local tumor invasion Consider nonoperative approach to palliation if able (e.g., Stent/PTC placement) [21] and biopsy Consider radiation/chemotherapy options

SMA superior mesenteric artery, *PTC* percutaneous transhepatic cholangiography/catheter

In extrahepatic cholangiocarcinoma, it has a definite mandatory role in determining margin status, unresectability, or the presence of metastases. Frozen section margin status in intrahepatic cholangiocarcinoma is largely academic, as technical limitations dictate whether further margins are possible.

- *Role of Transplant in Hilar Cholangiocarcinoma:*
  - *Mayo Protocol* for patients with unresectable hilar cholangiocarcinoma or cholangiocarcinoma arising de novo in the setting of PSC is offered at UHN.
  - *Exclusion Criteria*—patients with intrahepatic cholangiocarcinoma, intrahepatic or extrahepatic metastases, gall bladder/below cystic duct involvement, tumor size ≥3 cm, age ≥ 65 years old, Hx of malignancy within 5 years, Hx of prior RT in upper abdo, prior hilar dissection within 12 months, any patients who underwent transperitoneal biopsy within 12 months.
  - *Original Mayo protocol*; Preoperative Radiation—40–45 Gy, with concurrent 5-FU, followed by 20–30 Gy transcatheter irradiation with iridium. Capecitabine until transplantation.
  - *UHN Mayo protocol*; Preoperative Radiation—Conformal RT boost, local regional 45 Gy + Boost 54–75 Gy, with concurrent Capecitabine, Gemcitabine + Cisplatin until transplantation.
  - *Preoperative Assessment*—staging laparotomy (patients must be node negative, negative for metastases and no evidence of locally advanced disease). Liberal endoscopic ultrasound and fine needle aspiration of regional nodes have identified occult metastatic disease prior to neoadjuvant therapy.
  - 5-year survival for patients who entered Mayo protocol is 54% and for patients transplanted is 73% [18].
  - Fallout rate is about 30% and median survival after fall out is 6.8 months [19].
- *Role of Medical Oncology*: All patients with a good performance status should be referred to a medical oncologist following resection for consideration of adjuvant systemic chemotherapy. Recent data from the phase III BILCAP trial in the United Kingdom revealed an improvement in median overall survival to 53 months with adjuvant capecitabine compared to 36 months with observation alone (Primose abstract, Ghidini et al.). Subgroup analysis reveals the benefit was present in R0 resections (HR 0.73) and R1 resections (HR 0.90) as well as node negative or node positive disease (2-year OS of 80% vs. 50%). Furthermore, those with perihilar tumors did not benefit from adjuvant therapy in this trial.
- *Quality Indicators*: Margin: tumor margin of at least 5 mm or more [13]. Pathological analysis: regional lymphadenectomy includes 12 or more LN.

Landmark Publications

Prospective RCTs regarding surgical management of this disease are few, due to the relative rarity of the disease. Surgical management is largely dictated by consensus statements formed by large high volume centers (see Table 5.6).

Table 5.6 Landmark publications

Consensus guidelines	*ESMO Clinical Practice guidelines: Biliary Cancer* Eckel et al. [22]		European guidelines
	Clinical Practice Guidelines: JSHBPS Kondo et al. [23]		Japanese guidelines
	AHPBA Summary statement: Hilar Cholangiocarcinoma Clary et al. [24]		North American guidelines
	SIGE/AIGO/AIOM/AIRO Position Paper Alvaro et al. [1]		Italian guidelines
	Study	*Methods*	*Results*
Medical oncology management	*UK-ABC-02* Valle et al. [25] *BILCAP* Primrose et al. [26] *PRODIGE 12-ACCORD 18 UNICANCER GI* Edeline et al. [27]	RCT phase 3 Conducted in 37 centers in the UK *N* = 410 patients Non-resectable, recurrent, or metastatic biliary cancer (included intra–/extrahepatic cholangiocarcinoma, ampullary, gallbladder cancer) RCT phase 3 Conducted in 44 centers in the UK *N* = 447 patients Resected gallbladder cancer or cholangiocarcinoma (included intra–/extrahepatic cholangiocarcinoma) Two groups, adjuvant Capecitibine for 24 weeks or observation alone RCT phase 3 Conducted in 33 centers in France *N* = 196 patients Resected gallbladder cancer or cholangiocarcinoma (included intra–/extrahepatic cholangiocarcinoma) Two groups, adjuvant GEMOX or observation alone for 12 weeks	Median survival was 11.7 vs. 8.1 months for the Gemcitabine–Cisplatin and Gemcitabine-alone groups, respectively (HR 0.64) Significant improvement in progression-free survival, 8 months vs. 5 months Gem-Cis vs. Gem, respectively (HR 0.63) The combination of Gem-Cis chemotherapy for advanced/metastatic disease gave an average of 3.6 months longer life than gemcitabine alone, with limited toxicity, and represents an appropriate option for treatment in these patients In the per-protocol analysis, median overall survival was 53 vs. 36 months for the capecitabine and observation groups respectively (HR 0.75) Median recurrence-free survival (ITT) was 24.4 months for capecitabine and 17.5 months for observation with a difference in months 0–24 after randomization (HR 0.75). No difference in recurrence-free survival, 30.4 vs. 18.5 months for the GEMOX and observation groups, respectively (HR 0.88) No difference in overall survival, 75.8 vs. 50.4 months for the GEMOX and observation groups, respectively (HR 1.08)

RCT randomized controlled trial, ITT intention-to-treat, GEMOX gemcitabine and oxaliplatinin

Referring to Medical Oncology

1. Resectable and unresectable disease with good performance status.

Referring to Radiation Oncology

1. R1 resection.
2. Palliative patients for consideration of symptomatic control/photodynamic therapy.
3. Locally advanced disease.

Referring to Multidisciplinary Cancer Conference (MCC)

1. R1 resection.
2. Locally advanced disease.
3. Unresectable disease.
4. All potentially resectable cases should be reviewed and treated at a high-volume HPB surgical oncology center.
5. Patients with PSC.
6. Mayo protocol candidate.

Toronto Pearls

- Strongly consider biliary decompression of future remnant liver for hilar tumor preoperatively and wait for near normal bilirubin levels if possible.
- Biliary decompression should occur prior to portal vein embolization (if required).
- Future remnant liver volume > 40% may be required.
- Caudate lobe resection should be considered in all cases, unless drainage of caudate duct into unaffected duct can be confirmed on MRCP and will not compromise surgical margin.
- Biliary infection/sepsis must be treated prior to proceeding to resection.
- Early and aggressive management of biliary infections in the postoperative period, considering drug resistant organisms if patient has had previous preopereative cholangitis and longer term antibiotic treatment AND never request a percutaneous biopsy in unresectable Klatskin's tumors if considering Mayo protocol.

References

1. Alvaro D, Cannizzaro R, Labianca R, et al. Cholangiocarcinoma: a position paper by the Italian Society of Gastroenterology (SIGE), the Italian Association of Hospital Gastroenterology (AIGO), the Italian Association of Medical Oncology (AIOM) and the Italian Association of Oncological Radiotherapy (AIRO). Dig Liver Dis. 2010;42:831–8.
2. Burak K, Angulo P, Pasha TM, et al. Incidence and risk factors for cholangiocarcinoma in primary sclerosing cholangitis. Am J Gastroenterol. 2004;99:523–6.

3. Broome U, Olsson R, Loof L, et al. Natural history and prognostic factors in 305 Swedish patients with primary sclerosing cholangitis. Gut. 1996;38:610–5.
4. Hakamada K, Sasaki M, Endoh M, et al. Late development of bile duct cancer after sphincteroplasty: a ten-to twenty-two year follow up study. Surgery. 1997;1215:488–92.
5. Roukounakis NE, Kuhn JA, McCarty TM. Association of an abnormal pancreaticobiliary junction with biliary tract cancers. Proc (Bayl Univ Med Cent). 2000;13:11–3.
6. Shaib YH, El-Serag HB, Davila JA, et al. Risk factors of intrahepatic cholangiocarcinoma in the United States: a case control study. Gastroenterology. 2005;128:620–6.
7. Alberts SR, Gores GJ, Kim GP, et al. Treatment options for hepatobiliary and pancreatic cancer. Mayo Clin Proc. 2007;82:628–37.
8. Burke EC, Jarnagin WR, Hochwald SN, et al. Hilar cholangiocarcinoma: patterns of spread, the importance of hepatic resection for curative operation, and a pre-surgical clinical staging system. Ann Surg. 1998;228:385–94.
9. Bismuth H, Corlette MB. Intrahepatic cholangioenteric anastomosis in carcinoma of the hilum of the liver. Surg Gynecol Obstet. 1975;140:170–8.
10. Bergquist A, Ekbom A, Olsson R, et al. Hepatic and extrahepatic malignancies in primary sclerosing cholangitis. J Hepatol. 2002;36:321–7.
11. Cleary SP, Knox J, Dawson L. Carcinoma of the biliary tract. In: Blanke CD, Rodel C, Talamonti MS, editors. Gastrointestinal oncology: a practical guide. Berlin: Springer; 2010. p. 251–99.
12. Stain SC, Guthrie CR, Yellin AE, Donovan AJ. Choledochal cyst in the adult. Ann Surg. 1995;222:128–33.
13. Khan SA, Davidson BR, Goldin R, et al. Guidelines for the diagnosis and treatment of cholangiocarcinoma: consensus document. Gut. 2002;51 Suppl 6:vi1–9.
14. Bridgewater J, Galle PR, Khan SA, et al. Guidelines for the diagnosis and management of intrahepatic cholangiocarcinoma. J Hepatol. 2014;60:1268–89.
15. Kondo N, Murakami Y, Uemura K, et al. Elevated perioperative serum CA19-9 levels are independent predictors of poor survival in patients with resectable cholangiocarcinoma. J Surg Oncol. 2014;110:422–9.
16. Chapman R, Fevery J, Kalloo A, et al. Diagnosis and management of primary sclerosing cholangitis. Hepatology. 2010;51:660–78.
17. Cleary SP, Dawson LA, Knox JJ, Gallinger S. Cancer of the gallbladder and extrahepatic bile ducts. Curr Probl Surg. 2007;44:396–482.
18. Rosen CB, Heimbach JK, Gores GJ. Liver transplantation for cholangiocarcinoma. Transpl Int. 2010;23:692–7.
19. Sio TT, Martenson JA, Haddock MG, et al. Outcome of transplant-fallout patients with unresectable cholangiocarcinoma. Am J Clin Oncol. 2014. [Epub ahead of print].
20. Jarnagin WR, Fong Y, DeMatteo RP, et al. Staging, resectability, and outcome in 225 patients with hilar cholangiocarcinoma. Ann Surg. 2001;234:507–17.
21. Baron TH. Expandable metal stents for the treatment of cancerous obstruction of the gastrointestinal tract. N Engl J Med. 2001;344:1681–7.
22. Eckel F, Brunner T, Jelic S. On behalf of the ESMO Guidelines Working Group Biliary cancer: ESMO clinical practice guidelines for diagnosis, treatment and follow-up. Ann Oncol. 2010;21(Suppl 5):v65–9.
23. Kondo S, Takada T, Miyazaki M, et al. Guidelines for the management of biliary tract and ampullary carcinomas: surgical treatment. J Hepato-Biliary-Pancreat Surg. 2008;15:41–54.
24. Clary B, Jarnigan W, Pitt H, et al. Hilar cholangiocarcinoma. J Gastrointest Surg. 2004;8:298–302.
25. Valle J, Wasan H, Palmer D, et al. Cisplatin plus gemcitabine versus gemcitabine for biliary tract cancer. N Engl J Med. 2010;362:1273–81.
26. Primrose JN, Fox RP, Palmer DH, et al. Capecitabine compared with observation in resected biliary tract cancer (BILCAP): a randomised, controlled, multicentre, phase 3 study. Lancet Oncol. 2019;20(5):663–73.
27. Edeline J, Benabdelghani M, Bertaut A, et al. Gemcitabine and oxaliplatin chemotherapy or surveillance in resected biliary tract cancer (PRODIGE 12-ACCORD 18-UNICANCER GI): a randomized phase III study. J Clin Oncol. 2019;37(8):658–67.

Colon Cancer

6

Sepehr Khorasani, Aman Pooni, Usmaan Hameed,
Robert Gryfe, Shady Ashamalla, Fayez A. Quereshy,
and Nancy N. Baxter

Introduction

Colorectal cancer (CRC) is the second most common cancer in Canada, with an estimated 26,900 new cases diagnosed in 2020 [1]. It is also the second leading cause of death from cancer in Canada with an estimated 9700 deaths (5300 men and 4400 women) in 2020 [1, 2]. Although the age-standardized incidence for CRC has been declining in males and females, this decline appears to be confined to older adults as the incidence has been rising in those younger than age 50 [1].

The most common stage of CRC at the time of diagnosis is stage III [1]. There is a strong association between cancer stage at time of diagnosis and survival (Table 6.1).

The current recommended staging system is the American Joint Committee on Cancer (AJCC) eighth edition.

S. Khorasani · A. Pooni
Colorectal Surgery, University of Toronto, Toronto, ON, Canada
e-mail: sepehr.khorasani@mail.utoronto.ca; aman.pooni@mail.utoronto.ca

U. Hameed · R. Gryfe · S. Ashamalla · F. A. Quereshy
Department of Surgery, University of Toronto, Toronto, ON, Canada
e-mail: Usmaan.Hameed@nygh.on.ca; rgryfe@mtsinai.on.ca; Shady.ashamalla@sunnybrook.ca; fayez.quereshy@uhn.ca

N. N. Baxter (✉)
Department of Surgery, University of Toronto, Toronto, ON, Canada

Melbourne School of Population and Global Health, University of Melbourne, Melbourne, Victoria, Australia
e-mail: nancy.baxter@unimelb.edu.au

F. C. Wright et al. (eds.), *Surgical Oncology Manual*,
https://doi.org/10.1007/978-3-030-48363-0_6

Table 6.1 Incidence and associated 5-year survival based on stage of colorectal cancer

Presentation	Average annual number [1]	Incidence (%) [1, 3]	5-year survival (%) [1, 2]
Localized colorectal cancer (stage I, II)	4008	47.1	90
Regional colorectal cancer (stage III)	2118	29.1	71
Metastatic colorectal cancer (stage IV)	1676	19.9	13

Table 6.2 Screening recommendations

Patient population	Recommendation
Average risk: Age 50–74, asymptomatic, no first-degree family history, no personal history of precancerous polyps, no IBD	gFOBT or FIT (preferred) beginning at age 50 with colonoscopy if positive Repeat FOBT q2 years with flexible sigmoidoscopy q5 years Colonoscopy also reasonable as initial test with repeat q10 years if normal
Increased risk: First-degree relative with CRC	Colonoscopy at age 50 or 10 years earlier than youngest affected relative If negative, repeat q5 years (if first-degree relative diagnosed before age 60) or q10 years (if diagnosed after age 60)

gFOBT guaiac fecal occult blood test; *FIT* fecal immunochemical test, *IBD* inflammatory bowel disease

Screening and Surveillance for Average and High-Risk Patients

Screening

Special Notes

- There is good quality evidence that population screening using either FOBT or flexible sigmoidoscopy reduces colorectal cancer mortality [4, 5] (Table 6.2).
- FOBT has been shown to reduce relative risk of CRC mortality by 16% [4, 5].
- FIT has been shown to have superior sensitivity in detecting CRC and advanced adenoma when compared to gFOBT [6]. It is also anticipated that the reduction in CRC-related death through FIT screening is at least equivalent to that through gFOBT. However, direct comparison between gFOBT and FIT in terms of CRC-related mortality is lacking.
- A randomized trial from Norway showed that population screening with flexible sigmoidoscopy decreased colorectal cancer mortality (11.7/100,000 deaths per person-years absolute risk reduction) [7].
- At least four randomized controlled trials and ten observational studies have shown that screening with flexible sigmoidoscopy reduces incidence and mortality in distal, but not proximal colorectal cancer [8].

- A systematic review and meta-analysis showed decreased mortality for proximal cancers with colonoscopy compared to flexible sigmoidoscopy based on observational data [8].
- Colonoscopy is recommended by the American College of Gastroenterology for screening, although there are no randomized trials demonstrating a reduction in mortality [9].
- A population-based study in Ontario of 2,412,077 people demonstrated that the colonoscopy rate was inversely proportional to death from CRC [10]. A case–control study in Ontario has demonstrated a significant association between colonoscopy and fewer deaths from CRC; specifically left-sided cancers [11].
- Colonoscopy is the most sensitive of available screening options at detecting cancer or polyps and is thus an acceptable modality; however, it is associated with the highest risk and cost.
- A shorter interval between testing or repeat colonoscopy should be performed if the first colonoscopy is sub-optimal.
- Quality indicators for colonoscopy:
  - Cecal intubation rate > 90%, adequate bowel preparation, post polypectomy bleeding rate of <0.5%, and perforation rate of <0.1% [12, 13].
  - Polypectomy and adenoma detection rates (ADR) are also important quality indicators. Some studies have suggested ADR ≥ 25% may be associated with lower incidence of interval cancer [14]; however, there is no consensus on what the appropriate target should be [12, 13].
  - There is insufficient evidence to suggest a minimum withdrawal time from the cecum of 6 min improves quality of endoscopy or improves ADR [10, 11]. However, shorter mean withdrawal times have been independently associated with lower ADR [14].

Surveillance

Special Notes

- Table 6.3 is adapted from Ontario ColonCancerCheck Guidelines.
- Patients with multiple colorectal adenomas (>10) should be considered for germline genetic testing of *APC*, *MUTYH*, and *MMR*.
- Above surveillance interval assumes (1) no family history of CRC in a first-degree relative with an age of onset <60, (2) colonoscopy was complete and adequate, and all visible polyps were completely removed.

Hereditary Colorectal Cancer Syndromes

Lynch Syndrome and Microsatellite Instability

- Lynch syndrome is the most common hereditary CRC syndrome with a lifetime colorectal cancer risk of 40–80% (Table 6.4). This genetic disease results from mutations in DNA mismatch repair (MMR) genes leading to microsatellite instability (MSI).

Table 6.3 Surveillance of patients with polyps identified at colonoscopy [15]

Initial colonoscopy finding	Timing/type of next test	Subsequent colonoscopy finding	Timing/type of next test
No polyps or hyperplastic polyps[a] in sigmoid/rectum	10 years/FIT	N/A	
LRA	5 years/FIT	N/A	
HRA	3 years/colonoscopy	No polyps/hyperplastic polyps in sigmoid or rectum/LRA	5 years/ colonoscopy
		HRA	3 years/ colonoscopy
>10 adenomas[b]	<1 year/clearing colonoscopy	<3 years at endoscopist's discretion	
SSA <10 mm without dysplasia	5 years/colonoscopy	At endoscopist's discretion[c]	
SSA ≥10 mm or with dysplasia or TSA	3 years/colonoscopy		
Large sessile polyp removed piecemeal	≤6 m/colonoscopy to check site		
Serrated polyposis syndrome[d]	1 year/colonoscopy	1–2 years at endoscopist's discretion	

FIT fecal immunochemical test, *N/A* not applicable, *LRA* low-risk adenoma (1–2 tubular adenomas <10 mm and without high-grade dysplasia), *HRA* high-risk adenoma/advanced adenoma (one or more tubular adenomas ≥10 mm, three or more adenomas of any size, villous adenomas, adenomas with high-grade dysplasia), *SSA* sessile serrated adenoma/sessile serrated polyp (if dysplasia, considered advanced); *TSA* traditional serrated adenoma (uncommon, often protrubrant and left-sided polyps)

[a]Usually diminutive (<5 mm) nondysplastic polyps in rectum/sigmoid and are not associated with increased risk of CRC (i.e., not screening-relevant)

[b]Genetic testing for FAP should be offered. If no FAP and colon cleared, surveillance colonoscopy should be in <3 years

[c]Both SSA and TSA require surveillance; however, evidence to suggest specific surveillance interval is lacking

[d]At least 5 serrated polyps proximal to sigmoid, two of which >10 mm, or first-degree relative with serrated polyposis and having any number of serrated polyps proximal to sigmoid, or more than 20 serrated polyps of any size and in any location

Table 6.4 Gene mutations and colorectal cancer risk in hereditary colorectal cancer syndromes

Colorectal cancer syndrome	Pattern of inheritance	Mutated germline gene	Colorectal cancer risk
Adenomatous			
Lynch syndrome	AD	*MLH1, MSH2, MSH6, PMS2, EPCAM/TACSTD1*	40–80% by age 75
Familial adenomatous polyposis (FAP)	AD	*APC*	90% by age 45
Attenuated FAP (AFAP)	AD	*APC*	70% by age 80
MUTYH-associated polyposis (MAP)	AR	*MUTYH*	35–55%
Hamartomatous			
Peutz–Jeghers	AD	*STK1*	40% by age 70
Juvenile polyposis	AD	*SMAD4, BMPR1A*	15–70% by age 60

AD autosomal dominant, *AR* autosomal recessive

- MSI is identified in approximately 15% of all CRC and is a feature of Lynch syndrome.
- Majority of cases of MSI are sporadic, due to methylation of an MMR gene, rather than a germline mutation found in Lynch syndrome. Revised Bethesda Guidelines provide criteria for testing of individuals at risk for Lynch syndrome [16].
- MSI may be screened for in all colorectal cancers via PCR or Immunohistochemistry (IHC) for defective MMR.

Revised Bethesda Guidelines

- CRC diagnosed in a patient < age 50.
- Synchronous or metachronous CRC or other Lynch-related tumor.
- CRC diagnosed in a first-degree relative with a Lynch-related tumor, one diagnosed < age 50.
- CRC diagnosed in two or more first- or second-degree relatives with Lynch-related tumors.
- CRC with MSI-high (MSI-H) histology in patient < age 60:
  - Tumor infiltrating lymphocytes.
  - Crohn's-like lymphocytic reaction.
  - Medullary growth pattern.
  - Mucinous/Signet ring differentiation.

Special Notes

- In stage II patients, IHC testing should be considered as MSI-H status has been shown to predict lack of benefit from fluorouracil-based adjuvant chemotherapy [7, 18].
- Extracolonic manifestations of Lynch syndrome include cancers of the uterus (30–60%), ovary (4–12%), urinary tract (5–12%), stomach (8–10%), small bowel, pancreas (4%), biliary tract, brain, and skin [15].
- Testing guidelines based on age and family history miss a significant proportion of patients with MSI-H tumors. Universal testing of patients with CRC is a more sensitive method of identifying MSI-H patients and may be more cost-effective than traditional guidelines [19–21].
- The proposed ASCO/ESMO guidelines suggest (1) universal testing of all patients with CRC or (2) testing of all patients <70 and patients >70 who fulfill any of the revised Bethesda guidelines [19].
- Tumor testing for MMR deficiency with IHC ± MSI:
  - If loss of MLH1/PMS2 protein expression is observed in the tumor, analysis of BRAF V600E mutation and/or analysis of methylation of the MLH1 promoter should be carried out first to rule out a sporadic case.
  - If tumor is MMR deficient and somatic BRAF mutation is not detected or MLH1 promoter methylation is not identified, testing for germline mutations is indicated.

- If loss of any of the other proteins (MSH2/MSH6/PMS2) is identified, test for corresponding genes to the absent protein (e.g., MSH2, MSH6, EPCAM, PMS2, MLH1).
- Full germline testing for Lynch should include DNA sequencing and large re-arrangement analysis.

Polyposis Syndromes

Familial Adenomatous Polyposis (FAP)

- >100–1000s of adenomas distributed in the colon and rectum at presentation.
- Accounts for <1% of all CRC cancers. Polyps often manifest in adolescents or young adults.
- Extracolonic manifestations of FAP: gastric and duodenal polyps, desmoid tumors, thyroid and brain tumors, congenital hypertrophy of the retinal pigmented epithelium (CHRPE), supernumerary teeth, osteomas, and epidermoid cysts.
- Duodenal/ampullary adenocarcinomas follow CRC as the major cause of cancer death in patients with FAP.
- Desmoid tumors are found in up to 30% of patients with FAP and are the third most common cause of death in FAP. They peak around age 30 or 2–3 years after surgery. Depending on the location and symptoms, management includes observation (10% resolve spontaneously), medical therapy (NSAIDS, tamoxifen, vinblastine/methotrexate, or chemotherapy), or surgical resection.

Attenuated Familial Adenomatous Polyposis (AFAP)

- 10–99 colorectal adenomas at presentation, preponderance for right colon. Polyps tend to develop later in life compared to FAP.

MUTYH-Associated Polyposis (MAP)

- Autosomal recessive inheritance, phenotype characterized by <100 adenomas. Average age of onset mid-50s. Up to 1/3 of biallelic MUTYH-mutation carriers may develop CRC in the absence of colorectal polyposis. Heterozygote individuals are also at a slightly increased risk of CRC (Table 6.4).

Germline Testing for APC and MUTYH [15]

- Should be considered in all patients with multiple colorectal adenomas (>10).
- APC germline testing should include DNA sequencing and large re-arrangement analysis.

Management

Primary Localized Colon Cancer

Special Notes

- *Polyps*
  - Endoscopic management of sessile and pedunculated polyps is appropriate provided they are removed as a single specimen and lack high-risk features [28–30].
  - High-risk features of malignant polyps include poorly differentiated histology, lymphovascular invasion, tumor budding, piecemeal excision, and positive margin [28, 29].
  - Data regarding surveillance following successful endoscopic resection is lacking. Repeat endoscopic evaluation for local recurrence is recommended 3–6 months post resection. There is no defined role for routine imaging (Table 6.5); however, in high-risk patients not undergoing resection, enrollment in a surveillance program may be considered [28–30].
  - Given that lymph node involvement has been reported in 5–17% of malignant polyps [28–31], practice at the University of Toronto has included radiographic staging at diagnosis.
- *Adjuvant Treatment*
  - Adjuvant chemotherapy should begin within 8 weeks of surgery. If delayed beyond 12 weeks, there is limited to no clinical benefit [32, 33].
  - The benefit of adjuvant chemotherapy is clearest in patients with stage III disease where ~30% decrease in risk of recurrence and mortality has been demonstrated [34].
  - The role of adjuvant chemotherapy among patients with high-risk stage II disease (perforation, obstruction, nodal harvest <12 nodes, T4, poorly differentiated histology) is more controversial [34].
  - When adjuvant chemotherapy is administered for stage II disease, oxaliplatin is often omitted due to adverse side effects and unclear benefit. Additionally, as noted previously, MIS-H status predicts lack of benefit from fluorouracil-based adjuvant chemotherapy in stage II disease [17, 18].
  - Six months of adjuvant therapy remains the standard of care; however, given the small absolute difference in DFS and the reduced rates of toxicity, adjuvant therapy may be limited to 3 months in patients with T1-T3 and N1 disease [35].
- *Technical Considerations*
  - A minimally invasive approach is recommended in all suitable patients. Evidence suggests that the principal benefits are reduction in length of stay and postoperative pain with equivalent oncological outcomes [28, 36–40].
  - Several retrospective studies and one prospective randomized trial have evaluated the use of robotic surgery. While feasibility and safety compared to laparoscopy has been demonstrated, to date there is no convincing evidence to favor the use of robotics over conventional laparoscopic techniques [28, 44–47].

Table 6.5 Management and surveillance protocol for primary localized colon cancer

Clinical scenario	Workup	Surgical management	Adjuvant therapy	Follow-up (FU)/ surveillance
Malignant polyp	History and physical exam Colonoscopy With tattoo of site Pathology review Consider imaging: CT Chest/abdo/ pelvis Consider CEA	If incompletely resected or any high-risk features: resection with appropriate nodal basin	None	Clinical assessment Q3–6 months × 5 years Colonoscopy at 1 year, then q5 years if normal
Stage I, low-risk stage II	History and physical exam Labs: CBC, CEA Imaging: CT chest/ abdo/pelvis Colonoscopy	Resection with appropriate nodal basin	None	Clinical assessment, Colonoscopy at 1 year; if no advanced adenoma, repeat in 3 years then q5 years if normal Stage II: annual CT chest/ abdomen/pelvis [22–24] CEA Q3-6months x 5 years
High-risk stage II	As above	As above	Consider 5-FU, capecitabine Less benefit for MSI-H tumors [16, 17]	As above
Stage III	As above	As above	Recommend FOLFOX [25, 26] Capecitabine may be given as alternative to 5-FU/LV [27]	As above

Adapted from: Cancer Care Ontario Program in Evidence-Based Care: Follow-up Care, Surveillance Protocol, and Secondary Prevention Measures for Survivors of Colorectal Cancer

- Routine extended lymphadenectomy is not standard of care. At present, no randomized trials have compared complete mesocolic excision surgery to conventional colectomy [28].
- Quality Indicators:

  Uninvolved radial resection margin [28, 41].

  A minimum of 12 lymph nodes in the resected specimen [28, 42, 43].

  A minimum of 5 cm proximal and distal margins recommended [28, 42, 43].

- *Surveillance*
  - If a preoperative assessment was not performed, colonoscopy should be performed within 6 months of surgery or as soon as possible after the completion of adjuvant therapy. Frequency of colonoscopies thereafter should be dictated by the findings [24, 48].
  - Of patients who recur, 80% are within the first 2–2.5 years, and 95% recur by 5 years [48]
  - Any new and persistent or worsening symptoms warrant the consideration of a recurrence.
  - The general practice at the University of Toronto is to perform CT of the chest/abdomen/pelvis every 6 to 12 months for the first 2 years then annually up to 5 years.
  - The American Society of Clinical Oncology (ASCO) 2013 endorsement of CCO practice guidelines suggests considering CT chest/abdomen every 6–12 months for 3 years in patients at a higher risk of recurrence [48].
  - The intensity of postoperative surveillance should depend on the likelihood that additional therapy would be recommended in the setting of recurrent disease.

Management of Patient Populations at High Risk for Colon Cancer

Special Notes

- Lynch syndrome: Segmental resection may be considered in cases of significant comorbidity, advanced age, or advanced disease. Detailed discussion of risk/benefits and need for close endoscopic surveillance should be emphasized if segmental resection is to be performed.
- FAP: The choice between colectomy + IRA and TPC-IPAA must be balanced with patient age, degree of rectal polyposis, wish to bear children, risk of developing desmoids, and possibly the site of mutation in the APC gene.
- AFAP/MAP: Preservation of the rectum may be considered when rectal clearance is possible (Table 6.6). The risk of recurrence in rectal stump must be balanced against the alteration in function with proctocolectomy and pelvic pouch.
- IBD: Nomenclature and management of dysplasia in IBD is evolving. Recent SCENIC [49] guidelines advocate chromoendoscopy for surveillance. Consider referral to an IBD center if dysplasia is identified on random biopsy. Endoscopic management of dysplasia associated mass lesions (DALM) should be done at expert centers.

Locally Advanced Colon Cancer or Locoregional Recurrence

Special Notes

- Histologically negative margins should be the goal of en bloc resection [50, 51]. Relevant margins should be marked on the specimen by the surgeon.
- Neoadjuvant chemoradiotherapy may improve resectability and negative margin rates (Table 6.7) [52, 53].

Table 6.6 Screening, management, and surveillance protocols for high-risk populations

Clinical scenario	Screening	Surgical management	Surveillance
Lynch syndrome	Colonoscopy q1–2 years beginning at age 20–25 or 10 years prior to youngest case in family	Total colectomy at time of cancer diagnosis Consider prophylactic TAH-BSO >35 years after childbearing is complete	Endoscopic assessment of remaining colon/rectum q1–2 years Gynecologic exam with transvaginal US and aspiration biopsy annually
FAP	Flexible sigmoidoscopy (or colonoscopy) q1–2 years from age 10 to 12 OGD with regular and side-viewing scope for duodenal adenomas from age 20–25 or when colonic polyposis diagnosed	Surgery after development of large number of polyps or HGD: Colectomy + IRA TPC-IPAA TPC with end ileostomy	Colonoscopy q1–2 years for life in mutation carriers Rectum present: endoscopic assessment q6–12 months Ileal pouch: evaluation q1–3 years for pouch polyps OGD interval depending on Spigelman stage
AFAP	Colonoscopy (preponderance of right-sided adenomas) q1–2 years starting age 18–20 OGD with regular and side-viewing scope for duodenal adenomas from age 20–25 or when colonic polyposis diagnosed	As above for FAP Extent of surgery depends on extent of polyposis and rectal involvement	Surveillance interval depends on extent of polyposis Colonoscopy q1–2 years in mutation carriers Colonoscopy and polypectomy q1 year once adenomas are detected
MAP	As above for FAP or AFAP, depending on extent of polyposis and family history	As above for AFAP	As above for AFAP
Ulcerative colitis/ Crohn's colitis	HD colonoscopy q1–2 years beginning 8 years after diagnosis Four quadrant biopsies every 10 cm Chromoendoscopy if available	Malignancy or high grade dysplasia on random biopsy: TPC ± IPAA Expert pathology review advisable for dysplasia	Endoscopic assessment of rectal stump/reservoir q1–2 years

FAP familial adenomatous polyposis, *AFAP* attenuated FAP, *MAP MUTYH-associated polyposis*, *APC* adenomatous polyposis coli, *TAH-BSO* total abdominal hysterectomy + bilateral salpingo-oophorectomy, *TPC* total proctocolectomy, *IRA* ileorectal anastomosis, *IPAA* ileal pouch-anal anastomosis

Adapted from Hereditary colorectal cancer syndromes: American Society of Clinical Oncology clinical practice guideline endorsement of the familial risk-colorectal cancer: European society for medical oncology clinical practice guidelines [19] and SCENIC guideline [49]

Table 6.7 Management and follow-up of locally advanced/locoregional recurrence

Workup	Surgical management	Adjuvant therapy	Follow-up (F/U)
History and physical exam Labs: CBC, CEA Imaging: CT chest/abdomen/pelvis Consider MRI Colonoscopy Multidisciplinary review	En bloc resection with adjacent structures and negative margins Consider neoadjuvant chemoradiotherapy to facilitate R0 resection (negative microscopic margins)	Recommend FOLFOX; Capecitabine as alternative to 5-FU/LV Adjuvant therapy for recurrence individualized based on previous regimen	Clinical assessment at least q6 monthly for 3 years, then annually Colonoscopy at 1 year, then q3–5 years Consider CEA, imaging of liver/lungs

Table 6.8 Management and follow-up of colon cancer with distant metastasis

Workup	Surgery (referral to appropriate surgical sub-specialty)	Systemic management	Follow-up (F/U)
History and physical exam Labs: CEA Imaging: CT chest/abdo/pelvis Consider US or MRI liver as indicated Consider US for ovarian metastases CT head/bone scan for symptoms	Liver: Surgical resection with modern chemotherapy offers a 5-year OS up to 58% Lung: Surgical resection with modern chemotherapy offers a 5-year OS up to 40% Peritoneum: Referral to peritoneal malignancy program for evaluation Ovary: Bilateral oophorectomy should be considered if one ovary is involved Brain: Consider resection for solitary metastases	FOLFOX or FOLFIRI with bevacizumab recommended [54–56] Cetuximab/panitumumab can be considered for K-Ras wild type [57] Consider a clinical trial	Patients receiving chemotherapy with potentially resectable metastatic disease should have imaging every three cycles to assess response to therapy Patients in palliative care should only have blood tests and or imaging as dictated by clinical condition

Colon Cancer with Distant Metastases

Special Notes

- Resection of the primary tumor should be considered in symptomatic patients or in those with potentially resectable metastatic disease.
- First-line chemotherapy should be strongly considered in asymptomatic patients with unresectable metastatic disease (Table 6.8).
- If a synchronous metastasis is resectable, the timing of surgery and chemotherapy should be individualized for each patient. Options include synchronous or staged colectomy with metastasectomy vs. neoadjuvant chemotherapy followed by synchronous or staged colectomy and metastasectomy vs. colectomy followed by chemotherapy and staged metastasectomy or vice versa.

- Patients with unresected primaries should be followed as up to 20% need surgical resection during the course of their treatment.
- Bevacizumab administration has been associated with delayed wound healing and GI perforation [54, 58, 59]. The bevacizumab product monograph states it should be discontinued ≥28 days before elective surgery and should not be initiated for ≥28 days after surgery.
- However, while patients on bevacizumab therapy undergoing surgery have been shown to experience significant morbidity and mortality, the risk of complications has not been detectably associated with time since exposure in population-based studies [59].
- There may be a survival advantage in resection of the primary tumor in patients with unresectable metastatic disease [60]. Randomized trials investigating this topic are ongoing [61, 62].

Landmark Publications (Table 6.9)

Referring to Medical Oncology (See Tables 6.7 and 6.8)

1. High-risk stage II.
2. Stage III, IV.
3. Locally advanced or recurrent disease.

Table 6.9 Summary of landmark publications

Topic	Study	Methods	Results
Laparoscopic vs Open resection	COST Trial [37] Fleshman et al., 2007 update [63]	RCT $N = 872$ Colon cancer only	No significant difference in time to recurrence or OS, median F/U 7 years Shorter median hospital stay
	CLASSIC Trial Jayne et al. [38] Green et al., 2013 update [64]	RCT $N = 794$ (526 laparoscopic, 48% rectal cancer)	No significant difference in OS, DFS or recurrence, median F/U 62.9 months
	COLOR Trial Buunen et al. [65] Deijen et al. 2016 update [66]	RCT $N = 1248$ (excluded BMI >30) Colon cancer only	A 3-year difference in OS could not be ruled out in favor of open colectomy 10-year follow-up of Dutch patients showed no difference in OS, DFS and recurrence
	Barcelona Trial Lacy et al. [39] Lacey et al. update [67]	RCT $N = 219$ Colon cancer only	Trend toward higher cancer-related survival in laparoscopic, median F/U 95 months Shorter hospital stay

Table 6.9 (continued)

Topic	Study	Methods	Results
Chemotherapy	NSABP C-07 Kuebler et al. [25] Yothers et al., 2011 update [68]	RCT *N* = 2407 Stage II/III resected with curative intent 5-FU/LV alone (FUFA) vs. 5-FU/LV+ Oxaliplatin (FLOX)	4-year DFS (stage II and III): 73.2% FLOX 67% FUFA 8 year DFS (stage II and III) 69.4% FLOX 64.2% FUFA
	MOSAIC Andre et al. [26] Andre et al., 2009 update [69] Tournigand et al. [70] (sub-group analysis) Andre et al., 2015 update [71]	RCT *N* = 2246 Stage II/III colon cancer resected with curative intent FOLFOX4 vs. 5-FU/LV	5-year DFS (stage II and III): 73.3% FOLFOX4 67.4% 5-FU/LV 6-year OS (stage III): 72.9% FOLFOX4 68.7% 5-FU/LV 10 year OS (stage III) 67.1% FOLFOX4 59.0% 5-FU/LV Stage II: No improvement in DFS/OS No difference in DFS/OS in low vs. high risk
	X-ACT Twelves et al. [27] Twelves et al., Update 2012 [72]	RCT *N* = 1987 Capecitabine vs. Bolus 5-FU/LV in resected stage III colon cancer	Equivalent DFS and OS for capecitabine and 5-FU/LV, with few adverse events Median follow-up 6.9 years
	IDEA Collaboration Grothey et al. [35]	Preplanned pooled analysis of 6 RCTs (N = 12,834) 3 vs. 6 months of oxaliplatin-based chemotherapy in resected stage III colon cancer	Noninferiority of 3 months regime not confirmed in the overall study population (HR=, 1.07; 95% CI: 1.00–1.15) Noninferiority of shorter regime seen in CAPOX but not FOLFOX Among T1, T2, or T3 and N1 cancers, 3 months of therapy was noninferior to 6 months, 3-year DFS 83.1% vs. 83.3%

OS overall survival, *F/U* follow-up, *LR* local recurrence, *DFS* disease-free survival, *RCT* randomized controlled trial

Referring to Radiation Oncology (See Tables 6.7 and 6.8)

1. Consider for locally advanced or recurrent disease.
2. Palliative management of symptomatic lesions with unresectable metastatic disease.

Referring to Multidisciplinary Cancer Conference (MCC)

1. Locally advanced or recurrent disease.
2. Metastatic disease in fit patients (synchronous and metachronous).

Toronto Pearls

- Neoadjuvant chemoradiotherapy for locally advanced or recurrent colon cancer may improve resectability and negative margin rates. Careful preoperative planning and multidisciplinary approach are necessary to achieve the goal of R0 resection.

References

1. Canadian Cancer Statistics Advisory Committee. Canadian Cancer Statistics 2020. Toronto: Canadian Cancer Society; 2020. Available at: https://www.cancer.ca/~/media/cancer.ca/CW/cancer%20information/cancer%20101/Canadian%20cancer%20statistics%20supplementary%20information/2020/2020_cancer-specific-stats.pdf?la=en. Accessed 21 June 2020.
2. Canadian Cancer Society's Steering Committee on Cancer Statistics. Canadian cancer statistics 2014. Toronto: Canadian Cancer Society; 2014.
3. Colorectal Cancer Staging and Survival. Toronto: Canadian Partnership Against Cancer; 2010.
4. Hewitson P, Glasziou P, Watson E, et al. Cochrane systematic review of colorectal cancer screening using the fecal occult blood test (hemoccult): an update. Am J Gastroenterol. 2008;103(6):1541–9.
5. Holme O, Bretthauer M, Fretheim A, Odgaard-Jensen J, Hoff G. Flexible sigmoidoscopy versus faecal occult blood testing for colorectal cancer screening in asymptomatic individuals. Cochrane Database of Syst Rev. 2013;9:CD009259.
6. Tinmouth J, Vella ET, Baxter NN, et al. Colorectal cancer screening in average risk populations: evidence summary. Can J Gastroenterol Hepatol. 2016;2016:2878149.
7. Holme O, Loberg M, Kalager M, Bretthauer M, Hernan MA, Aas E, et al. Effect of flexible sigmoidoscopy screening on colorectal cancer incidence and mortality: a randomized clinical trial. JAMA. 2014;312(6):606–15.
8. Brenner H, Stock C, Hoffmeister M. Effect of screening sigmoidoscopy and screening colonoscopy on colorectal cancer incidence and mortality: systematic review and meta-analysis of randomised controlled trials and observational studies. BMJ. 2014;348:g2467.
9. Rex DK, Johnson DA, Anderson JC, et al. American College of Gastroenterology guidelines for colorectal cancer screening 2009 [corrected]. Am J Gastroenterol. 2009;104(3):739–50.
10. Rabeneck L, Paszat LF, Saskin R, Stukel TA. Association between colonoscopy rates and colorectal cancer mortality. Am J Gastroenterol. 2010;105(7):1627–32.
11. Baxter NN, Goldwasser MA, Paszat LF, et al. Association of colonoscopy and death from colorectal cancer. Ann Intern Med. 2009;150(1):1–8.
12. Tinmouth J, Kennedy EB, Baron D, Burke M, Feinberg S, Gould M, et al. Colonoscopy quality assurance in Ontario: systematic review and clinical practice guideline. Can J Gastroenterol Hepatol. 2014;28(5):251–74.
13. Lieberman DA, Rex DK, Winawer SJ, Giardiello FM, Johnson DA, Levin TR, et al. Guidelines for colonoscopy surveillance after screening and polypectomy: a consensus update by the US Multi-Society Task Force on Colorectal Cancer. Gastroenterology. 2012;143(3):844–57.

14. Shaukat A, Rector TS, Church TR, et al. Longer withdrawal time is associated with a reduced incidence of interval cancer after screening colonoscopy. Gastroenterology. 2015;149:952–7.
15. Dubé C, McCurdy BR, Bronstein T, et al. ColonCancerCheck: recommendations for post polypectomy surveillance. 2019. https://www.cancercareontario.ca/en/content/coloncancercheck-recommendations-post-polypectomy-surveillance.
16. Umar A, Boland CR, Terdiman JP, et al. Revised Bethesda guidelines for hereditary nonpolyposis colorectal cancer (Lynch syndrome) and microsatellite instability. J Natl Cancer Inst. 2004;96(4):261–8.
17. Ribic CM, Sargent DJ, Moore MJ, et al. Tumor microsatellite-instability status as a predictor of benefit from fluorouracil-based adjuvant chemotherapy for colon cancer. N Engl J Med. 2003;349(3):247–57.
18. Sargent DJ, Marsoni S, Monges G, et al. Defective mismatch repair as a predictive marker for lack of efficacy of fluorouracil-based adjuvant therapy in colon cancer. J Clin Oncol. 2010;28(20):3219–26.
19. Stoffel EM, Mangu PB, Gruber SB, Hamilton SR, Kalady MF, Lau MW, et al. Hereditary colorectal cancer syndromes: American Society of Clinical Oncology clinical practice guideline endorsement of the familial risk-colorectal cancer: European society for medical oncology clinical practice guidelines. J Clin Oncol. 2015;33(2):209–17.
20. Matloff J, Lucas A, Polydorides AD, Itzkowitz SH. Molecular tumor testing for Lynch syndrome in patients with colorectal cancer. J Natl Compr Cancer Netw. 2013;11(11):1380–5.
21. Perez-Carbonell L, Ruiz-Ponte C, Guarinos C, Alenda C, Paya A, Brea A, et al. Comparison between universal molecular screening for Lynch syndrome and revised Bethesda guidelines in a large population-based cohort of patients with colorectal cancer. Gut. 2012;61(6):865–72.
22. Jeffery M, Hickey BE, Hider PN. Follow-up strategies for patients treated for non-metastatic colorectal cancer. Cochrane Database Syst Rev. 2007;1:002200.
23. Figueredo A, Rumble RB, Maroun J, et al. The members of the Gastrointestinal Cancer Disease Site Group. Follow-up of patients with curatively resected colorectal cancer. Practice Guideline Report #2–9. June 16, 2010.
24. Members of the Colorectal Cancer Survivorship Group. Follow-up care, surveillance protocol, and secondary prevention measures for survivors of colorectal cancer. Toronto: Cancer Care Ontario; 2012 [Being Updated 2018 Jun]. Program in Evidence-based Care Evidence-Based Series No.: 26–2 Version 2.
25. Kuebler JP, Wieand HS, O'Connell MJ, et al. Oxaliplatin combined with weekly bolus fluorouracil and leucovorin as surgical adjuvant chemotherapy for stage II and III colon cancer: results from NSABP C-07. J Clin Oncol. 2007;25(16):2198–204.
26. Andre T, Boni C, Mounedji-Boudiaf L, et al. Multicenter international study of oxaliplatin/5-Fluorouracil/Leucovorin in the Adjuvant Treatment of Colon Cancer (MOSAIC) Investigators. Oxaliplatin, fluorouracil, and leucovorin as adjuvant treatment for colon cancer. N Engl J Med. 2004;350(23):2343–51.
27. Twelves C, Wong A, Nowacki MP, et al. Capecitabine as adjuvant treatment for stage III colon cancer. N Engl J Med. 2005;352(26):2696–704.
28. Vogel JD, Eskicioglu C, Weiser MR, et al. The American Society of Colon and Rectal Surgeons clinical practice guidelines for the treatment of colon cancer. Dis Colon Rectum. 2017;60:999–1017.
29. Williams JG, Pullan RD, Hill J, et al. Management of the malignant colorectal polyp: ACPGBI position statement. Color Dis. 2013;15(Suppl 2):1–38.
30. Rutter MD, Chattree A, Barbour JA, et al. British Society of Gastroenterology/ Association of Coloproctologists of Great Britain and Ireland guidelines for the management of large non-pedunculated colorectal polyps. Gut. 2015;64:1847–73.
31. Suzuki T, Sadahiro S, Mukoyama S, et al. Risk of lymph node and distant metastases in patients with early invasive colorectal cancer classified as Haggitt's level 4 invasion: image analysis of submucosal layer invasion. Dis Colon Rectum. 2003;45(2):203–8.

32. Biagi JJ, Raphael MJ, Mackillop, et al. Association between time to initiation of adjuvant chemotherapy and survival in colorectal cancer: a systematic review and meta-analysis. JAMA. 2011;305(22):2335–42.
33. Lima IS, Yasui Y, Scarfe A, Winget M. Association between receipt and timing of adjuvant chemotherapy and survival for patients with stage III colon cancer in Alberta. Canada Cancer. 2011;117:3833–40.
34. Meyers B, Cosby R, Quereshy F, Jonker D. Adjuvant systemic chemotherapy for stage II and III colon cancer following complete resection. Toronto: Cancer Care Ontario; 2015. [In Review 2017 Nov]. Program in Evidence-based Care Evidence-based Series No.: 2-29 Version 2.
35. Grothey A, Sobrero AF, Shields AF, et al. Duration of adjuvant chemotherapy for stage III colon cancer. N Engl J Med. 2018;378:1177–88.
36. Smith A, Rumble RB, Langer B, et al. Laparoscopic surgery for cancer of the colon. Toronto: Cancer Care Ontario; 2005. Program in Evidence-Based Care. Evidence-based Series #2-20-2.
37. Clinical Outcomes of Surgical Therapy Study Group. A comparison of laparoscopically assisted and open colectomy for colon cancer. N Engl J Med. 2004;350(20):2050–9.
38. Jayne DG, Guillou PJ, Thorpe H, et al. Randomized trial of laparoscopic-assisted resection of colorectal carcinoma: 3-year results of the UK MRC CLASICC Trial Group. J Clin Oncol. 2007;25(21):3061–8.
39. Lacy AM, Garcia-Valdecasas JC, Delgado S, et al. Laparoscopy-assisted colectomy versus open colectomy for treatment of non-metastatic colon cancer: a randomised trial. Lancet. 2002;359(9325):2224–9.
40. Kuhry E, Schwenk W, Gaupset R, et al. Long-term outcome of laparoscopic surgery for colorectal cancer: a cochrane systematic review of randomised controlled trials. Cancer Treat Rev. 2008;34(6):498–504.
41. Amri R, Bordeianou LG, Sylla P, Berger DL. Association of radial margin positivity with colon cancer. JAMA Surg. 2015;150:890–8.
42. Le Voyer TE, Sigurdson ER, Hanlon AL, et al. Colon cancer survival is associated with increasing number of lymph nodes analyzed: a secondary survey of intergroup trial INT-0089. J Clin Oncol. 2003;21(15):2912–9.
43. Smith AJ, Driman DK, Spithoff K, et al. Guideline for optimization of colorectal cancer surgery and pathology. J Surg Oncol. 2010;101(1):5–12.
44. Park JS, Choi GS, Park SY, Kim HJ, Ryuk JP. Randomized clinical trial of robot-assisted versus standard laparoscopic right colectomy. Br J Surg. 2012;99:1219–26.
45. Lorenzon L, Bini F, Balducci G, et al. Laparoscopic versus robotic-assisted colectomy and rectal resection: a systematic review and meta-analysis. Int J Color Dis. 2016;31(2):161–73.
46. Juo YY, Hyder O, Haider AH, Camp M, Lidor A, Ahuja N. Is minimally invasive colon resection better than traditional approaches?: First comprehensive national examination with propensity score matching. JAMA Surg. 2014;149(2):177–84.
47. Pinar I, Fransgaard T, Thygesen LC, et al. Long-term outcomes of robot-assisted surgery in patients with colorectal cancer. Ann Surg Oncol. 2018;25(13):3906–12.
48. Meyerhardt JA, Mangu PB, Flynn PJ, Korde L, Loprinzi CL, Minsky BD, et al. Follow-up care, surveillance protocol, and secondary prevention measures for survivors of colorectal cancer: American Society of Clinical Oncology clinical practice guideline endorsement. J Clin Oncol. 2013;31(35):4465–70.
49. Laine L, Kaltenbach T, Barkun A, et al. SCENIC international consensus statement on surveillance and management of dysplasia in inflammatory bowel disease. Gastrointest Endosc. 2015;81:489–501.
50. Bowne WB, Lee B, Wong WD, et al. Operative salvage for locoregional recurrent colon cancer after curative resection: an analysis of 100 cases. Dis Colon Rectum. 2005;48(5):897–909.
51. Smith AJ, Driman DK, Spithoff K, McLeod R, Hunter A, Rumble RB, et al. Optimization of surgical and pathological quality performance in radical surgery for colon and rectal cancer: margins and lymph nodes. Toronto: Cancer Care Ontario; 2008. [In review 2013 Dec]. Program in Evidence-based Care Evidence-based Series No.: 7–14.

52. Cukier M, Smith AJ, Milot L, et al. Neoadjuvant chemoradiotherapy and multivisceral resection for primary locally advanced adherent colon cancer: a single institution experience. Eur J Surg Oncol. 2012;38(8):677–82.
53. Hallet J, Zih FS, Lemke M, et al. Neo-adjuvant chemoradiotherapy and multivisceral resection to optimize R0 resection of locally recurrent adherent colon cancer. Eur J Surg Oncol. 2014;40(6):706–12.
54. Hurwitz H, Fehrenbacher L, Novotny W, et al. Bevacizumab plus irinotecan, fluorouracil, and leucovorin for metastatic colorectal cancer. N Engl J Med. 2004;350(23):2335–42.
55. Giantonio BJ, Catalano PJ, Meropol NJ, et al. Bevacizumab in combination with oxaliplatin, fluorouracil, and leucovorin (FOLFOX4) for previously treated metastatic colorectal cancer: results from the Eastern Cooperative Oncology Group Study E3200. J Clin Oncol. 2007;25(12):1539–44.
56. Saltz LB, Clarke S, Diaz-Rubio E, et al. Bevacizumab in combination with oxaliplatin-based chemotherapy as first-line therapy in metastatic colorectal cancer: a randomized phase III study. J Clin Oncol. 2008;26:2013–9. Erratum appears in J Clin Oncol. 2009;27(4):653.
57. Van Cutsem E, Kohne CH, Hitre E, et al. Cetuximab and chemotherapy as initial treatment for metastatic colorectal cancer. N Engl J Med. 2009;360(14):1408–17.
58. Hapani S, Chu D, Wu S. Risk of gastrointestinal perforation in patients with cancer treated with bevacizumab: a meta-analysis. Lancet Oncol. 2009;10:559–68.
59. Baxter N, Fischer HD, Richardson D, et al. A population-based study of complications after colorectal surgery in patients who have received Bevacizumab. Dis Colon Rectum. 2018;61(3):306–13.
60. Faron M, Pignon JP, Malka D, Bourredjem A, Douillard JY, Adenis A, et al. Is primary tumour resection associated with survival improvement in patients with colorectal cancer and unresectable synchronous metastases? A pooled analysis of individual data from four randomised trials. Eur J Cancer. 2015;51(2):166–76.
61. Jorine't Lam-Boer J, Mol L, Verhoef C, et al. The CAIRO4 study: the role of surgery of the primary tumour with few or absent symptoms in patients with synchronous unresectable metastases of colorectal cancer – a randomized phase III study of the Dutch Colorectal Cancer Group (DCCG). BMC Cancer. 2014;14:741.
62. Rahbari NN, Lordick F, Fink C, et al. Resection of the primary tumour versus no resection prior to systemic therapy in patients with colon cancer and synchronous unresectable metastases (UICC stage IV): SYNCHRONOUS – a randomised controlled multicentre trial (ISRCTN30964555). BMC Cancer. 2012;12:142.
63. Fleshman J, Sargent DJ, Green E, et al. Laparoscopic colectomy for cancer is not inferior to open surgery based on 5-year data from the COST Study Group trial. Ann Surg. 2007;246(4):655–62. discussion 662–4.
64. Green BL, Marshall HC, Collinson F, et al. Long-term follow-up of the Medical Research Council CLASICC trial of conventional versus laparoscopically assisted resection in colorectal cancer. Br J Surg. 2013;100(1):75–82.
65. Colon Cancer Laparoscopic or Open Resection Study Group, Buunen M, Veldkamp R, Hop WC, Kuhry E, Jeekel J, et al. Survival after laparoscopic surgery versus open surgery for colon cancer: long-term outcome of a randomised clinical trial. Lancet Oncol. 2009;10(1):44–52.
66. Deijen CL, Vasmel JE, de Lange-de Klerk ESM, et al. Ten-year outcomes of a randomised trial of laparoscopic versus open surgery for colon cancer. Surg Endosc. 2016;31(6):2607–15.
67. Lacy AM, Delgado S, Castells A, et al. The long-term results of a randomized clinical trial of laparoscopy-assisted versus open surgery for colon cancer. Ann Surg. 2008;248(1):1–7.
68. Yothers G, O'Connell MJ, Allegra CJ, et al. Oxaliplatin as adjuvant therapy for colon cancer: updated results of NSABP C-07 trial, including survival and subset analyses. J Clin Oncol. 2011;29(28):3768–74.
69. Andre T, Boni C, Navarro M, et al. Improved overall survival with oxaliplatin, fluorouracil, and leucovorin as adjuvant treatment in stage II or III colon cancer in the MOSAIC trial. J Clin Oncol. 2009;27(19):3109–16.

70. Tournigand C, Andre T, Bonnetain F, Chibaudel B, Lledo G, Hickish T, et al. Adjuvant therapy with fluorouracil and oxaliplatin in stage II and elderly patients (between ages 70 and 75 years) with colon cancer: subgroup analyses of the Multicenter International Study of Oxaliplatin, Fluorouracil, and Leucovorin in the Adjuvant Treatment of Colon Cancer trial. J Clin Oncol. 2012;30(27):3353–60.
71. André T, de Gramont A, Vernerey D, et al. Adjuvant Fluorouracil, Leucovorin, and Oxaliplatin in stage II to III Colon Cancer: updated 10-year survival and outcomes according to BRAF mutation and mismatch repair status of the MOSAIC Study. J Clin Oncol. 2015;33:4176–87.
72. Twelves C, Scheithauer W, McKendrick J, Seitz JF, Van Hazel G, Wong A, et al. Capecitabine versus 5-fluorouracil/folinic acid as adjuvant therapy for stage III colon cancer: final results from the X-ACT trial with analysis by age and preliminary evidence of a pharmacodynamic marker of efficacy. Ann Oncol. 2012;23(5):1190–7.

Colorectal Liver Metastases

7

Michail N. Mavros, Shiva Jayaraman, Melanie E. Tsang, Paul J. Karanicolas, and Alice C. Wei

Introduction

The liver is the most common site of metastases from colorectal cancer (CRC) [1]. Approximately 15% of patients with CRC present with synchronous liver metastases, and 15% of patients will develop metachronous metastases to the liver [2]. Of the patients who develop liver metastases, up to 80% have unresectable disease at presentation [3, 4]. Modern systemic chemotherapy has increased the median survival of non-resected patients to 22 months [5], but patients who undergo complete resection can achieve 5-year survival up to 47–58% [3, 6–8], with 10-year survival up to 28% [3, 9, 10].

Prognostic Variables

Various clinical risk scores have been developed to help clinicians estimate survival outcomes for individual patients (see Table 7.1). One of the most commonly used is the Clinical Risk Score (Fong Criteria) which takes into account the size and number of CRLM, serum CEA, primary tumor nodal status, and disease-free interval [11, 12]. This was recently modified to include the CRLM RAS status [13], which

M. N. Mavros
Complex General Surgical Oncology & HPB Surgery, University of Toronto, Toronto, ON, Canada
e-mail: michail.mavros@mail.utoronto.ca

S. Jayaraman · M. E. Tsang · P. J. Karanicolas
Department of Surgery, University of Toronto, Toronto, ON, Canada
e-mail: Shiva.Jayaraman@unityhealth.to; Melanie.Tsang@unityhealth.to; Paul.Karanicolas@sunnybrook.ca

A. C. Wei (✉)
Department of Surgery, Memorial Sloan Kettering Cancer Center, New York, NY, USA
e-mail: weia@mskcc.org

F. C. Wright et al. (eds.), *Surgical Oncology Manual*,
https://doi.org/10.1007/978-3-030-48363-0_7

Table 7.1 Risk scores predicting survival and recurrence in patients with CRLM

Study	Variables	Score	5-year OS (%)
Clinical risk score Fong et al., 1999 [11]	Node positive primary Size > 5 cm >1 lesion CEA level > 200 ng/mL Disease-free interval < 12 months	0 1 2 3 4 5	60 44 40 20 25 14
Modified clinical score Brudvik et al., 2019 [13]	Node positive primary Size > 5 cm RAS mutation	0 1 2 3	78 46 23 17
Basingstoke predictive index Rees et al., 2008 [22]	Node positive primary (2 points) Primary tumor differentiation (moderate: 2; poor: 4 points) CEA level, ng/mL (6–60:1; >60: 3 points) Size, cm (5–10: 2; >10: 7 points) Positive resection margin (11 points) Extrahepatic metastasis (4 points)	0 5 10 15 20 25 30	64 49 34 21 11 5 2
Nordlinger et al., 1996 [23]	Age > 60 years		2-year OS (%)
	Size > 5 cm Extension of primary into serosa Lymphatic spread Disease-free interval ≤ 2 years ≥4 lesions Resection margin < 1 cm	0–2 3–4 5–7	79 60 43

Abbreviations: *OS* overall survival, *CEA* carcinoembryonic antigen

has been consistently shown to predict earlier systemic recurrence and shorter overall survival [14–16]. Additional prognostic variables that have recently emerged include the following:

- Embryologic origin of primary tumor: Midgut-derived colon cancers (SMA distribution; right colon and hepatic flexure) are more often of mucinous histology and likely to harbor BRAF mutations compared to tumors arising from the hindgut (IMA distribution; left colon, sigmoid, rectum) [17]. Midgut origin is also associated with worse response to preoperative chemotherapy and shorter overall and recurrence-free survival; this association may persist even after controlling for RAS mutation status [6, 18].
- Response to chemotherapy: Poor pathologic response to preoperative chemotherapy has been consistently associated with shorter overall and recurrence-free survival, and is considered a relative contraindication to surgery [19, 20]. A similar trend is now emerging for patients who respond to chemotherapy, but exhibit disease progression shortly after chemotherapy cessation [21].

Table 7.2 Overview of work-up and follow-up of patients with CRLM

Work-up	Follow-up
Labs: Serum CEA LFTs **Imaging**: CT chest, abdomen, pelvis Consider MRI with liver-specific contrast agent (e.g., gadoxetic acid) **Colonoscopy** within the preceding 18 months	Every 3–6 months for the first 2 years then every 6 months thereafter: CT chest, abdomen, pelvis Serum CEA Colonoscopy at 1 year

Abbreviations: *CEA* carcino-embryonic antigen, *LFT* liver function test

Management of CRLM

Initial Work-Up

Initial liver imaging usually consists of CT (ideally 4-phase: precontrast, arterial, portal, and delayed venous; see Table 7.2). MRI (especially with hepatocyte-specific contrast, i.e., gadoxetic acid) may be beneficial for macrosteatotic livers, the detection of subcentimeter nodules, and in the post-chemotherapy setting [24]. PET does not result in change in management in >90% of cases and is not routinely recommended [25]. Ultrasound is routinely performed intra-operatively to confirm extent of disease and delineate transection margins [26]. Further, ultrasound may have enhanced diagnostic value with the addition of IV contrast [27, 28].

Surgical Considerations in Resectable CRLM

The goal of surgical resection in CRLM is to remove all the tumors with ≥1 mm margin, while preserving as much liver remnant as possible [8]. Compared to anatomic liver resection, parenchymal-sparing resection has similar long-term oncologic outcomes, while maximizing the functional liver remnant, and is now considered standard of care [29–32].

- Intra-operative ultrasound (IOUS) is crucial for planning of a liver resection. IOUS is sensitive and specific (98% and 95%, respectively) for the detection of CRLM ≥5 mm [33], and it is also used to precisely characterize the intrahepatic vascular anatomy and delineate the transection margins in parenchymal-sparing resections [26, 34].
- Laparoscopic resection in selected patients in centers with expertise in minimally invasive surgery [35, 36] is oncologically similar to open hepatectomy, with potential improvement in some perioperative outcomes [37–39].
- Every attempt should be made to minimize perioperative transfusions [40, 41] and postoperative complications [42, 43], as they have been associated with poor oncologic outcomes.

Table 7.3 Overview of sequencing of surgical management for synchronous CRLM

Strategy	Management [48]
Simultaneous resection	1. Uncomplicated colon resection + liver resection 2. Complicated colon resection + limited liver resection
Staged resection	1. Complicated rectal resection, extensive colon resection 2. Major liver resection (>3 segments)
Primary first	Traditional approach **Advantage**: Avoids potential complications from primary disease (bleeding, perforation) **Disadvantage**: Postoperative complications can delay resection of hepatic disease
Liver resection first	Consider in Extensive hepatic disease with asymptomatic primary Patients with rectal primary who have received radiation (due to planned wait time of 8–12 weeks after chemoradiation before primary is resected) **Advantages**: Early control of CRLM with opportunity to eradicate all hepatic disease. Complications from primary resection will not delay/prevent resection of metastatic disease **Disadvantages**: Primary may progress to unresectability or complications from progression may develop. Patient may have unnecessary liver resection, delaying palliative systemic treatment

- Enhanced Recovery After Surgery (ERAS) protocols allow for earlier recovery and shorter length of hospital stay after liver resection [44–46]. The use of medial open transversus abdominis plane (MOTAP) catheters results in decreased opioid requirements and shorter length of stay [47].

Management of Synchronous CRLM

The presence of synchronous CRLM (diagnosed at or before diagnosis of primary) portends worse prognosis than metachronous, especially late metachronous (>12 months of diagnosis of primary) disease. The selection and sequence of therapies in the treatment of colorectal cancer with synchronous CRLM is a complicated process and should be discussed in a multidisciplinary cancer setting (see Table 7.3). General considerations include the following:

- Is the primary symptomatic?
- Are the CRLM resectable?
- Where is the bulk of the disease?

Assessment of Resectability of CRLM [24]

The assessment for resectability of CRLM is based on oncologic (tumor biology) and technical (tumor location/size/number) criteria (see Table 7.4).

Table 7.4 Assessment of resectability of CRLM

Oncologic criteria	Technical criteria
1. Prior to considering resection of CRLM, pretreatment radiological staging is required to assess for the presence and extent of intrahepatic and extrahepatic disease. 2. Patients harboring limited extrahepatic disease, particularly in the lungs, or with reasonable expectations for long-term control should be considered for a liver resection. 3. For patients with significant progression of metastatic disease during treatment with optimal systemic therapy, consider deferring surgical resection until disease control is achieved with other systemic or regional therapies.	1. Resectability is defined by the ability to achieve an R0 margin with acceptable morbidity/mortality. 2. The technical feasibility of liver resection is based on three criteria related to the liver remnant after resection: (a) The anticipated ability to preserve adequate future liver remnant (FLR) volume (20% in normal liver and 30% in pretreated liver with chemotherapy). (b) The anticipated ability to preserve adequate vascular inflow, outflow, and biliary drainage. (c) The demonstrated ability of the FLR to adequately function based on the appropriate regenerative response after portal vein embolization in patients with a marginal FLR volume and/or underlying liver disease.

Expanding Resectability of CRLM

One of the major factors that precludes resectability of CRLM is inadequate liver remnant, and therefore several strategies have been developed in an attempt to maximize the future liver remnant (FLR) and shrink tumor burden [49]. The FLR is calculated using volumetric CT or MRI and is a function of anticipated remnant liver volume and body surface area, a surrogate of total liver volume [50, 51]. Systemic chemotherapy is usually administered in conjunction with these strategies.

- Local ablation (microwave or radiofrequency) can be employed at the time of liver resection for lesions that are not amenable to resection. Overall the evidence on long-term oncologic outcomes is conflicting in retrospective series, but outcomes appear similar when applied to small lesions [52–54].
- Portal vein embolization (PVE) is a percutaneous modality to increase the FLR. In principle, embolization of the right portal vein induces hypertrophy of the left hemiliver and atrophy of the right hemiliver. This is typically performed in anticipation of an extended right hepatectomy [55].
- Two-stage hepatectomy is a strategy employed in patients with significant bilobar disease, and has gained wider acceptance when used in conjunction with PVE [56]. During the first stage, parenchymal-sparing resections of the left lobe are aimed to clear the left hemiliver of any disease. This is followed by right PVE (or right portal vein ligation), and the left hemiliver is then allowed to hypertrophy for 4–6 weeks. If on repeat volumetric CT the new FLR is deemed adequate, a right hepatectomy is then performed. This strategy allowed complete resection of the CRLM in 69–75% of patients in retrospective series, and 5-year survival reached 32–51% [57–60].

- Associating liver partition with portal vein ligation for staged hepatectomy (ALPPS) is an unproven technique performed in few centers [61]. During the first stage, parenchymal-sparing resections of the left lobe are aimed to clear the left hemiliver of any disease. At the same time, the right portal vein is ligated/embolized and the parenchyma between segments 4A/B and the left lateral segment is divided. This induces accelerated hypertrophy of the remnant liver and the patient receives volumetric CT at regular intervals postoperatively until the FLR reaches 30%; at that time the deportalized right lobe is removed [61]. While this technique may result in faster and perhaps greater left lobe hypertrophy, it has not been widely adopted due to preliminary results of high morbidity and mortality, as well as poor oncologic outcomes [61–63]. A recent RCT from Norway (LIGRO trial) showed promising short-term outcomes (better resection rates than two-stage hepatectomy/PVE with comparable morbidity/mortality), but long-term results are pending [64]. ALPPS can also be considered as a salvage option in patients who do not achieve adequate FLR after PVE [65].

Management of Unresectable CRLM

The primary treatment for patients with unresectable CRLM is systemic chemotherapy. Rarely, unresectable patients may be downsized to resectable/borderline resectable disease with chemotherapy alone (see below, "Role of systemic chemotherapy") [66]. In selected patients with liver-only metastatic disease that is unresectable due to the location or extent of the lesions, the following liver-directed strategies can be employed:

- Hepatic artery infusion pump (HAIP) therapy is used in specialized centers [67]. A catheter is surgically placed in the proper hepatic artery (via the gastroduodenal artery), connected to a subcutaneous reservoir, and FUDR is administered through the pump, typically in combination with systemic chemotherapy. This combination can convert unresectable to resectable/ablatable disease in 25–50% of patients [68, 69].
- Liver transplantation is currently being revisited as an option in patients with unresectable liver-only metastatic disease [70]. Small series reported 5-year OS 50–56% with acceptable morbidity [71–73], and there are currently 4 open trials investigating this topic.

Role of Systemic Chemotherapy

In the setting of resectable CRLM, the role of systemic chemotherapy is controversial (see Table 7.5). The EORTC Intergroup Trial 40,983 reported marginally better PFS, but no difference in OS with perioperative FOLFOX [74, 75]. Pseudo-neoadjuvant chemotherapy can also be used as a test for the biology of the disease

Table 7.5 RCTs examining perioperative chemotherapy for CRLM

Study	Methods	Results
EORTC intergroup trial 40,983 Nordlinger et al. [74, 75]	RCT – Perioperative FOLFOX (6 + 6 cycles) vs surgery alone (*N* = 364)	Perioperative chemotherapy increased PFS (3-year PFS: 38.2% vs 30.3%); no difference in OS (5-year OS: 51.2% vs 47.8%) [intention-to-treat population]. The chemotherapy arm had more postoperative complications (25% vs 16%)
EPOC trial, Primrose et al. [79, 80]	RCT – Perioperative chemotherapy (FOLFOX, CAPOX, or FOLFIRI) with vs without cetuximab in KRAS wild-type patients (*N* = 336)	Terminated early. Addition of cetuximab to perioperative chemotherapy decreased PFS (median 14.1 vs 20.5 months); no difference in OS (39.1 months vs not reached). On longer follow-up [80], the cetuximab group had shorter OS (median 55.4 vs 81 months) but similar PFS (15.5 vs 23.9 months)
EXPERT trial, Mise et al. [81]	RCT – Perioperative FOLFOX + cetuximab (6 + 6 cycles) vs adjuvant FOLFOX (12 cycles) in KRAS wild-type patients	Terminated early due to slow accrual (*N* = 77). No difference in PFS (3-year PFS 30% vs 35%) or OS (3-year OS 74% vs 86%)

Abbreviations: *RCT* randomized controlled trial, *PFS* progression-free survival, *OS* overall survival

and possibly prevent an operation in patients with overly aggressive disease. On the other hand, pseudo-neoadjuvant chemotherapy could render treated metastases invisible to imaging ("ghost" metastases) [76], and the chemotherapy-induced hepatotoxicity (especially if >6 cycles or pre-existing liver disease) may increase perioperative morbidity and mortality [77]. In this context, pseudo-neoadjuvant chemotherapy should be mostly considered in patients at higher risk of progression to assess biology of the disease.

The addition of epidermal growth factor receptor (EGFR) inhibitors (cetuximab, panitumumab) has generally improved oncologic outcomes in RAS and BRAF wild-type patients with metastatic colorectal cancer [78]. In the setting of resectable CRLM, the new EPOC trial initially showed shorter PFS (no difference in OS) when cetuximab was added to perioperative chemotherapy in mostly RAS wild-type patients; on longer follow-up the cetuximab group had shorter OS [79, 80]. Another similar trial from Japan (EXPERT trial) showed no difference in OS or PFS, but was terminated early due to slow accrual [81].

The use of chemotherapy in the adjuvant setting is also controversial. A pooled analysis of 2 small RCTs explored the benefit of systemic FU-based chemotherapy and suggested a trend towards longer progression-free (median 27.9 vs 18.8 months,

Table 7.6 RCTs comparing pseudo-neoadjuvant chemotherapy regimens with intent to convert unresectable/not optimally resectable CRLM to resectable

Study	Methods	Results
OLIVIA trial Gruenberger et al. [83]	RCT phase II – Pseudo-neoadjuvant bevacizumab + FOLFOX vs FOLFOXIRI ($N = 80$)	R0 resection rate of 23% vs 49%, median PFS 11.5 vs 18.6 months
CELIM trial Folprecht et al. [84, 85]	RCT phase II – Pseudo-neoadjuvant cetuximab + FOLFOX vs FOLFIRI ($N = 111$)	R0 resection rate of 38% vs 30%, KRAS WT patients had higher response rate. Median PFS 11.2 vs 10.5 months, median OS 35.8 vs 29 months (no difference)
Ye et al. [86]	RCT – Pseudo-neoadjuvant chemotherapy (FOLFIRI/FOLFOX) with vs without cetuximab in KRAS WT patients ($N = 138$)	Addition of cetuximab increased objective response rates (57.1% vs 29.4%) and R0 resection rate (25.7% vs 7.4%)

Resection rates should be interpreted with caution as the criteria of upfront unresectability were variable and no longer apply

Abbreviations: *RCT* randomized controlled trial, *WT* wild type, *OS* overall survival, *PFS* progression-free survival

$p = 0.058$) and overall survival (median 62.2 vs 47.3 months, $p = 0.095$) in the chemotherapy arm [82]. Although the difference was not statistically significant, these trials used suboptimal regimens by modern standards. Pending future randomized studies, adjuvant chemotherapy is usually considered in patients with high risk for recurrence despite inconclusive evidence.

In the setting of unresectable CRLM, systemic chemotherapy is the primary treatment. Several studies have investigated different regimens with intent to convert unresectable CRLM to resectable, but the results have been inconsistent, and the interpretation of conversion rates should take into consideration the variability in the definition of "unresectable" and "not optimally resectable" CRLM among the studies (see Table 7.6) [83–90]. In this setting, the addition of EGFR (for RAS/BRAF wild-type patients) or vascular endothelial growth factor (VEGF) inhibitors (bevacizumab) to standard doublet chemotherapy may improve objective response and R0 resection rates.

Special Notes

- Hold chemotherapy 3–4 weeks prior to liver resection.
- Hold bevacizumab for 6 weeks prior to liver resection to reduce the risk of bleeding [91].

Table 7.7 Local therapy modalities for CRLM

Local therapy.	Mechanism	Advantage	Disadvantage
Radiofrequency ablation (RFA) [54]	Direct current transmission into tissue	Can be used for selected patients with otherwise unresectable disease (due to patient or disease factors) or to clear liver to extend resectability	Unpredictable results as functions on impedance which changes during ablation Incomplete ablation with lesions >3 cm. Cannot be used near large vessels or portal structures due to heat sink and potential damage to structures
Microwave ablation (MWA) [94]	Microwave energy agitates water molecules to create heat	As above. More uniform/predictable ablation zone and shorter time than RFA	Limit on size of treatable lesions
Stereotactic ablative radiotherapy (SABR/SBRT) [95–97]	Delivery of high doses of radiation to a focused target. Role in patients unfit for surgery with oligometastatic CRLM	Limited evidence – Retrospective series of patients with oligometastatic CRLM reported median OS 31.5 months with acceptable morbidity. No randomized data available	Not widely available
Irreversible electroporation (IRE) [98]	Electric pulses cause permeabilization of membranes of tumor and parenchymal cells. Role under investigation	Limited evidence – Retrospective series report IRE is safe in perivascular liver tumors. No efficacy data available	Not used in patients with pacemakers or arrhythmias. Requires general anesthesia

Local Therapies

Local therapies can be used in conjunction with liver resection for borderline resectable CRLM (discussed above), or in the setting of unresectable CRLM, usually in combination with systemic chemotherapy (see Table 7.7) [92]. A recent phase II trial (EORTC 40004 CLOCC) randomized 119 patients with up to 9 unresectable CRLM to systemic chemotherapy vs chemotherapy and aggressive local therapies (radiofrequency ablation ± wedge liver resections), and reported a survival benefit in the combined therapy arm (5- and 8-year OS 43.1% and 35.9% vs 30.3% and 8.9%, respectively) [93].

Regional Therapies

Regional therapies are geared towards treating the entire liver. The indications include unresectable CRLM, technically resectable CRLM in patients unfit for hepatectomy, and second-line treatment after progression of the liver disease through systemic chemotherapy. There are varying degrees of evidence supporting the use of different regional therapies (see Table 7.8).

Table 7.8 Regional therapy modalities for CRLM

Regional therapy	Technique & setting	Evidence	Disadvantages
Hepatic artery infusion pump (HAIP) therapy [67]	Surgically placed catheter into proper hepatic artery with subcutaneous reservoir. Role in unresectable CRLM and in the adjuvant setting	HAIP with systemic chemotherapy can convert 25–50% of unresectable CRLM to resectable/ablatable [68, 69]. HAIP in the adjuvant setting is controversial; small trials reported a survival benefit with the addition of HAIP to systemic chemotherapy (older regimens) [99, 100], especially in patients in high risk for recurrence [101], but whether HAIP offers any benefit in conjunction with modern chemotherapy has not been thoroughly evaluated [102]	Requires multidisciplinary team with expertise in hepatobiliary surgery, medical oncology, interventional radiology, nuclear medicine, and nursing. Not widely available
DEBIRI (drug-eluting bead, irinotecan) TACE (transarterial chemotherapy) [103–105]	Transarterial embolization with drug-eluting beads with irinotecan. Role in unresectable CRLM	In a phase III RCT, patients with unresectable CRLM treated with DEBIRI vs FOLFIRI had longer OS (median 22 vs 15 months), with a sustained improvement in quality of life [105]	Not widely available

Table 7.8 (continued)

Regional therapy	Technique & setting	Evidence	Disadvantages
Yttrium-90 radioembolization [106–108] (SIRT, selective internal radiotherapy)	High-dose radiation delivered via the hepatic artery with microspheres. Role in unresectable CRLM	A phase III RCT reported no benefit in OS with the addition of Y-90 to FU in patients with unresectable CRLM (median OS 10 vs 7.3 months) [107]. A combined analysis of 3 multicenter phase III RCTs reported no benefit in OS with the addition of Y-90 to FOLFOX in patients with unresectable CRLM (median OS 22.6 vs 23.3 months) [108]	Short-term restriction in patient exposure to friends/family due to radiation. Not widely available

Abbreviations: *RCT* randomized controlled trial, *OS* overall survival, *FU* fluorouracil

Extrahepatic Metastases (EHM)

The presence of EHM used to be a contraindication for liver resection for concurrent CRLM, but this is no longer the case. Several series and a phase II trial have demonstrated long-term survival in selected patients with EHM who undergo complete resection of the CRLM and the EHM (see Table 7.9) [109–111]. All cases of CRLM with limited EHM should be reviewed at a multidisciplinary cancer conference and preoperative/perioperative systemic chemotherapy should be considered. Surgical management and outcomes vary depending on the site of EHM:

- Lungs: Subcentimeter pulmonary nodules (SPN) do not alter long-term prognosis, and therefore should not preclude liver resection. Lung metastases have an indolent course; for larger pulmonary nodules, staged resection of tumors in the liver and lung if they are resectable with R0 intent (liver resection first, followed by lung resection) [112]. Selected patients may achieve long-term survival (5-year OS 32–74%) [7, 111, 113, 114].
- Peritoneum: Peritoneal metastases have variable biologic behavior. Potential liver resection should be assessed in conjunction with a peritoneal malignancy program. Selected patients may achieve long-term survival (5-year OS 26–42%) [111, 114].
- Ovaries: Ovarian metastases are considered equivalent to limited peritoneal disease. Resection should be considered if complete resection can be achieved. Selected patients may achieve long-term survival (5-year OS 34%) [111].

Table 7.9 Surgical management of extrahepatic metastases

Study	Methods	Results
Toronto phase II trial, Wei et al. [109]	Phase II trial ($N = 26$) CRLM and EHM resection (lung, portal LN, peritoneum, adrenals, other)	Median OS and RFS 38 and 5 months, respectively. Major morbidity 19%, mortality 4%, QoL returned to baseline 1 year post-treatment
MSKCC study, Leung et al. [111]	Retrospective review ($N = 219$) CRLM and synchronous EHM resection (lung, portal/ retroperitoneal LN, peritoneum, ovaries, other)	Median OS and RFS 34.4 and 8 months, respectively. 3 poor prognostic factors: CRLM >3 cm, >5 CRLM, and unfavorable EHM site; 5-year OS ranged from 43% (0 factors) to 0% (3 factors)
French study, Adam et al. [7]	Retrospective review ($N = 186$) Liver resection and EHM resection (lung, LN, peritoneum, other)	5 poor prognostic factors: EHM other than lung, EHM concomitant to CRLM recurrence, CEA ≥ 10 ng/mL, ≥ 6 CRLM, and right colon; 5-year OS ranged from 64% (0 factors) to 0% (>3 factors). Overall 5-year OS 28% (33% for isolated lung mets)
International study, Pulitano et al. [114]	Retrospective review ($N = 171$) CRLM and EHM resection (lung, peritoneum, portal LN, aortocaval LN, other)	5-year OS 26%; OS worse with R1 resection, multiple sites of EHM and location (aortocaval LN worst)

Abbreviations: *EHM* extrahepatic metastases, *LN* lymph node, *OS* overall survival, *RFS* recurrence-free survival, *QoL* quality of life

- Portal and retroperitoneal lymph nodes: Metastasis to portal and retroperitoneal lymph nodes is believed to represent a re-metastasis from the CRLM and thus an indicator of more aggressive biological behavior. Long-term outcomes are generally poor (5-year OS 14–21%) [111, 115–117]. It is often considered a relative contraindication to liver resection, although resection can be considered in patients with limited lymph node involvement (especially for portal rather than para-aortic nodes) and good response to systemic chemotherapy [112, 115–118].

Toronto Pearls

- If there is any doubt about the volume of future liver remnant, obtain formal volumetrics and consider preoperative portal vein embolization.
- When performing liver resections, use the principle of parenchyma-sparing surgery as a guide.
- Resection of all visible disease is the goal: use systemic therapy sparingly and with this ultimate goal always in mind.

- Subcentimeter pulmonary nodules are very common and do not affect prognosis; ignore them.
- Blood loss and transfusion are associated with adverse perioperative outcomes and long-term disease recurrence: incorporate preoperative, operative, and postoperative strategies to reduce bleeding and transfusion.
- The role of pseudo-neoadjuvant therapy is to assess biology of disease; select agents to minimize hepatotoxicity (FOLFOX) and limit the duration to 4 cycles.

References

1. Hugen N, van de Velde CJ, de Wilt JH, Nagtegaal ID. Metastatic pattern in colorectal cancer is strongly influenced by histological subtype. Ann Oncol. 2014;25(3):651–7.
2. Manfredi S, Lepage C, Hatem C, Coatmeur O, Faivre J, Bouvier AM. Epidemiology and management of liver metastases from colorectal cancer. Ann Surg. 2006;244(2):254–9.
3. Wei AC, Greig PD, Grant D, Taylor B, Langer B, Gallinger S. Survival after hepatic resection for colorectal metastases: a 10-year experience. Ann Surg Oncol. 2006;13(5):668–76.
4. Adam R, Delvart V, Pascal G, Valeanu A, Castaing D, Azoulay D, et al. Rescue surgery for unresectable colorectal liver metastases downstaged by chemotherapy: a model to predict long-term survival. Ann Surg. 2004;240(4):644–57; discussion 57–8
5. Gallagher DJ, Kemeny N. Metastatic colorectal cancer: from improved survival to potential cure. Oncology. 2010;78(3–4):237–48.
6. Creasy JM, Sadot E, Koerkamp BG, Chou JF, Gonen M, Kemeny NE, et al. The impact of primary tumor location on long-term survival in patients undergoing hepatic resection for metastatic colon cancer. Ann Surg Oncol. 2018;25(2):431–8.
7. Adam R, de Haas RJ, Wicherts DA, Vibert E, Salloum C, Azoulay D, et al. Concomitant extrahepatic disease in patients with colorectal liver metastases: when is there a place for surgery? Ann Surg. 2011;253(2):349–59.
8. Pawlik TM, Scoggins CR, Zorzi D, Abdalla EK, Andres A, Eng C, et al. Effect of surgical margin status on survival and site of recurrence after hepatic resection for colorectal metastases. Ann Surg. 2005;241(5):715–22, discussion 22–4
9. Choti MA, Sitzmann JV, Tiburi MF, Sumetchotimetha W, Rangsin R, Schulick RD, et al. Trends in long-term survival following liver resection for hepatic colorectal metastases. Ann Surg. 2002;235(6):759–66.
10. Tomlinson JS, Jarnagin WR, DeMatteo RP, Fong Y, Kornprat P, Gonen M, et al. Actual 10-year survival after resection of colorectal liver metastases defines cure. J Clin Oncol. 2007;25(29):4575–80.
11. Fong Y, Fortner J, Sun RL, Brennan MF, Blumgart LH. Clinical score for predicting recurrence after hepatic resection for metastatic colorectal cancer: analysis of 1001 consecutive cases. Ann Surg. 1999;230(3):309–18.. discussion 18-21
12. Kattan MW, Gönen M, Jarnagin WR, DeMatteo R, D'Angelica M, Weiser M, et al. A nomogram for predicting disease-specific survival after hepatic resection for metastatic colorectal cancer. Ann Surg. 2008;247(2):282–7.
13. Brudvik KW, Jones RP, Giuliante F, Shindoh J, Passot G, Chung MH, et al. RAS mutation clinical risk score to predict survival after resection of colorectal liver metastases. Ann Surg. 2019;269(1):120–6.
14. Vauthey JN, Zimmitti G, Kopetz SE, Shindoh J, Chen SS, Andreou A, et al. RAS mutation status predicts survival and patterns of recurrence in patients undergoing hepatectomy for colorectal liver metastases. Ann Surg. 2013;258(4):619–26; discussion 26–7

15. Brudvik KW, Kopetz SE, Li L, Conrad C, Aloia TA, Vauthey JN. Meta-analysis of KRAS mutations and survival after resection of colorectal liver metastases. Br J Surg. 2015;102(10):1175–83.
16. Passot G, Denbo JW, Yamashita S, Kopetz SE, Chun YS, Maru D, et al. Is hepatectomy justified for patients with RAS mutant colorectal liver metastases? An analysis of 524 patients undergoing curative liver resection. Surgery. 2017;161(2):332–40.
17. Loupakis F, Yang D, Yau L, Feng S, Cremolini C, Zhang W, et al. Primary tumor location as a prognostic factor in metastatic colorectal cancer. J Natl Cancer Inst. 2015;107(3):dju427.
18. Yamashita S, Brudvik KW, Kopetz SE, Maru D, Clarke CN, Passot G, et al. Embryonic origin of primary Colon Cancer predicts pathologic response and survival in patients undergoing resection for Colon Cancer liver metastases. Ann Surg. 2018;267(3):514–20.
19. Adam R, Pascal G, Castaing D, Azoulay D, Delvart V, Paule B, et al. Tumor progression while on chemotherapy: a contraindication to liver resection for multiple colorectal metastases? Ann Surg. 2004;240(6):1052–61.. discussion 61-4
20. Blazer DG, Kishi Y, Maru DM, Kopetz S, Chun YS, Overman MJ, et al. Pathologic response to preoperative chemotherapy: a new outcome end point after resection of hepatic colorectal metastases. J Clin Oncol. 2008;26(33):5344–51.
21. Vigano L, Darwish SS, Rimassa L, Cimino M, Carnaghi C, Donadon M, et al. Progression of colorectal liver metastases from the end of chemotherapy to resection: a new contraindication to surgery? Ann Surg Oncol. 2018;25(6):1676–85.
22. Rees M, Tekkis PP, Welsh FK, O'Rourke T, John TG. Evaluation of long-term survival after hepatic resection for metastatic colorectal cancer: a multifactorial model of 929 patients. Ann Surg. 2008;247(1):125–35.
23. Nordlinger B, Guiguet M, Vaillant JC, Balladur P, Boudjema K, Bachellier P, et al. Surgical resection of colorectal carcinoma metastases to the liver. A prognostic scoring system to improve case selection, based on 1568 patients. Association Française de Chirurgie. Cancer. 1996;77(7):1254–62.
24. Adams RB, Aloia TA, Loyer E, Pawlik TM, Taouli B, Vauthey JN, et al. Selection for hepatic resection of colorectal liver metastases: expert consensus statement. HPB (Oxford). 2013;15(2):91–103.
25. Moulton CA, Gu CS, Law CH, Tandan VR, Hart R, Quan D, et al. Effect of PET before liver resection on surgical management for colorectal adenocarcinoma metastases: a randomized clinical trial. JAMA. 2014;311(18):1863–9.
26. Rifkin MD, Rosato FE, Branch HM, Foster J, Yang SL, Barbot DJ, et al. Intraoperative ultrasound of the liver. An important adjunctive tool for decision making in the operating room. Ann Surg. 1987;205(5):466–72.
27. Leen E, Ceccotti P, Moug SJ, Glen P, MacQuarrie J, Angerson WJ, et al. Potential value of contrast-enhanced intraoperative ultrasonography during partial hepatectomy for metastases: an essential investigation before resection? Ann Surg. 2006;243(2):236–40.
28. Pandey P, Lewis H, Pandey A, Schmidt C, Dillhoff M, Kamel IR, et al. Updates in hepatic oncology imaging. Surg Oncol. 2017;26(2):195–206.
29. Moris D, Ronnekleiv-Kelly S, Rahnemai-Azar AA, Felekouras E, Dillhoff M, Schmidt C, et al. Parenchymal-sparing versus anatomic liver resection for colorectal liver metastases: a systematic review. J Gastrointest Surg. 2017;21(6):1076–85.
30. Sarpel U, Bonavia AS, Grucela A, Roayaie S, Schwartz ME, Labow DM. Does anatomic versus nonanatomic resection affect recurrence and survival in patients undergoing surgery for colorectal liver metastasis? Ann Surg Oncol. 2009;16(2):379–84.
31. Gold JS, Are C, Kornprat P, Jarnagin WR, Gönen M, Fong Y, et al. Increased use of parenchymal-sparing surgery for bilateral liver metastases from colorectal cancer is associated with improved mortality without change in oncologic outcome: trends in treatment over time in 440 patients. Ann Surg. 2008;247(1):109–17.
32. Mise Y, Aloia TA, Brudvik KW, Schwarz L, Vauthey JN, Conrad C. Parenchymal-sparing hepatectomy in colorectal liver metastasis improves salvageability and survival. Ann Surg. 2016;263(1):146–52.

33. Schmidt J, Strotzer M, Fraunhofer S, Boedeker H, Zirngibl H. Intraoperative ultrasonography versus helical computed tomography and computed tomography with arterioportography in diagnosing colorectal liver metastases: lesion-by-lesion analysis. World J Surg. 2000;24(1):43–7.. discussion 8
34. Castaing D, Emond J, Kunstlinger F, Bismuth H. Utility of operative ultrasound in the surgical management of liver tumors. Ann Surg. 1986;204(5):600–5.
35. Buell JF, Cherqui D, Geller DA, O'Rourke N, Iannitti D, Dagher I, et al. The international position on laparoscopic liver surgery: the Louisville Statement, 2008. Ann Surg. 2009;250(5):825–30.
36. Abu Hilal M, Aldrighetti L, Dagher I, Edwin B, Troisi RI, Alikhanov R, et al. The Southampton consensus guidelines for laparoscopic liver surgery: from indication to implementation. Ann Surg. 2018;268(1):11–8.
37. Fretland Å, Dagenborg VJ, Bjørnelv GMW, Kazaryan AM, Kristiansen R, Fagerland MW, et al. Laparoscopic versus open resection for colorectal liver metastases: the OSLO-COMET randomized controlled trial. Ann Surg. 2018;267(2):199–207.
38. Castaing D, Vibert E, Ricca L, Azoulay D, Adam R, Gayet B. Oncologic results of laparoscopic versus open hepatectomy for colorectal liver metastases in two specialized centers. Ann Surg. 2009;250(5):849–55.
39. Nguyen KT, Laurent A, Dagher I, Geller DA, Steel J, Thomas MT, et al. Minimally invasive liver resection for metastatic colorectal cancer: a multi-institutional, international report of safety, feasibility, and early outcomes. Ann Surg. 2009;250(5):842–8.
40. Kooby DA, Stockman J, Ben-Porat L, Gonen M, Jarnagin WR, Dematteo RP, et al. Influence of transfusions on perioperative and long-term outcome in patients following hepatic resection for colorectal metastases. Ann Surg. 2003;237(6):860–9; discussion 9–70
41. Hallet J, Tsang M, Cheng ES, Habashi R, Kulyk I, Hanna SS, et al. The impact of perioperative red blood cell transfusions on long-term outcomes after hepatectomy for colorectal liver metastases. Ann Surg Oncol. 2015;22(12):4038–45.
42. Ito H, Are C, Gonen M, D'Angelica M, Dematteo RP, Kemeny NE, et al. Effect of postoperative morbidity on long-term survival after hepatic resection for metastatic colorectal cancer. Ann Surg. 2008;247(6):994–1002.
43. Mavros MN, de Jong M, Dogeas E, Hyder O, Pawlik TM. Impact of complications on long-term survival after resection of colorectal liver metastases. Br J Surg. 2013;100(5): 711–8.
44. Melloul E, Hübner M, Scott M, Snowden C, Prentis J, Dejong CH, et al. Guidelines for perioperative care for liver surgery: enhanced recovery after surgery (ERAS) society recommendations. World J Surg. 2016;40(10):2425–40.
45. Schultz NA, Larsen PN, Klarskov B, Plum LM, Frederiksen HJ, Christensen BM, et al. Evaluation of a fast-track programme for patients undergoing liver resection. Br J Surg. 2013;100(1):138–43.
46. van Dam RM, Hendry PO, Coolsen MM, Bemelmans MH, Lassen K, Revhaug A, et al. Initial experience with a multimodal enhanced recovery programme in patients undergoing liver resection. Br J Surg. 2008;95(8):969–75.
47. Karanicolas PJ, Cleary S, McHardy P, Kiss A, Sawyer J, Behman R, et al. Medial Open Transversus Abdominis Plane (MOTAP) catheters reduce opioid requirements and improve pain control following open liver resection: a multicenter, blinded, randomized controlled trial. Ann Surg. 2018;268(2):233–40.
48. Adam R, de Gramont A, Figueras J, Kokudo N, Kunstlinger F, Loyer E, et al. Managing synchronous liver metastases from colorectal cancer: a multidisciplinary international consensus. Cancer Treat Rev. 2015;41(9):729–41.
49. Qadan M, D'Angelica MI. Complex surgical strategies to improve resectability in borderline-resectable disease. Curr Colorectal Cancer Rep. 2015;11(6):369–77.
50. Abdalla EK, Denys A, Chevalier P, Nemr RA, Vauthey JN. Total and segmental liver volume variations: implications for liver surgery. Surgery. 2004;135(4): 404–10.

51. Chun YS, Ribero D, Abdalla EK, Madoff DC, Mortenson MM, Wei SH, et al. Comparison of two methods of future liver remnant volume measurement. J Gastrointest Surg. 2008;12(1):123–8.
52. Abdalla EK, Vauthey JN, Ellis LM, Ellis V, Pollock R, Broglio KR, et al. Recurrence and outcomes following hepatic resection, radiofrequency ablation, and combined resection/ablation for colorectal liver metastases. Ann Surg. 2004;239(6):818–25; discussion 25–7
53. Gleisner AL, Choti MA, Assumpcao L, Nathan H, Schulick RD, Pawlik TM. Colorectal liver metastases: recurrence and survival following hepatic resection, radiofrequency ablation, and combined resection-radiofrequency ablation. Arch Surg. 2008;143(12):1204–12.
54. Karanicolas PJ, Jarnagin WR, Gonen M, Tuorto S, Allen PJ, DeMatteo RP, et al. Long-term outcomes following tumor ablation for treatment of bilateral colorectal liver metastases. JAMA Surg. 2013;148(7):597–601.
55. Farges O, Belghiti J, Kianmanesh R, Regimbeau JM, Santoro R, Vilgrain V, et al. Portal vein embolization before right hepatectomy: prospective clinical trial. Ann Surg. 2003;237(2):208–17.
56. Adam R, Laurent A, Azoulay D, Castaing D, Bismuth H. Two-stage hepatectomy: a planned strategy to treat irresectable liver tumors. Ann Surg. 2000;232(6):777–85.
57. Wicherts DA, Miller R, de Haas RJ, Bitsakou G, Vibert E, Veilhan LA, et al. Long-term results of two-stage hepatectomy for irresectable colorectal cancer liver metastases. Ann Surg. 2008;248(6):994–1005.
58. Jaeck D, Oussoultzoglou E, Rosso E, Greget M, Weber JC, Bachellier P. A two-stage hepatectomy procedure combined with portal vein embolization to achieve curative resection for initially unresectable multiple and bilobar colorectal liver metastases. Ann Surg. 2004;240(6):1037–49; discussion 49–51
59. Narita M, Oussoultzoglou E, Jaeck D, Fuchschuber P, Rosso E, Pessaux P, et al. Two-stage hepatectomy for multiple bilobar colorectal liver metastases. Br J Surg. 2011;98(10):1463–75.
60. Brouquet A, Abdalla EK, Kopetz S, Garrett CR, Overman MJ, Eng C, et al. High survival rate after two-stage resection of advanced colorectal liver metastases: response-based selection and complete resection define outcome. J Clin Oncol. 2011;29(8):1083–90.
61. Schnitzbauer AA, Lang SA, Goessmann H, Nadalin S, Baumgart J, Farkas SA, et al. Right portal vein ligation combined with in situ splitting induces rapid left lateral liver lobe hypertrophy enabling 2-staged extended right hepatic resection in small-for-size settings. Ann Surg. 2012;255(3):405–14.
62. Adam R, Imai K, Castro Benitez C, Allard MA, Vibert E, Sa Cunha A, et al. Outcome after associating liver partition and portal vein ligation for staged hepatectomy and conventional two-stage hepatectomy for colorectal liver metastases. Br J Surg. 2016;103(11):1521–9.
63. Shindoh J, Vauthey JN, Zimmitti G, Curley SA, Huang SY, Mahvash A, et al. Analysis of the efficacy of portal vein embolization for patients with extensive liver malignancy and very low future liver remnant volume, including a comparison with the associating liver partition with portal vein ligation for staged hepatectomy approach. J Am Coll Surg. 2013;217(1):126–33; discussion 33–4
64. Sandström P, Røsok BI, Sparrelid E, Larsen PN, Larsson AL, Lindell G, et al. ALPPS improves resectability compared with conventional two-stage hepatectomy in patients with advanced colorectal liver metastasis: results from a Scandinavian Multicenter Randomized Controlled Trial (LIGRO Trial). Ann Surg. 2018;267(5):833–40.
65. Enne M, Schadde E, Björnsson B, Hernandez Alejandro R, Steinbruck K, Viana E, et al. ALPPS as a salvage procedure after insufficient future liver remnant hypertrophy following portal vein occlusion. HPB (Oxford). 2017;19(12):1126–9.
66. Lam VW, Spiro C, Laurence JM, Johnston E, Hollands MJ, Pleass HC, et al. A systematic review of clinical response and survival outcomes of downsizing systemic chemotherapy and rescue liver surgery in patients with initially unresectable colorectal liver metastases. Ann Surg Oncol. 2012;19(4):1292–301.

67. Karanicolas PJ, Metrakos P, Chan K, Asmis T, Chen E, Kingham TP, et al. Hepatic arterial infusion pump chemotherapy in the management of colorectal liver metastases: expert consensus statement. Curr Oncol. 2014;21(1):e129–36.
68. Ammori JB, Kemeny NE, Fong Y, Cercek A, Dematteo RP, Allen PJ, et al. Conversion to complete resection and/or ablation using hepatic artery infusional chemotherapy in patients with unresectable liver metastases from colorectal cancer: a decade of experience at a single institution. Ann Surg Oncol. 2013;20(9):2901–7.
69. D'Angelica MI, Correa-Gallego C, Paty PB, Cercek A, Gewirtz AN, Chou JF, et al. Phase II trial of hepatic artery infusional and systemic chemotherapy for patients with unresectable hepatic metastases from colorectal cancer: conversion to resection and long-term outcomes. Ann Surg. 2015;261(2):353–60.
70. Gorgen A, Muaddi H, Zhang W, McGilvray I, Gallinger S, Sapisochin G. The new era of transplant oncology: liver transplantation for nonresectable colorectal cancer liver metastases. Can J Gastroenterol Hepatol. 2018;2018:9531925.
71. Hagness M, Foss A, Line PD, Scholz T, Jørgensen PF, Fosby B, et al. Liver transplantation for nonresectable liver metastases from colorectal cancer. Ann Surg. 2013;257(5):800–6.
72. Dueland S, Guren TK, Hagness M, Glimelius B, Line PD, Pfeiffer P, et al. Chemotherapy or liver transplantation for nonresectable liver metastases from colorectal cancer? Ann Surg. 2015;261(5):956–60.
73. Toso C, Pinto Marques H, Andres A, Castro Sousa F, Adam R, Kalil A, et al. Liver transplantation for colorectal liver metastasis: survival without recurrence can be achieved. Liver Transpl. 2017;23(8):1073–6.
74. Nordlinger B, Sorbye H, Glimelius B, Poston GJ, Schlag PM, Rougier P, et al. Perioperative chemotherapy with FOLFOX4 and surgery versus surgery alone for resectable liver metastases from colorectal cancer (EORTC Intergroup trial 40983): a randomised controlled trial. Lancet. 2008;371(9617):1007–16.
75. Nordlinger B, Sorbye H, Glimelius B, Poston GJ, Schlag PM, Rougier P, et al. Perioperative FOLFOX4 chemotherapy and surgery versus surgery alone for resectable liver metastases from colorectal cancer (EORTC 40983): long-term results of a randomised, controlled, phase 3 trial. Lancet Oncol. 2013;14(12):1208–15.
76. Benoist S, Brouquet A, Penna C, Julié C, El Hajjam M, Chagnon S, et al. Complete response of colorectal liver metastases after chemotherapy: does it mean cure? J Clin Oncol. 2006;24(24):3939–45.
77. Vauthey JN, Pawlik TM, Ribero D, Wu TT, Zorzi D, Hoff PM, et al. Chemotherapy regimen predicts steatohepatitis and an increase in 90-day mortality after surgery for hepatic colorectal metastases. J Clin Oncol. 2006;24(13):2065–72.
78. Allegra CJ, Rumble RB, Hamilton SR, Mangu PB, Roach N, Hantel A, et al. Extended RAS gene mutation testing in metastatic colorectal carcinoma to predict response to anti-epidermal growth factor receptor monoclonal antibody therapy: American Society of Clinical Oncology provisional clinical opinion update 2015. J Clin Oncol. 2016;34(2):179–85.
79. Primrose J, Falk S, Finch-Jones M, Valle J, O'Reilly D, Siriwardena A, et al. Systemic chemotherapy with or without cetuximab in patients with resectable colorectal liver metastasis: the New EPOC randomised controlled trial. Lancet Oncol. 2014;15(6):601–11.
80. Bridgewater J, Pugh S, Whitehead A, Stanton L, Eminton Z, Mellor J, et al. Perioperative chemotherapy with or without cetuximab in patients (pts) with resectable colorectal liver metastasis (CRLM): mature analysis of overall survival (OS) in the new EPOC randomised controlled trial. Ann Oncol. 2017;28:162.
81. Mise Y, Hasegawa K, Oba M, Yamaguchi K, Uetake H, Yoshino T, et al. EXPERT study: randomized phase III trial of radical surgery and postoperative mFOLFOX6 versus perioperative mFOLFOX6 plus cetuximab in patients with KRAS wild-type resectable colorectal liver metastases (CLMs). J Clin Oncol. 2019;37:652.
82. Mitry E, Fields AL, Bleiberg H, Labianca R, Portier G, Tu D, et al. Adjuvant chemotherapy after potentially curative resection of metastases from colorectal cancer: a pooled analysis of two randomized trials. J Clin Oncol. 2008;26(30):4906–11.

83. Gruenberger T, Bridgewater J, Chau I, García Alfonso P, Rivoire M, Mudan S, et al. Bevacizumab plus mFOLFOX-6 or FOLFOXIRI in patients with initially unresectable liver metastases from colorectal cancer: the OLIVIA multinational randomised phase II trial. Ann Oncol. 2015;26(4):702–8.
84. Folprecht G, Gruenberger T, Bechstein WO, Raab HR, Lordick F, Hartmann JT, et al. Tumour response and secondary resectability of colorectal liver metastases following neoadjuvant chemotherapy with cetuximab: the CELIM randomised phase 2 trial. Lancet Oncol. 2010;11(1):38–47.
85. Folprecht G, Gruenberger T, Bechstein W, Raab HR, Weitz J, Lordick F, et al. Survival of patients with initially unresectable colorectal liver metastases treated with FOLFOX/cetuximab or FOLFIRI/cetuximab in a multidisciplinary concept (CELIM study). Ann Oncol. 2014;25(5):1018–25.
86. Ye LC, Liu TS, Ren L, Wei Y, Zhu DX, Zai SY, et al. Randomized controlled trial of cetuximab plus chemotherapy for patients with KRAS wild-type unresectable colorectal liver-limited metastases. J Clin Oncol. 2013;31(16):1931–8.
87. Wong R, Cunningham D, Barbachano Y, Saffery C, Valle J, Hickish T, et al. A multicentre study of capecitabine, oxaliplatin plus bevacizumab as perioperative treatment of patients with poor-risk colorectal liver-only metastases not selected for upfront resection. Ann Oncol. 2011;22(9):2042–8.
88. Ji JH, Park SH, Lee J, Kim TW, Hong YS, Kim KP, et al. Prospective phase II study of neoadjuvant FOLFOX6 plus cetuximab in patients with colorectal cancer and unresectable liver-only metastasis. Cancer Chemother Pharmacol. 2013;72(1):223–30.
89. Takahashi T, Shibata Y, Tojima Y, Tsuboi K, Sakamoto E, Kunieda K, et al. Multicenter phase II study of modified FOLFOX6 as neoadjuvant chemotherapy for patients with unresectable liver-only metastases from colorectal cancer in Japan: ROOF study. Int J Clin Oncol. 2013;18(2):335–42.
90. Ychou M, Rivoire M, Thezenas S, Quenet F, Delpero JR, Rebischung C, et al. A randomized phase II trial of three intensified chemotherapy regimens in first-line treatment of colorectal cancer patients with initially unresectable or not optimally resectable liver metastases. The METHEP trial. Ann Surg Oncol. 2013;20(13):4289–97.
91. Gruenberger B, Tamandl D, Schueller J, Scheithauer W, Zielinski C, Herbst F, et al. Bevacizumab, capecitabine, and oxaliplatin as neoadjuvant therapy for patients with potentially curable metastatic colorectal cancer. J Clin Oncol. 2008;26(11):1830–5.
92. Johnston FM, Mavros MN, Herman JM, Pawlik TM. Local therapies for hepatic metastases. J Natl Compr Cancer Netw. 2013;11(2):153–60.
93. Ruers T, Van Coevorden F, Punt CJ, Pierie JE, Borel-Rinkes I, Ledermann JA, et al. Local treatment of unresectable colorectal liver metastases: results of a randomized phase II trial. J Natl Cancer Inst. 2017;109(9):djx015.
94. Correa-Gallego C, Fong Y, Gonen M, D'Angelica MI, Allen PJ, DeMatteo RP, et al. A retrospective comparison of microwave ablation vs. radiofrequency ablation for colorectal cancer hepatic metastases. Ann Surg Oncol. 2014;21(13):4278–83.
95. Comito T, Cozzi L, Clerici E, Campisi MC, Liardo RL, Navarria P, et al. Stereotactic Ablative Radiotherapy (SABR) in inoperable oligometastatic disease from colorectal cancer: a safe and effective approach. BMC Cancer. 2014;14:619.
96. Chang DT, Swaminath A, Kozak M, Weintraub J, Koong AC, Kim J, et al. Stereotactic body radiotherapy for colorectal liver metastases: a pooled analysis. Cancer. 2011;117(17):4060–9.
97. Petrelli F, Comito T, Barni S, Pancera G, Scorsetti M, Ghidini A, et al. Stereotactic body radiotherapy for colorectal cancer liver metastases: a systematic review. Radiother Oncol. 2018;129(3):427–34.
98. Kingham TP, Karkar AM, D'Angelica MI, Allen PJ, Dematteo RP, Getrajdman GI, et al. Ablation of perivascular hepatic malignant tumors with irreversible electroporation. J Am Coll Surg. 2012;215(3):379–87.

99. Kemeny N, Huang Y, Cohen AM, Shi W, Conti JA, Brennan MF, et al. Hepatic arterial infusion of chemotherapy after resection of hepatic metastases from colorectal cancer. N Engl J Med. 1999;341(27):2039–48.
100. Kemeny MM, Adak S, Gray B, Macdonald JS, Smith T, Lipsitz S, et al. Combined-modality treatment for resectable metastatic colorectal carcinoma to the liver: surgical resection of hepatic metastases in combination with continuous infusion of chemotherapy–an intergroup study. J Clin Oncol. 2002;20(6):1499–505.
101. Kemeny NE, Gonen M. Hepatic arterial infusion after liver resection. N Engl J Med. 2005;352(7):734–5.
102. Groot Koerkamp B, Sadot E, Kemeny NE, Gönen M, Leal JN, Allen PJ, et al. Perioperative hepatic arterial infusion pump chemotherapy is associated with longer survival after resection of colorectal liver metastases: a propensity score analysis. J Clin Oncol. 2017;35(17):1938–44.
103. Martin RC, Joshi J, Robbins K, Tomalty D, Bosnjakovik P, Derner M, et al. Hepatic intra-arterial injection of drug-eluting bead, irinotecan (DEBIRI) in unresectable colorectal liver metastases refractory to systemic chemotherapy: results of multi-institutional study. Ann Surg Oncol. 2011;18(1):192–8.
104. Richardson AJ, Laurence JM, Lam VW. Transarterial chemoembolization with irinotecan beads in the treatment of colorectal liver metastases: systematic review. J Vasc Interv Radiol. 2013;24(8):1209–17.
105. Fiorentini G, Aliberti C, Tilli M, Mulazzani L, Graziano F, Giordani P, et al. Intra-arterial infusion of irinotecan-loaded drug-eluting beads (DEBIRI) versus intravenous therapy (FOLFIRI) for hepatic metastases from colorectal cancer: final results of a phase III study. Anticancer Res. 2012;32(4):1387–95.
106. Saxena A, Bester L, Shan L, Perera M, Gibbs P, Meteling B, et al. A systematic review on the safety and efficacy of yttrium-90 radioembolization for unresectable, chemorefractory colorectal cancer liver metastases. J Cancer Res Clin Oncol. 2014;140(4):537–47.
107. Hendlisz A, Van den Eynde M, Peeters M, Maleux G, Lambert B, Vannoote J, et al. Phase III trial comparing protracted intravenous fluorouracil infusion alone or with yttrium-90 resin microspheres radioembolization for liver-limited metastatic colorectal cancer refractory to standard chemotherapy. J Clin Oncol. 2010;28(23):3687–94.
108. Wasan HS, Gibbs P, Sharma NK, Taieb J, Heinemann V, Ricke J, et al. First-line selective internal radiotherapy plus chemotherapy versus chemotherapy alone in patients with liver metastases from colorectal cancer (FOXFIRE, SIRFLOX, and FOXFIRE-Global): a combined analysis of three multicentre, randomised, phase 3 trials. Lancet Oncol. 2017;18(9):1159–71.
109. Wei AC, Coburn NG, Devitt KS, Serrano PE, Moulton CA, Cleary SP, et al. Survival following resection of intra- and extra-hepatic metastases from colorectal cancer: a phase II trial. Ann Surg Oncol. 2016;23(8):2644–51.
110. Passot G, Kim BJ, Glehen O, Mehran RJ, Kopetz SE, Goere D, et al. Impact of RAS mutations in metastatic colorectal cancer after potentially curative resection: does site of metastases matter? Ann Surg Oncol. 2018;25(1):179–87.
111. Leung U, Gönen M, Allen PJ, Kingham TP, DeMatteo RP, Jarnagin WR, et al. Colorectal cancer liver metastases and concurrent extrahepatic disease treated with resection. Ann Surg. 2017;265(1):158–65.
112. Gallinger S, Biagi JJ, Fletcher GG, Nhan C, Ruo L, McLeod RS. Liver resection for colorectal cancer metastases. Curr Oncol. 2013;20(3):e255–65.
113. Shah SA, Haddad R, Al-Sukhni W, Kim RD, Greig PD, Grant DR, et al. Surgical resection of hepatic and pulmonary metastases from colorectal carcinoma. J Am Coll Surg. 2006;202(3):468–75.
114. Pulitanò C, Bodingbauer M, Aldrighetti L, de Jong MC, Castillo F, Schulick RD, et al. Liver resection for colorectal metastases in presence of extrahepatic disease: results from an international multi-institutional analysis. Ann Surg Oncol. 2011;18(5):1380–8.
115. Pulitanò C, Bodingbauer M, Aldrighetti L, Choti MA, Castillo F, Schulick RD, et al. Colorectal liver metastasis in the setting of lymph node metastasis: defining the benefit of surgical resection. Ann Surg Oncol. 2012;19(2):435–42.

116. Nanji S, Tsang ME, Wei X, Booth CM. Regional lymph node involvement in patients undergoing liver resection for colorectal cancer metastases. Eur J Surg Oncol. 2017;43(2):322–9.
117. Adam R, de Haas RJ, Wicherts DA, Aloia TA, Delvart V, Azoulay D, et al. Is hepatic resection justified after chemotherapy in patients with colorectal liver metastases and lymph node involvement? J Clin Oncol. 2008;26(22):3672–80.
118. Okuno M, Goumard C, Mizuno T, Kopetz S, Omichi K, Tzeng CD, et al. Prognostic impact of perihepatic lymph node metastases in patients with resectable colorectal liver metastases. Br J Surg. 2018;105(9):1200–9.

Desmoid Fibromatosis and Dermatofibrosarcoma Protuberans

8

Ricky Jrearz, Samir Fasih, Brendan C. Dickson, Abha A. Gupta, and Rebecca A. Gladdy

Introduction

Desmoid tumors (DTs, also known as desmoid-type fibromatosis) and dermatofibrosarcoma protuberans (DFSP) are rare mesenchymal neoplasms of fibroblastic/myofibroblastic derivation.

DT can be locally invasive, but has no metastatic potential. They account for 0.03% of all neoplasms with an annual incidence of 2–4 per 1,000,000 individuals [3, 10, 37]. The peak age of presentation is between 30 and 40 years of age. In contrast to its superficial counterpart, palmer/planter fibromatosis, DT typically occurs in the deep soft tissues. Most desmoids arise sporadically, although some may be associated with trauma or pregnancy. Approximately 5–10% of desmoids occur in patients that have familial adenomatous polyposis (FAP); 10–20% of FAP patients will develop DT [52]. Nuchal fibromas (Gardner's syndrome) can occasionally transform into desmoids [53].

R. Jrearz
General Surgical Oncology, University of Toronto, Toronto, ON, Canada

S. Fasih
Medical Oncology, University of Toronto, Toronto, ON, Canada
e-mail: samir.fasih@uhn.ca

B. C. Dickson
Department of Laboratory Medicine and Pathobiology, University of Toronto, Toronto, ON, Canada
e-mail: BDickson@mtsinai.on.ca

A. A. Gupta
Division of Medical Oncology, University of Toronto, Toronto, ON, Canada
e-mail: abha.gupta@sickkids.ca

R. A. Gladdy (✉)
Department of Surgery, University of Toronto, Toronto, ON, Canada
e-mail: rgladdy@mtsinai.on.ca

F. C. Wright et al. (eds.), *Surgical Oncology Manual*,
https://doi.org/10.1007/978-3-030-48363-0_8

DFSP is a soft tissue neoplasm that is locally invasive and a subset have metastatic potential. They account for less than 0.1% of all malignancies, but are the most common sarcoma of the skin [54]. The annual incidence of DFSP is 1–4 per 1,000,000 individuals [6, 7]. It is most commonly seen between 20 and 50 years of age. Most DFSPs are low grade tumors. However, fibrosarcomatous transformation (FS-DFSP) occurs in 5–15% of tumors. FS-DFSP is an intermediate grade sarcoma that has a 10–15% chance of metastasis [8]. The presence of a positive surgical margin significantly increases the risk of local recurrence in DFSP [9, 24, 40].

Histology and Molecular Genetics

DT

DTs are characterized histologically by infiltrative fascicles of monomorphic spindle cells. The majority (85%) of sporadic tumors contain mutations in exon 3 of the CTNNB1 gene which encodes for β-catenin [1, 2, 22]. Recent studies have shown that many of the so-called "wild-type" (15%) DT will actually contain mutations in *CTNNB1* with deeper sequencing [55]. Familial DT and a subset of sporadic DT display mutations in the adenomatous polyposis coli (*APC*) gene [56, 57].

DFSP

DFSP originates superficially in the dermis or subcutis. Histologically it is characterized by storiform whorls of monomorphic spindle cells [58]. FS-DFSP is associated with architectural transformation into a herringbone pattern, and greater pleomorphism and mitotic activity; frequently, these tumors will also lose expression of CD34, an immunohistochemical marker typical of DFSP. Greater than 90% of tumors exhibit a translocation resulting in *COL1A1-PDGFB* gene fusion [5], which renders the tumor sensitive to imatinib.

Staging and Prognosis (See Table 8.1)

DT

DT is not included in the most recent American Joint Committee on Cancer AJCC 8th edition staging system as it is considered a benign neoplasm. Staging systems

Table 8.1 Prognosis of DT and DFSP

	Prognosis [9–17]	
	5-year overall survival (OS) (%)	5-year local recurrence (LR) (%)
DT	76[a] – 100	20–47
DFSP	98–100	3–25

[a]Intra-abdominal DT in FAP patients – deaths due to complications of DT treatment or other causes

for intra-abdominal DT in the context of FAP has been proposed based on size, symptoms, growth, and complications [59].

DFSP

The AJCC 8th edition is the current recommended staging system for DFSP. Staging differs based on location of the primary tumor; extremities and trunk vs. head and neck.

Management (See Table 8.2)

DT

There has been a paradigm shift in the management of DT from upfront surgical resection to upfront active surveillance [18, 19, 25, 65]. A large recent prospective French

Table 8.2 Management, workup, and follow-up for DT

Workup	Management	Follow-up

History and physical exam
Imaging:
  MRI preferred for abdominal wall, trunk, and extremity (CT if MRI not available)
CT for intra-abdominal lesions
Investigations:
  Percutaneous core biopsy
  MCC discussion
  Consider colonoscopy to r/o FAP (higher risk in <40, multifocal, intra-abdominal/ retroperitoneal DT, family hx of colon cancer)
	Trial of active surveillance to assess growth rate (1–2 years)
	  Ensure discontinuation of all exogenous estrogen (i.e., oral contraception)
	Consider active treatment if:
	  Progression over at least 2 subsequent assessments
	  Increase of symptom burden
	  Disease close to critical structure (mesentery, head and neck)
	Initial medical treatment on progression:
	  Intra-abdominal/retroperitoneal DT
	  Head and neck, extremity, chest wall DT
	  Abdominal wall DT
	Medical treatment options:
	  Consider targeted agents[a] or cytotoxic chemotherapy[b] [26–31]
	  Consider for a clinical trial or trial of NSAIDs[c] or antiestrogens[d] if the above options not possible
	Surgical resection can be considered at all DT sites if progression on medical treatment; the aim is for gross resection with preservation of function
	Radiotherapy can be first-line alternative in highly selective cases (age, comorbidities, etc.)
		History and physical exam every 3–6 months to establish pattern of growth MRI or CT every 3–6 months for first 2 years
		If stabilization/ regression ➔ active surveillance with annual MRI/ physical exam
		Can consider US if demonstrated long-term stability
		In case of progression, consider medical or surgical treatment

ER/PR estrogen receptor/progesterone receptor, MCC multidisciplinary cancer conference, NSAIDs nonsteroidal anti-inflammatory drugs, US ultrasound, TKIs tyrosine kinase inhibitors

[a]For example, sorafenib, pazopanib

[b]For example, Methotrexate plus vinca alkaloid, doxorubicin, liposomal doxorubicin, dacarbazine

[c]For example, sulindac, indomethacin

[d]For example, tamoxifen, raloxifene, toremifene

study showed no difference in surgery vs. active surveillance in 2-year event-free survival [60]. Similar results have been observed in studies comparing initial active surveillance to upfront medical therapy [63]. Studies have demonstrated through multivariate analysis and predictive nomograms that age (<37), tumor site (non-abdominal wall), and tumor size (>7 cm) are independent risk factors for local recurrence after resection [20, 21]. Specific mutations in exon 3 such as S45T have also been associated with increased risk of recurrence after resection [22, 23]; whether this mutation is associated with tumor progression during active surveillance is currently being prospectively studied.

Special Notes

Recurrence:

- Recurrent DT should be managed in a similar fashion to primary DT with consideration to previous therapies, tumor location, and biology
- Patients with multiple recurrences after adequate resections should be considered for medical therapy

Margins:

- The aim of surgical resection should be negative histologic margins with preservation of function. Despite this, 25% of cases with negative margins will recur locally.
- The evidence is controversial on margin status and recurrence. Therefore, unlike sarcomas, positive margins should be followed and not necessarily re-excised [65].

Imaging:

- A baseline MRI and assessment of T2 hyperintensity within the tumor may be predictive of desmoid progression during active surveillance [64].

Medical Therapy:
Several options and considerations for medical therapy are listed in Table 8.3. The discussion of pros/cons of various therapies with the patient will aid in decision-making.

Regression:

- Spontaneous regression has been reported in 19–28% of cases [20, 32]; this is seen predominately in abdominal wall DT.

FAP:

- Younger patients (<40 years) with a new diagnosis of DT should be screened for FAP with colonoscopy.
- Intra-abdominal or retroperitoneal DT, multifocal disease, and positive family history are associated with FAP.

Table 8.3 Type of medical therapy for DT

Type of therapy	Number of patients	Objective response rates	Considerations	Reference
Targeted therapy			Total duration of therapy remains unclear	Gounder MM; 2018 [41] Maud T; 2018 [42] Chugh R; 2010 [43]
1. Sorafenib 2. Pazopanib 3. Imatinib	87 72 51	33% 37% 5%		
Cytotoxic chemotherapy			1. Intravenous therapy, prolonged course 2. Hair loss with doxorubicin	Azzarelli A; 2001 [44] Patel S; 1993 [45] Constantinidou A; 2010 [46]
1. Metho-trexate/vinblastine or vinorelbine 2. Doxorubicin/dacarbazine 3. Pegylated liposomal doxorubicin (PLD)	30 11 14	40% 54% 33%		
Nonsteroidal anti-inflammatory drugs (NSAIDs)			May be considered in patients with FAP	Nishida Y; 2012 [47] Tsukada K; 1992 [48]
1. Meloxicam 2. Sulindac	20 14	40% 57%		
Antiestrogen therapy			Use with caution in premenopausal women due to ovarian cyst development	Brooks M; 1992 [49] Fiore M; 2011 [50]
1. Toremifene or tamoxifen 2. Toremifene	20 27	65% 26%		
Gamma-secretase inhibitors			Duration of therapy unclear. Diarrhea can be problematic.	Kummar S; 2017 [51]
1. Nirogacestat	17	29%		

- FAP patients with DT have a higher rate of recurrence and nonsurgical options should be strongly considered prior to resection [11].

Pregnancy:

- Disease progression often occurs during pregnancy but can generally be managed safely with close observation with serial US in most cases [33].
- The risk of adverse obstetric events is not increased in DT [33].
- DT should not be a contraindication to future pregnancies [33].
- Tumors arise in previous caesarian-section sites.

Table 8.4 Workup, management, and follow-up for DFSP

Workup	Management	Follow-up [62]
History and physical exam Investigations: Percutaneous or excisional biopsy MRI in selected cases to assess extent/depth/multifocality Routine staging not indicated unless: Clinical signs of metastases Recurrent disease Fibrosarcomatous transformation MCC discussion	Surgical resection Wide local excision (WLE) 2–3 cm Plastic surgery consultation if primary closure is anticipated to be challenging[a] Medical treatment: Imatinib (inoperable tumors or preoperative downstaging to preserve function, limit extent of soft tissue reconstruction)	Low risk DFSP (wide R0, no FS changes) Routine self-examination Np formal follow-up Low risk DFSP (close R0, R1, no FS, difficult to examine locations, i.e., axilla, perineum, etc.) Annual clinical exam × 10 years No routine imaging High risk DFSP (FS changes) Clinical exam + CXR q3–6 months × 2–3 years then annually × 10 years total

[a]Approximately 30% of reconstructions require plastic surgery techniques [35]

- 17% of pregnancy induced DT experience spontaneous regression [33].
- Discontinue the use of exogenous hormones as they can impact growth.

Radiation Therapy:

- In selected circumstances such as age, patient intolerance/preference to surgical/medical therapy, comorbidities, rapidly growing lesion threatening vital structures (head and neck, limb salvage, etc.), radiation can be considered in as a treatment for DT [65].
- May be considered in patients with multiple local recurrences or unresectable disease, but MCC discussion should be conducted prior to treatment [34].

Primary DFSP (See Table 8.4)

The primary treatment modality for localized DFSP is surgical resection with negative margins. Local recurrence has been associated with depth of invasion, anatomical location, margin status [40], and FS status [61].

Special Notes

Imatinib:

- Consider neoadjuvant imatinib for large, borderline resectable, or complex recurrent lesions in order to downsize prior to surgery.
- Can also use imatinib to help with function preservation.

Resection:

- Wide local excision is preferred, 2–3 cm in non-critical areas. Margins may be limited in facial resections.
- Mohs micrographic surgery (MMS) is not recommended in the treatment of DFSP.

Margins:
- Negative histologic margins should be the goal of surgical resection (R0).
- The ideal planned margins are 2–3 cm radially in the dermis with fascial clearance deep to tumor.

Reconstruction:
- Delayed definitive reconstruction for complex resections until margin status is confirmed can be considered in some cases.

Recurrence:
- Treat with surgical resection if possible.
- Local recurrence rates have been reported between 1% and 22% [35, 40, 61].

Lymph Nodes:
- Assessment of regional lymph nodes is not required in the absence of clinically or radiologically apparent disease.

FS-DFSP:
- Approximately 10–15% of DFSP contain fibrosarcomatous progression that behaves more aggressively (i.e., widespread metastasis) than classic DFSP [36].

Radiation Therapy:
- May be useful for recurrent tumors when surgical morbidity limits ability to re-excise. Delivery of radiation is considered only after multidisciplinary discussion [62].

Metastatic DFSP (See Table 8.5)

Special Notes

Metastases
- Most commonly occur in lungs.
- Can also occur in pancreas, liver, and bone [61].

Medical Therapy:
- Imatinib can be used for unresectable, recurrent, or metastatic disease.
- >90% of DFSP are characterized by the t(17;22) chromosomal translocation and may be susceptible to targeted platelet-derived growth factor inhibition [38].
- Response rate has been reported at 50%.

Table 8.5 Workup, management, and follow-up for metastatic DFSP

Workup	Management	Follow-up
History and physical exam CT chest/abdo/pelvis Case discussion at MCC	Systemic therapy with imatinib Consider resection (lung, liver) if: R0 resection can be achieved Favorable biology (slow growing, long disease-free interval) Primary tumor is resected or resectable Isolated/few metastases Radiation therapy for unresectable, progressive, or bony metastases	As clinically warranted

- There is limited data on cytotoxic chemotherapy and its utility in DFSP; when transformation has occurred, traditional cytotoxic therapies may be considered in the palliative setting.

Landmark Publications

There are limited prospective randomized control trials (RCT) on the management of DT (see Table 8.6) or DFSP (see Table 8.7). Management is largely dictated by consensus statements formed by expert, high-volume centers [65].

DT

DFSP

Referring to Medical Oncology

DT

1. Patients with progressive or recurrent disease.
2. Multifocal disease.
3. FAP patients.

Table 8.6 Landmark publications for DT

Study	Methods	Results
Burtenshaw et al. [15]	Retrospective review $n = 213$ Abdo wall DTs Primary DT with no prior treatment (Group A) vs. previously resected DT (Group B) vs. recurrent DT (Group C)	Abdo wall (48%) or intra-abdominal (43%) Group A ($n = 176$) 93% of patients who underwent observation alone (54/58) had stable disease or spontaneous regression 38% (67) overall required surgery (primary treatment or second line after observation/medical tx) 24% recurrence after surgery (med f/u 22 months) Abdo wall DT >7 cm and intra-abdo DT more likely to recur Group B ($n = 19$) 95% managed with upfront observation despite 63% having had R1/R2 resection Group C ($n = 18$) 61% managed non-operatively
Gronchi et al. [39]	Retrospective review $n = 203$ All patients treated with surgical resection All patients had complete macroscopic resection	DFS better in primary disease than recurrent disease (76% vs. 59% at 10 years)
Nieuwenhuis Et al. [4]	Retrospective population-based review $n = 519$ All Dutch patients with DT over a 10-year period	7.5% of DT associated with FAP factors identified with FAP-associated DT: Male, age < 60, intra-abdominal location
Gounder et al. [41]	Phase III RCT $n = 87$ Progressive, recurrent, or symptomatic DT Sorafenib vs. placebo	2-year PFS 81% vs. 36% Of note, objective response in placebo arm of 30%, consistent with spontaneous regression rates
Penel et al. [60]	Prospective randomized study Initial surgery vs. initial observation $n = 771$	Overall 2-year EFS 53% vs. 58% Favorable location DT (abdo wall, intra-abdo, breast, digestive viscera, lower limb) similar 2-year EFS (70% vs. 63%) Unfavorable location (chest wall, upper limb, head and neck) 2-year EFS significantly better in observation group (25% vs. 52%)
Salas et al. [20]	Multi-institution retrospective review $n = 426$ All patients had sporadic DT	Subgroup of patients treated with wait-and see (policy 19% spontaneous remission) Age, tumor size, tumor site (extra-abdominal) predictive of PFS on multivariate analysis

RT radiation therapy, *DFS* disease-free survival, *PFS* progression-free survival, *EFS* event-free survival

Table 8.7 Landmark publications for DFSP

Study	Methods	Results
Bowne et al. [9]	Retrospective review $N = 159$ All patients treated with WLE 16% had FS-DFSP	Positive margins and FS-DFSP predictors of poor outcome 2% of patients developed metastases and died of disease
Fiore et al. [16]	Retrospective review $N = 218$ All patients treated with WLE	Low rate of LR at 5 years (3%) Rate of distant metastases at 5 years (2%)
Huis in't Veld et al. [61]	Retrospective review $N = 357$ 87.5% treated with WLE 11.5% treated with MMS 17.4% presented with local recurrence 11.4% had FS-DFSP	LR rate 22.7% Median time to recurrence 55.5 months FS-DFSP and positive margins prognostic for recurrence 61.7% of LR identified by self-examination Rate of distant metastases 1.1% at median time of 68 months
Fields et al. [40]	Retrospective review $N = 244$ All patients treated with WLE	Depth and margin status predictive of DFS Low LR with WLE (92% DFS at 5 years)

FS-DFSP DFSP with fibrosarcomatous transformation, *DFS* disease-free survival, *WLE* wide local excision, *LR* local recurrence

DFSP

1. All patients with metastatic, recurrent, or unresectable disease.
2. Patients considered for neoadjuvant therapy to downstage bulk of disease or to preserve function.

Referring to Radiation Oncology

DT

1. Patients with multiple local recurrences for consideration of combined pre- or postoperative treatment.
2. Patients with unresectable disease that has progressed on medical therapy.
3. Patients with progressive disease not amenable to frontline medical or surgical therapy due to comorbidities/preferences.

DFSP

1. Patients with positive margins after maximal surgical resection.
2. Patients with DFSP-FS progression not amenable to surgery.
3. Patients with disease not amenable to frontline medical or surgical therapy due to comorbidities/preferences.

Referring to Multidisciplinary Cancer Conference (MCC)

DT

All cases should be discussed.

DFSP

All cases should be discussed.

Toronto Pearls

DT

- The biology and behavior of DT can be greatly varied between growth, stabilization, or regression. Non-aggressive interventions including active observation are increasingly employed in DT patients. Systemic therapy choices must balance quality of life, drug access, and symptoms.
- Percutaneous core biopsies should ideally be done with image guidance at sarcoma centers with specialized radiologists. A minimum of 4 good quality tissue cores should be obtained for accurate diagnosis.
- Pathology review should be performed by expert pathologists experienced in sarcoma.
- DT is commonly seen in young patients and has no metastatic potential. Surgical resection, if undertaken, should focus on preservation of function to avoid significant morbidity.
- DT is rarely a cause for mortality except in large, recurrent intra-abdominal tumors (particularly in FAP). Consequently, a multidisciplinary approach should be considered before embarking on extensive surgical resection.

DFSP

- Pathology review should be performed by expert pathologists experienced in sarcoma with access to appropriate molecular diagnostic techniques for accurate diagnosis.
- Definitive treatment is surgical resection in DFSP. A wide local excision should be performed to minimize local recurrence.
- Patients with DFSP-FS progression should be followed closely as they have a higher propensity for metastatic disease.
- Consider the use of imatinib in the neoadjuvant setting for locally advanced disease or in the management of metastatic disease.

References

1. Fletcher CDM, Bridge JA, Hogendoorn PCW, Mertens F. WHO classification of tumours of soft tissue and bone. 4th ed. Lyon: IARC; 2013.
2. Huss S, Nehles J, Binot E, et al. β-Catenin (CTNNB1) mutations and clinicopathologic features of mesenteric desmoid-type fibromatosis. Histopathology. 2013;62(2):294–304.
3. Reitamo JJ, Hayry P, Nykyri E, et al. The desmoid tumor I: incidence, sex-, age- and anatomical distribution in the Finnish population. Am J Clin Pathol. 1982;77(6):665–73.
4. Nieuwenhuis MH, Casparie M, Mathus-Vliegen LM, et al. A nation-wide study comparing sporadic and familial adenomatous polyposis-related desmoid-type fibromatoses. Int J Cancer. 2011;129:256–61.
5. Patel KU, Szabo SS, Hernandez VS, et al. Dermatofibrosarcoma protuberans COL1A1-PDGFB fusion is identified in virtually all dermatofibrosarcoma protuberans cases when investigated by newly developed multiplex reverse transcription polymerase chain reaction and fl uorescence in situ hybridization assays. Hum Pathol. 2008;39:184–93.
6. Koh CK, Ko CB, Bury HP, et al. Dermatofibrosarcoma protuberans. Int J Dermatol. 1995;34(4):256–60.
7. Criscione VD, Weinstock MA. Descriptive epidemiology of dermatofibrosarcoma protuberans in the United States, 1973 to 2002. J Am Acad Dermatol. 2007;56(6):968–73.
8. Stacchiotti S, Pedeutour F, Negri T, et al. Dermatofibrosarcoma protuberans-derived fibrosarcoma: clinical history, biological profile and sensitivity to imatinib. Int J Cancer. 2011;129:1761–72.
9. Bowne WB, Antonescu CR, Leung DH, et al. Dermatofibrosarcoma protuberans: a clinicopathologic analysis of patients treated and followed at a single institution. Cancer. 2000;88(12):2711–20.
10. Quintini C, Ward G, Shatnawei A, et al. Mortality of intra-abdominal desmoid tumors in patients with familial adenomatous polyposis: a single center review of 154 patients. Ann Surg. 2012;255:511–6.
11. Clark SK, Neale JC, Landgrebe JC, et al. Desmoid tumours complicating familial adenomatous polyposis. Br J Surg. 1999;86:1185–9.
12. Spear MA, Jennings LC, Mankin HJ, et al. Individualizing management of aggressive fibromatoses. Int J Radiat Oncol Biol Phys. 1998;40(3):637–45.
13. Lev D, Kotilingam D, Wei C, et al. Optimizing treatment of desmoid tumors. J Clin Oncol. 2007;25(13):1785–91.
14. Peng PD, Hyder O, Mavros MN, et al. Management and recurrence patterns of desmoids tumors: a multi-institutional analysis of 211 patients. Ann Surg Oncol. 2012;19:4036–42.

15. Burtenshaw SM, Cannell AJ, Mcalister ED, Siddique S, Kandel R, Blackstein ME, et al. Toward observation as first-line management in abdominal desmoid tumors. Ann Surg Oncol. 2016;23(7):2212–9.
16. Fiore M, Miceli R, Mussi C, et al. Dermatofibrosarcoma protuberans treated at a single institution: a surgical disease with a high cure rate. J Clin Oncol. 2005;23(30):7669–75.
17. Chang CK, Jacobs IA, Salti GI. Outcomes of surgery for dermatofibrosarcoma protuberans. Eur J Surg Oncol. 2004;30:341–5.
18. Bonvalot S, Edlweny H, Haddad V, et al. Extra-abdominal primary fibromatosis: aggressive management could be avoided in a subgroup of patients. Eur J Surg Oncol. 2008;34:462–8.
19. Fiore M, Rimareix F, Mariani L, et al. Desmoid-type fibromatosis: a front-line conservative approach to select patients for surgical treatment. Ann Surg Oncol. 2009;16:2587–93.
20. Salas S, Dufresne A, Bui B, et al. Prognostic factors influencing progression-free survival determined from a series of sporadic desmoid tumors: a wait-and-see policy according to tumor presentation. J Clin Oncol. 2011;29(26):3553–8.
21. Crago AM, Denton B, Salas S, et al. A prognostic nomogram for prediction of recurrence in desmoid fibromatosis. Ann Surg. 2013;258(2):347–53.
22. Lazar AJF, Tuvin D, Hajibashi S, et al. Specific mutations in the β-catenin gene (CTNNB1) correlate with local recurrence in sporadic desmoid tumors. Am J Pathol. 2008;173(5):1518–27.
23. Colombo C, Miceli R, Lazar AJ, et al. CTNNB1 45F mutation is a molecular prognosticator of increased postoperative primary desmoid tumor recurrence. Cancer. 2013;119:3696–702.
24. Cates JM, Stricker TP. Surgical resection margins in desmoid-type fibromatosis: a critical reassessment. Am J Surg Pathol. 2014;38(12):1707–14.
25. Gronchi A, Colombo C, Le Pechoux C, et al. Sporadic desmoid-type fibromatosis: a stepwise approach to a non-metastasising neoplasm – a position paper from the Italian and the French sarcoma group. Ann Oncol. 2014;25:578–83.
26. Janinis J, Patriki M, Vini L, et al. The pharmacological treatment of aggressive fibromatosis: a systematic review. Ann Oncol. 2003;14:181–90.
27. Garbay D, Cesne AL, Penel N, et al. Chemotherapy in patients with desmoid tumors: a study from the French sarcoma group (FSG). Ann Oncol. 2012;23:182–6.
28. de Camargo VP, Keohan ML, D'Adamo DR, et al. Clinical outcomes of systemic therapy for patients with deep fibromatosis (desmoid tumors). Cancer. 2010;116(9):2258–65.
29. Gega M, Yanagi H, Yoshikawa R, et al. Successful chemotherapeutic modality of doxorubicin plus dacarbazine for the treatment of desmoid tumors in association with familial adenomatous polyposis. J Clin Oncol. 2006;24(1):102–5.
30. Heinrich MC, McArthur GA, Demetri GD, et al. Clinical and molecular studies of the effect of Imatinib on advanced aggressive fibromatosis (desmoid tumor). J Clin Oncol. 2006;24(7):1195–203.
31. Gounder MM, Lefkowitz RA, Keohan ML, et al. Activity of Sorafenib against desmoid tumor/deep fibromatosis. Clin Cancer Res. 2011;17:4082–90.
32. Bonvalot S, Ternes N, Fiore M, et al. Spontaneous regression of primary abdominal wall desmoid tumors: more common than previously thought. Ann Surg Oncol. 2013;20:4096–102.
33. Fiore M, Coppola S, Cannell AJ, et al. Desmoid-type fi bromatosis and pregnancy: a multiinstitutional analysis of recurrence and obstetric risk. Ann Surg. 2014;259:973–8.
34. Gluck I, Griffith KA, Biermann JS, et al. Role of radiotherapy in the management of desmoid tumors. Int J Radiat Oncol Biol Phys. 2011;80(3):787–92.
35. Farma JM, Ammori JB, Zager JS, et al. Dermatofibrosarcoma protuberans: how wide should we resect? Ann Surg Oncol. 2010;17:2112–8.
36. Mendenhall WM, Zlotecki RA, Scarborough MT. Dermatofibrosarcoma protuberans. Cancer. 2004;101:2503–8.
37. Shields CJ, Winter DC, Kirwan WO, Redmond HP. Desmoid tumours. Eur J Surg Oncol. 2001;27:701–6.
38. McArthur GA, Demetri GD, van Oosterom A, et al. Molecular and clinical analysis of locally advanced dermatofibrosarcoma protuberans treated with imatinib: imatinib target exploration consortium study B2225. J Clin Oncol. 2005;23(4):866–73.

39. Gronchi A, Casali PG, Mariani L, et al. Quality of surgery and outcome in extra-abdominal aggressive fibromatosis: a series of patients surgically treated at a single institution. J Clin Oncol. 2003;21(7):1390–7.
40. Fields RC, Hameed M, Qin L, et al. Dermatofibrosarcoma protuberans (DFSP): predictors of recurrence and the use of systemic therapy. Ann Surg Oncol. 2011;18:328–36.
41. Gounder MM, Mahoney MR, Van Tine BA, Ravi V, Attia S, Deshpande HA, et al. Sorafenib for advanced and refractory desmoid tumors. N Engl J Med. 2018;379(25):2417–28.
42. Toulmonde M, Ray-Coquard IL, Pulido M, Andre T, Isambert N, Chevreau C, et al. DESMOPAZ pazopanib (PZ) versus IV methotrexate/vinblastine (MV) in adult patients with progressive desmoid tumors (DT) a randomized phase II study from the French Sarcoma Group. J Clin Oncol. 2018;36(15_suppl):11501.
43. Chugh R, Wathen JK, Patel SR, Maki RG, Meyers PA, Schuetze SM, et al. Efficacy of imatinib in aggressive fibromatosis: results of a phase II multicenter Sarcoma Alliance for Research through Collaboration (SARC) trial. Clin Cancer Res. 2010;16(19):4884–91.
44. Azzarelli A, Gronchi A, Bertulli R, Tesoro JD, Baratti D, Pennacchioli E, et al. Low-dose chemotherapy with methotrexate and vinblastine for patients with advanced aggressive fibromatosis. Cancer. 2001;92(5):1259–64.
45. Patel SR, Evans HL, Benjamin RS. Combination chemotherapy in adult desmoid tumors. Cancer. 1993;72(11):3244–7.
46. Constantinidou A, Jones RL, Scurr M, Al-Muderis O, Judson I. Advanced aggressive fibromatosis: effective palliation with chemotherapy. Acta Oncol (Madr). 2011;50(3):455–61.
47. Nishida Y, Tsukushi S, Shido Y, Urakawa H, Arai E, Ishiguro N. Transition of treatment for patients with extra-abdominal desmoid tumors: Nagoya university modality. Cancers (Basel). 2012;4(1):88–99.
48. Tsukada K, Church JM, Jagelman DG, Fazio VW, McGannon E, George CR, et al. Noncytotoxic drug therapy for intra-abdominal desmoid tumor in patients with familial adenomatous polyposis. Dis Colon Rectum. 1992;35(1):29–33.
49. Edmonson JH, Ryan LM, Blum RH, Brooks JS, Shiraki M, Frytak S, et al. Randomized comparison of doxorubicin alone versus ifosfamide plus doxorubicin or mitomycin, doxorubicin, and cisplatin against advanced soft tissue sarcomas. J Clin Oncol. 1993;11(7):1269–75.
50. Fiore M, Colombo C, Radaelli S, Prestianni P, Sanfilippo R, Morosi C, et al. Activity of toremifene in sporadic desmoid-type fibromatosis. J Clin Oncol [Internet]. 2011;29(15_suppl):10033.
51. Kummar S, O'Sullivan Coyne G, Do KT, Turkbey B, Meltzer PS, Polley E, et al. Clinical activity of the γ-secretase inhibitor PF-03084014 in adults with desmoid tumors (aggressive fibromatosis). J Clin Oncol. 2017;35(14):1561–9.
52. Righetti AEM, Jacomini C, Parra RS, De Almeida ALNR, JJR R, Féres O. Familial adenomatous polyposis and desmoid tumors. Clinics. 2011;66(10):1839–42.
53. Allen PW, Hasan N, Thorburn M. Nuchal-type fibroma appearance in a desmoid fibromatosis. Am J Surg Pathol. 2001;25(6):828–9.
54. Mullen JT. Dermatofibrosarcoma protuberans. Surg Oncol Clin N Am. 2016;25(4):827–39.
55. Crago AM, Chmielecki J, Rosenberg M, Oconnor R, Byrne C, Wilder FG, et al. Near universal detection of alterations inCTNNB1and Wnt pathway regulators in desmoid-type fibromatosis by whole-exome sequencing and genomic analysis. Genes Chromosom Cancer. 2015;54(10):606–15.
56. Zreik RT, Fritchie KJ. Morphologic spectrum of desmoid-type fibromatosis. Am J Clin Pathol. 2016;145(3):332–40.
57. Salas S, Chibon F, Noguchi T, Terrier P, Ranchere-Vince D, Lagarde P, et al. Molecular characterization by array comparative genomic hybridization and DNA sequencing of 194 desmoid tumors. Genes Chromosom Cancer. 2010;49(6):560–8.
58. Choi JH, Ro JY. Cutaneous spindle cell neoplasms: pattern-based diagnostic approach. Arch Pathol Lab Med. 2018;142(8):958–72.

59. Church J, Berk T, Boman BM, et al. Staging intra-abdominal desmoid tumors in familial adenomatous polyposis: a search for a uniform approach to a troubling disease. Dis Colon Rectum. 2005;48(8):1528–34.
60. Penel N, Cesne AL, Bonvalot S, Giraud A, Bompas E, Rios M, et al. Surgical versus non-surgical approach in primary desmoid-type fibromatosis patients: a nationwide prospective cohort from the French Sarcoma Group. Eur J Cancer. 2017;83:125–31.
61. Eva A, In'T Veld H, Coevorden FV, Grünhagen DJ, Smith MJ, ACJV A, MWJM W, et al. Outcome after surgical treatment of dermatofibrosarcoma protuberans: is clinical follow-up always indicated? Cancer. 2019;125(5):735–41.
62. Gladdy RA, Wunder JS. Risk-stratified surveillance in dermatofibrosarcoma protuberans: less is more. Cancer. 2019;125(5):670–2.
63. Colombo C, Miceli R, Le Pechoux C, et al. Sporadic extra abdominal wall desmoid-type fibromatosis: surgical resection can be safely limited to a minority of patients. Eur J Cancer. 2015;51:186–92.
64. Cassidy MR, Lefkowitz RA, Long N, Qin L-X, Kirane A, Sbaity E, et al. Association of MRI T2 signal intensity with desmoid tumor progression during active observation. Ann Surg. 2018;271:748.
65. Kasper B, Gronchi A, et al. The management of desmoid tumours: A joint global consensus-based guideline approach for adult and paediatric patients. Desmoid Tumor Working Group. Eur J Cancer. 2020;127:96–107. https://doi.org/10.1016/j.ejca.2019.11.013. PMID: 32004793.

Esophageal Cancer

9

Nicolas Devaud, Vaibhav Gupta, Eran Shlomovitz, Jonathan C. Yeung, Michael Ko, and Gail Darling

Introduction

Esophageal cancer is an ominous disease worldwide, with a 5-year survival ranging from 4 to 40%, depending on stage, and an 18% overall 5-year survival [1].

In recent years, a sixfold increase in incidence for adenocarcinoma in the United States and Canada from 1975 to 2000 has been documented, making it the most rapidly increasing cancer in North America [2].

Because early esophageal cancer (EC) is frequently asymptomatic, the majority (about 60%) of patients have advanced cancer when diagnosed, with dysphagia as the most common presenting symptom.

The most common histologic types of EC are squamous cell carcinoma (SCC) and esophageal adenocarcinoma (EAC), with the majority in the Western world being EAC. Less than 2% of all esophageal cancers are mesenchymal tumors (GIST, leiomyosarcoma) or small cell carcinoma. Lymphoma, neuroendocrine tumor, and melanoma can also develop in the esophagus, but with even lower incidence [3].

N. Devaud
Complex General Surgical Oncology, University of Toronto, Toronto, ON, Canada
e-mail: Nicolas.devaud@uhn.ca

V. Gupta
General Surgery Resident, University of Toronto, Toronto, ON, Canada
e-mail: vaibhav.gupta@mail.utoronto.ca

E. Shlomovitz · J. C. Yeung · M. Ko · G. Darling (✉)
Department of Surgery, University of Toronto, Toronto, ON, Canada
e-mail: eran.shlomovitz@uhn.ca; jonathan.yeung@uhn.ca;
mko@stjoestoronto.ca, michael.ko@unityhealth.to; gail.darling@uhn.ca

F. C. Wright et al. (eds.), *Surgical Oncology Manual*,
https://doi.org/10.1007/978-3-030-48363-0_9

Epidemiology

- EC is the eighth most common cancer worldwide and the sixth leading cause of cancer-related mortality [4].
- Its incidence varies greatly geographically. Squamous cell carcinoma (SCC) is the most prevalent histological type worldwide, particularly in countries of East Asia, Eastern Africa, and South America. In Western countries such as the United States, Canada, United Kingdom, Finland, France, and Australia, there is a predominance of esophageal adenocarcinoma (EAC).
- Asia represents 75% of the world's burden of EC, with an age-standardized rate for incidence (ASR-I) in Eastern Asia of 11/100000. China alone accounts for 50% of the world's EC incidence [1].
- The overall incidence for SCC increases with age, reaching a peak in the seventh decade. Major risk factors for SCC are alcohol consumption and tobacco use. Smoking, in combination with alcohol, has been proven to have a synergistic effect and increases the relative risk with an OR for combined alcohol and tobacco use of 3.28 (95% confidence interval (CI), $P = 0.05$) [5].
- Race and gender are also known risk factors. The relative risk in men who use both heavy tobacco and alcohol is 35.4 in white males and 149.2 in black males, compared to men of the same race and region who were non-smokers or drinkers [6]. The average male:female ratio for SCC is 2.5, and for EAC the ratio is 4.4 [1].
- From 1975 to 2004, the incidence of EAC among white American males increased by more than 460% and by 355% among white American females [7].
- Obesity and gastroesophageal reflux (GERD) have a distinct link to EAC. Therefore, adenocarcinoma of the esophagus occurs predominantly in the distal esophagus or gastroesophageal junction, compared to SCC which occurs mostly in the cervical, proximal, and mid thoracic esophagus. GERD is related to the development of Barrett's esophagus (BE) and the risk of developing EC is 50–100 times more likely in those with BE [8]. However, less than 5% of patients diagnosed with adenocarcinoma of the esophagus have a prior diagnosis of BE [9].

Diagnosis and Staging

Progressive dysphagia, initially to solids and later to soft and liquid diet, is usually the presenting symptom and is associated with general signs of malignancy such as weight loss and anemia. As dysphagia to solids is a relatively late symptom, EC is usually diagnosed in advanced stages. The incidence by stage defined as localized, regional, and distant disease in Eastern countries is 33%, 37.8%, and 17.3%, respectively, mostly for SCC [10]. In the Western population, particularly North America, localized disease accounts for 24%, 36% is regional and 40% presents with distant disease at the time of diagnosis with 67% of patients presenting with EAC [11, 12].

Diagnosis at the early stage is usually the result of a fortuitous incidental finding after an upper endoscopy for other symptoms.

Clinical staging is critical for deciding whether a patient is a candidate for endoscopic resection, upfront surgery, induction therapy, or palliation. The staging workup may include esophagogastroduodenoscopy (EGD) + biopsy, barium swallow, endoscopic ultrasound (EUS), CT, and FDG PET/CT. In upper and middle thoracic tumors, a bronchoscopy should be considered to rule out bronchial/tracheal involvement. Involvement of these structures would be a contraindication for radiation due to the high risk of post-radiation fistula and also precludes surgical therapy.

EGD and Barium Swallow

- Endoscopy allows for an anatomic evaluation of the tumor in relation to the hiatus and squamo-columnar junction, along with tumor length, degree of circumferential involvement, degree of obstruction, and presence of Barrett's esophagus.
- Endoscopy also allows for histological diagnosis by biopsy. Histopathologic cell type and grade markedly influence survival and guide management.
- Barium swallow has been used as the initial diagnostic test in the past but has largely been supplanted by endoscopy.

Endoscopic Ultrasonography (EUS)

- EUS is the most sensitive test for locoregional staging in EC. EUS can determine the depth of tumor invasion (cT), as well as confirm nodal involvement of suspicious paraesophageal or perigastric lymph nodes through fine-needle aspiration (cN). EUS is however a costly and operator-dependent procedure which may not be available in all centers.
- The greatest impact of EUS is defining those who will benefit from neoadjuvant chemoradiotherapy and surgery versus early-stage patients who may only require surgery. It cannot reliably differentiate between T1a and T1b, limiting its effectiveness in defining patients who may be candidates for endoscopic therapy.
- The accuracy of EUS for evaluating primary tumor and nodal status has been reported to be 85% and 75% respectively, while the sensitivity has been reported to be in the range of 85–95% for primary tumor evaluation and 70–80% for nodal evaluation [13].
- Obstructing lesions limit the passage of the EUS scope, precluding evaluation in patients with advanced disease. However, such patients generally have locally advanced disease (T3 or T4) and have a high probability of N+ disease. Therefore they will be candidates for combined modality therapy on this basis alone.

CT

- CT of the chest and abdomen is useful in initial staging for evaluating the primary tumor, regional nodes, and metastatic disease. Identification of distant metastatic disease on CT obviates the need for PET-CT. CT is also useful to determine the location of the tumor as well as involvement of adjacent structures.

- CT angiogram may be useful to determine the patency and quality of the right gastroepiploic artery, especially in situations where the patient has evidence of atherosclerosis elsewhere.

FDG-PET/CT

- FDG-PET CT is useful to determine a) the baseline FDG uptake of the primary tumor prior to induction therapy, b) the presence of locoregional disease, c) the presence of distant metastatic disease, and d) response to therapy (post-treatment).
- SCC and EAC have differential uptake in FDG-PET. Most studies have found a high degree of FDG-avidity in SCC at the primary tumor site. The majority of false negatives appear to be in small-volume tumors [14]. In contrast, insufficient or absent FDG uptake by the primary tumor is more frequently encountered in EAC. However, this depends on tumor growth type, differentiation, and mucus content.
- Non-avid EAC tumors are often poorly differentiated, showing a diffuse, non-intestinal growth type and mucus-containing tumor type (signet ring variant) [15].
- FDG-PET is superior to contrast-enhanced CT for the detection of metastatic nodes [10]. The sensitivity, specificity, and accuracy of PET-CT is 52%, 94%, and 84%, respectively, compared to 15%, 97%, and 77%, respectively, for CT [16].
- PET has also been shown to have higher accuracy (82% vs 64%) and sensitivity (74% vs 47%) when compared to CT and EUS for the detection of distant metastatic disease [17].
- The degree of FDG-avidity may potentially be used to assess response to induction therapy [18].
- One limitation of FDG-PET is the difficulty of detecting nodes close to the primary tumor (3 cm or less). Intense FDG uptake by the primary tumor can often obscure the detection of nearby associated nodal metastasis, leading to false negatives.
- False positives can also be the result of inflammatory disease causing increased FDG uptake, such as sarcoidosis.

Staging, AJCC, Eighth Edition

For the purpose of staging, the esophagus is usually divided in three anatomic compartments: cervical, thoracic, and abdominal esophagus. The thoracic esophagus is also divided arbitrarily into equal thirds: upper, middle, and lower.

The cervical esophagus anatomically lies in the neck, bordered superiorly by the hypopharynx and inferiorly by the thoracic inlet at the level of the sternal notch. It extends from 15 to 20 cm measured from the incisors. Cancers located in the cervical esophagus are staged as upper thoracic esophageal cancers and not as head and neck cancers [19].

For staging purposes, the AJCC, Eighth Edition, includes gastroesophageal junction tumors which have an epicenter within 2 cm of the cardia (Siewert types I/II). Tumors with an epicenter more than 2 cm distal to the cardia are staged as gastric cancers (Tables 9.1, 9.2, 9.3, 9.4, 9.5, 9.6).

AJCC, Eighth Edition, staging system includes cTNM, yTNM for post-neoadjuvant treatment restaging, pTNM for pathologic staging after esophagectomy alone, and ypTNM for pathologic staging after esophagectomy with induction therapy, where histology and tumor location are included. SCC staging pTNM includes tumor location.

Table 9.1 Primary tumor (T): all carcinomas

T category	T criteria
TX	Tumor cannot be assessed
T0	No evidence of primary tumor
Tis	High-grade dysplasia, defined as malignant cells confined to the epithelium by the basement membrane
T1	Tumor invades the lamina propria, muscularis mucosae, or submucosa
T1a	Tumor invades lamina propria or muscularis mucosae
T1b	Tumor invades the submucosa
T2	Tumor invades the muscularis propria
T3	Tumor invades adventitia
T4	Tumor invades adjacent structures
T4a	Tumor invades the pleura, pericardium, azygos vein, diaphragm, or peritoneum
T4b	Tumor invades other adjacent structures, such as the aorta, vertebral body, or airway

Table 9.2 Regional lymph nodes (N): all carcinomas

N category	N criteria
NX	Regional lymph nodes cannot be assessed
N0	No regional lymph node metastasis
N1	Metastasis in 1–2 regional lymph nodes
N2	Metastasis in 3–6 regional lymph nodes
N3	Metastasis in ≥7 regional lymph nodes

Table 9.3 Distant metastasis (M): all carcinomas

M category	M criteria
M0	No distant metastasis
M1	Distant metastasis

Table 9.4 Histologic grade: all carcinomas

G	G definition
GX	Grade cannot be assessed
G1	Well differentiated
G2	Moderately differentiated
G3	Poorly differentiated

Table 9.5 Definition of location: squamous cell carcinoma

Location category	Location criteria
X	Unknown
Upper	Cervical esophagus to lower border of azygos vein
Middle	Lower border of azygos vein to lower border of pulmonary vein
Lower	Lower border of inferior pulmonary vein to stomach, including GE junction

Table 9.6 SCC and adenocarcinoma post-neoadjuvant treatment stages (ypTNM)

ypT	ypN	ypM	Stage
T0–2	N0	M0	I
T3	N0	M0	II
T0–2	N1	M0	IIIA
T3	N1	M0	IIIB
T0–3	N2	M0	IIIB
T4a	N0	M0	IIIB
T4a	N1–2	M0	IVA
T4a	NX	M0	IVA
T4b	N0–2	M0	IVA
Any T	N3	M0	IVA
Any T	AnyN	M1	IVB

Treatment

Treatment of EC is based on a multimodal approach that is determined by the histologic subtype, location, and clinical staging (cTNM). This approach may include upfront resection for early-stage disease (endoscopic or surgical), neoadjuvant therapy (chemoradiotherapy or chemotherapy) followed by surgery, definitive chemoradiotherapy, or palliative systemic treatment.

The treatment of thoracic esophageal cancer is generally determined by cTNM; however, many centers would alter the approach for locally advanced disease depending on SCC or EAC, in some cases with a preference toward definitive chemoradiotherapy for SCC and trimodality therapy for EAC.

Cervical Esophagus

- Pharyngo-laryngo-esophagectomy (PLE) was considered the gold standard of treatment for cervical SCC for many years. However, it is associated with a high incidence of postoperative morbidity and mortality. Anastomotic leakage and operative mortality are both described at ~9% [20]. It also causes a significantly compromised quality of life.
- Definitive chemoradiation (CRT) has evolved as a curative treatment modality for cervical esophageal SCC. Studies have shown similar overall survival with

definitive CRT compared to surgery, with a superior post-therapeutic quality of life compared to PLE, particularly because laryngectomy is avoided.

- Definitive CRT includes a three-dimensional conformal approach with a total radiation dose of 60–68 Gy. Cisplatin and 5-FU based chemotherapy is given concurrently for a total of four cycles [21].

High-volume institutions treating esophageal SCC have reported their results comparing PLE to definitive CRT in cervical esophageal cancer. Median overall survival for patients treated with PLE was 19.9 months vs 24.9 months among those treated with CRT. After stratifying for intent of resection (R-category) in the PLE patients and response to chemotherapy in the CRT, patients with curative PLE (R0) had a median survival of 22.4 months vs 28.6 months in CRT responders [21]. Therefore, definitive chemoradiation has emerged as the treatment of choice for patients with cervical SCC.

Thoracic Esophagus

Clinical Stage 0-I

Endoscopic Resection

- Lesions that do not infiltrate beyond the mucosa or lamina propria (cT1a) are rarely accompanied by lymph-node metastasis (<5%) [22]. Endoscopic resection is therefore a potentially curative treatment for such lesions.
- Lesions that reach the muscularis mucosae or infiltrate the upper submucosa (up to 200 μm: SM1) are associated with a 10% rate of lymph-node metastasis. Endoscopic resection remains feasible for selected patients with no clinical or radiologic evidence of lymph-node metastasis. However, surgical resection is also an appropriate option for fit patients with T1b SM1, given the lymph node metastasis rate. The decision to proceed with endoscopic resection versus upfront surgery requires a careful discussion with the patient regarding benefits of either treatment.
- Lesions showing deep invasion of the submucosa (more than 200 μm; SM2, SM3) are associated with a 25–50% rate of lymph-node metastasis and therefore fit patients should be offered upfront surgical resection.
- Lesions requiring a circumferential mucosal resection exceeding two-thirds of the circumference of the esophagus are relative contraindication for endoscopic treatment, considering the high rate of postoperative stenosis [23]. These patients are considered for upfront surgery.

Definitive Chemoradiotherapy in SCC

- Can be an alternative for patients with mucosal cancers that are too wide to be resected endoscopically.
- A phase II study of definitive chemoradiotherapy for stage I SCC of the esophagus (JCOG 9708) demonstrated a complete response rate of 96% and a 2-year

survival rate of 93% [24]. These results, comparable to radical surgery in Japan, are currently being studied in a phase III study JCOG 0502.

Clinical Stage II-III (except cT4)

Neoadjuvant Chemoradiotherapy Followed by Radical Surgery

A number of different regimens for preoperative induction therapy with chemotherapy or chemoradiotherapy have been described (Table 9.7). Prior to 2015,

Table 9.7 Randomized clinical trials (RCT) comparing neoadjuvant chemoradiation treatment and surgery vs surgery alone in esophageal cancer

Study	Methods	Results
Urba et al. 2001 [25]	RCT, $N = 100$ Surgery alone vs chemoradiation followed by surgery. Chemoradiation: Cisplatin +5FU + vinblastine Radiation: 1.5 Gy twice/day × 21 days Surgery: Transhiatal esophagectomy, day 42	Median follow-up = 8.2 years Median OS = 17.6 months vs 16.9 months 3-year OS = 16% vs 30% [HR 0.73 (95% CI, 0.48–1.12) $p = 0.15$]
Medical Research Council Oesophageal Cancer Working Party 2002 [26]	RCT, $N = 802$ CS arm ($N = 400$): Cisplatin +5FU +/– radiation followed by surgery S arm ($N = 402$): Surgery alone Primary endpoint: Survival time by intention to treat	OS was better in the CS group (hazard ratio 0.79; 95% CI 0·67–0·93; $p = 0·004$). Median survival was 512 days (16·8 months) in the CS group vs 405 days (13·3 months) in the S group (difference 107 days; 95% CI 30–196). 2-year survival rates were 43% and 34% (difference 9%; 3–14).
RTOG trial 2007 [27]	RCT, $N = 443$ Preoperative chemotherapy followed by surgery vs surgery alone Pre-op chemo ($N = 216$): 3 cycles of cisplatin +5FU Radiation therapy not part of preoperative treatment plan Primary endpoint: Overall survival	No difference in overall survival for patients receiving perioperative chemotherapy compared with the surgery-only group
CROSS trial 2015 [28]	RCT, $N = 368$ Weekly neoadjuvant chemoradiotherapy (intravenous carboplatin and intravenous paclitaxel for 23 days) with concurrent radiotherapy followed by surgery, or surgery alone Primary endpoint was overall survival, analyzed by intention-to-treat	Median OS for chemoradiation plus surgery vs surgery alone SCC: 81.6 vs 21.1 months (HR 0·48 [95% CI 0·28–0·83]) EAC: 43.2 vs 27.1 months (HR 0·73 [95% CI 0·55–0·98]; log-rank $p = 0·038$).

most induction therapy was being performed with cisplatin/5FU followed by surgery for resectable clinical stage II-III esophageal cancer. However, the CROSS trial introduced a new regimen of neoadjuvant chemoradiation of intravenous carboplatin [AUC 2 mg/mL per min] and paclitaxel [50 mg/m2 of body-surface area for 23 days] with concurrent radiotherapy (41.4 Gy, given in 23 fractions of 1.8 Gy on 5 days per week). This regimen has shown the highest survival benefit for resectable stage II/III EC. The median overall survival for SCC was 81.6 vs. 21.1 months for trimodality therapy vs. surgery alone. For EAC, median overall survival was 43.2 vs. 27.1 months in the experimental arm vs. surgery alone [28].

Surgery

McKeown vs Akiyama: For SCC of the thoracic esophagus, a two- vs. three-field lymph-node dissection has long been a matter of discussion between the East (Japan) and the West.

The McKeown esophagogastrectomy may be used for SCC or EAC. It includes 1) an initial thoracic approach with esophageal dissection and radical lymphadenectomy, including nodes over the level of the azygous vein and recurrent laryngeal nerve, 2) a subsequent abdominal approach for construction of the gastric conduit and abdominal lymph node dissection, and 3) a third cervical approach to complete the cervical esophagogastric anastomosis in the neck. The Akiyama operation follows the same steps as the McKeown, though it includes a radical cervical lymph node dissection at the time of the cervical anastomosis.

In Japan, the radical cervical lymph node dissection improved outcomes slightly in patients with SCC of the thoracic esophagus, though the 5-year survival rate did not reach 70% [22]. Patients included in the CROSS trial had a two-field lymph-node dissection with a similar 5-year overall survival close to 70%. Overall, morbidity described for the Akiyama approach is 58%, with pulmonary complications occurring in 32.8%, cardiac dysrhythmias in 10.9%, and persistent recurrent laryngeal nerve problems in 2.6% [29].

Ivor Lewis: This two-field operation is primarily used for EAC located below the level of the carina. An abdominal approach is used to fashion the gastric conduit and to perform a radical lymph node dissection of the left gastric, common hepatic, and splenic arteries. Many surgical groups include a pyloroplasty as a standard to prevent delayed gastric emptying of the conduit, although this is decreasing in frequency. The second step in the operation is the thoracic approach for the thoracic esophageal dissection and radical lymph node dissection including inferior mediastinal nodes as well as the infracarinal lymph nodes. The anastomosis is completed above the azygous vein, with mechanical surgical staples or hand-sewn.

A Chinese trial published in 2015 compared Ivor Lewis esophagectomy (midline abdominal dissection followed by right thoracic dissection and anastomosis in the chest) with Sweet esophagectomy (left thoracoabdominal incision) for esophageal SCC [30]. It showed less morbidity, shorter hospital stay, fewer reoperations, greater lymph node yield, and a trend toward lower in-hospital mortality for the Ivor Lewis group.

Resection margins and en-bloc lymph node dissection: Many studies have compared transhiatal esophagectomy (THE) with the transthoracic esophagectomy (TTE), either McKeown or Ivor Lewis approach.

Both TTE and THE for thoracic esophageal cancer consider an abdominal and mediastinal lymph node dissection. The abdominal lymphadenectomy includes perigastric stations 1, 2, and 3 dissected en bloc with the specimen, left gastric nodes (station 7), celiac trunk, and common hepatic and splenic artery nodes (stations 8, 9, and 11).

TTE approach, however, enables an en-bloc dissection of the mediastinal nodes and a better control of the circumferential radial margin (CRM) compared to THE [31, 32].

Locoregional recurrences are predominant failure patterns in CRM-positive patients. In the first study of CRM involvement by Sagar et al., significantly more patients with a positive CRM (55%) developed a local recurrence as compared to those without involvement of the CRM (13%) [33]. Chao et al. found a significant influence of an involved CRM not only on locoregional but also on distant recurrences, while an involvement of the CRM of less than 1 mm was associated with early locoregional recurrences [34].

Longitudinal resection margin for thoracic esophageal cancer has not been as clearly defined as it has for distal/GEJ tumors. However, >3 cm proximal margin for SCC would render less than a 5% risk of margin involvement. For EAC, 7–10 cm proximal and 5 cm distal margins would be considered adequate.

TTE enables a better lymph node dissection compared to THE [32]. The optimum number of lymph nodes dissected will be dependent on T and N(+) stage. In pN + M0 cancers and 1 to 6 nodes positive, optimum lymphadenectomy is 10 for pT1, 15 for pT2, and 29 to 50 for pT3/T4 [35].

However, it is still unclear whether the more extensive removal of regional (metastatic or not) nodes contributes to the cure of patients with esophageal cancer.

Definitive Chemoradiotherapy and SCC

Chemoradiotherapy is a good definitive alternative for patients; however, neoadjuvant chemotherapy plus radical surgery has demonstrated the best long-term survival.

- In Japan, a phase II study was conducted to assess the effectiveness of definitive chemoradiotherapy in patients with stage II or III esophageal SCC (JCOG 9906). This study demonstrated a CR rate of 62% and a median survival time of 29 months, with 3- and 5-year survival rates of 44.7% and 36.8%, respectively [36].
- In a French trial comparing definitive chemoradiotherapy to neoadjuvant chemoradiotherapy followed by radical surgery, 259 patients with operable T3N0-1 M0 thoracic esophageal cancer, who had received two cycles of fluorouracil (5-FU) and cisplatin (days 1 to 5 and 22 to 26) and either conventional (46 Gy in 4.5 weeks) or split-course (15 Gy, days 1 to 5 and 22 to 26) concomitant radiotherapy, were randomized to surgery (arm A) or continuation of chemoradiation

(arm B; three cycles of FU/cisplatin and either conventional [20 Gy] or split-course [15 Gy] radiotherapy). Two-year survival rate was 34% in arm A versus 40% in arm B (hazard ratio for arm B vs. arm A = 0.90; adjusted $P = 0.44$). Median survival time was 17.7 months in arm A compared with 19.3 months in arm B. Two-year local control rate was 66.4% in arm A compared with 57.0% in arm B, and stents were required less often in the surgery arm (5% in arm A vs. 32% in arm B; $P < 0.001$). The 3-month mortality rate was 9.3% in arm A compared with 0.8% in arm B ($P = 0.002$) [37]. Neoadjuvant chemoradiation followed by radical surgery demonstrated a better local disease control; however, a higher perioperative mortality and similar overall survival were shown compared to definitive chemoradiation for SCC.

Clinical Stage III-IVa

Patients who fall in this clinical stage include those with cT4a, cN3, and cM0. They are usually treated with definitive chemoradiotherapy because survival outcomes after surgical treatment are generally poor. Phase II studies with cisplatin, 5-FU, and 60 Gy of radiotherapy in advanced thoracic esophageal cancer demonstrated a CR rate of 15–33% with a median survival time of 9–10 months [38, 39]. The addition of taxanes such as docetaxel to cisplatin plus 5-FU with concurrent radiotherapy (DCF-R) demonstrated a median progression-free survival of 11.1 months, and a median survival of 29.0 months with a survival rate of 43.9% at 3 years [40].

However, surgery may be still offered to patients with cT4aN1–2, given a more durable palliation with similar OS compared to definitive chemoradiation [41].

Clinical Stage IVb or Recurrent Disease

Palliation Chemotherapy in the setting of metastatic or recurrent disease is designed to improve survival and quality of life. Cisplatin plus 5-FU are the most commonly used regimens for combination palliative chemotherapy. Paclitaxel has demonstrated good results with acceptable toxicity as second-line treatment after platinum-based chemotherapy [42].

Palliation of symptoms such as dysphagia, pain, and bleeding can be treated with expandable endoscopic stents or radiotherapy including brachytherapy.

- When compared head-to-head, a 2004 randomized trial of brachytherapy versus self-expanding metal stents showed that long-term dysphagia relief was better with brachytherapy, with fewer complications and better quality of life scores [43].
- A 2005 study similarly showed more durable results with brachytherapy, although it is recognized that stents offer more immediate relief [44].

Abdominal Esophagus and Gastroesophageal Junction Adenocarcinoma (EAC)

Neoadjuvant and Adjuvant Therapies

- Induction therapy for EAC of the gastroesophageal junction (GEJ) remains controversial. This is because these tumors are often grouped together with proximal gastric cancers for the purposes of trial inclusion. This has led to a broad heterogeneity in practice. The main protocols that have been established are known as the MAGIC, POET, CROSS, and FLOT trials (Table 9.8).
- The MAGIC and CROSS regimens were considered to be standard of care until the presentation of FLOT. Longer-term follow-up and survival data with FLOT are highly anticipated and pending, but many centers adopted FLOT as standard of care when the results were presented, even prior to publication.

Table 9.8 Randomized clinical trials (RCT) comparing neoadjuvant or perioperative treatment in GEJ and gastric adenocarcinoma

Study	Methods	Results
MAGIC trial (2006) [45]	503 patients with gastric and GEJ cancer patients 25% of the population consisted of lower esophagus and GEJ tumors Compared 3 preoperative and 3 postoperative cycles of epirubicin, cisplatin, and fluorouracil (ECF) chemotherapy to surgery alone	5-year OS benefit with perioperative chemotherapy compared to surgery alone (36% vs 23%)
CROSS trial (2015) [28]	368 patients with esophageal and GEJ tumors (24%) Compared preoperative chemoradiotherapy (carboplatin, paclitaxel, and concurrent radiotherapy) to surgery alone	5-year OS of 47% in the chemoradiotherapy group, compared to 34% with surgery alone
FLOT trial (2019) [46]	716 patients with locally advanced, resectable gastric or GEJ adenocarcinoma Compared perioperative chemotherapy using fluorouracil, leucovorin, oxaliplatin, and docetaxel to the MAGIC regimen	Significant improvement in median overall survival of 50 months with FLOT compared to 35 months with ECF/ECX, giving a hazard ratio of 0.77 (95% CI 0.63–0.94)
POET trial (2009) [47]	119 patients with locally advanced AC of the lower esophagus or gastric cardia Randomized to 15 weeks of chemotherapy (n = 59) or 12 weeks of chemotherapy followed by 3 weeks of chemoradiotherapy (n = 60), followed by surgery	The study was closed early because of poor accrual, but showed a non-significant trend toward higher rates of complete response, lower recurrence, and improved survival with chemoradiotherapy

Based on the above data, patients with GEJ tumors should be offered preoperative chemoradiotherapy, with preoperative chemotherapy as an alternative. Ongoing trials will help define the optimal perioperative treatment of these cancers.

- Genomic characterization is identifying new options for biologic and targeted therapies to improve response rates and survival for gastroesophageal cancers.
- For patients with unresectable disease, the ToGa trial established a role for trastuzumab in the treatment of advanced HER2-positive GEJ AC (18% of study population) [48].
- Ramucirumab was also shown to increase overall survival for patients with advanced, pre-treated GEJ adenocarcinoma in the RAINBOW and REGARD trials [49, 50].
- Immune checkpoint inhibitors are actively being investigated for targeted therapy. Programmed death-ligand 1 (PD-L1) upregulation is seen in approximately 40% of gastroesophageal cancers, and PD-L1 inhibitors are showing encouraging results in select patients [51].
- It is likely that future neoadjuvant and adjuvant therapies will be guided by specific somatic genomic alternations and gene expression [52].

Surgical Therapy

The surgical approach has varied for GEJ tumors as well, and part of that variability comes from overlap in treatment by thoracic surgeons and upper GI surgeons.

- Resection is a mainstay in the treatment of GEJ cancer for fit patients who do not have disease involving distant sites or extra regional (para-aortic or mesenteric) lymph nodes. It is usually performed 4–6 weeks following preoperative therapy as part of the treatment plan.
- The surgical approach for Siewert 1 and 2 would be an Ivor Lewis esophagogastrectomy. However, the treatment for Siewert 2 EAC is a matter of debate since many upper GI surgeons would also treat with a D2 total gastrectomy and partial esophagectomy with a high intra-mediastinal esophago-jejunal anastomosis [53].
- The goals of surgery include complete (R0) resection of the primary tumor, with approximately a 7–10 cm proximal margin considering longitudinal intramural lymphatic progression. The optimum lymphadenectomy defined by pTNM is 10 to 12 nodes for pT1, 15 to 22 for pT2, and 31 to 42 for pT3/T4, depending on histopathologic cell type. In pN + M0 cancers with 1 to 6 nodes positive, optimum lymphadenectomy is 10 for pT1, 15 for pT2, and 29 to 50 for pT3/T4, but this remains debated in the literature [35].

Transthoracic Versus Transhiatal Esophagectomy

There is still controversy and limited evidence about the optimal surgical approach to tumors of the esophagogastric junction.

- A Dutch randomized trial in 2002 compared transhiatal esophagectomy to transthoracic McKeown esophagectomy for Siewert types 1 and 2 tumors. All patients

received partial gastrectomy and extended en-bloc lymphadenectomy. Less morbidity was observed with the transhiatal approach, but no difference in postoperative mortality [54]. However, there was a non-significant trend toward improved 5-year survival for Siewert type 1 tumors treated with the transthoracic approach [55].
- A Japanese trial in 2006 compared left thoracoabdominal to transhiatal partial esophagectomy with total gastrectomy and D2 lymphadenectomy in both groups, for Siewert types 2 and 3 tumors [56]. The left thoracoabdominal group had a thorough mediastinal lymph node dissection below the left inferior pulmonary vein. The trial closed early after a planned interim analysis because it seemed unlikely that the thoracoabdominal approach would yield improved survival compared to the transhiatal approach and had greater morbidity and mortality.

Patients with Siewert types 1 and 2 tumors are thus preferentially treated with transthoracic esophagectomy and partial gastrectomy with D2 lymphadenectomy (Ivor Lewis) to ensure an adequate 7–10 cm proximal esophageal and 5 cm distal gastric margin. Siewert types 2 and 3 tumors can be treated with total gastrectomy, transhiatal partial esophagectomy, and D2 lymphadenectomy. If there is concern about achieving an adequate proximal margin, the transthoracic approach should be used.

Extent of Lymphadenectomy

For tumors at the GEJ, an adequate regional lymph node dissection involves periesophageal nodes and a D2 lymphadenectomy, which entails removing perigastric nodes and those along the hepatic, left gastric, celiac, and splenic arteries.

- Mediastinal lymph node dissection appears to be more important for type 1 tumors, where up to 85% of lymph node metastases occur in the mediastinum, compared to 30% for type 2 and 10% for type 3 tumors [57, 58].
- Types 2 and 3 tumors do not appear to benefit from mediastinal lymph node dissection as those with positive nodes in the mediastinum already have significant abdominal lymphadenopathy [57, 59]. This may be the rationale to avoid the transthoracic approach for type 3 tumors.
- The rate of cervical lymph node metastases for adenocarcinoma of the GEJ has not been well studied and the role of cervical lymphadenectomy remains to be elucidated. However, similar to the above scenario, patients with cervical lymphadenopathy generally already have mediastinal lymphadenopathy and further dissection may not impact outcome.

Optimum lymphadenectomy for esophageal cancer continues to be debated, but it is clear that lymphadenectomy is associated with better staging and improved survival. A 2010 study of over 4600 patients from the Worldwide Esophageal Cancer Collaboration published by Rizk and colleagues looked at the optimum lymphadenectomy to maximize survival by stage and suggested resecting 10 nodes for pT1, 20 for pT2, and > 30 for pT3/4 [35].

However, in the developing era of multimodal neoadjuvant treatment for locoregional control and tumor downstaging, recent studies have questioned the survival benefit of extended lymphadenectomy for esophageal cancer. Lagergren et al., in a Swedish cohort of 606 patients with esophageal cancer (83% EAC), were unable to prove a significant difference in 5-year all-cause or disease-specific survival comparing extended lymphadenectomy (21–52 nodes) to limited lymph node dissection (0–10 nodes) (HR, 0.98; 95% CI, 0.57–1.66) [60].

Minimally Invasive Approach

Esophagectomy, gastrectomy, and lymphadenectomy can be performed with an open or minimally-invasive approach (thoracoscopic and laparoscopic). The advantages of minimally invasive approach can include smaller incisions, less pain, fewer complications, and shorter admissions, while achieving equivalent lymphadenectomy and resection margins [61–63]. Experience is being gained with robotic esophagectomy at specialized centers. Early reports show its safety and feasibility, but definitive evidence regarding its utility over laparoscopic and thoracoscopic esophagectomy is currently unavailable [64].

Summary

Classification of tumors at the GEJ continues to evolve and remains somewhat controversial. Future genomic alteration analyses will likely impact classification of these tumors as esophageal or gastric. Multiple modalities are now available to clinically stage patients and those with locally advanced tumors should be considered for neoadjuvant and adjuvant therapies to improve survival. Surgical resection is a mainstay in curative-intent treatment and should involve an adequate lymphadenectomy for accurate staging. Postoperative outcomes are improving with advances in minimally invasive techniques, enhanced recovery programs, and centralization of esophageal surgery to high-volume centers. Survival for resectable disease continues to improve with multimodality treatment, and future targeted, biological, and immuno-therapies may improve prognosis for esophageal cancer.

References

1. Malhotra GK, Yanala U, Ravipati A, Follet M, Vijayakumar M, Are C. Global trends in esophageal cancer. J Surg Oncol. 2017;115(5):564–79.
2. DaVee T, Ajani JA, Lee JH. Is endoscopic ultrasound examination necessary in the management of esophageal cancer? World J Gastroenterol. 2017;23(5):751–62.
3. Napier KJ, Scheerer M, Misra S. Esophageal cancer: a review of epidemiology, pathogenesis, staging workup and treatment modalities. World J Gastrointest Oncol. 2014;6(5):112–20.
4. Ferlay J, Soerjomataram I, Dikshit R, Eser S, Mathers C, Rebelo M, et al. Cancer incidence and mortality worldwide: sources, methods and major patterns in GLOBOCAN 2012. Int J Cancer. 2015;136(5):E359–86.

5. Prabhu A, Obi KO, Rubenstein JH. The synergistic effects of alcohol and tobacco consumption on the risk of esophageal squamous cell carcinoma: a meta-analysis. Am J Gastroenterol. 2014;109(6):822–7.
6. Lm S, Ep Q, Rh W. The next wave: confexting. J Digit Imaging. 2012;25(1):25–9.
7. Brown LM, Devesa SS, Chow WH. Incidence of adenocarcinoma of the esophagus among white Americans by sex, stage, and age. J Natl Cancer Inst. 2008;100(16):1184–7.
8. Mao WM, Zheng WH, Ling ZQ. Epidemiologic risk factors for esophageal cancer development. Asian Pac J Cancer Prev. 2011;12(10):2461–6.
9. Dulai GS, Guha S, Kahn KL, Gornbein J, Weinstein WM. Preoperative prevalence of Barrett's esophagus in esophageal adenocarcinoma: a systematic review. Gastroenterology. 2002;122(1):26–33.
10. Shin A, Won YJ, Jung HK, Kong HJ, Jung KW, Oh CM, et al. Trends in incidence and survival of esophageal cancer in Korea: analysis of the Korea Central Cancer Registry Database. J Gastroenterol Hepatol. 2018;33(12):1961–8.
11. Patel N, Benipal B. Incidence of esophageal cancer in the United States from 2001–2015: a United States cancer statistics analysis of 50 states. Cureus. 2018;10(12):e3709.
12. Hur C, Miller M, Kong CY, Dowling EC, Nattinger KJ, Dunn M, et al. Trends in esophageal adenocarcinoma incidence and mortality. Cancer. 2013;119(6):1149–58.
13. Romagnuolo J, Scott J, Hawes RH, Hoffman BJ, Reed CE, Aithal GP, et al. Helical CT versus EUS with fine needle aspiration for celiac nodal assessment in patients with esophageal cancer. Gastrointest Endosc. 2002;55(6):648–54.
14. Flamen P. Positron emission tomography in gastric and esophageal cancer. Curr Opin Oncol. 2004;16(4):359–63.
15. Stahl A, Ott K, Weber WA, Becker K, Link T, Siewert JR, et al. FDG PET imaging of locally advanced gastric carcinomas: correlation with endoscopic and histopathological findings. Eur J Nucl Med Mol Imaging. 2003;30(2):288–95.
16. Kim K, Park SJ, Kim BT, Lee KS, Shim YM. Evaluation of lymph node metastases in squamous cell carcinoma of the esophagus with positron emission tomography. Ann Thorac Surg. 2001;71(1):290–4.
17. Flamen P, Lerut A, Van Cutsem E, De Wever W, Peeters M, Stroobants S, et al. Utility of positron emission tomography for the staging of patients with potentially operable esophageal carcinoma. J Clin Oncol. 2000;18(18):3202–10.
18. Schroer-Gunther M, Scheibler F, Wolff R, Westwood M, Baumert B, Lange S. The role of PET and PET-CT scanning in assessing response to neoadjuvant therapy in esophageal carcinoma. Dtsch Arztebl Int. 2015;112(33–34):545–52.
19. Rice TW, Gress DM, Patil DT, Hofstetter WL, KelsenDP, Blackstone EH. Cancer of the esophagus and esophagogastric junction- Major changes in the American Joint Committee on Cancer eight edition cancer staging manual. Ca Cancer J Clin. 2017;67:304–17. https://doi.org/10.332/caac.21399.
20. Wei WI, Lam LK, Yuen PW, Wong J. Current status of pharyngolaryngo-esophagectomy and pharyngogastric anastomosis. Head Neck. 1998;20(3):240–4.
21. Tong DK, Law S, Kwong DL, Wei WI, Ng RW, Wong KH. Current management of cervical esophageal cancer. World J Surg. 2011;35(3):600–7.
22. Higuchi K, Koizumi W, Tanabe S, Sasaki T, Katada C, Azuma M, et al. Current management of esophageal squamous-cell carcinoma in Japan and other countries. Gastrointest Cancer Res. 2009;3(4):153–61.
23. Katada C, Muto M, Manabe T, Boku N, Ohtsu A, Yoshida S. Esophageal stenosis after endoscopic mucosal resection of superficial esophageal lesions. Gastrointest Endosc. 2003;57(2):165–9.
24. Kato H, Sato A, Fukuda H, Kagami Y, Udagawa H, Togo A, et al. A phase II trial of chemoradiotherapy for stage I esophageal squamous cell carcinoma: Japan Clinical Oncology Group Study (JCOG9708). Jpn J Clin Oncol. 2009;39(10):638–43.

25. Urba SG, Orringer MB, Turrisi A, Iannettoni M, Forastiere A, Strawderman M. Randomized trial of preoperative chemoradiation versus surgery alone in patients with locoregional esophageal carcinoma. J Clin Oncol. 2001;19(2):305–13.
26. Medical Research Council Oesophageal Cancer Working Group. Surgical resection with or without preoperative chemotherapy in oesophageal cancer: a randomised controlled trial. Lancet. 2002;359(9319):1727–33.
27. Kelsen DP, Winter KA, Gunderson LL, Mortimer J, Estes NC, Haller DG, et al. Long-term results of RTOG trial 8911 (USA intergroup 113): a random assignment trial comparison of chemotherapy followed by surgery compared with surgery alone for esophageal cancer. J Clin Oncol. 2007;25(24):3719–25.
28. Shapiro J, van Lanschot JJB, Hulshof MCCM, van Hagen P, van Berge Henegouwen MI, Wijnhoven BPL, et al. Neoadjuvant chemoradiotherapy plus surgery versus surgery alone for oesophageal or junctional cancer (CROSS): long-term results of a randomised controlled trial. Lancet Oncol. 2015;16(9):1090–8.
29. Lerut T, Nafteux P, Moons J, Coosemans W, Decker G, De Leyn P, et al. Three-field lymphadenectomy for carcinoma of the esophagus and gastroesophageal junction in 174 R0 resections: impact on staging, disease-free survival, and outcome. Ann Surg. 2004;240(6):962–74.
30. Li B, Xiang J, Zhang Y, Li H, Zhang J, Sun Y, et al. Comparison of Ivor-Lewis vs Sweet esophagectomy for esophageal squamous cell carcinoma: a randomized clinical trial. JAMA Surg. 2015;150(4):292–8.
31. Karstens KF, Izbicki JR, Reeh M. Does the margin matter in esophageal cancer. Dig Surg. 2018;35(3):196–203.
32. Pennathur A, Gibson MK, Jobe BA, Luketich JD. Oesophageal carcinoma. Lancet. 2013;381(9864):400–12.
33. Sagar PM, Johnston D, McMahon MJ, Dixon MF, Quirke P. Significance of circumferential resection margin involvement after oesophagectomy for cancer. Br J Surg. 1993;80(11):1386–8.
34. Chao YK, Yeh CJ, Chang HK, Tseng CK, Chu YY, Hsieh MJ, et al. Impact of circumferential resection margin distance on locoregional recurrence and survival after chemoradiotherapy in esophageal squamous cell carcinoma. Ann Surg Oncol. 2011;18(2):529–34.
35. Rizk NP, Ishwaran H, Rice TW, Chen LQ, Schipper PH, Kesler KA, et al. Optimum lymphadenectomy for esophageal cancer. Ann Surg. 2010;251(1):46–50.
36. Kato K, Muro K, Minashi K, Ohtsu A, Ishikura S, Boku N, et al. Phase II study of chemoradiotherapy with 5-fluorouracil and cisplatin for Stage II-III esophageal squamous cell carcinoma: JCOG trial (JCOG 9906). Int J Radiat Oncol Biol Phys. 2011;81(3):684–90.
37. Bedenne L, Michel P, Bouche O, Milan C, Mariette C, Conroy T, et al. Chemoradiation followed by surgery compared with chemoradiation alone in squamous cancer of the esophagus: FFCD 9102. J Clin Oncol. 2007;25(10):1160–8.
38. Ohtsu A, Boku N, Muro K, Chin K, Muto M, Yoshida S, et al. Definitive chemoradiotherapy for T4 and/or M1 lymph node squamous cell carcinoma of the esophagus. J Clin Oncol. 1999;17(9):2915–21.
39. Ishida K, Ando N, Yamamoto S, Ide H, Shinoda M. Phase II study of cisplatin and 5-fluorouracil with concurrent radiotherapy in advanced squamous cell carcinoma of the esophagus: a Japan Esophageal Oncology Group (JEOG)/Japan Clinical Oncology Group trial (JCOG9516). Jpn J Clin Oncol. 2004;34(10):615–9.
40. Higuchi K, Komori S, Tanabe S, Katada C, Azuma M, Ishiyama H, et al. Definitive chemoradiation therapy with docetaxel, cisplatin, and 5-fluorouracil (DCF-R) in advanced esophageal cancer: a phase 2 trial (KDOG 0501-P2). Int J Radiat Oncol Biol Phys. 2014;89(4):872–9.
41. Makino T. DY. Treatment of T4 esophageal cancer. Definitive chemo-radiotherapy vs chemoradiotherapy followed by surgery. Ann Thorac Cardiovasc Surg. 2011;17(3):221–8.
42. Tahara M, Minami H, Hasegawa Y, Tomita K, Watanabe A, Nibu K, et al. Weekly paclitaxel in patients with recurrent or metastatic head and neck cancer. Cancer Chemother Pharmacol. 2011;68(3):769–76.

43. Homs MY, Steyerberg EW, Eijkenboom WM, Tilanus HW, Stalpers LJ, Bartelsman JF, et al. Single-dose brachytherapy versus metal stent placement for the palliation of dysphagia from oesophageal cancer: multicentre randomised trial. Lancet. 2004;364(9444):1497–504.
44. Bergquist H, Wenger U, Johnsson E, Nyman J, Ejnell H, Hammerlid E, et al. Stent insertion or endoluminal brachytherapy as palliation of patients with advanced cancer of the esophagus and gastroesophageal junction. Results of a randomized, controlled clinical trial. Dis Esophagus. 2005;18(3):131–9.
45. Cunningham D, Allum WH, Stenning SP, Thompson JN, Van de Velde CJ, Nicolson M, et al. Perioperative chemotherapy versus surgery alone for resectable gastroesophageal cancer. N Engl J Med. 2006;355(1):11–20.
46. Al-Batran S-E, Homann N, Pauligk C, Goetze TO, Meiler J, Kasper S, et al. Perioperative chemotherapy with fluorouracil plus leucovorin, oxaliplatin, and docetaxel versus fluorouracil or capecitabine plus cisplatin and epirubicin for locally advanced, resectable gastric or gastro-oesophageal junction adenocarcinoma (FLOT4): a randomised, phase 2/3 trial. Lancet. 2019;393(10184):1948–57.
47. Stahl M, Walz MK, Stuschke M, Lehmann N, Meyer HJ, Riera-Knorrenschild J, et al. Phase III comparison of preoperative chemotherapy compared with chemoradiotherapy in patients with locally advanced adenocarcinoma of the esophagogastric junction. J Clin Oncol. 2009;27(6):851–6.
48. Bang YJ, Van Cutsem E, Feyereislova A, Chung HC, Shen L, Sawaki A, et al. Trastuzumab in combination with chemotherapy versus chemotherapy alone for treatment of HER2-positive advanced gastric or gastro-oesophageal junction cancer (ToGA): a phase 3, open-label, randomised controlled trial. Lancet. 2010;376(9742):687–97.
49. Wilke H, Muro K, Van Cutsem E, Oh SC, Bodoky G, Shimada Y, et al. Ramucirumab plus paclitaxel versus placebo plus paclitaxel in patients with previously treated advanced gastric or gastro-oesophageal junction adenocarcinoma (RAINBOW): a double-blind, randomised phase 3 trial. Lancet Oncol. 2014;15(11):1224–35.
50. Fuchs CS, Tomasek J, Yong CJ, Dumitru F, Passalacqua R, Goswami C, et al. Ramucirumab monotherapy for previously treated advanced gastric or gastro-oesophageal junction adenocarcinoma (REGARD): an international, randomised, multicentre, placebo-controlled, phase 3 trial. Lancet. 2014;383(9911):31–9.
51. Raufi AG, Klempner SJ. Immunotherapy for advanced gastric and esophageal cancer: preclinical rationale and ongoing clinical investigations. J Gastrointest Oncol. 2015;6(5):561–9.
52. Rice TW, Kelsen DP, Blackstone EH, Ishwaran H, Patil DT, Bass AJ, et al. Esophagus and esophagogastric junction. In: Amin MB, Edge SB, Greene FL, editors. AJCC Cancer staging manual. 8th ed. New York, NY: Springer; 2017. p. 185–202.
53. Barbour AP, Rizk NP, Gonen M, Tang L, Bains MS, Rusch VW, et al. Adenocarcinoma of the gastroesophageal junction: influence of esophageal resection margin and operative approach on outcome. Ann Surg. 2007;246(1):1–8.
54. Hulscher JB, van Sandick JW, de Boer AG, Wijnhoven BP, Tijssen JG, Fockens P, et al. Extended transthoracic resection compared with limited transhiatal resection for adenocarcinoma of the esophagus. N Engl J Med. 2002;347(21):1662–9.
55. Omloo JM, Lagarde SM, Hulscher JB, Reitsma JB, Fockens P, van Dekken H, et al. Extended transthoracic resection compared with limited transhiatal resection for adenocarcinoma of the mid/distal esophagus: five-year survival of a randomized clinical trial. Ann Surg. 2007;246(6):992–1000; discussion -1.
56. Sasako M, Sano T, Yamamoto S, Sairenji M, Arai K, Kinoshita T, et al. Left thoracoabdominal approach versus abdominal-transhiatal approach for gastric cancer of the cardia or subcardia: a randomised controlled trial. Lancet Oncol. 2006;7(8):644–51.
57. Dresner SM, Lamb PJ, Bennett MK, Hayes N, Griffin SM. The pattern of metastatic lymph node dissemination from adenocarcinoma of the esophagogastric junction. Surgery. 2001;129(1):103–9.

58. Pedrazzani C, de Manzoni G, Marrelli D, Giacopuzzi S, Corso G, Minicozzi AM, et al. Lymph node involvement in advanced gastroesophageal junction adenocarcinoma. J Thorac Cardiovasc Surg. 2007;134(2):378–85.
59. Kurokawa Y, Sasako M, Sano T, Yoshikawa T, Iwasaki Y, Nashimoto A, et al. Ten-year follow-up results of a randomized clinical trial comparing left thoracoabdominal and abdominal transhiatal approaches to total gastrectomy for adenocarcinoma of the oesophagogastric junction or gastric cardia. Br J Surg. 2015;102(4):341–8.
60. Lagergren J, Mattsson F, Zylstra J, Chang F, Gossage J, Mason R, et al. Extent of lymphadenectomy and prognosis after esophageal cancer surgery. JAMA Surg. 2016;151(1):32–9.
61. Biere SS, van Berge Henegouwen MI, Maas KW, Bonavina L, Rosman C, Garcia JR, et al. Minimally invasive versus open oesophagectomy for patients with oesophageal cancer: a multicentre, open-label, randomised controlled trial. Lancet. 2012;379(9829):1887–92.
62. Dantoc M, Cox MR, Eslick GD. Evidence to support the use of minimally invasive esophagectomy for esophageal cancer: a meta-analysis. Arch Surg. 2012;147(8):768–76.
63. Burdall OC, Boddy AP, Fullick J, Blazeby J, Krysztopik R, Streets C, et al. A comparative study of survival after minimally invasive and open oesophagectomy. Surg Endosc. 2015;29(2):431–7.
64. Bongiolatti S, Annecchiarico M, Di Marino M, Boffi B, Borgianni S, Gonfiotti A, et al. Robot-sewn Ivor-Lewis anastomosis: preliminary experience and technical details. Int J Med Robot. 2016;12(3):421–6.

Gallbladder Cancer

10

Nicolas Devaud, Natalie G. Coburn, and Melanie E. Tsang

Introduction

Gallbladder cancer (GBC) is an adenocarcinoma developing from the gallbladder mucosa. It is a relatively uncommon disease, with an incidence in North America from 1 to 2 cases per 100,000 population.

Incidence may significantly differ geographically, as in regions of East Asia, East Europe, and South America. Residents of the Indo-Gangetic belt, particularly females of northern India (21.5/100000) and south Karachi Pakistan (13.8/100000), have been reported as one of the highly affected population in the world. In southern Chile, the rate of GBC reaches 12.3/100000 for males and 27.3/100000 for females [1].

GBC is often found incidentally after an elective or emergent laparoscopic cholecystectomy for gallstone disease or cholecystitis. The main risk factors associated with the development of cancer include the following:

- Female:male ratio (1.3–3.5:1) [2]
- History of gallstones/cholecystitis [3–8]
- Ethnic groups: Native American, Mexican, East Asian, Hispanic [9]
- Obesity and a high carbohydrate diet [10, 11]
- Anomalous pancreaticobiliary duct junction (APBDJ) [12, 13]
- Chronic GB infection (*S. typhi*) [14]
- Age (increased incidence) [15]
- Previous gastric surgery [16]

N. Devaud
Complex General Surgical Oncology, University of Toronto, Toronto, ON, Canada
e-mail: nicolas.devaud@uhn.ca

N. G. Coburn · M. E. Tsang (✉)
Department of Surgery, University of Toronto, Toronto, ON, Canada
e-mail: natalie.coburn@sunnybrook.ca; Melanie.Tsang@unityhealth.to

F. C. Wright et al. (eds.), *Surgical Oncology Manual*,
https://doi.org/10.1007/978-3-030-48363-0_10

Definitions/Terminology

- *Simple cholecystectomy (SC)*: removal of the gall bladder and a portion of the cystic duct performed laparoscopically or open. Simple cholecystectomy is conducted in a subserosal plane.
- *Radical cholecystectomy (RC)*: removal of the gallbladder including a subsegmental or segmental 4B/5 liver resection, removal of the portal/hepatoduodenal lymph nodes and possible common bile duct excision (depending upon cystic duct margin status) with appropriate reconstruction.

Incidental Gallbladder Cancer (IGBC)

Almost 50% of all patients who present with gallbladder cancer are detected incidentally during or after elective/emergent cholecystectomy. Cancers detected at the time of surgery are referred to as incidental gallbladder cancer (IGBC). In most cases, cancer is diagnosed by a pathologist after the initial cholecystectomy (index cholecystectomy, IC). Following this IC, patients undergo clinical staging to complete later an oncologic extended resection and ensure removal of any local residual cancer.

There is conflicting data whether non-oncologic index cholecystectomy leading to discovery of IGBC negatively impacts survival. Early studies showed that long-term survival was not worse for patients with IGBC who undergo oncologic extended resection after prior simple cholecystectomy than for patients with non-IGBC who undergo upfront radical cholecystectomy [17–19].

However, recent data suggests that tumor disruption, such as in patients with the tumor in the dissection plane of a routine cholecystectomy (T2b, hepatic- side tumors), has a negative survival impact from IC [20]. Therefore, in trying to favor a single-time oncologic operation, a high level of suspicion should be kept before index cholecystectomy in patients with thickened gallbladder/chronic inflammatory changes in the preoperative imaging. Surgeons may change their approach (laparoscopic to open) if there is a high preoperative level of suspicion and be prepared for frozen section to decide upon completion of radical surgery favoring a single-time operation.

Staging

Unfortunately, less than 25% of patients will present with disease amenable for curative intent surgery at the time of diagnosis [21–24]. The high incidence of patients presenting with advanced disease, spillage of bile and tumor cells during initial cholecystectomy, evidence of rapid progression, and dismal prognosis when important residual disease is left after the first operation highlight the role of accurate restaging before oncologic extended resection.

The role of routine staging laparoscopy and paraaortic lymph node biopsy is a matter of debate to prevent a futile radical (most commonly open) surgery.

CT and MRI

- CT and MRI are the most common imaging techniques used to evaluate local and distant extension of disease and recognize the relationship between localized or residual tumor and nearby vascular structures and the biliary tree.
- MRI has a higher yield in detecting smaller liver metastatic lesions and their relationship with intrahepatic ducts. However, it has well-recognized limitations for the detection of tumor recurrence mostly related to difficulty in differentiating residual/recurrent tumor from surgically induced scarring or inflammatory changes.

PET-CT

- Limitations of cross-sectional imaging studies to restage patients with residual disease have prompted exploration of the added diagnostic value of FDG PET-CT. Functional imaging prior to attempted curative intervention could improve the pre-treatment selection of patients who might potentially benefit from such interventions.
- FDG PET-CT has been reported to improve the sensitivity to detect non-clinically evident metastatic disease. FDG PET-CT may change management by identifying metastatic disease not seen in previous studies in 23–25% of cases [25, 26].
- However, other studies have proven that sensitivity and positive predictive values of FDG PET-CT for residual disease may be as low as 28.5% and 20%, respectively, particularly among those patients with small volume carcinomatosis and signet ring cell tumors [25].
- These studies showed that the use of PET is definitively helpful in 5% and confirmatory in 15% of cases. However, in 3% of patients it may underestimate signs of unresectable disease. In the majority of patients, CT and PET were completely concordant and PET did not add any information [27].
- With modern high-quality cross-sectional imaging, it is uncommon for PET findings to be the sole determinant of resectability [27]. FDG PET-CT is therefore not routinely recommended unless there is persistent imaging uncertainty.

Staging Laparoscopy

- Staging laparoscopy identifies metastatic disease/locally advanced deemed unresectable in 27.6% of patients with suspected GBC [28].
- The yield of staging laparoscopy for identifying metastatic disease is higher among poorly differentiated, T3 or positive-margin gallbladder tumors [29].

Routine Paraaortic (Station 16b1) Lymph Node Biopsy.

- Involvement of paraaortic (16b1) lymph node in GBC is a sign of advanced disease with a prognosis equivalent to that of distant metastases [30].
- The appearance (size >10 mm and heterogeneous internal architecture) of the 16b1 lymph nodes on CT of the abdomen has been reported to be useful in predicting metastatic involvement in some studies; however, others have not found these factors to be good predictors of metastatic disease [31, 32].
- Routine 16b1 LN biopsy has proven to prevent non-therapeutic radical resection in 18.6% of patients deemed resectable on preoperative staging [33].

AJCC Eighth Edition

The recommended staging system is the International Union Against Cancer and American Joint Committee on Cancer (UICC/AJCC), eighth edition, with some changes introduced to the previous edition [34] (Tables 10.1, 10.2, 10.3, 10.4, 10.5).

The main change of this classification was the novel definition of T2a and T2b which effectively stratified the prognosis of patients with T2 GBC. Furthermore,

Table 10.1 Primary tumor (T)

T category	T criteria
TX	Primary tumor cannot be assessed
T0	No evidence of primary tumor
T1a T1b	Tumor invades lamina propria Tumor invades the muscular layer
T2a	Tumor invades the perimuscular connective tissue on the peritoneal side, without involvement of the serosa (visceral peritoneum)
T2b	Tumor invades the perimuscular connective tissue on the hepatic side, with no extension into the liver
T3	Tumor perforates serosa (visceral peritoneum) and/or directly invades the liver and/or other adjacent organ or structure, such as stomach, duodenum, colon, pancreas, omentum, or extrahepatic bile duct
T4	Tumor invades main portal vein or hepatic artery or invades two or more extrahepatic organs or structures

Table 10.2 Regional lymph node (N)

N category	N criteria
NX	Regional lymph nodes cannot be assessed
N0	No regional lymph node metastasis
N1	Metastases to 1–3 regional lymph nodes
N2	Metastases ≥4 regional lymph nodes

Table 10.3 Distant metastasis (M)

M category	M criteria
M0	No distant metastasis
M1	Distant metastasis

Table 10.4 AJCC prognostic stage groups

T	N	M	Stage
Tis	N0	M0	0
T1	N0	M0	I
T2a	N0	M0	IIA
T2b	N0	M0	IIB
T3	N0	M0	IIIA
T1–3	N1	M0	IIIB
T4	N0–1	M0	IVA
Any T	N2	M0	IVB
Any T	Any N	M1	IVB

Table 10.5 Survival by AJCC stage group

Presentation (AJCC staging system)	Prognosis (5-year overall survival (OS))
Early (stage 0–1)	50–100%
Advanced/regional (stage 2A-4A)	4–30%
Metastatic (stage 4B)	2%

patients with stage IIa tumors also obtained significantly improved overall survival time compared with patients with stage IIb tumors (Table 10.1). Additionally, the new N category stratified the survival of patients effectively based on the number of positive lymph nodes and not on their anatomical distribution (Table 10.2).

Management

Special Notes: (See Tables 10.6, 10.7, 10.8)

- In Ontario, all patients with known or suspected GBC should be referred for management at a high-volume hepatopancreatobiliary surgical oncology center.
- Bile spillage is estimated to occur in up to 20–40% of elective laparoscopic cholecystectomy [37–39]. Bile spillage that has occurred during laparoscopic cholecystectomy in the setting of a high-grade tumor should not delay or act as a deterrent for definitive surgery. Patients should be evaluated and treated according to the pathology of the tumor, and fitness of the patient for surgery, although they are likely at higher risk of recurrence.
- Further resection for T1b cancers has not been shown to improve overall survival but may decrease rate of recurrence [40, 41]. In reasonable operative candidates, recommendation is to proceed with segment 4B/5 resection and lymphadenectomy (Table 10.6).

Table 10.6 General approach

Gallbladder Polyps/ adenoma	Incidental finding Intraoperative diagnosis/ pathologic diagnosis	Suspected resectable GBC	Unresectable GBC
History and physical exam Ultrasound imaging Diagnostic workup should proceed as for suspected GBC if suggested by abnormal features on initial imaging For polyps of a size ≥1 cm, surgery is advised Consider laparoscopic cholecystectomy including cystic duct LN for 1–2 cm polyps, and if the polyp position is favorable (on the contralateral wall to the bare area of the liver) All specimens should be removed in a bag including cystic lymph node Gallbladder perforation and bile spillage should be avoided Open cholecystectomy for larger polyps [35, 36] where preoperative imaging or intraoperative frozen section will dictate whether adjacent liver is removed en bloc	0.3–2% of laparoscopic cholecystectomies Intraoperative finding [2]: Intraoperative staging Frozen section of gallbladder sent after extraction of entire specimen in a bag Remove cystic lymph node Alert the pathologist as the specimen will be processed differently Evaluate for definitive surgery, depending on surgeon experience and tumor resectability If in doubt, close and refer to HPB Cancer Centre Postoperative finding: History and physical exam Pathology/operative note review If T in situ or T1a No further evaluation needed, clinical surveillance only. No consensus on imaging follow-up If T1b or higher Labs – Liver function, Ca 19–9, CEA Imaging – CT chest, abdomen, pelvis; MRI Radical cholecystectomy	History and physical exam Labs: Including liver function tests, Ca 19–9, CEA Imaging: CT chest and triphasic liver MRI/MRCP liver Consider staging laparoscopy (if ≥T2, equivocal imaging) Avoid biopsy if lesion is deemed surgically resectable ⇒ Jaundice is frequently a dismal prognostic indicator, and many would preclude surgery ⇒ Consider ERCP if drainage required, although percutaneous approach usually allows better access to proximal hepatic ducts	History and physical exam Labs: Including liver function tests, Ca 19–9, CEA Imaging: CT chest, abdomen, pelvis MRI/MRCP Consider biopsy of distant disease (percutaneous) Decompression if jaundice present (PTC with internalization if central obstruction, ERCP if distal obstruction) Medical/ radiation oncology referral

GBC gallbladder cancer, *ERCP* endoscopic retrograde cholangiopancreatography, *EUS* endoscopic ultrasound, *PTC* percutaneous transhepatic cholangiography/catheter

- A negative frozen section of the cystic duct margin is mandatory during all radical cholecystectomies if the extrahepatic bile duct is not being resected.
- Jaundice is a poor prognostic marker (median disease-specific survival was 6 months vs 16 months in non-jaundiced patients; no jaundiced patients were alive at 3 years). Surgery exploration may not be warranted in this patient population [42].
- The presence of residual cancer after incidental cholecystectomy (pT2b or higher, positive cystic duct margin or pN+) is associated with poor disease-

Table 10.7 Management of advanced GB tumors

Clinical scenario	Surgical management
T2: Penetrates perimuscular connective tissue, no extension beyond serosa or into liver *T2a*: Peritoneal side, without involvement of the serosa *T2b*: Hepatic side, with no extension into the liver *T3: perforates serosa and/or directly invades the liver or other adjacent structure*	T2: LN metastases 20–62% (portal node involvement), 20% celiac and peripancreatic nodes [50] Segment 4b/5 non-anatomic liver resection, with a 2 cm clear margin, recommended for T2 and T3 lesions LN harvest recommended to include porta hepatis, gastrohepatic ligament, retroduodenal nodes
T4: invades main portal vein/hepatic artery or invades two or more extra hepatic structures	Radical hepatectomy (extended right hepatectomy or right trisectionectomy) +/− PVR in very selected cases (see note) LN harvest recommended to include porta hepatic, gastrohepatic ligament, retroduodenal nodes

LN lymph nodes, *PVR* portal vein resection

Table 10.8 Unresectable/metastatic disease

Criteria of unresectability	Surgical management
Metastatic disease: To liver, lung, peritoneum, distant lymph nodes (celiac, SMA nodes) Patient factors: Comorbidities rendering patient unable to tolerate potentially curative surgery Anatomical factors: There is no consensus for local extension of tumor that precludes resection. Tumor encasement of bilateral hepatic arteries or the common hepatic artery, however, is a contraindication to surgery	Consider non-operative approach to palliation if able (e.g., endoscopic stent/PTC placement) [59]

SMA superior mesenteric artery, *PTC* percutaneous transhepatic cholangiography/catheter

specific survival even when R0 resection is achieved after oncologic extended resection. Median disease-free survival (DFS) is 11.2 vs. 93.4 months, ($p < 0.0001$) and disease-specific survival (DSS) 25.2 months vs. not reached, ($p < 0.0001$), when compared to no-residual cancer after IC [43–45].

- Extended lymphadenectomy is required for IGBC, independent of cystic duct lymph node status. Cystic duct node positivity has been associated with positive perihilar nodes (odds ratio 5.2, $p = 0.012$), but not with common hepatic artery, pancreaticoduodenal nor paraaortic lymph nodes, which have an OS comparable to M1 disease [46].
- Port/Trocar site metastases, the implantation of disease at any of the port sites (not limited to the extraction site), was originally estimated to occur in 10–18% cases after laparoscopic cholecystectomy [47]. More recent data suggests, however, that the incidence of abdominal wall recurrence after laparoscopic procedure is low (7%) and comparable to open technique (5.1%) [48].

Port-site excision during re-resection for IGBC has been proven in more recent data not to be associated with improved overall survival and has the same distant disease recurrence compared to no port-site excision; therefore, it is no longer recommended routinely [49].

- Patients without residual cancer at oncologic extended resection and positive incidental cystic duct node may have similar DSS to patients with negative nodes, 70 vs 60% ($p = 0.337$) [46].
- *Quality Indicators*:
  - *Pathologic review* should include location and size of tumor, depth of invasion, presence of perineural/vascular/lymphatic invasion, cystic duct node involvement, surgical margin status (particularly cystic duct margin), and evidence of perforation of gall bladder.
  - *Operative note* should include whether gallbladder was removed intact, evidence of perforation or spillage of bile, excision of cystic node, removal of gallbladder using a bag with identification of the port site used, and use of wound protector.

Special Notes:
- Early re-exploration for patients with incidentally found T2 lesions [51] (Table 10.7).
- Adequacy of tumor resection (R0 status), rather than the extent of resection, predicts survival. Therefore, surgical resection should be tailored to obtaining complete oncologic clearance of the tumor and adequate lymphadenectomy [52].
- Extent of surgery for formal resection is determined by the location and stage of the tumor, as well as the intrahepatic anatomy and cystic duct margin.
- Right trisectionectomy is necessary for cancers involving the right hepatic artery and advanced lesions. PVE may be useful in these cases (Table 10.7).
- Pancreaticoduodenectomy has been reported for distal lesions, although 5-year survival is reported at 9–10% in two small series and median survival of 21 months (one alive at 42 months) in another [53–55] series. The main limitation of a local (segment 4b/5) resection is the distance between the GB and the segment 8 portal pedicle, which can be as little as 2 mm away. Limited 4b/5 resections should only be considered in T2 lesions located in the fundus where an adequate (2 cm) margin can be obtained by ligation of the segment 5 portal pedicle with preservation of the segment 8 portal branches.
- Routine bile duct resection does not improve overall survival [56, 57]. Resection of the extrahepatic biliary duct (EHBD), however, is indicated in cases where the cystic duct margin is positive for cancer or high-grade dysplasia [58].
- Extrahepatic bile duct resection may be indicated in cases of cystic duct and Hartman's pouch cancers, as well as cases where resection of the EHBD is required to achieve adequate oncologic clearance due to proximity of GB or tumor infiltration of the EHBD.
- The presence of metastatic disease during exploration is considered unresectable (Table 10.8).

Landmark Publications

Prospective randomized control trials (RCTs) regarding surgical management of this disease are few due to the relative rarity of the disease. Surgical management is largely dictated by consensus statements formed by high-volume centers. Most data have been developed from retrospective series with limited number of patients. Any reference to staging refers to the eighth edition of UICC staging (Table 10.9).

Table 10.9 Restropective reviews and RCTs in GBC

Topic	Study	Methods	Results
Stage 1	Wagholikar et al., 2002 [60]	Retrospective review $n = 14$ patients Early stage 12 patients treated with SC 2 patients treated with RC	Median survival ($n = 14$): 42 months 5-yr survival ($n = 14$): 68% LR in 5/12 patients: All had pT1b cancer treated with SC pT1a lesions can be treated with SC Recommend T1b be treated with RC
	Wakai et al., 2001 [61]	Retrospective review $n = 25$ patients Patients with T1b cancer 13 patients treated with SC 12 patients treated with RC	10-yr survival ($n = 25$): 87% No difference in survival in patients with SC (100%) vs. RC (87%) No LR in either group pT1b lesions can be treated with SC without impact on survival
Stage 2	Taner et al., 2008 [62]	Retrospective review $n = 131$ patients 45 patients treated with SC 60 patients treated with RC 25% patients had T2	Median survival($n = 131$): 11 months RC associated with longer survival than SC (HR 0.42) for pT2 or higher RC for patients with pT2 tumors or greater (achieves longer term survival, whether administered as the initial surgery or after incidental discovery)

(continued)

Table 10.9 (continued)

Topic	Study	Methods	Results
Stage 3/stage 4A	Sasaki et al., 2006 [63]	Retrospective review $n = 65$ patients Advanced GBC 27 patients with N1 disease 6 underwent PD with hepatectomy	Overall 5-yr survival, N1 disease ($n = 21$): 46.8% 16 patients recurred after curative OR (lymph node and distant metastases) Surgical resection recommended only if R0 margin possible High morbidity and mortality rates associated with extensive surgery, to be avoided in patients with para-aortic nodal disease
Medical oncology	UK-ABC-02 Valle et al., 2010 [64]	RCT phase 3, conducted in 37 centers in the UK $n = 410$ patients Unresectable, recurrent, or metastatic biliary cancer (included intra−/extrahepatic cholangiocarcinoma, ampullary, gallbladder cancer) Gemcitabine + cisplatin vs. gemcitabine alone for 24 weeks	Median survival was 11.7 vs. 8.1 mos for the Gem-Cis vs Gem-alone groups, respectively (HR 0.64) Significant improvement in progression-free survival, 8 mos vs. 5 mos Gem-Cis vs. Gem groups, respectively (HR 0.63) The combination of Gem-Cis chemotherapy for advanced/metastatic disease gave an average of 3.6 mos longer life than gemcitabine alone, with limited toxicity, and represented an appropriate option for treatment in these patients

Table 10.9 (continued)

Topic	Study	Methods	Results
	BILCAP Primrose et al., 2019 [65]	RCT phase 3, conducted in 44 centers in the UK $n = 447$ patients Histologically confirmed cholangiocarcinoma or muscle-invasive gallbladder cancer who had undergone a macroscopically complete resection with curative intent Patients were randomly assigned 1:1 to receive oral capecitabine or observation commencing within 16 weeks of surgery	The prespecified per-protocol analysis (210 patients in the capecitabine group and 220 in the observation group): Median overall survival was 53 months (95% CI: 40 to not reached) in the capecitabine group and 36 months (30–44) in the observation group (adjusted HR 0·75, 95% CI 0·58–0·97; $p = 0{\cdot}028$) Median recurrence-free survival was 25·9 months (95% CI 19·8–46·3) in the capecitabine group and 17.4 months (12.0–23.7) in the observation group
Radiation oncology	Kresl et al., 2002 [66]	Retrospective review $n = 21$ patients (stage III-IV) Adjuvant CRT (5-FU + EBRT 54Gy)	5-yr OS = 33% (21 patients), 64% if R0 resection with the addition of radiation When compared to historical surgical control group, improved 5-yr OS with R0 resection and addition of radiation (33% vs. 64%)

OS overall survival, *SC* simple cholecystectomy, *RC* radical cholecystectomy, *GBC* gallbladder cancer, *LR* locoregional recurrence, *PD* pancreaticoduodenectomy, *R0*: negative microscopic margins, *CRT* chemoradiotherapy, *EBRT* external beam radiotherapy

Referring to Medical Oncology

1. All patients who are stage 2 or higher for adjuvant chemotherapy [65].
2. All metastatic patients considered for palliative therapy.

Referring to Radiation Oncology

1. All patients who are T2 or higher and considered for adjuvant therapy (though there is limited evidence for this). Adjuvant treatment can be considered for R1 resection.
2. Palliative patients for consideration of symptomatic control.

Referring to MCC

1. All patients with T1b disease or higher.

Toronto Pearls

- All incidental T1b and higher cancers should be considered for re-resection. Aggressive surgery in early-stage disease is associated with potential for cure.
- Laparoscopic radical cholecystectomy has been reported with reasonable oncologic outcomes, but the data is not robust enough for it to be routinely recommended [67, 68].
- Formal resection should be tailored to achieve complete oncologic (R0) clearance of the tumor.
- Limited resection (seg4b/5) should be used selectively in T1b/T2 and T3 tumors located in the fundus where adequate tumor clearance can be achieved at the bifurcation of the right portal structures.
- Bile duct resection may be performed selectively based on cystic duct margin or oncologic clearance of the tumor.
- Portal lymphadenectomy should be performed for all cases with T1b and higher tumors.
- Adjuvant therapy should be considered for stage 2 disease and higher.

References

1. Sharma A, et al. Gallbladder cancer epidemiology, pathogenesis and molecular genetics: recent update. World J Gastroenterol. 2017;23(22):3978–98.
2. Wernberg JA, Lucarelli DD. Gallbladder cancer. Surg Clin North Am. 2014;94(2):343–60.
3. Diehl AK. Epidemiology of gallbladder cancer: a synthesis of recent data. J Natl Cancer Inst. 1980;65(6):1209–14.

4. Lowenfels AB, et al. Gallstones and risk of gallbladder cancer. J Natl Cancer Inst. 1985;75(1):77–80.
5. Lowenfels AB, et al. Gallstone growth, size, and risk of gallbladder cancer: an interracial study. Int J Epidemiol. 1989;18(1):50–4.
6. Zatonski WA, et al. Epidemiologic aspects of gallbladder cancer: a case-control study of the SEARCH Program of the International Agency for Research on Cancer. J Natl Cancer Inst. 1997;89(15):1132–8.
7. Lowenfels AB, et al. Epidemiology of gallbladder cancer. Hepato-Gastroenterology. 1999;46(27):1529–32.
8. Serra I, Diehl AK. Number and size of stones in patients with asymptomatic and symptomatic gallstones and gallbladder carcinoma. J Gastrointest Surg. 2002;6(2):272–3.
9. Randi G, Franceschi S, La Vecchia C. Gallbladder cancer worldwide: geographical distribution and risk factors. Int J Cancer. 2006;118(7):1591–602.
10. Moller H, et al. Obesity and cancer risk: a Danish record-linkage study. Eur J Cancer. 1994;30A(3):344–50.
11. Calle EE, et al. Overweight, obesity, and mortality from cancer in a prospectively studied cohort of U.S. adults. N Engl J Med. 2003;348(17):1625–38.
12. Kimura K, et al. Association of gallbladder carcinoma and anomalous pancreaticobiliary ductal union. Gastroenterology. 1985;89(6):1258–65.
13. Nuzzo G, et al. Papillary carcinoma of the gallbladder and anomalous pancreatico-biliary junction. Report of three cases and review of the literature. Hepato-Gastroenterology. 2005;52(64):1034–8.
14. Dutta U, et al. Typhoid carriers among patients with gallstones are at increased risk for carcinoma of the gallbladder. Am J Gastroenterol. 2000;95(3):784–7.
15. Misra S, et al. Carcinoma of the gallbladder. Lancet Oncol. 2003;4(3):167–76.
16. Caygill C, et al. Increased risk of biliary tract cancer following gastric surgery. Br J Cancer. 1988;57(4):434–6.
17. Fong Y, Jarnagin W, Blumgart L. Gallbladder cancer: comparison of patients presenting initially for definitive operation with those presenting after prior noncurative intervention. Ann Surg. 2000;232:4.
18. Goetze TO, Paolucci V. Prognosis of incidental gallbladder carcinoma is not influenced by the primary access technique: analysis of 837 incidental gallbladder carcinomas in the German Registry. Surg Endosc. 2013;27(8):2821–8.
19. Foster JM, et al. Gallbladder cancer: defining the indications for primary radical resection and radical re-resection. Ann Surg Oncol. 2007;14(2):833–40.
20. Vega EA, et al. Incidental versus non-incidental gallbladder cancer: index cholecystectomy before oncologic re-resection negatively impacts survival in T2b tumors. HPB (Oxford). 2019;21(8):1046–56.
21. Alexander F, et al. Biliary carcinoma. A review of 109 cases. Am J Surg. 1984;147(4):503–9.
22. Oertli D, Herzog U, Tondelli P. Primary carcinoma of the gallbladder: operative experience during a 16 year period. Eur J Surg. 1993;159(8):415–20.
23. Wade TP, et al. Experience with distal bile duct cancers in U.S. Veterans Affairs hospitals: 1987-1991. J Surg Oncol. 1997;64(3):242–5.
24. de Groen PC, et al. Biliary tract cancers. N Engl J Med. 1999;341(18):1368–78.
25. Shukla PJ, et al. Does PET-CT scan have a role prior to radical re-resection for incidental gallbladder cancer? HPB (Oxford). 2008;10(6):439–45.
26. Corvera CU, et al. 18F-fluorodeoxyglucose positron emission tomography influences management decisions in patients with biliary cancer. J Am Coll Surg. 2008;206(1):57–65.
27. Leung U, et al. Impact of pre-operative positron emission tomography in gallbladder cancer. HPB (Oxford). 2014;16(11):1023–30.
28. Tian Y, et al. Diagnostic role of staging laparoscopy in a subset of biliary cancers: a meta-analysis. ANZ J Surg. 2017;87(1–2):22–7.
29. Butte JM, et al. The role of laparoscopic staging in patients with incidental gallbladder cancer. HPB (Oxford). 2011;13(7):463–72.

30. Kondo S, et al. Regional and para-aortic lymphadenectomy in radical surgery for advanced gallbladder carcinoma. Br J Surg. 2000;87(4):418–22.
31. Ohtani T, Shirai Y, Tsukada K, Muto T, Hatakeyama K. Spread of gallbladder carcinoma: CT evaluation with pathologic correlation. Abdom Imaging. 1996;21(3):195–201.
32. Noji T, et al. CT evaluation of paraaortic lymph node metastasis in patients with biliary cancer. J Gastroenterol. 2005;40(7):739–43.
33. Agarwal AK, et al. Role of routine 16b1 lymph node biopsy in the management of gallbladder cancer: an analysis. HPB (Oxford). 2014;16(3):229–34.
34. Amin MB, editor. *AJCC Cancer Staging Manual.* 8th ed: Switzerland: Springer; 2017.
35. Koga A, et al. Diagnosis and operative indications for polypoid lesions of the gallbladder. Arch Surg. 1988;123(1):26–9.
36. Park JY, et al. Long-term follow up of gallbladder polyps. J Gastroenterol Hepatol. 2009;24(2):219–22.
37. Ouchi K, Mikuni J, Kakugawa Y. Laparoscopic cholecystectomy for gallbladder carcinoma: results of a Japanese survey of 498 patients. J Hepato-Biliary-Pancreat Surg. 2002;9(2):256–60.
38. Weiland ST, et al. Should suspected early gallbladder cancer be treated laparoscopically? J Gastrointest Surg. 2002;6(1):50–6.
39. Cleary SP, et al. Cancer of the gallbladder and extrahepatic bile ducts. Curr Probl Surg. 2007;44(7):396–482.
40. Ouchi K, et al. Laparoscopic cholecystectomy for gallbladder carcinoma: results of a Japanese survey of 498 patients. J Hepato-Biliary-Pancreat Surg. 2002;9(2):256–60.
41. Lee SE, et al. Practical guidelines for the surgical treatment of gallbladder cancer. J Korean Med Sci. 2014;29(10):1333–40.
42. Hawkins WG, et al. Jaundice predicts advanced disease and early mortality in patients with gallbladder cancer. Ann Surg Oncol. 2004;11(3):310–5.
43. Vega EA, et al. Positive cystic duct margin at index cholecystectomy in incidental gallbladder cancer is an important negative prognosticator. Eur J Surg Oncol. 2019;45(6):1061–68.
44. Butte JM, et al. Residual disease predicts outcomes after definitive resection for incidental gallbladder cancer. J Am Coll Surg. 2014;219(3):416–29.
45. Vinuela E, et al. Incidental gallbladder cancer: residual cancer discovered at oncologic extended resection determines outcome: a report from high- and low-incidence countries. Ann Surg Oncol. 2017;24(8):2334–43.
46. Vega EA, et al. Extended lymphadenectomy is required for incidental gallbladder cancer independent of cystic duct lymph node status. J Gastrointest Surg. 2018;22(1):43–51.
47. Wakai T, Shirai Y, Hatakeyama K. Radical second resection provides survival benefit for patients with T2 gallbladder carcinoma first discovered after laparoscopic cholecystectomy. World J Surg. 2002;26(7):867–71.
48. Paolucci V, Neckell M, Gotze T. Unsuspected gallbladder carcinoma--the CAE-S/CAMIC registry. Zentralbl Chir. 2003;128(4):309–12.
49. Ethun CG, et al. Routine port-site excision in incidentally discovered gallbladder cancer is not associated with improved survival: a multi-institution analysis from the US Extrahepatic Biliary Malignancy Consortium. J Surg Oncol. 2017;115(7):805–11.
50. Fong Y, Heffernan N, Blumgart LH. Gallbladder carcinoma discovered during laparoscopic cholecystectomy: aggressive reresection is beneficial. Cancer. 1998;83(3):423–7.
51. Muratore A, et al. Gallbladder cancer invading the perimuscular connective tissue: results of reresection after prior non-curative operation. J Surg Oncol. 2003;83(4):212–5.
52. Pawlik TM, et al. Incidence of finding residual disease for incidental gallbladder carcinoma: implications for re-resection. J Gastrointest Surg. 2007;11(11):1478–86; discussion 1486-7.
53. Nimura Y, et al. Hepatopancreatoduodenectomy for advanced carcinoma of the biliary tract. Hepato-Gastroenterology. 1991;38(2):170–5.
54. Wakai T, et al. Combined major hepatectomy and pancreaticoduodenectomy for locally advanced biliary carcinoma: long-term results. World J Surg. 2008;32(6):1067–74.
55. Doty JR, et al. Cholecystectomy, liver resection, and pylorus-preserving pancreaticoduodenectomy for gallbladder cancer: report of five cases. J Gastrointest Surg. 2002;6(5):776–80.

56. Choi SB, et al. Surgical strategy for T2 and T3 gallbladder cancer: is extrahepatic bile duct resection always necessary? Langenbeck's Arch Surg. 2013;398(8):1137–44.
57. Wiggers JK, et al. Patterns of recurrence after resection of gallbladder cancer without routine extrahepatic bile duct resection. HPB (Oxford). 2014;16(7):635–40.
58. Shukla PJ, Barreto SG. Systematic review: should routine resection of the extra-hepatic bile duct be performed in gallbladder cancer? Saudi J Gastroenterol. 2010;16(3):161–7.
59. Baron TH. Expandable metal stents for the treatment of cancerous obstruction of the gastrointestinal tract. N Engl J Med. 2001;344(22):1681–7.
60. Wagholikar GD, et al. Early gallbladder cancer. J Am Coll Surg. 2002;194(2):137–41.
61. Wakai T, et al. Early gallbladder carcinoma does not warrant radical resection. Br J Surg. 2001;88(5):675–8.
62. Taner CB, Nagorney DM, Donohue JH. Surgical treatment of gallbladder cancer. J Gastrointest Surg. 2004;8(1):83–9.
63. Sasaki R, et al. Significance of extensive surgery including resection of the pancreas head for the treatment of gallbladder cancer—from the perspective of mode of lymph node involvement and surgical outcome. World J Surg. 2006;30(1):36–42.
64. Valle J, et al. Cisplatin plus gemcitabine versus gemcitabine for biliary tract cancer. N Engl J Med. 2010;362(14):1273–81.
65. Primrose JN, et al. Capecitabine compared with observation in resected biliary tract cancer (BILCAP): a randomised, controlled, multicentre, phase 3 study. Lancet Oncol. 2019;20(5):663–73.
66. Kresl JJ, et al. Adjuvant external beam radiation therapy with concurrent chemotherapy in the management of gallbladder carcinoma. Int J Radiat Oncol Biol Phys. 2002;52(1):167–75.
67. Cho JY, et al. Laparoscopic approach for suspected early-stage gallbladder carcinoma. Arch Surg. 2010;145(2):128–33.
68. Shirobe T, Maruyama S. Laparoscopic radical cholecystectomy with lymph node dissection for gallbladder carcinoma. Surg Endosc. 2014;29(8):2244–50.

Gastric Adenocarcinoma

11

Mohammadali Khorasani, Savtaj S. Brar, and Natalie G. Coburn

Introduction

In 2017, the Canadian Cancer Society estimated gastric adenocarcinoma to be the 14th most commonly diagnosed malignancy, with 3500 new cases and 2100 deaths. The age-standardized incidence and mortality rate for gastric cancer have decreased from 19.0/100,000 cases and 15.5/100,000 deaths in 1980 to 8.6/100,000 and 5.1/100,000 deaths, respectively, in 2017 [1]. Enormous geographic variation in the incidence of gastric cancer exists with the highest incidence being observed in East Asia. Similarly, wide geographic variation in treatment outcomes is observed with overall 5-year survival rates of 40–60% reported in Asia and Europe, compared to 25–29% in Canada and the USA [1–3].

Risk Factors

Established risk factors for gastric cancer (GC) include *Helicobacter pylori* infection, smoking, alcohol, and dietary factors (such as processed meats and salt-preserved foods). Hereditary gastric cancers represent <5% of all gastric cancers. Main gastric cancer familial predispositions are hereditary diffuse gastric cancer

M. Khorasani
General Surgical Oncology, University of Toronto, Toronto, ON, Canada
e-mail: Mohammadali.Khorasani@alumni.ubc.ca

S. S. Brar
Department of Surgery, University of Toronto, Toronto, ON, Canada
e-mail: sbrar@mtsinai.on.ca

N. G. Coburn (✉)
Department of Surgery, Sunnybrook Health Sciences Centre, University of Toronto, Toronto, ON, Canada
e-mail: Natalie.Coburn@sunnybrook.ca

F. C. Wright et al. (eds.), *Surgical Oncology Manual*,
https://doi.org/10.1007/978-3-030-48363-0_11

(HDFC), gastric adenocarcinoma and proximal polyposis of stomach (GAPPS), familial intestinal gastric cancer (FIGC). Other hereditary cancer syndromes associated with increased risk of gastric cancer include Lynch syndrome, Peutz-Jeghers syndrome (PJS), familial adenomatous polyposis (FAP), Li-Fraumeni syndrome, and BRCA syndromes (BReast CAncer) (see Table 11.1 below).

Table 11.1 Selected familial predispositions to gastric cancer

	Gene mutation	Risk of gastric cancer	Notes
HDGC [4–9]	*CDH-1*[a] (codes for E-cadherin)	70% men, 56% females (by 80 years of age) Average 37 years of age	Autosomal dominant Diffuse-type GCA Prophylactic total gastrectomy + D1 LND recommended at age 20–30 years if CDH-1 positive 87% have microscopic adenocarcinoma on prophylactic gastrectomy specimen CDH-1 positive women: 42% risk of lobular breast cancer by age of 80 years
GAPPS [10, 11]	*APC* promoter IB Variants[a]	12 families have been described with GAPPS to date Youngest reported age of gastric adenocarcinoma is 23 years	Autosomal dominant FGP sparing the antrum. No significant colorectal or duodenal polyps Guidelines not well defined for surveillance or timing of prophylactic gastrectomy
FAP [12, 13]	*APC*	1–2% lifetime risk	Duodenal/peri-ampullary cancer most common extracolonic manifestation ~50% non-adenomatous FGP, ~10% of gastric polyps adenomatous (mostly in antrum) and need to be removed Guidelines recommend surveillance starting at 25–30 years of age Incidence of gastric cancer in FAP patients may be rising [14]
Lynch syndrome [15, 16]	*MMR*, *EPCAM*	Cumulative risk of 7–8%, mean age of 56 years	Autosomal dominant After endometrial cancer, one of the most common extra-colonic manifestations of Lynch syndrome Mostly intestinal type Benefit of surveillance for gastric cancer is unknown[a]
PJS[a] [17, 18]	*STK11*	29% lifetime risk, mean age of 42	Autosomal dominant Surveillance recommended to start in late teens

HDGC hereditary diffuse gastric cancer, *GCA* gastric cancer, *LND* lymph node dissection, *GAPPS* gastric adenocarcinoma and proximal polyposis of stomach syndrome, *APC* adenomatous polyposis coli, *FGP* fundic gland polyps, *FAP* familial adenomatous polyposis, *MMR* mismatch repair, *EPCAM* epithelial cell adhesion molecule, *PJS* Peutz-Jeghers syndrome

[a]See Special Notes below

Special Notes

- *Hereditary Diffuse Gastric Cancer:* criteria for diagnosis of HDGC and genetic testing for *CDH1* mutation are as mentioned below [8]. Of note, in countries with low incidence of sporadic gastric cancer (such as Canada), approximately 10–18% are identified with *CDH-1* mutation.
  1. Two gastric cancer cases in first- or second-degree relatives regardless of age, at least one confirmed to be diffuse gastric cancer (DGC) or
  2. One case of DGC diagnosed below the age of 40 years in a first- or second-degree relative or
  3. Personal or family history of DGC and LBC, one diagnosed below the age of 50 years.
- *Gastric Adenocarcinoma and Proximal Polyposis of Stomach Syndrome*: Proposed criteria for diagnosis are [11] as follows:
  1. Gastric polyps restricted to the body and fungus with no evidence of colorectal or duodenal polyposis
  2. More than 100 polyps in the proximal stomach of the affected patient (or more than 30 polyps in the first-degree relative)
  3. Some FGPs having regions of dysplasia (or a family member with FGP and adenocarcinoma)
  4. Autosomal dominant inheritance
- *Peutz-Jeghers Syndrome*: Clinical diagnosis of PJS is made when any of the following criteria are present [18]:
  1. Two or more histological confirmed Peutz-Jeghers (PJ) polyps
  2. Any number of PJ polyps detected in someone with family history of PJS
  3. Any number of PJ polyps in someone with characteristic mucocutaneous pigmentation
- *Lynch Syndrome* [19–21]:
  1. Patients are at risk of extra-colonic malignancies of endometrium, stomach, ovaries, hepatobiliary, renal pelvis/ureteric, brain and skin
  2. Consensus guidelines for gastric cancer surveillance are variable. In general, a baseline upper GI scope at age of 30–35 years and subsequent scopes every 1–5 years are recommended, especially in patients with risk factors such as intestinal metaplasia, gastric atrophy, family history of gastric cancer, and immigration from countries with high incidence of gastric cancer. In addition, *H. pylori* testing and eradication are recommended.

Classification and Staging

Histopathology

Gastric adenocarcinomas are classified histologically according to the Lauren classification as (1) intestinal (well-differentiated) or (2) diffuse (undifferentiated) histologic subtypes [22]. Such classification can have clinical implications with respect to prognosis and management decision-making.

Intestinal-type adenocarcinoma of stomach is more sporadic and believed to be causally related to *H. pylori* and environmental risk factors of gastric cancer (GC) [23]. Whereas intestinal-type GC is believed to follow sequential progression of dysplasia to invasive carcinoma, the development of diffuse-type GC is not believed to follow defined preneoplastic stages [23]. Diffuse-type GC has defective intercellular adhesions and tend to spread within deeper layers of gastric wall and in a less coherent fashion [24, 25]. Fashion, which can lead to underestimation of its extent by visual assessment of gastric mucosa. As such, wider gross surgical resection margins may be needed in patients with diffuse-type GC, and if intra-operative frozen sections are being done, full gastric wall thickness assessment of the resection margin should be considered by the pathology team.

In addition, multiple retrospective studies suggest prognostic and predictive value in Lauren classification of gastric adenocarcinoma. Diffuse-type GC has been shown to be associated with worse disease-free survival (DFS) and overall survival (OS) rates [24–26]. Furthermore, in phase 2/3 of the prospective randomized FLOT4 study, comparing pathological response to two different perioperative chemotherapy regimens (ECF/ECX vs. FLOT), analysis of the pooled population of both groups showed that patients with intestinal-type GC had 16% complete pathological response vs. only 3% in patients with diffuse-type GC ($p = 0.004$) [27]. In this study, it was also shown that oxaliplatin-based chemotherapy (FLOT) resulted in more frequent partial tumor response in patients with intestinal-type GC compared to diffuse type (42% vs. 23%, $P = 0.04$), but tumor response between the two Lauren classification subtypes was similar in the non-oxaliplatin group (ECF/ECX).

Molecular Classification

Recently, as part of the Cancer Genome Atlas (TCGA), a molecular classification for gastric cancer has been developed, dividing gastric cancer into four subtypes: Epstein-Barr virus (EBV) positive, microsatellite unstable (MSI), genomically stable tumors (GS), and those with chromosomal instability (CIN) [28]. These molecular subtypes have been shown to have distinct salient genomic features which may provide guidance in using targeted agents in the future. In Fig. 11.1 below, salient features associated with each subtype, and their distribution in the stomach, are summarized.

Molecular classification is emerging, as potential biomarkers to explore personalized treatment strategies in gastric cancer are in the experimental stages at this time. For instance, studies have shown that EBV-positive and MSI high, gastric cancers have higher PD-L1 expression, making them potential candidates for immunotherapy [28, 29]. In addition, there is data to support prognostic value in this

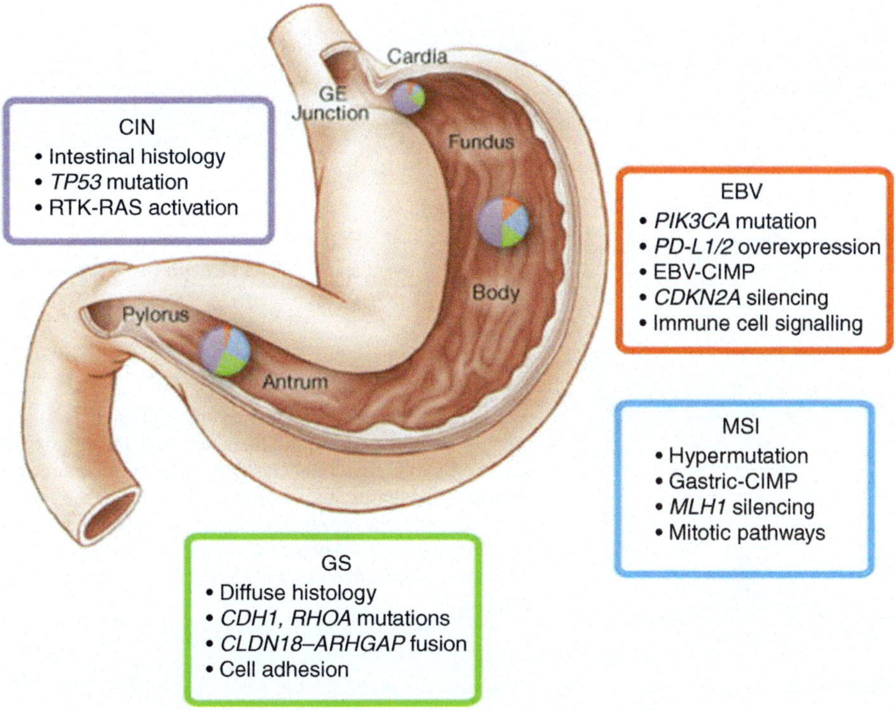

Fig. 11.1 Molecular subtypes of gastric cancer and their distribution within the stomach [28]. (Permission for use of this figure was obtained from Macmillan Publishers Limited)

molecular classification, suggesting EBV-positive tumors have the best prognosis and GS subtype is associated with the worst outcomes [29]. There is also preliminary evidence to suggest that MSI high status may be a negative prognostic marker in patients treated with perioperative chemotherapy [30]. Ongoing research is needed to better define the role of molecular classification in clinical practice.

Staging

Staging of gastric adenocarcinoma is according to the American Joint Committee on Cancer (AJCC), eighth edition. Gastroesophageal junction tumors with their epicenter located less than 2 cm into proximal stomach are classified, staged, and treated as esophageal cancers [31]. This most recent edition of AJCC has separated clinical from pathological staging and has incorporated post-neoadjuvant staging for gastric cancer (see Table 11.2 below).

Table 11.2 Gastric cancer patient outcomes according to the eighth edition of AJCC [32, 33]

Pathological stage[a]	5-year survival (%)
Stage 1a	93.6
Stage 1b	88.0
Stage 2a	81.8
Stage 2b	68.0
Stage 3a	54.2
Stage 3b	36.2
Stage 3c	17.9

Post-neoadjuvant stage[a]	5-year survival (%)
Stage 1	76.5
Stage 2	46.3
Stage 3	18.3
Stage 4	5.7

[a]Pathological stage group patients are without neoadjuvant therapy prior to resection; their survival information is based on the International Gastric Cancer Association data (mostly Japanese and Korean patient data); post-neoadjuvant stage group had either systemic therapy or radiotherapy prior to surgery, and their survival rates in this table are based on the National Cancer Database (US-based database)

Table 11.3 Diagnostic tool accuracy when used for assessment of gastric cancer [34, 35]

	EUS	CT	MRI	PET
T-stage (overall accuracy in %)	75	72	83	–
N-stage (%)				
Overall accuracy	64	66	53	60
Sensitivity	74	77	85	40
Specificity	80	78	75	98
M-stage (overall accuracy (%))	–	81	–	88

Staging Workup

The initial treatment plans are made based on the clinical stage of the patient. There are multiple tools that can be considered to improve the accuracy of the clinical stage and guide clinical decisions. CT scan, MRI, PET scan, endoscopic ultrasound (EUS), and staging laparoscopy ± peritoneal washings are some of these tools.

To evaluate the extent of locoregional disease, diagnostic tools have different accuracies, as summarized in Table 11.3.

According to a meta-analysis [35], EUS was most accurate for T3 disease (85%), followed by T4 and T1 (79% and 77%, respectively). Pooled accuracy of EUS in staging T2 lesions was only 65% in this meta-analysis. CT scan accuracy in assessment of T stage was suggested to be lowest in T1 lesions, being only

63% [34]. When comparing CT against MRI for assessment of T stage [34], MRI's accuracy is statistically significantly higher overall (83% vs. 72%) and when identifying T1 lesions (86% vs. 63%). When assessing for N-Stage, meta-analysis results suggest that both CT and MRI are statistically significantly more sensitive than PET scan, but PET was shown to be more specific than both other techniques [34].

Early vs. Advanced Gastric Cancer

One clinically useful way of classifying gastric cancer is *early* vs. *advanced.* This classification can help guide the management strategy:

Early Gastric Cancer (EGC) tumors confined to the mucosa (Tis or T1a) or submucosa (T1b), independent of the presence of lymph node involvement [36]. EGC is predominately identified by subtle changes in color, vascularity, or texture and is rarely diagnosed outside areas where population-based screening is offered, such as in Japan and Korea.

Advanced Gastric Cancer (AGC) T2 to T4 (invading muscularis propria, subserosa, perforating serosa, or invading adjacent structures), without distant metastasis.

Management

In this section, we discuss the management of gastric cancer classified into *early gastric cancer* and *advanced gastric cancer* (see above for definitions of this classification). Below are definitions of some of the terminologies that are used in the chapter.

Endoscopic Mucosal Resection (EMR) employs endoscopic techniques to elevate (e.g., injection and suction) and resect (e.g., cautery and banding) mucosal lesions en bloc.

Endoscopic Submucosal Dissection (ESD) a variation of EMR that employs submucosal injection and a specialized needle-knife to permit en bloc resection of mucosal and submucosal lesions.

Subtotal Gastrectomy (SG) removal of one-half to three-fourths of the gastric tissue, including omentum and all associated lymph nodes appropriate for a D1 or D2 lymphadenectomy. For distal gastric cancers, SG has been shown to have an equivalent oncological outcome and lesser morbidity when compared to total gastrectomy. SG is also associated with a better nutritional status and quality of life [37].

Total Gastrectomy (TG) removal of all of the gastric tissue and distal esophagus, including omentum and all associated lymph nodes appropriate for a D1 or D2 lymphadenectomy. TG is preferred for tumors confined to the proximal one-third of the stomach.

Palliative Gastrectomy (PG) gastrectomy performed with the intent to alleviate symptoms from the primary gastric cancer in the context of metastatic disease. A gastrectomy performed otherwise in a patient with metastatic disease is considered a non-curative gastrectomy [38].

D1 Lymph Node Dissection includes removal of the omentum with perigastric lymph nodes (stations 1–6) and lymph nodes along the left gastric artery (station 7). *It is important to note that station 1 (right paracardial) is part of a D1 LND, but station 2 (left paracardial) is not removed for SG* [39]. See Fig. 11.2 for schematic of the lymph node stations.

D2 Lymph Node Dissection D1 nodes and lymph nodes along the common hepatic artery (station 8a), celiac axis (station 9), splenic artery (stations 10 and 11), and hepatic artery proper (station 12a) [39]. Clearance of station 10 and 11 nodes may require splenectomy (See Special Notes – Extent of Lymphadenectomy) (Fig. 11.2) [39].

Bursectomy Removal of anterior leaflet of the transverse mesocolon and the pancreatic capsule, along with total omentectomy.

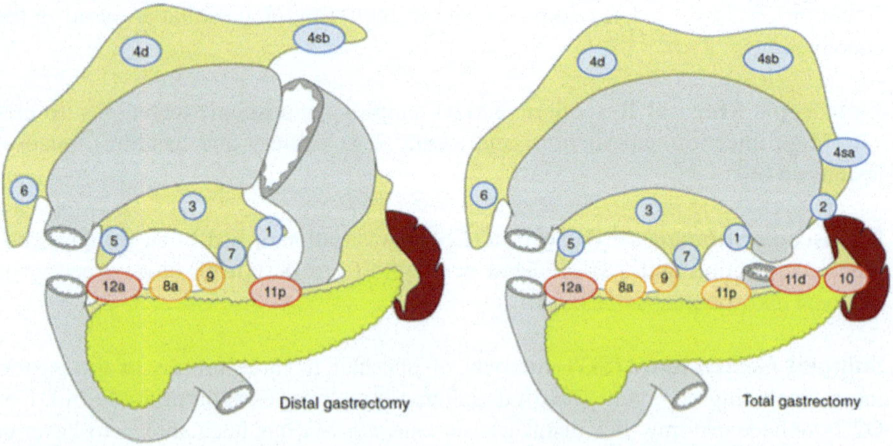

Fig. 11.2 Lymph node stations according to the Japanese gastric cancer treatment guidelines. (Figure adopted from 2014 Japanese gastric cancer treatment guidelines, Springer publications [40]). Numbers in *blue* color: D1 lymphadenectomy stations; numbers in *orange* color: D1+ lymphadenectomy stations; numbers in *red* color: D2 lymphadenectomy stations

Early Gastric Cancer (EGC)

Workup	Surgery	Adjuvant therapy	Follow-up (f/u)
Recommended: History and physical exam Upper endoscopy Imaging: CT abdomen/ pelvis EUS Staging laparoscopy[a] *Optional:* CT chest PET is not indicated for EGC	*Gastrectomy* with D1 lymph node dissection[a] OR *Endoscopic resection* can be considered for lesions fulfilling all of the following [41][a]: Intestinal type Confined to mucosa (Tis or T1a) and cN0 Elevated lesions <20 mm or flat lesions <10 mm in diameter Absence of high-risk features (ulceration, poorly differentiated, lymphovascular invasion) Clear lateral and deep margins after excision	Indicated for all node-positive disease, and those who are found to be T2 or higher after resection (please see section on "Advanced Gastric Cancer")	*Recommended:* Iron, B12, calcium supplements Every 3–6 months for 1–2 years, then every 6–12 months for 3–5 years, and yearly thereafter with: History and physical exam B12, Fe, bone density if TG was performed *Optional:* CT abdomen/pelvis[a] EGD[a]

EGC early gastric cancer, *EUS* endoscopic ultrasound, *EMR* endoscopic mucosal resection, *ESD* endoscopic submucosal dissection, *SG* subtotal gastrectomy, *TG* total gastrectomy, *RCT* randomized controlled trials, *EGD* esophago-gastro duodenoscopy

[a]See Special Notes

Special Notes: Early Gastric Cancer

Endoscopic resection EMR/ESD may be used in appropriately selected lesions amenable to en bloc resection that have minimal or no risk of nodal metastasis by experienced providers. Expanded criteria for ESD outside of the criteria listed above are considered investigational. ESD expertise and regional outcomes should be considered when choosing ESD as the treatment strategies, as recent meta-analysis has suggested worse endoscopic outcomes in Western countries compared to Eastern countries [42]. If after endoscopic resection it is revealed that the lesion is outside of the above-mentioned criteria (i.e. non-curative endoscopic resection), further treatment with gastrectomy and lymphadenectomy should be considered [43].

In the case of T upstage after endoscopic resection, management as per recommendations in the section "Advanced Gastric Cancer" should be considered.

Staging Laparoscopy (SL) Limited use in EGC. In cases where the tumor is reliably felt to be clinically T1 and N0, then SL can be omitted.

Extent of Lymphadenectomy Considerable controversy surrounds the role of extended lymphadenectomy (D1 vs. D2 resection) in early gastric cancer. Adequate staging requires 15 or more lymph nodes to be harvested. For cT1N0 tumors, D1 with splenopancreatic preservation is generally recommended. Worse outcomes have been associated with D2 lymphadenectomy in patients with EGC [44]. If clinically node positive, the staging should be reassessed to ensure not AGC.

Resection Margin (Early and Advanced Gastric Cancer) Positive microscopic margins after gastrectomy are associated with inferior outcomes when compared to those in whom R0 status was achieved [45–48]. When subtotal gastrectomy is performed, in general a gross proximal margin of at least 4 cm is recommended to ensure R0 resection [48–50]; however, guidelines differ in their recommendation (see table below). Likely, smaller gross margins can be used in resection of EGC (T1), advocated by Japanese gastric cancer treatment guidelines, suggesting a 2 cm gross proximal margin in such cases [36]. Of note, diffuse or signet ring cell subtypes are at higher risk of positive margin, and in these cases a greater gross resection margin can be considered. Recommendations from three different guidelines for surgical resection margins in gastric cancer are outlined in Table 11.4 below.

Intra-operative frozen sections of resection margin can be considered selectively, and in retrospective studies, they have been shown to be associated with low (1.7%) false-negative rates [52]. However, patients with signet ring cell or diffuse-type histology are at higher risk of false-negative intra-operative frozen section assessment [52].

To address a microscopically positive margin (R1 resection), consideration for re-resection *or* post-op CRT is recommended by clinical guidelines [50, 51] in selected cases.

Table 11.4 Recommended gastric cancer macroscopic proximal resection margin based on guidelines

	Recommended proximal gross margin
JGCG [40]	EGC: 2 cm AGC: 3–5 cm (depending on the growth pattern)
NCCN [50]	4 cm
ESMO [51]	5 cm (stage 1b-3) Consider 8 cm in diffuse type

JGCG Japanese Gastric Cancer Treatment Guidelines, *NCCN* National Comprehensive Cancer Network, *ESMO* European Society for Medical Oncology, *EGC* early gastric cancer, *AGC* advanced gastric cancer

- Decision to re-resect in this scenario is complex and requires careful consideration of anatomical feasibility, patient factors, and disease factors. Microscopically positive margins in gastric cancer may not be an independent predictor of outcomes in patients with more advanced disease [45, 48, 53]; therefore, re-resection after a microscopically positive margin, when technically feasible, may only be considered in patients who have favorable stage of disease.
- Demonstrated recurrence and survival benefits of post-operative CRT after R1 resection are based on retrospective studies only [54–57], and its potential risks/benefits should be carefully discussed in multidisciplinary cancer conferences on a case by case basis.

Laparoscopic Gastrectomy (LG) LG is appropriate for EGC in experienced, high-volume centers, where results are monitored and assessed against international benchmarks [58]. It is safe and improved short-term outcomes have been demonstrated, but oncologic outcomes are currently being evaluated with ongoing RCTs [59].

Follow-Up Surveillance
Evidence to support the benefit of early detection of recurrence is lacking. Most providers perform surveillance with serial CT scans. Surveillance EGD should be offered to patients at risk of local recurrence (e.g., following endoscopic resection) when complete gastrectomy would be considered.

Advanced Gastric Cancer

Workup	Surgery	Perioperative/adjuvant therapy	Follow-up (f/u)
Recommended tests: History and physical exam Upper endoscopy Imaging: CT abdomen/pelvis Staging laparoscopy[a] *Optional tests*: CT chest EUS[a] PET is not indicated	*Gastrectomy* D2 LND SG or TG depending on location of tumor[a] Consider intraoperative margin assessment[a] Multi-visceral resection should be performed if the patient is considered a candidate for curative resection	Options are: Perioperative FLOT chemo (preferred) [56, 60] *OR*[a] Adjuvant 5-FU-based CRT (if D1 LND or less) [61] *OR*[a] If no pre-op therapy, consider adjuvant chemo after D2 LND (If N+ may consider addition of CRT to the post-op regimen) Each of the options above has been shown to be superior to resection alone in RCTs [62]. For guidance on choice of multimodality therapy, see Special Notes below	Every 3–6 months for 1–2 years, then every 6–12 months for 3–5 years, and yearly thereafter with: History and physical exam B12, Fe, bone density if TG was performed *Optional tests:* CT abdomen/pelvis[a] EGD[a]

EUS endoscopic ultrasound, *SG* subtotal gastrectomy, *TG* total gastrectomy, *RCT* randomized controlled trial, *ECF* epirubicin, cisplatin and fluorouracil (5-FU), FLOT docetaxel, oxaliplatin, fluorouracil, and leucovorin, *CRT* chemoradiotherapy, *EGD* esophago-gastro duodenoscopy

[a]See Special Notes

Special Notes: Advanced Gastric Cancer

Staging Laparoscopy (SL) Radiologically occult peritoneal metastases are found in 20–30% of patients with T2 or higher disease [63]. SL is indicated in patients with clinical T2 or higher, or node positive on clinical staging to rule out radiologically occult peritoneal metastasis or positive peritoneal cytology [50]. Patients with positive peritoneal washings experience outcomes comparable to those with overt metastatic disease and should be considered palliative [64]. In patients who are being considered for preoperative therapy, SL with peritoneal washings should be obtained prior to preoperative therapy. Even though there are some data to suggest that patients who are converted from cytology positive to negative with systemic therapy have better outcomes [50, 65], role of surgery (gastric resection ± intra-peritoneal chemotherapy) is considered experimental and not the standard of care. Further studies are ongoing to better define the role of surgery in patients with peritoneal disease [66, 67].

Endoscopic Ultrasound (EUS) EUS is valuable in the distinction between EGC and AGC and is critical if considering EMR/ESD. In patients with an established diagnosis of AGC, EUS is unlikely to change management and is not routinely required.

Resection Margin:
Please refer to the "Resection Margin" section under Early Gastric Cancer management.

Extent of Lymphadenectomy Evidence suggests improved cancer-specific outcomes with D2 resection, particularly in higher staged tumors (T2–4) [44, 68]. Splenopancreatectomy is clearly associated with higher operative morbidity and is avoided unless required to achieve R0 resection margins [39, 69]. Involvement of nodes beyond a D2 resection (i.e., mesenteric, para-aortic, retroperitoneal) is classified as distant metastases [31]. The role of "D3" resections is not supported in the management of gastric cancer [70].

Bursectomy Bursectomy was routinely considered/performed for serosa-positive gastric cancers according to Japanese guidelines, but has been studied further in JCOG 1001 randomized control trial in patients with resectable cT3/T4a GC [60]. The results of the study were published early, after second interim analysis in 2017, on the basis of futility. Based on these results, bursectomy did not provide survival advantage over non-bursectomy and was significantly associated with more pancreatic fistula [60]. A recent meta-analysis also was consistent with the results of JCOG

1001, but did not demonstrate superior overall or recurrence-free survival in patients with resectable cT3/T4 GC who received bursectomy [71].

Laparoscopic Gastrectomy (LG) LG is not recommended for AGC due to limited available evidence on oncologic outcome [40, 50]. A Korean RCT is investigating oncologic outcomes of LG in AGC [72].

Combined Modality Treatment:
Strong evidence exists to support adding systemic therapy or chemoradiotherapy (CRT) to surgical resection as part of the treatment for patients with advanced GC improves outcomes [61, 73–75]. Below, we discuss peri-operative vs. postoperative therapy treatment strategies, as well as roles of chemotherapy and CRT in treatment of advanced GC. This is followed by Fig. 11.3, which summaries this discussion.

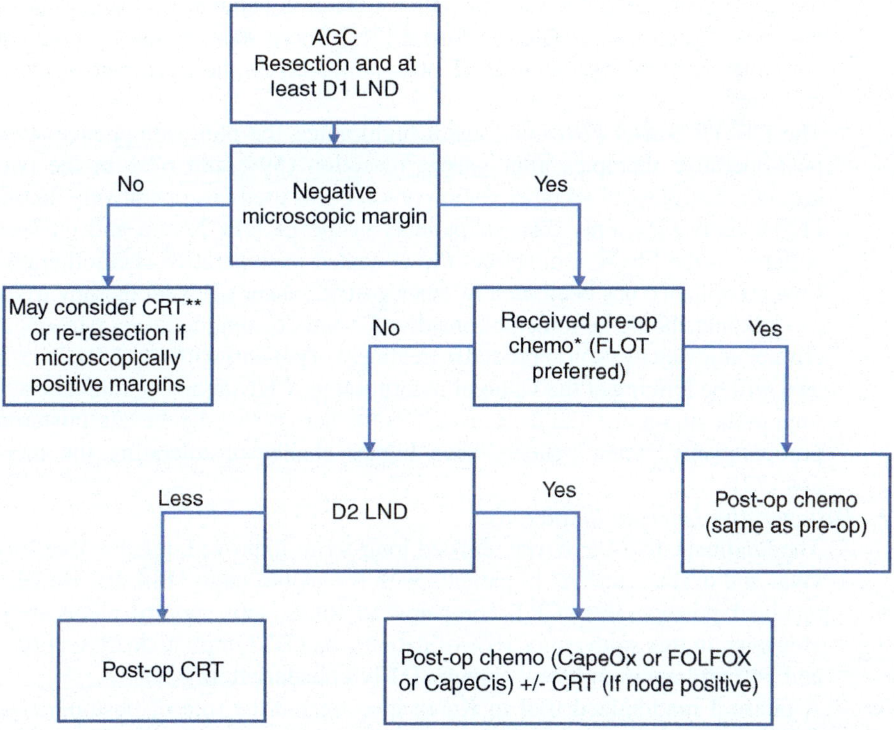

Fig. 11.3 Peri-operative/postoperative therapy decision tree for advanced gastric cancer (AGC). Please see section above on "Combined Modality Treatment" for further details. *For treatment of AGC, we advocate for peri-operative chemotherapy approach over adjuvant therapy only, given low compliance rate with adjuvant therapy post-gastric surgery. **The benefit of post-op CRT in this scenario is only demonstrated in retrospective studies. Its risk/benefit or indication should be discussed on a case-by-case basis in multidisciplinary rounds. *R1 resection* microscopically positive margin, *CRT* chemoradiotherapy, *LND* lymphadenectomy, *AGC* advanced gastric cancer, *FLOT* docetaxel, oxaliplatin, fluorouracil, and leucovorin, *CapeOx* capecitabine and oxaliplatin, *CapeCis* capecitabine and cisplatin, *FOLFOX* FOLinic acid, fluorouracil, oxaliplatin

- *Peri-operative Chemotherapy*
  - Currently, in North America, peri-operative chemotherapy is the favored multi-modality approach for treatment of AGC. Peri-operative FLOT has been recently adopted as the standard of care in North America for management of patients with cT2 or greater and/or cN-positive patients [75].
  - Three preoperative and three postoperative cycles of ECF/ECX were compared against four pre- and 4 postoperative cycles of FLOT in a phase 3 randomized trial. The results showed that FLOT was associated with improved OS and PFS, with no increased complications rates [75]. More patients in the FLOT arm were able to complete all allocated treatment cycles compared to ECF/ECX. Peri-operative FLOT also resulted in improved R0 resection rates.
  - In the phase 2 of the same trial, four cycles of preoperative FLOT was associated with significantly higher rates of pathological complete regression (16%) compared to three cycles of preoperative ECF/ECX (6%) [27].
  - The role of replacing postoperative chemotherapy with CRT after preoperative chemo and adequate surgery (at least D1+) in patients with stage 1B-4a was investigated in the CRITICS trial [76]. There was no improvement in outcomes with incorporating CRT postoperatively in the treatment of these patients.
  - The CRITICS trial [76] once again highlighted the poor compliance with post-operative therapies after gastric resection (59% and 62% in the two groups) regardless of whether chemo or CRT was used postoperatively. In the FLOT study [75], only 52% of patients in the ECF/ECX arm and 60% of patients in the FLOT arm started the allocated postoperative chemotherapy. Low compliance has been seen in other gastric cancer adjuvant therapy trials as well, and should be a factor considered when deciding between peri-operative or adjuvant therapy approach in treatment of patients with GC. CRITICS-2 trial will be looking at the value of incorporating CRT in the neoadjuvant setting, in an attempt to find the most effective therapy that can be administered preoperatively, when patients have higher chance of tolerating the therapy [77].
- *Postoperative Chemoradiotherapy*
  - The landmark INT-0116 trial showed long-term, improved, relapse-free survival and overall survival in patients with resectable stage 1B-4 disease who received postoperative CRT compared to those with surgery alone [61]. However, in this study, only 10% of patients had D2 lymph node dissections, and 54% did not even have complete D1 lymphadenectomy [19].
  - A phase 3 randomized trial in Korea investigated the role of postoperative CRT after curative resection of advanced gastric cancer with D2 lymphadenectomy, and did not demonstrate benefit with addition of adjuvant CRT in this group of patients compared to adjuvant chemotherapy alone [78, 79]. Unplanned subgroup analysis [79] suggested improved disease-free survival in node-positive patients who received concurrent adjuvant CRT compared to

adjuvant chemotherapy alone. Benefits of adjuvant CRT in this subset of patients will be explored further in ARTIST-2 trial.
  - There may be a role for considering postoperative radiation in the case of microscopically positive resection margins. Please see the section “Resection Margin” above for more details.
  - To summarize the role of radiotherapy, patients with resected advanced GC who had curative resection but only D1 lymphadenectomy and no neoadjuvant chemo should be considered for adjuvant CRT [61]. In patients who receive neoadjuvant chemo followed by curative resection and at least D1 lymphadenectomy, no clear benefit has been demonstrated in post-op CRT compared to post-op chemo [76]. Lastly, in node-positive patients with completely resected gastric cancer and D2 lymphadenectomy who did not receive preoperative chemotherapy, there may be benefit in incorporating CRT in their adjuvant regimen [79].
- *Postoperative Chemotherapy:*
  - Following curative resection (R0) and D2 lymphadenectomy of advanced GC, in patients who did not receive preoperative chemo, the results of phase 3 randomized trials as well as meta-analysis support use of adjuvant chemotherapy over surgery alone, when possible [74, 78, 80–83]. However, the role of adjuvant chemotherapy in this patient population who have received D1 lymphadenectomy (or less) is not well defined, and adjuvant CRT tends to be the treatment of choice [50, 61].

Unresectable or Metastatic Gastric Cancer

Workup	Management	Follow-up (F/U)
Recommended tests: History and physical exam Upper endoscopy HER-2 status Imaging: CT abdomen/pelvis *Optional tests:* Staging laparoscopy[a] CT chest	Consider chemotherapy, radiotherapy, and nonoperative management for symptomatic patients Palliative gastrectomy should be avoided and only performed for symptomatic patients, for whom all nonsurgical and less morbid options have been considered Stenting is associated with less morbidity than resection or bypass for palliation of obstruction and is typically preferred Radiation or angioembolization can be effective for transfusion-dependent bleeding	As symptoms warrant

[a]See Special Notes

Special Notes: Unresectable or Metastatic Gastric Cancer

Staging Laparoscopy may have utility in confirming metastatic disease, especially carcinomatosis, if suspected on imaging.

Criteria for Nonoperative Management

- Unresectable
  - Level 3 or 4 suspicious nodes on imaging or confirmed by biopsy. Level 3 nodes include the posterior surface of the pancreas (nodal station 13), superior mesenteric artery, and vein (station 14). Level 4 nodes are middle colic vessels (station 15) and the para-aortic nodes (station 16).
  - Invasion or encasement of major vascular structures, such as celiac axis and its branches, is considered unresectable. Isolated left gastric artery involvement can be treated with curative intent if an R0 margin is obtainable.
- Metastatic spread or peritoneal seeding (including positive peritoneal cytology) identified at surgical resection is considered incurable. Unless symptoms exist, systemic therapy should be considered rather than resection.
- Non-curative gastrectomy has been demonstrated to impart no benefit in the setting of metastatic disease and exposes patients to unnecessary surgical procedures and risks of complications. In a phase 3 trial, survival of gastrectomy (followed by postoperative chemotherapy) in patients with advanced gastric cancer and one non-curative factor was compared against modern chemotherapy only, showing no survival benefit from gastrectomy and higher serious adverse events [84].

Landmark Surgical Publications (D1 vs. D2 Lymphadenectomy)

Study	Methods	Results
Dutch Trial Bonenkamp et al. [69]	RCT $N = 711$ D1 vs. D2 resection D2 resection included distal pancreatectomy (30%) and splenectomy (38%)	Morbidity: 43% D2 vs. 25% D1 ($p < 0.001$) Mortality: 10% D2 vs. 4.0% D1 ($p = 0.004$) Median postoperative stays: D2 25 days vs. D1 18 days; $p < 0.001$ *5-year update* [39]: No difference in 5-year OS rates: 35% D1 vs. 33% D2 *15-year update* [68]: Overall 15-year survival: 22% D1 vs. 28% D2; $p = 0.34$ Deaths from gastric cancer: 48% D1 vs. 37% D2; $p = 0.01$

Study	Methods	Results
Medical Research Council (MRC) ST01 Cuschieri et al. [85]	RCT $N = 400$ D1 vs. D2 resection D2 resection includes distal pancreatectomy and splenectomy (56%), or only splenectomy (66%)	Morbidity: 46% D2 vs. 28% D1; $p < 0.001$ Mortality: 13% D2 vs. 6.5% D1; $p = 0.04$ *5-year update* [86]*:* No difference in 5-year OS rates: 35% D1 vs. 33% D2
Italian Gastric Cancer Surgical Group (IGCSG) Degiuli et al. [87]	RCT $N = 267$ D1 vs. D2 resection In the D2 arm, spleen and pancreas were preserved unless direct tumor extension. Splenectomy was performed for T1 or higher tumors on the greater curvature of the proximal or middle one-third of the stomach	No difference in 5-year OS: 66.5% D1 vs. 64.2% D2 Morbidity: 10.5% D1 vs. 16.3% D2; $p < 0.29$ In-hospital mortality: 0% D2 vs. 1.3% D1; not statistically significant *5-year update* [44]*:* Trend toward improved 5-year OS for advanced disease (T2-4; N+): 59% D2 vs. 38% D1; $p = 0.055$ 5-year DSS for pT1 cancers were worse in the D2 arm compared to the D1 group (83% vs. 98%; $p = 0.015$)

CRT chemoradiotherapy, *OS* overall survival, *RCT* randomized control trial

Landmark Chemotherapy and Chemoradiation Publications

Study	Methods	Results
FLOT Trial Al-Batran et al. [75]	RCT $N = 716$ Stage ≥cT2 and/or cN+, M0 resectable gastric and GEJ adenocarcinoma 3 preoperative and 3 postoperative 3-week cycles of ECF/ECX or 4 preoperative and 4 postoperative 2-week cycles of FLOT	*Peri-op FLOT improved overall survival and progression-free survival compared to peri-op ECF/ECX* Median OS 50 months vs. 35 months (HR 0.77 [0.63–0.94]; $p = 0.012$) PFS 30 vs. 18 months (HR 0.75 [0.62–0.91]; $p = 0.004$) More grade 3 and 4 nausea/vomiting within ECF/ECX group compared to FLOT

Study	Methods	Results
CRITICS Trial Cats et al. [76]	RCT $N = 788$ Stage 1B-4. Induction. 3 cycles of pre-op ECX, then curative gastrectomy and at least D1 LND, then randomized to post-op chemo (3 cycles of ECX) or CRT (45 Gy + weekly and daily capecitabine) Post-op only 59% of chemo group and 62% of CRT group started post-op therapy	*Post-op CRT did not improve overall survival* vs. *post-op chemo* Median OS 43 months (95% CI 31–57) in chemo group and 37 months (30–48) in CRT group (HR 1.01 m, 95% CI 0.84–1.22; $p = 0.90$). Median follow-up 61.4 months No mortality in post-op period. Grade 3 and 4 complications during post-op were 48% and 9% in chemo group vs. 41% and 4% in CRT group
INT-0116 Trial MacDonald et al. [61]	RCT $N = 556$ Surgery plus adjuvant CRT vs. surgery alone Adjuvant treatment was 5-FU + leucovorin followed by 4500 cGy All patients received curative-intent surgery: Only 10% received D2 resection 54% received D0 resection	*Improved overall and relapse-free survival with adjuvant CRT* Median OS: 36-month CRT vs. 27-month surgery alone; $p = 0.005$ Median RFS: 30-month CRT vs. 19-month surgery alone; $p < 0.001$ 3-year OS: 50% CRT vs. 41% surgery alone; $p = 0.005$
MAGIC Trial Cunningham et al. [73]	RCT $N = 503$, T2 or higher Surgery with perioperative ECF vs. surgery alone ECF was administered for 3 cycles preoperatively and 3 cycles postoperatively	*Improved PFS and OS with perioperative ECF* 5-year OS: 36% ECF vs. 23% surgery alone; HR 0.75 (95% CI 0.60–0.93), $p = 0.009$ PFS: HR 0.66 (95% CI 0.53–0.81), $p < 0.001$
GASTRIC Study Paoletti et al. [74]	Patient-level meta-analysis of 17 RCTs $N = 3838$ Chemotherapy after complete resection vs. surgery alone	*Improved OS and DFS with adjuvant chemotherapy in resectable gastric cancer* OS: HR = 0.82 (95% CI 0.76–0.90; $P < 0.001$) DFS: HR = 0.82 (95% CI 0.75–0.90; $P < 0.001$)
CLASSIC Trial Noh et al. [80]	Multicenter RCT $n = 1035$ patients, stage II–IIIB Surgery plus adjuvant capecitabine and oxaliplatin vs. surgery alone All patients underwent D2 resection	*Improved DFS and OS with chemo* 5-year DFS: 68% vs. 53%; HR 0.58 (95% CI 0.47–0.72) 5-year OS: 78% vs. 69%; HR 0.66 (95% CI 0.51–0.85)

Study	Methods	Results
ARTIST-I Trial Park et al. [78, 79]	RCT $n = 458$ All patients underwent D2 gastrectomy Chemotherapy alone (6 cycles capecitabine + cisplatin) vs. CRT (4 cycles chemo; 45 Gy with concurrent capecitabine)	*No difference in DFS and OS at 7years of median follow-up* 5-year DFS: HR 0.74 (95% CI 0.52–1.05; $p = 0.092$) 5-year OS: 73% vs. 75%, HR 1.13 (95% CI 0.78–1.65; $p = 0.53$) Subgroup analysis suggests benefit of CRT for node-positive disease and intestinal subtype (awaiting results of ARTIST-II trial)

CRT chemoradiotherapy, *OS* overall survival, *RFS* relapse-free survival, *PFS* progression-free survival, *DFS* disease-free survival, *HR* hazard ratio, *RCT* randomized control trial, *ECF* epirubicin/cisplatin/5-fluorouracil, *FLOT* docetaxel, oxaliplatin, fluorouracil, and leucovorin

Landmark Palliative Publications

Study	Methods	Results
Chemotherapy vs. best supportive care in non-curable gastric cancer Glimelius et al. [88]	RCT $N = 61$, unresectable Chemotherapy + best supportive care vs. best supportive care alone Chemotherapy was ELF-regimen consisting of 5-fluorouracil, leucovorin, and etoposide	*Improved or prolonged high-quality life at 4 months*: 45% chemotherapy group vs. 20% best supportive care group; $p < 0.05$
TOGA Trial Bang et al. [89]	RCT $N = 584$, inoperable or metastatic, HER-2+ gastric cancer Chemotherapy alone (capecitabine or 5-FU + cisplatin) vs. chemotherapy + trastuzumab	*Improved median OS in HER2+ patients treated with trastuzumab*: median OS 13.8-month trastuzumab vs. 11.1-month chemotherapy alone ($p = 0.0046$) 22% of patients assessed were HER2+
REGATTA Trial Fujitani et al. 2016 [84]	RCT $N = 175$ (planned $N = 330$) Eligibility: gastric cancer (cT1-3), single non-curable site of disease confined to liver, peritoneum or para-aortic lymph node, PS 0-1 Gastrectomy (D1 without resection of metastases) followed by chemotherapy (S-1 plus cisplatin) vs. chemotherapy alone	Terminated early by DSMC based on futility: 2-year OS 25.1% for gastrectomy followed by chemotherapy vs. 31.7% for chemotherapy alone ($p = 0.68$)

OS overall survival, *RCT* randomized control trial, *5-FU* fluorouracil, *PS* performance status, *DSMC* data safety monitoring committee

Referral to Medical Oncology and Radiation Oncology

- As the decision regarding adjuvant treatments should be made preoperatively, all patients should be referred to medical oncology and radiation oncology prior to resection and discussed at a multidisciplinary care conference.
- Relative contraindications to chemotherapy [62]
  - Impaired cardiac function such as congestive heart failure, baseline left ventricular ejection fraction less than 50%, transmural myocardial infarction, valvular heart disease, high-risk arrhythmias
  - Impaired renal function (Cr clearance of <60 ml/min)
  - Disorders of the nervous system and diabetes are relative contraindications for chemotherapy with neuropathic agents (e.g., platinums)
- Relative contraindications to radiation
  - Prohibitive toxicities anticipated due to volume or adjacent structures
  - Connective tissue disease
  - Previous irradiation to area

Referral to Multidisciplinary Cancer Conference

- All cases of advanced gastric cancer should be discussed at a Multidisciplinary Cancer Conference (MCC), before surgical intervention to devise an individual plan for each patient.
- Gastric cancer cases that were not discussed at MCC preoperatively should be discussed if the final pathology is >T1N0.

References

1. Canadian Cancer Society. Canadian Cancer Society's Steering Committee: Canadian Cancer Statistics 2018. http://www.cancer.ca/~/media/cancer.ca/CW/cancer%20information/cancer%20101/Canadian%20cancer%20statistics/Canadian-Cancer-Statistics-2018-EN.pdf?la=en.
2. Kim JP. Surgical results in gastric cancer. Semin Surg Oncol. 1999;17:132–8.
3. Jim MA, Pinheiro PS, Carreira H, et al. Stomach cancer survival in the United States by race and stage (2001-2009): findings from the CONCORD-2 study. Cancer. 2017;123(Suppl):4994–5013.
4. Fitzgerald RCCC. Clinical implications of E-Cadherin associated hereditary diffuse gastric cancer. Gut. 2004;53:775–8.
5. Gayther SA, Gorrini's KL, Ramos SJ, et al. Identification of germ-line E-Catherine mutations in gastric cancer families of European Origin. Cancer Res. 1998;58:4086–9.
6. Seevaratnam R, Coburn N, Cardozo R, et al. A systematic review of the indications for genetic testing and prophylactic gastrectomy among patients with hereditary diffuse gastric cancer. Gastric Cancer. 2012;15(Suppl 1):S153–63.
7. Pharoah PD, Guilford PCC. Incidence of gastric cancer and breast cancer in CDH1 (E-cadherin) mutation carriers from hereditary diffuse gastric cancer families. Gastroenterology. 2001;121:1348–53.

8. van der Post RS, Vogelaar IP, Carneiro F, et al. Hereditary diffuse gastric cancer: updated clinical guidelines with an emphasis on germline CDH1 mutation carriers. J Med Genet. 2015;52(6):361–74.
9. Caldas C, Carneiro F, Lynch HT, et al. Familial gastric cancer: overview and guidelines for management. J Med Genet. 1999;36:873.
10. Rudloff U. Gastric adenocarcinoma and proximal polyposis of the stomach: diagnosis and clinical perspectives. Clin Exp Gastroenterol. 2018;11:447–59.
11. Worthley DL, Phillips KD, Wayte N, et al. Gastric adenocarcinoma and proximal polyposis of the stomach (GAPPS): a new autosomal dominant syndrome. Gut. 2012;61(5):774–9.
12. Anaya DA, Chang GJ, Rodriguez-bigas MA. Extracolonic manifestation of hereditary colorectal cancer syndrome. Clin Colon Rectal Surg. 2008;21(4):263–72.
13. Syngal S, Brand RE, Church JM, et al. ACG clinical guideline: genetic testing and management of hereditary gastrointestinal cancer syndromes. Am J Gastroenterol. 2015;110:223.
14. Mankaney G, Leone P, Cruise M, et al. Gastric cancer in FAP: a concerning rise in incidence. Familial Cancer. 2017;16:371–6.
15. Møller P, Seppaia TT, Bernstein I, et al. Cancer risk and survival in path_MMR carriers by gene and gender up to 75 years of age: a report from the prospective lynch syndrome database. Gut. 2018;67(7):1306–16.
16. Vasen HF, Blanco I, Astana-Collin K, et al. Revised guidelines for the clinical management of Lynch syndrome (HNPCC): recommendations by a group of European experts. Gut. 2013;62(6):812–23.
17. Tomlinson IP, Houlston RS. Peutz-Jeghers Syndrome. J Med Genet. 1997;34:1007–11.
18. Van Lier MG, Wagner A, Mathus-Vliegen EM, et al. High cancer risk in Peutz-Jeghers syndrome: a systematic review and surveillance recommendations. Am J Gastroenterol. 2010;105(6):1258–64.
19. Gupta S, Provenzale D, Regenbogen SE, et al. NCCN guidelines ® insights: genetic/familial high-risk assessment: colorectal, version 3.2017 featured updates to the NCCN guidelines. J Natl Compr Canc Netw. 2017;15:1465–75.
20. Balmaña J, Balaguer F, Cervantes A, Arnold D. Familial risk-colorectal cancer: ESMO clinical practice guidelines. Ann Oncol. 2013;24(Suppl 6):vi73–80.
21. Stoffel EM, Mangu PB, Gruber SB, et al. Hereditary colorectal cancer syndromes: American society of clinical oncology clinical practice guideline endorsement of familial risk-colorectal cancer: European Society for medical oncology clinical practice guidelines. J Clin Oncol. 2015;33:209–17.
22. Lauren P. The two histological main types of gastric carcinoma: diffuse and so-called intestinal-type carcinoma. An attempt at a histo-clinical classification. Acta Pathol Microbiol Scand. 1965;64:31–49.
23. Correa P. Human gastric carcinogenesis: a multistep and multifactorial process--First American Cancer Society Award Lecture on Cancer Epidemiology and Prevention. Cancer Res. 1992;52(24):6735–40.
24. Qiu M, Cai M, Zhang D, et al. Clinicopathological characteristics and prognostic analysis of Lauren classification in gastric adenocarcinoma in China. J Transl Med. 2013;11:58.
25. Chen YC, Fang WL, Wang RF, et al. Clinicopathological variation of Lauren classification in gastric cancer. Pathol Oncol Res. 2016;22(1):197–202.
26. Kung PL, Gubens M, Fisher GA, Ford JM, et al. Long-term survivors of gastric cancer: a California population-based study. J Clin Oncol. 2012;30(28):3507–15.
27. Al-Bartan SE, Hofheinz RD, Pauligk C, et al. Histopathological regression after neoadjuvant docetaxel, oxaliplatin, fluorouracil, and leucovorin versus epirubicin, cisplatin, and fluorouracil or capecitabine in patients with resectable gastric or gastro-oesophageal junction adenocarcinoma (FLOT4-AIO): results from the phase 2 part of a multicentre, open-label, randomised phase 2/3 trial. Lancet Oncol. 2016;17(12):1697–708.

28. Cancer Genome Atlas Research Network, Bass AJ, Thorsson V, Shmulevich I, et al. Comprehensive molecular characterization of gastric adenocarcinoma. Nature. 2014;513(7517):202–9.
29. Sohn BH, Hwang JE, Jang HJ, et al. Clinical significance of four molecular subtypes of gastric cancer identified by the cancer genome atlas project. Clin Cancer. 2017. https://doi.org/10.158/1078-0432.CCR-16-2211.
30. Smyth EC, Wotherspoon A, Peckitt C, et al. Mismatch repair deficiency, microsatellite instability, and survival: an exploratory analysis of the Medical Research Council adjuvant gastric infusional chemotherapy (MAGIC) trial. JAMA Oncol. 2017;3(9):1197–203.
31. Amin MB, Edge S, Greene F, et al. American Joint Committee Cancer staging manual. New York: Springer; 2017.
32. Sano T, Coit DG, Kim HH, et al. Proposal of a new stage grouping of gastric cancer for TNM classification: International Gastric Cancer Association staging project. Gastric Cancer. 2017;20:2017.
33. In H, Ravetch E, Langdon-Embry M, et al. The newly proposed clinical and post-neoadjuvant treatment staging classifications for gastric adenocarcinoma for the American Joint Committee on Cancer (AJCC) staging. Gastric Cancer. 2018;21(1):1–9.
34. Seevaratnam R, Cardoso R, Mcgregor C, et al. How useful is preoperative imaging for tumor, node, metastasis (TNM) staging of gastric cancer? A meta-analysis. Gastric Cancer. 2012;15(Suppl):S3–S18.
35. Cardoso R, Coburn N, Seevaratnam R, et al. A systematic review and meta-analysis of the utility of EUS for preoperative staging for gastric cancer. Gastric Cancer. 2012;15(Suppl):S19–26.
36. Association Gastric Cancer Association. Japanese classification of gastric carcinoma – 2nd English edition. Gastric Cancer. 1998;1(1):10–24.
37. Gouzi JL, et al. Total versus subtotal gastrectomy for adenocarcinoma of the gastric antrum. A French prospective controlled study. Ann Surg. 1989;209:162–6.
38. Mahar AL, et al. A systematic review of surgery for non-curative gastric cancer. Gastric Cancer. 2012;15(Suppl 1):S125–37.
39. Bonenkamp JJ, et al. Extended lymph-node dissection for gastric cancer. N Engl J Med. 1999;340:908–14.
40. Association JGC. Japanese gastric cancer treatment guidelines 2014 (ver. 4). Gastric Cancer. 2017;20:1–19.
41. Gotoda T. Endoscopic resection of early gastric cancer: the Japanese perspective. Curr Opin Gastroenterol. 2006;22(5):561–9.
42. Daoud DC, Suter N, Durand M, et al. Comparing outcomes for endoscopic submucosal dissection between Eastern and Western countries: a systematic review and meta-analysis. World J Gastroenterol. 2018;24(23):2518–36.
43. Jeon MY, Park JC, Hahn KY, et al. Long-term outcomes after noncurative endoscopic resection of early gastric cancer: the optimal time for additional endoscopic treatment. Gastrointest Endosc. 2018;87(4):1003–1013.e2.
44. Degiuli M, et al. Randomized clinical trial comparing survival after D1 or D2 gastrectomy for gastric cancer. Br J Surg. 2014;101:23–31.
45. Morgagni P, La Barba G, Colciago E, et al. Resection line involvement after gastric cancer treatment: handle with care. Updat Surg. 2018;70(2):213–23.
46. Bria E, De Manzoni G, Beghelli S, et al. A clinical-biological risk stratification model for resected gastric cancer: prognostic impact of Her2, Fhit, and APC expression status. Ann Oncol. 2013;24(3):693–701.
47. Songun I, Bonenkamp JJ, Hermans J, et al. Prognostic value of resection-line involvement in patients undergoing curative resections for gastric cancer. Eur J Cancer. 1996;32A:433–7.
48. Kim SH, Karpeh MS, Klimstra DS, et al. Effect of microscopic resection line disease on gastric cancer survival. J Gastrointest Surg. 1999;3:24–33.
49. Ito H, Clancy TE, Osleen RT, et al. Adenocarcinoma of the gastric cardia: what is the optimal surgical approach? J Am Coll Surg. 2004;199(6):880–6.

50. National Comprehensive Cancer Network. NCCN clinical practice guideline in oncology gastric cancer. v2.2018. http://www.nccn.org/professionals/physician_gls/pdf/gastric.pdf http://www.nccn.org/professionals/physician_gls/pdf/gastric.pdf.
51. Smyth EC, Verheij M, Allum W, et al. Gastric cancer: ESMO Clinical Practice Guidelines for diagnosis, treatment and follow-up. Ann Oncol. 2016;27(Suppl 5):38–49.
52. McAuliffe JC, Tang LH, Kamrani K, et al. Prevalence of false-negative results of intraoperative consultation on surgical margins during resection of gastric and gastroesophageal adenocarcinoma. JAMA Surg. 2018;154:126.
53. Squires MH 3rd, Kooby DA, Pawlik TM, et al. Utility of the proximal margin frozen section for resection of gastric adenocarcinoma: a 7-Institution Study of the US Gastric Cancer Collaborative. Ann Surg Oncol. 2014;21(13):4202–10.
54. Stiekema J, Trip AK, Jansen EPM, et al. Does adjuvant chemoradiotherapy improve the prognosis of gastric cancer after an R1 resection? Results from a Dutch cohort study. Ann Surg Oncol. 2015;22:581–8.
55. Stiekema J, Trip AK, Jansen EPM, Boot H, Cats A, Ponz OB, et al. The prognostic significance of an R1 resection in gastric cancer patients treated with adjuvant chemoradiotherapy. Ann Surg Oncol. 2014;21:1107–14.
56. Rhome RM, Moshier E, Sarpel U, et al. Predictors of positive margins after definitive resection for gastric adenocarcinoma and impact of adjuvant therapies. Int J Radiat Oncol Biol Phys. 2017;98:1106–15.
57. Dikken JL, Jansen EPM, Cats A, Bakker B, Hartgrink HH, Kranenbarg EMK, et al. Impact of the extent of surgery and postoperative chemoradiotherapy on recurrence patterns in gastric cancer. J Clin Oncol. 2010;28:2430–6.
58. Brar S, Law C, McLeod R, et al. Defining surgical quality in gastric cancer: a RAND/UCLA appropriateness study. J Am Coll Surg. 2013;217(2):347–57.e1.
59. Kim W, Kim HH, Han SU, et al. Decreased morbidity of laparoscopic distal gastrectomy compared with open distal gastrectomy for stage I gastric cancer: short-term outcomes from a multicenter randomized controlled trial (KLASS-01). Ann Surg. 2016;263:28–35.
60. Kurokawa Y, Doki Y, Mizusawa J, et al. Bursectomy versus omentectomy alone for resectable gastric cancer (JCOG1001): a phase 3, open-label, randomised controlled trial. Lancet Gastroenterol Hepatol. 2018;3(7):460–8.
61. Macdonald JS, Smalley SR, Benedetti J, et al. Chemoradiotherapy after surgery compared with surgery alone for adenocarcinoma of the stomach or gastroesophageal junction. N Engl J Med. 2001;345:725–30.
62. Knight G, Earle CC, Cosby R, TGCDSG, et al.. Neoadjuvant or adjuvant therapy for resectable gastric cancer, Evidence-based series 2–14 version 3. Toronto Cancer Care Ontario; 2011.
63. Lowy AM, Mansfield PF, Leach SD, et al. Laparoscopic staging for gastric cancer. Surgery. 1996;119:611–4.
64. Oh CA, Bae JM, Oh SJ, et al. Long-term results and prognostic factors of gastric cancer patients with only positive peritoneal lavage cytology. J Surg Oncol. 2012;105:393–9.
65. Mezhir JJ, Shah MA, Jacks LM, et al. Positive peritoneal cytology in patients with gastric cancer: natural history and outcome of 291 patients. Ann Surg Oncol. 2010;17(12):3173–80.
66. Newhook TE, Agnes A, Blum M, et al. Laparoscopic hyperthermic intraperitoneal chemotherapy is safe for patients with peritoneal metastases from gastric cancer and may Lead to gastrectomy. Ann Surg Oncol. 2019;26(5):1394–400.
67. Badgwell B, Blum M, Das P, et al. Phase II trial of laparoscopic hyperthermic intraperitoneal chemoperfusion for peritoneal carcinomatosis or positive peritoneal cytology in patients with gastric adenocarcinoma. Ann Surg Oncol. 2017;24(11):3338–44.
68. Songun I, Putter H, Kranenbarg EM, et al. Surgical treatment of gastric cancer: 15-year follow-up results of the randomised nationwide Dutch D1D2 trial. Lancet Oncol. 2010;11:439–49.
69. Bonenkamp JJ, Songun I, Hermans J, et al. Randomised comparison of morbidity after D1 and D2 dissection for gastric cancer in 996 Dutch patients. Lancet. 1995;345:745–8.

70. Sasako M, Sano T, Yamamoto S, et al. D2 lymphadenectomy alone or with para-aortic nodal dissection for gastric cancer. N Engl J Med. 2008;359:453–62.
71. Xiong B, Ma L, Huang W, et al. Efficiency of bursectomy in patients with resectable gastric cancer: an updated meta-analysis. Eur J Surg Oncol. 2019;45:1483.
72. Kim HI, Hur H, Kim YN, et al. Standardization of D2 lymphadenectomy and surgical quality control (KLASS-02-QC): a prospective, observational, multicenter study [NCT01283893]. BMC Cancer. 2014;14:209.
73. Cunningham D, Allum WH, Stenning SP, et al. Perioperative chemotherapy versus surgery alone for resectable gastroesophageal cancer. N Engl J Med. 2006;355:11–20.
74. GASTRIC, Paoletti X, Oba K, et al. Benefit of adjuvant chemotherapy for resectable gastric cancer: a meta-analysis. JAMA. 2010;303:1729–37.
75. Al-Bartan SE, Homann N, Pauligk C, et al. Perioperative chemotherapy with fluorouracil plus leucovorin, oxaliplatin, and docetaxel versus fluorouracil or capecitabine plus cisplatin and epirubicin for locally advanced, resectable gastricor gastro-oesophageal junction adenocarcinoma (FLOT4): a randomised, phase 2/3 trial. Lancet. 2019;393:1948.
76. Cats A, Jansen EPM, van Grieken NCT, et al. Chemotherapy versus chemoradiotherapy after surgery and preoperative chemotherapy for resectable gastric cancer (CRITICS): an international, open-label, randomised phase 3 trial. Lancet Oncol. 2018;19(5):616–28.
77. Slagter AE, Jansen EPM, van Laarhoven HWM, et al. CRITICS-II: a multicentre randomised phase II trial of neo-adjuvant chemotherapy followed by surgery versus neo-adjuvant chemotherapy and subsequent chemoradiotherapy followed by surgery versus neo-adjuvant chemoradiotherapy followed by surgery in resectable gastric cancer. BMC Cancer. 2018;18(1):877.
78. Lee J, Lim DH, Kim S, et al. Phase III trial comparing capecitabine plus cisplatin versus capecitabine plus cisplatin with concurrent capecitabine radiotherapy in completely resected gastric cancer with D2 lymph node dissection: the ARTIST trial. J Clin Oncol. 2012;30:268–73.
79. Park SH, Sohn TS, Lee J, et al. Phase III trial to compare adjuvant chemotherapy with capecitabine and cisplatin versus concurrent chemoradiotherapy in gastric cancer: final report of the adjuvant chemoradiotherapy in stomach Tumors trial, including survival and subset analyses. J Clin Oncol. 2015;33(28):3130–6.
80. Noh SH, Park SR, Yang HK, et al. Adjuvant capecitabine plus oxaliplatin for gastric cancer after D2 gastrectomy (CLASSIC): 5-year follow-up of an open-label, randomised phase 3 trial. Lancet Oncol. 2014;15:1389–96.
81. Diaz-Nieto R, Orti-Rodríguez R, Winslet M. Post-surgical chemotherapy versus surgery alone for resectable gastric cancer. Cochrane Database Syst Rev. 2013;(9):CD008415.
82. Grau JJ, Martín M, Fuster J, et al. Impact of adjuvant chemotherapy in the long-term outcome of patients with resected gastric cancer. J Surg Oncol. 2003;82(4):234–40.
83. Sasako M, Sakuramoto S, Katai H, et al. Five-year outcomes of a randomized phase III trial comparing adjuvant chemotherapy with S-1 versus surgery alone in stage II or III gastric cancer. J Clin Oncol. 2011;29:4387.
84. Fujita J, Yang HK, Mizusawa J, et al. Gastrectomy plus chemotherapy versus chemotherapy alone for advanced gastric cancer with a single non-curable factor (REGATTA): a phase 3, randomised controlled trial. Lancet Oncol. 2016;17(3):309–18.
85. Cuschieri A, Fayers P, Fielding J, et al. Postoperative morbidity and mortality after D1 and D2 resections for gastric cancer: preliminary results of the MRC randomised controlled surgical trial. The Surgical Cooperative Group. Lancet. 1996;347:995–9.
86. Cuschieri A, Weeden S, Fielding J, et al. Patient survival after D1 and D2 resections for gastric cancer: long-term results of the MRC randomized surgical trial. Surgical Co-operative Group. Br J Cancer. 1999;79:1522–30.
87. Degiuli M, Sasako M, Calgaro M, et al. Morbidity and mortality after D1 and D2 gastrectomy for cancer: interim analysis of the Italian Gastric Cancer Study Group (IGCSG) randomised surgical trial. Eur J Surg Oncol. 2004;30(3):303–8.

88. Glimelius B, Ekström K, Hoffman K, et al. Randomized comparison between chemotherapy plus best supportive care with best supportive care in advanced gastric cancer. Ann Oncol. 1997;8(2):163–8.
89. Bang YJ, Van Cutsem E, Feyereislova A, et al. Trastuzumab in combination with chemotherapy versus chemotherapy alone for treatment of HER2-positive advanced gastric or gastro-oesophageal junction cancer (ToGA): a phase 3, open-label, randomised controlled trial. Lancet. 2010;376(9742):687–97.

Gastrointestinal Stromal Tumor

12

Dario Callegaro, Richard Kirsch, Albiruni R. Abdul Razak, Fayez A. Quereshy, and Carol J. Swallow

Introduction

Epidemiology and Pathophysiology

Gastrointestinal stromal tumors (GISTs) are the most common mesenchymal neoplasms of the gastrointestinal tract with an incidence of approximately 10–15 per million population [1–4]. Although they can arise in any location throughout the gastrointestinal tract, they are found most commonly in the stomach (55.6%) and small intestine (31.8%, including the duodenum) [3, 5]. The median age at diagnosis is mid-60s, but GISTs can also present in the pediatric age group (older than 10 years, especially adolescents) and young adults. On average, 18% of GISTs are incidentally discovered, and this proportion has increased. Small asymptomatic gastric GISTs (micro-GIST) are common in the general population, especially in older adults. Pathologic studies have found micro-GIST in up to 35% of patients undergoing gastrectomy for other reasons [2, 3, 6].

The majority of GISTs (approximately 70%) are composed of spindle cells, about 20% are composed of epithelioid cells, while remaining 10% of mixed

D. Callegaro
General Surgical Oncology, University of Toronto, Toronto, ON, Canada
e-mail: dario.callegaro@one-mail.on.ca

R. Kirsch
Department of Pathology, University of Toronto, Toronto, ON, Canada
e-mail: Richard.Kirsch@sinaihealthsystem.ca

A. R. Abdul Razak
Department of Medicine, University of Toronto, Toronto, ON, Canada
e-mail: albiruni.razak@uhn.ca

F. A. Quereshy · C. J. Swallow (✉)
Department of Surgery, University of Toronto, Toronto, ON, Canada
e-mail: fayez.quereshy@uhn.ca; Carol.Swallow@sinaihealth.ca

F. C. Wright et al. (eds.), *Surgical Oncology Manual*,
https://doi.org/10.1007/978-3-030-48363-0_12

spindle-epithelioid morphology. Approximately 70–80% of GISTs result from activating mutations in the *KIT* (CD117) proto-oncogene while approximately 10% are associated with a platelet-derived growth factor receptor alpha gene (*PDGFRA*) mutation [7–10]. Immunohistochemical analysis has identified markers characteristic of GIST, facilitating its differentiation from other mesenchymal neoplasms. The most useful immunohistochemical markers for GIST are CD117 (KIT, positive in 95% of cases) and DOG1 (98%). Approximately 3% of GISTs of GI tract are negative for both DOG1 and KIT. Approximately 50% of KIT-negative GIST are positive for DOG1 and 50% of DOG1-negative GISTs are positive for KIT. Although DOG1 is highly specific for GIST, it can be positive also in uterine-type retroperitoneal leiomyomas, peritoneal leiomyomatosis, synovial sarcomas, and esophageal squamous cells and gastric carcinomas [11]. The cell of origin is the interstitial cell of Cajal [12]. Both KIT and DOG1 label GI Cajal cells.

Risk Stratification

The clinical behavior of GISTs is extremely variable, ranging from no growth over decades to highly aggressive with progression appreciable within weeks. The current AJCC Staging System for GIST (Eighth Edition, 2017) is based upon tumor size (with cutoffs at 2, 5, and 10 cm), lymph node metastasis, and distant metastasis, while grade is indicated by mitotic rate [13]. Other classification systems and prognostic tools have been shown to accurately predict the risk of GIST recurrence and survival after primary resection and these are in wider clinical use than the AJCC system.

The original NIH (National Institutes of Health) criteria [14] stratified GIST patients into four risk categories (very low risk, low risk, intermediate risk, and high risk) based upon tumor size and mitotic rate. Over the years, these criteria have been modified to additionally include primary tumor site and intraoperative tumor rupture (see Table 12.1) [15]. A widely applied risk stratification system in North America is that of Miettinen and colleagues (see Table 12.1) [5]. This is based upon tumor site, size, and mitotic count and is included in the College of American Pathologist protocol for the examination of specimens from patients with GIST [16].

In a comparative study, the modified NIH criteria proved to be the best instrument to identify a single high-risk group of patients for consideration of adjuvant therapy, while the highly sophisticated contour maps developed by Joensuu et al. provided the most accurate estimate of individualized patient outcome [17].

Molecular Classification

Approximately 85–90% of GIST harbor mutations in genes encoding receptor tyrosine kinases (RTK) c-KIT or PDGFR, with mutation type and location

Table 12.1 Risk stratification instruments for patients with GIST

Tumor characteristics		Modified NIH criteria		Miettinen and Lasota classification (% of patients with progressive disease during long-term follow-up)			
Tumor size (cm)[a]	Mitotic index (per 50 high-power fields, HPFs)[b]	Primary tumor site	Risk category	Gastric	Jejunal and ileal	Duodenal	Rectal
<2	≤5	Any	Very low	0	0	0	0
2.1–5.0	≤5	Any	Low	1.9	4.3	8.3	8.5
5.1–10.0	≤5	Gastric Nongastric	Intermediate High	3.6	24	/	/
>10.0	≤5	/	/	12	52	34	57
≤2	>5	/	/	0[c]	50[c]	/	54
2.1–5.0	>5	Gastric Nongastric	Intermediate High	16	73	50	52
< 5.0	6–10	Any	Intermediate	/	/	/	/
>5.0	>5	Any	High				
5.1–10.0	>5	/	/	55	85	/	/
>10	>5	/	/	86	90	86	71
>10.0	Any	Any	High	/	/	/	/
Any	>10	Any	High	/	/	/	/
Any	Any	Tumor rupture	High	/	/	/	/

Modified from Joensuu [15] and Miettinen and Lasota [5]
[a]Largest dimension
[b]Per 50 HPFs is a total of 5 mm^2. Field areas of different microscopes may vary substantially
[c]Small number of cases

associated with both clinical behavior and tyrosine kinase inhibitor (TKI) sensitivity (see the table below). Of the 10–15% of GISTs that are RTK wild type (WT), 20–40% are deficient in succinyl dehydrogenase (SDH) complex expression and approximately 10% harbor mutations in genes involved in RAS pathways (*BRAF*, *NF1*, or *RAS*). The terms "quadruple-negative" and "quadruple-WT" have been applied to GISTs that do not harbor any detectable mutation in the *KIT*, *PDGFRA*, *SDH*, or RAS pathway genes [18], which make up approximately 5% of all GISTs.

In the following section, the workup and management of patients with primary GIST according to the mutation status and the presence of genetic syndromes will be discussed (Tables 12.2, 12.3, and 12.4).

Table 12.2 GIST with *KIT* and *PDGFRA* mutation

Mutation site	Most common mutations	Tumor site	Oncological outcome	Response to imatinib	Clinical features
KIT exon 11 (90% of *KIT* mutations) [19–22]	Deletions (53% of exon 11 mutations): 46% of deletions affect codons 557-558 Missense mutations (30%) Duplications (14%)	Predominantly stomach	Median post-resection RFS (Z9000 trial): 42 months Median PFS with Im (advanced GIST): 40 months	Sensitive	Deletions: Higher-risk compared with other Ex11 mutation classes Deletions involving codons 557–558 are associated with worse RFS Better RFS if deletions of only one codon Codons 557-558 mutations are associated with the greatest sensitivity to Im (42%CR and 81%CR/PR in advanced patients) but also with a more rapid development of secondary resistance (median PFS 30.6mo vs >63mo for most distal Ex11 mutations in advanced patients) Substitution mutations: Some are associated with better RFS Duplications: Lower risk of recurrence than other Ex11 mutations
KIT exon 9 (8% of *KIT* mutations) [20, 21]	Duplication of AY502-503	Predominantly in small bowel	Median RFS post-resection (Z9000 trial): 19 months Median PFS with Im (advanced GIST): 12.6 months	Lower sensitivity to Im compared to Ex11 mutations	Unfavorable prognosis Higher Im dose (800 mg/day) may be indicated
PDGFRA exon 12 and exon 18 [21, 22]	Substitution of D842V (8% of all GIST)	Predominantly stomach	Better RFS post-resection than exon 11 and exon 9	D842V: resistant Other *PDGFRA* mutations: sensitive	Low mitotic rate Favorable prognosis D842V: superior RFS compared with *KIT* mutations (HR 0.34)

Table 12.3 Sporadic GIST without *KIT* or *PDGFRA* mutations

SDH status	Tumor site	Patient's age	Clinical features
Competent	Anywhere in GI tract but with small-intestine prevalence	Adults	Usually unifocal Tumor size and mitotic index predict outcome [23, 24]
Deficient	Mainly in the stomach	Young patients (see "Pediatric and Young Adults GIST" section)	Indolent course More prone to lymph node and liver metastases SDHA IHC can be useful to distinguish two different subgroups and might have therapeutic implications [24, 25]

Table 12.4 Syndromic GIST without KIT and PDGFRA mutations

SDH-status	Clinical scenario	Mutations and inheritance	Clinical features	Age at presentation with GIST
Deficient	Carney-Stratakis syndrome [26, 27]	Germline mutation in *SDHB*, *SDHC*, or *SDHD*. Inheritance: AD, incomplete penetrance	Multifocal gastric GISTs and multicentric paragangliomas GISTs: Epithelioid morphology Poor responses to traditional Im therapy	Median: third decade
Deficient	Carney triad [23, 28]	Lack of *SDH*-inactivating mutations (epigenetic modifications or mutations of other genes might be involved)	Multifocal gastric GISTs, paragangliomas and pulmonary chondromas Female predominance (95%) GISTs: Predominantly gastric in location Tend to be multifocal Epithelioid histology and plexiform growth pattern Unpredictable behavior	Median: 22

(continued)

Table 12.4 (continued)

SDH-status	Clinical scenario	Mutations and inheritance	Clinical features	Age at presentation with GIST
Competent	Neurofibromatosis type 1 [27, 29, 30]	Germline mutation in *NF1* Inheritance: AD	Cafè-au-lait spots, cutaneous neurofibromas, plexiform neurofibroma, armpit or inguinal freckling, eye's iris hamartomas (Lisch nodules) GISTs: Life-time risk: 7% Predominantly in the small bowel Often multifocal (43%). Spindle cell morphology, often background of Cajal cell hyperplasia Generally resistant to imatinib	Median: 49

A deficient SDH status is defined as the loss of SDHB at immunohistochemistry
SDH succinate dehydrogenase, *AD* autosomal dominant

Among GISTs without *KIT* or *PDGFRA* mutation (sometimes referred to as "wild type"), there are both sporadic and syndromic GISTs and SDH expression as assessed by immunohistochemistry is useful for further subcategorization.

Special Notes

- SDH-deficient GIST can be either sporadic (due to somatic mutations within the tumor) or familial (due to germline mutation). The vast majority are thought to be familial.
- Rare syndromes associated with germline mutation of *KIT* and *PDGFRA* have been described [31, 32].
- Mutation in RAS family genes have been identified in a subset of GIST. In particular, *BRAF* V600E mutations have been found in 7% of GISTs from adult patients that lack *KIT*/*PDGFRA* mutations. Mutation of *BRAF* may also represent a mechanism of imatinib resistance [9, 33].
- The terms "quadruple-negative" and "quadruple-WT" are used to refer to GISTs that do not harbor any detectable mutation in the *KIT*, *PDGFRA*, *SDH*, or *BRAF* genes [18].

Pediatric and Young Adults GIST

Pediatric GISTs are rare, and patients typically present in the second decade of life; there is a distinct female predominance (70%). The tumors can be sporadic or occur in the context of genetic syndromes (see above). Pediatric GISTs are located predominantly in the stomach, and they are usually epithelioid and tend to be multifocal or plexiform at presentation. Pediatric GISTs show a higher rate of lymphovascular invasion and higher propensity to spread to the lymph nodes, peritoneum, and liver compared to adult GISTs. In spite of often presenting with advanced disease, the natural course of pediatric GISTs is more indolent as compared with that in adults (10-year survival rate is 92–94%, despite disease recurrence post-resection in 70–80%). Modified NIH risk criteria do not apply. Almost all pediatric GISTs lack mutations in *KIT* and *PDGFRA*, and 88% of cases show either epigenetic silencing or mutation of one of the genes coding for the four subunits of the SDH complex. Management differs from other GIST (see section "Management of GIST in Children and Young Adults") [34].

Management of GIST in Adults

Overall, 13% of primary GISTs are <2 cm at presentation [3]. Their treatment (Table 12.5) differs from the treatment of larger GISTs (Table 12.6) since, overall, they are associated with a lower risk of disease recurrence. Principles of

Table 12.5 Workup and management of primary small GIST (<2 cm)

Clinical scenario	Workup	Management	Follow-up
Gastric GIST < 2 cm	History and physical exam Imaging: CT abdomen and pelvis (triple-phase contrast with gastric protocol) Upper GI endoscopy (if not already performed) EUS-guided biopsy	Surgical resection with negative microscopic margins is an option if anticipated surgical morbidity is low In the absence of high-risk histological and EUS features (irregular border, heterogeneity, cystic spaces and echogenic foci, ulceration), a watchful-waiting approach can be taken in shared decision-making with the patient [35] Small GISTs that increase in size or become symptomatic should be resected with negative histological margins	If not resected: CT abdomen/pelvis (gastric protocol) at 3 months then, if stable, q4-6 months; may lengthen follow-up interval over time, depending on patient circumstances If growing or becoming symptomatic: surgical resection If resected: physical exam and CT abdomen/pelvis with a schedule tailored to the specific risk of recurrence gleaned from histology

(continued)

Table 12.5 (continued)

Clinical scenario	Workup	Management	Follow-up
Non-gastric GIST <2 cm	History and physical exam Imaging: CT abdomen/pelvis (triple-phase contrast) MRI for duodenal and rectal location Endoscopy for duodenal and rectal locations EUS-guided biopsy Multidisciplinary consultation	Surgical resection with negative microscopic margins [35, 36]	History and physical exam and CT abdomen/pelvis with a schedule tailored to the specific risk of recurrence

EUS endoscopic ultrasound

Table 12.6 Workup and management of primary GIST (>2 cm)

Clinical scenario	Workup	Management	Follow-up
Localized, resectable with anticipated low morbidity and negative margins	History and physical exam Imaging: CT chest, abdomen, and pelvis (triple-phase contrast) MRI scan (rectal and duodenal locations) Endoscopy for gastric, duodenal, and rectal locations EUS-guided (preferable) or percutaneous biopsy Multidisciplinary consultation	Surgical resection with negative histological margins Adjuvant imatinib should be given to high-risk patients with sensitive mutations following R0/R1 resection for at least 3 years. In intermediate-risk patients, adjuvant therapy should be discussed	History and physical exam every 3–6 months CT abdomen/pelvis: high risk: every 3–6 months for 5 years low risk: every 6 months for 5 years annually after 5 years CT chest if new findings on CT abdomen/pelvis

(continued)

Table 12.6 (continued)

Clinical scenario	Workup	Management	Follow-up
Localized, resectable with anticipated high morbidity or risk for positive margins	History and physical exam Imaging: CT chest, abdomen, and pelvis (triple-phase) MRI scan (rectal and duodenal locations) Endoscopy for gastric, duodenal, and rectal locations EUS-guided (preferable) or percutaneous biopsy Multidisciplinary consultation	Mutation sensitive to imatinib: Neoadjuvant imatinib started at 400 mg/day (800 mg/day may be recommended for Exon 9 mutation) Early reassessment with CT scan abdomen/pelvis 1–3 months after starting imatinib. Continue reassessment with CT q 3 months Responders: Surgical resection with negative histological margins at time of desired response, which is judged by the surgeon. If GIST was originally of intermediate or high risk, adjuvant imatinib should be given for a minimum of 3 years in total Non-responders: Consider switching to Im 800 mg/day or second-line therapy if tumor remains technically unresectable vs. proceed with surgery Mutation not sensitive to imatinib: Upfront surgical resection vs. clinical trials	History and physical exam every 3–6 months CT abdomen/pelvis: high risk: every 3–6 months for 5 years low risk: every 6months for 5 years annually after 5 years CT chest if new findings on CT abdomen/pelvis

EUS endoscopic ultrasound

recommended practice for patients with unresectable, recurrent, or metastatic GIST are summarized in Table 12.7.

Special Notes

- A cutoff of 2 cm for the definition of small GIST is arbitrary and it is based upon the fact that many GIST<2 cm will be of either low risk or very low risk [36]. Nonetheless, tumor size and mitotic count should also be taken into account in the estimation of the specific risk of tumor recurrence and tumor spread, keeping

Table 12.7 Workup and management of unresectable, recurrent, or metastatic GIST

Workup	Management	Follow-up (F/U)
History and physical exam Imaging: CT chest/abdomen/pelvis (triple-phase) MRI scan (rectal and duodenal locations) Endoscopic (preferable) or percutaneous biopsy Multidisciplinary consultation	Imatinib mesylate at a starting dose of 400 mg/day. For exon 9 mutations, 800 mg/day may be considered. Close radiographic surveillance with CT scans every 3 months should be performed to assess tumor response Tumor response to imatinib: PR/CR: continue with Im vs surgery if completely resectable SD: continue with Im vs surgery if completely resectable Unifocal PD: Im dose escalation vs surgery of the local progression to delay switching to second-line TKI Generalized PD: dose escalation vs sunitinib, no elective surgery Resistance to both imatinib and sunitinib: third-line tyrosine-kinase inhibitors such as regorafenib. Consider enrollment in available clinical trials as appropriate. Currently, pan-Kit inhibitors such as BLU-285 (avapritinib) or DCC-2618 (ripretenib) are under evaluation in several Phase III trials in post-imatinib settings (2nd-, 3rd-, and 4th-line indications) [50] Radiation therapy may be considered for symptomatic bone metastases; for anemia due to bleeding Ablative therapies may be considered in localized, solid organ metastases Embolization may be effective in controlling hemorrhage	History and physical exam every 3–6 months CT abdomen/pelvis—the first CT scan following the initiation of imatinib should be at 3 months (or sooner based on clinical indication), then every 3–6 months for 5 years The interval between consecutive CT scans may be increased based on disease stability CT chest if new findings on CT abdomen/pelvis

FDG-PET 18F-fluorodeoxyglucose-positron emission tomography

in mind that mitotic counts from a biopsy may underestimate the actual mitotic count. In addition to tumor size and mitotic count, the presence of worrisome features on endoscopic ultrasound, patient's performance status, life expectancy, and preference should play a role in the decision to pursue further treatment vs. watchful waiting.

- Most GISTs of 2 cm or less are asymptomatic but bleeding is a possible complication [37].

- Histological confirmation of small GIST is advised. EUS-guided fine needle aspiration (FNA) or fine needle biopsy (FNB) is preferable. EUS-guided biopsy of gastric nodules <2 cm can be technically challenging. If biopsy is not technically feasible (or does not yield a pathological diagnosis) and the patient is asymptomatic, close follow-up is a reasonable option. A tissue biopsy that allows IHC staining is preferred over cytologic sampling. A study from Kagawa, Japan, showed that 25% of FNA samples were not large enough to allow mitotic index estimation [38]. In a study from Seoul, Korea, EUS-guided 19-gauge trucut biopsy had a higher diagnostic accuracy than 22-gauge FNA in gastric submucosal lesions larger than 2 cm, with similar complication rates [39]. Other techniques to obtain a larger amount of tissue for diagnosis in gastric subepithelial tumors such as mucosal incision and forceps biopsy [40] or drill needle aspiration biopsy [41] have recently been described.
- Endoscopic resection is an option for low-risk small gastric GIST in centers with advanced endoscopic skills. As compared to surgery, endoscopic resection is associated with a higher incidence of R1 margins but comparable local recurrence rate. Advantages of endoscopic resection include shorter procedure time and hospital stay, and accessibility to the GE junction location. Patient selection should take into consideration tumor size, site, and mobility of the lesion with respect to the gastric wall, with endophytic lesions being most favorable [42].
- Rectal GIST<2 cm should be resected due to the higher risk of tumor progression and worse prognosis.

Special Notes

- Every attempt should be made to obtain a histological diagnosis before planning any treatment. In particular, tumor biopsy is considered essential before starting neoadjuvant Im treatment to confirm the diagnosis and to test for mutations in *KIT* and *PDGFRA*. In the case of a locally advanced or complicated mass highly suspicious for GIST in a symptomatic patient, neoadjuvant Imatinib could be started while waiting for the pathology results, provided early imaging and clinical reassessment are planned.
- EUS-guided endoscopic biopsy is preferred. If not feasible, percutaneous biopsy is an option. An analysis of 47 patients enrolled in the SSG XVIII trial (1 vs 3 years of adjuvant Imatinib in patients surgically treated for high-risk GIST) who underwent a percutaneous biopsy showed no significant difference in RFS or OS as compared to patients who did not undergo a percutaneous biopsy. Of note, in this study, patients were treated with surgery and postoperative imatinib, and thus the results might not be generalizable to patients treated with surgery alone [43]. A Scandinavian study of 72 patients showed that recurrence rates were increased after major, but not minor, intraoperative tumor rupture, but did not take into consideration percutaneous core needle biopsy [44].
- Surgery is the primary and only curative therapy in localized GIST.

- Surgery should aim at R0 resection. A gross visceral margin of 1–2 cm will usually generate a negative microscopic margin; gross margin targets may be appropriately modified in areas of functional consequence such as the GE junction, second portion of the duodenum, and the low rectum, but these deliberations require expertise in GIST management. Tumor enucleation is not advisable since it is associated with a high risk of tumor recurrence [45]. En-bloc resection should be used as needed. Systematic regional lymphadenectomy is NOT indicated for adult-type GIST.
- The effect of R1 resection on the oncological outcome of GIST patients is unclear. A recent meta-analysis of 12 studies including 1985 patients concluded that a microscopically positive margin could significantly impact DFS (HR 1.6, p 0.09) but had no influence on OS. The meta-analysis showed that adjuvant imatinib could attenuate the risk of recurrence in R1 patients [46].
- In case of R1 resection on final pathology, early re-excision in an attempt to "clear the margin" is generally not advised.
- Intraoperative tumor rupture is associated with a much higher risk of tumor recurrence [47]. In particular, in a retrospective study on GIST of the small intestine, major defects in tumor integrity (tumor spillage, tumor fracture or piecemeal resection, bowel perforation at the tumor site, blood-tinged ascites, microscopic tumor infiltration into adjacent organs, surgical biopsy) were associated with a higher peritoneal (HR for major defect vs no defect: 4.98) and overall (HR for major defect vs no defect: 3.55) recurrence risk. However, minor defects (peritoneal tumor penetration or iatrogenic peritoneal laceration) and microscopically involved intestinal resection margins were not [44].
- Laparoscopic resection may be considered in select cases provided that oncologic principles are adhered to and that the tumor is handled carefully and rupture is prevented. The tumor should be removed intact, in an extraction bag and should not be morcellated.
- The purpose of neoadjuvant imatinib is tumor downsizing. In tumors that respond to imatinib, change in tumor density may precede tumor shrinkage and may even be associated with an initial increase in tumor size (pseudoprogression) [36].
- Neoadjuvant imatinib has been associated with higher rates of complete resection and improved organ preservation [48, 49].
- After neoadjuvant imatinib, a planned microscopically positive margin might be considered if obtaining a wider margin would entail a significantly more morbid procedure (i.e., small duodenal GIST close to the duodenal papilla, rectal GIST close to the sphincter) [36].

Special Notes

- In patients with metastatic GIST, imatinib is the standard treatment. Imatinib should not be stopped even in case of radiological complete response. Surgery as a frontline approach is not recommended either for the primary or for the metastases.
- A percutaneous or endoscopic biopsy of the metastatic site is sufficient to make the diagnosis and surgical exploration is not recommended.

- Cytoreductive surgery in patients with metastatic disease on imatinib should be viewed as experimental and generally considered only in patients with SD or PR in whom a complete resection of their GIST is achievable. TKI must be continued even if all gross disease is resected. It is unknown whether cytoreductive surgery combined with TKI ("adjuvant surgery") confers a survival advantage as compared to TKI alone. Two RCTs (EORTC 62062 and COMVIA trial) designed to answer this question were terminated early due to poor accrual [51]. The theoretical advantage to surgery in this setting would be by completely removing all macroscopic disease: prevention of development of secondary resistance mutations (benefit not proved) and prolongation of time to progression by eliminating resistant clones (benefit not proved). Cytoreductive surgery should not be offered to patients experiencing generalized progression due to the poor post-surgical outcome [51–53].
- Possible indications for surgical resection of one metastatic focus in patients on imatinib:
  - Management of complications (obstruction, bleeding)
  - Control of unifocal progression to delay the switch to second-line TKI
- Surgery in patients on sunitinib is associated with a high complication rate and a high rate of incomplete resection [54]. In this setting, surgery might be reserved to treat complications or in highly selected cases to treat focal progression.

Management of GIST in Children and Young Adults

Pediatric GISTs have different genetic background and clinical behavior. Principles of their management are summarized in Table 12.8.

Table 12.8 Workup and management of pediatric GIST

Clinical scenario	Work-up	Management	Follow-up
Pediatric GIST (diagnosis between 1 and 20 years old)	History and physical exam Imaging: CT abdomen and pelvis (triple-phase contrast, gastric protocol for gastric locations) Upper GI endoscopy (for upper GI locations) EUS-guided biopsy	Surgical resection with negative microscopic margins with an organ-sparing approach Consider D1 lymphadenectomy for gastric location, especially if known SDH deficient	Physical exam and CT abdomen/pelvis every 6 months for 5 years and yearly for further 5 years (long-term follow-up is required, particularly for syndromic GIST)

Special Notes

- Most pediatric GISTs are not responsive to imatinib. Unlike adults GISTs, they usually do not harbor *KIT* or *PDGFRA* mutations but generally demonstrate SDH alteration/deficiency. There are multiple trials investigating new target agents in this population.
- Patients with metastatic SDH-deficient GIST present with exceptionally long survival and, in the absence of clinical trials, anti-VEGF TKIs such as sunitinib or regorafenib have been used with limited efficacy [18].
- Aim of surgery should be to obtain an R0 resection with an organ-sparing approach whenever possible. The entire peritoneal cavity should be accurately inspected for metastatic deposits. Resection of metastatic foci can be considered if not associated with significant morbidity for staging purposes and to prevent future complications. There is no evidence in favor of an extended metastasectomy. Tumor spread to lymph nodes is much more common, and D1 lymphadenectomy is a reasonable treatment for pediatric GIST of the stomach. Careful inspection of the D2 lymph node stations should be performed and pathologic nodes should be removed. There is no evidence to support a D2 lymphadenectomy in pediatric gastric GIST patients. Retrospective data show that even in the metastatic setting, surgical resection of the primary tumor might be of value [55].

Landmark Trials

In this section, the landmark publications discussing surgical and medical management of GISTs are summarized (Table 12.9).

Table 12.9 Landmark publications – GIST

Topic	Study	Methods	Results
Neoadjuvant imatinib	RTOG 0132 Eisenberg et al.; Wang et al. [56, 57]	Single-arm Phase II trial $n = 63$:30 advanced primary (≥5 cm), 22 metastatic Neoadjuvant imatinib 600 mg/day for 8–12 weeks followed by surgery and adjuvant imatinib for 2 years	RECIST response to neoadjuvant imatinib in primary GIST: 7% partial, 83% stable, 0% progression, 10% unknown Median time of imatinib discontinuation prior to surgery: 2 days
Adjuvant imatinib in patients with resected localized GIST	ACOSOG Z9000 DeMatteo et al. [21, 58]	Single-arm Phase II trial $n = 106$ High-risk GIST (diameter > 10 cm, tumor rupture or ≤4 peritoneal implants) Imatinib 400 mg/day for 1 year	At a median FU of 7.7 years: 5-year OS 83%; 1-, 3-, and 5-year RFS 96%, 60% and 40%, respectively Tumor size, small bowel site, *KIT* exon 9 mutation, high mitotic rate, and age associated with lower RFS at multivariable analysis

(continued)

Table 12.9 (continued)

Topic	Study	Methods	Results
	ACOSOG Z9001 DeMatteo et al. [58]	Double-blind, placebo-controlled, Phase III RCT $N = 713$ GIST >3 cm 1 year of adjuvant Imatinib 400 mg/day vs placebo Crossover design	With a median FU of 19.7 months: Improved recurrence-free survival (RFS, primary endpoint) in the treatment arm (98% vs. 83% at 1 year, HR 0.35). No difference in OS (99.2% vs 99.7% at 1 year) among the two arms Long-term results (median FU 74 months): RFS remained superior in the imatinib arm (HR 0.6), no difference in OS
	SSG XVIII/AIO Joensuu et al. [59]	Open-label Phase III RCT $N = 400$ High-risk GIST (modified NIH Consensus Criteria) 1 vs 3 years of adjuvant imatinib 400 mg/day	Median follow-up of 54 months: Longer RFS (primary endpoint, 5-year RFS 65.6% vs. 47.9%, HR 0.46) and longer OS (5-year OS 92.0% vs. 81.7%, HR 0.45) in the 3-year group Discontinuation rates for reasons other than tumor recurrence were 12.6% and 25.8% in the 1- and 3-year groups, respectively Median FU of 90 months: Longer RFS (5-year RFS 71.1% vs. 52.3%, HR 0.60) and longer OS (5-year OS 91.9% vs. 85.3%, HR 0.60) in the 3-year group
	EORTC 62024 Casali et al. [60]	Open-label Phase III RCT $N = 908$ Intermediate- to high-risk GIST (2002 NIH consensus diagnosis) 2 years of adjuvant imatinib 400 mg/day vs. observation	At a median follow-up of 4.7 years: No difference in 5-year imatinib monotherapy failure-free survival (IFFS, primary endpoint) and 5-year OS among the two arms. Trend toward better IFFS in the treatment arm. Better RFS in the treatment arm (3-year RFS 84% vs 66%; 5-year RFS 69% vs 63%)

(continued)

Table 12.9 (continued)

Topic	Study	Methods	Results
	PERSIST-5 Raut et al. [61]	Single-arm Phase II trial *N* = 91, intermediate- to high-risk GIST Imatinib 400 mg/day for 5 years	5-year RFS 90% 5-year OS 95% Discontinuation rate before 5 years: 49%
	SSG XXII, NCT 02413736	Open-label Phase III RCT 3 years vs 5 years of imatinib 400 mg/day Estimated enrollment: 300 High-risk GIST (gastric GIST with mitotic count >10/50 HPFs, non-gastric GIST with mitotic count >5/50 HPFs, or tumor rupture)	Primary outcome: RFS Estimated primary completion date: May 2028
	ImadGist, NCT02260505	Open-label Phase III RCT 3 years vs. 6 years of imatinib 300 or 400 mg/day Estimated enrollment: 256 High-risk GIST	Primary outcome: DFS Estimated primary completion date: Dec 2020
Imatinib in unresectable or metastatic GIST	B2222 trial Demetri et al.; Blanke et al. [62, 63]	Open-label Phase II randomized trial Crossover design (+dose-escalation) *N* = 147, advanced unresectable or metastatic GIST Imatinib 400 mg/day vs. 600 mg/day	Long-term results (median FU 63 months): No difference in response rate, median PFS, median OS between the two arms Median survival for all patients: 4.75 years (5-year OS was 55% in responders and 9% in nonresponders) Median time to response: 2.7 months Tumor response (SWOG criteria): CR 1.4% PR 66.7% SD 15.6% PD 11.6%

(continued)

Table 12.9 (continued)

Topic	Study	Methods	Results
	EORTC 62005 Verweij et al. [64, 65]	Phase III RCT Crossover design *N* = 946, advanced or metastatic GIST 400 mg/day imatinib vs. 800 mg/day	With a median FU of 2 years: no difference in response or OS. PFS (primary endpoint) was better in the 800 mg/day group (HR 0.82) With a median FU of 10.9 years: No significant difference in PFS or OS (median PFS *1.9 years*, median OS 3.9 years) Long-term progression-free and overall survivors: 10% and 15% No difference in tumor response (CR 6.9%, PR 46.9%, SD 31.8%, PD 9.4%) Patients with a *KIT* exon 9 mutation had better PFS and OS with imatinib 800 mg/day Median PFS after cross-over: 2.8 months Predictive factor for response: genotype Predictive factor for duration of response: tumor burden
	S0033 trial Blanke et al. [66]	Phase III RCT Crossover design *N* = 746, unresectable or metastatic GIST Imatinib 400 mg/day vs. 800 mg/day	No significant differences in objective response rate (CR/PR in 45%), median PFS (18–20 months), or median OS (primary endpoint, 51–55 months) between the two arms Crossover to 800 mg/day after progression on 400 mg/day was associated with either an objective response or SD in 31%

(continued)

Table 12.9 (continued)

Topic	Study	Methods	Results
	BFR14 Blay et al.; LeCesne et al. [67, 68]	Phase III randomized trial Crossover design Metastatic GIST with tumor response or SD after 1, 3, or 5 years of imatinib 400 mg/day Randomization to treatment interruption vs. continuation at 1, 3, and 5 years	Randomization at 1, 3, and 5 years: Interruption results in progression in most patients Among patients who crossed over, the overall disease control rate (CR + PD + SD) after imatinib reintroduction was 96%, but quality of response upon reintroduction did not reach the tumor status observed at randomization No differences in OS or time to secondary resistance The longer the duration of imatinib treatment, the longer the median PFS after discontinuation After treatment discontinuation, the median PFS was 10.5, 6.2, and 3.2 months in patients with CR, PR, and SD at time of discontinuation, respectively Patients progressing rapidly after discontinuation had a poorer prognosis
	RIGHT trial Yoon-Ko K et al. [69]	Phase III double-blind RCT Crossover design $N = 81$ Metastatic or unresectable GIST with progression on at least imatinib and sunitinib who had initially benefited from first-line imatinib (response or SD for ≥6 months) Randomization to imatinib rechallenge 400 mg/day vs. placebo	Better PFS (primary endpoint) with rechallenge: *1.8 months* with imatinib, 0.9 months with placebo (HR for progression or death 0.46) Median PFS after crossover: 1.7 months 93% of patients in the placebo group crossed over to imatinib after PD. No difference in OS

(continued)

Table 12.9 (continued)

Topic	Study	Methods	Results
Sunitinib treatment	Demetri et al. [70]	Phase III double-blind RCT Crossover design *N* = 312 Metastatic or unresectable imatinib-resistant GIST Sunitinib (50 mg/day 4 weeks on, 2 weeks off) vs. placebo (2:1)	Median time-to-tumor-progression (primary endpoint) was *27.3 weeks* with sunitinib versus 6.4 weeks with placebo OS was better with sunitinib (HR 0.49) Tumor response with sunitinib: 7% PR, 58% SD, 19% PRO
Regorafenib treatment	GRID trial Demetri et al. [71]	Phase III double-blind RCT Crossover design *N* = 199 Metastatic or unresectable GIST resistant to imatinib and sunitinib Regorafenib (160 mg/day 3 weeks on, 1 week off) vs. placebo (2:1)	Improved median PFS (primary endpoint) with regorafenib (*4.8* vs. 0.9 *months*, HR 0.27) No difference in OS (but, after PD, 85% of patients assigned to placebo crossed over) Overall response rate with Regorafenib: 4.5%
Surgery in metastatic GIST on TKI	Du et al. [51]	Phase III randomized trial Target accrual: 210 patients. Study closed after 41 patients due to poor patient accrual Resectable metastatic GIST at 3–12 months from imatinib onset Imatinib alone vs surgery and postoperative imatinib	Nonsignificant trend toward better PFS in the surgery arm (2-year PFS 88% vs 58%)
	Raut et al. [52]	Retrospective single institution series *N* = 69 Patients who underwent surgery for advanced GIST while receiving TKI	Response to imatinib at time of surgery (SD vs limited progression vs generalized progression) correlates with completeness of surgery (78%, 25%, and 7%, respectively) and 12-month PFS (95%, 86%, and 0%, respectively).

(continued)

Table 12.9 (continued)

Topic	Study	Methods	Results
	Fairweather et al. [53]	Retrospective two institutional series $N = 323$ Patients who underwent surgery for advanced GIST while receiving TKI	Radiographic response categorized as responsive disease (RD, 16%), SD (25%), unifocal progressive disease (UPD, 33%), multifocal progressive disease (MPD, 26%) For patients on imatinib, radiographic response was predictive of postsurgery PFS (RD 36mo, SD 30mo, UPD 11mo, MPD 6mo) and OS Metastatic mitotic index≥5/50HPF, MPD and R2 resection were associated with worst PFS and OS
	Raut et al. [54]	Retrospective single institution series $N = 50$ Patients who underwent surgery for advanced GIST while receiving sunitinib	Completeness of resection did not correlate with preoperative response to sunitinib (unlike imatinib) Macroscopically complete resection: 50% Complication rate: 54% Reoperations: 16% Median PFS after surgery: 5.8 months Differences in PFS and OS based on response to SU were not significant Younger age was prognostic of survival

OS overall survival, *RFS* recurrence-free survival, *PFS* progression-free survival, *DSS* disease-specific survival, *PR* partial response

Referral to Medical Oncology

- All patients with histologically confirmed primary intermediate- or high-risk GISTs or metastatic GISTs should be referred to medical oncology. If any doubt exists regarding patient risk stratification, referral to medical oncology is warranted.

Referral to Radiation Oncology

- In the palliative setting, radiotherapy is an option in:
  - Patients with symptomatic bone metastases not responsive to TKI
  - Patients with gastrointestinal bleeding not responsive to TKI

- Beyond its palliative role, radiotherapy might play a role in:
  - Perioperative treatment of locally advanced primary GIST in difficult locations (i.e., rectum, esophagus)
  - Treatment of focal progression to TKI in the metastatic setting in combination with TKI
  - Treatment of primary tumor in patients who are not fit for surgery or when the tumor is unresectable [72, 73]

Referral to Multidisciplinary Cancer Team

- All patients with a diagnosis of GIST should be discussed before treatment begins at Multidisciplinary Cancer Conference (MCC) with a panel that routinely manages this disease.
- Patients on neoadjuvant imatinib should be followed closely by medical and surgical oncologists experienced on the management of GIST to establish the best time for surgery.
- Patients with metastatic GIST who experience limited progression after responding to TKI should be discussed again at MCC to re-evaluate the sequencing of multimodality treatment.

Toronto Pearls

- Neoadjuvant imatinib is not associated with risk of bleeding. In fact, surgical experience is that GISTs become less vascular and less friable and, therefore, less prone to intraoperative rupture after neoadjuvant imatinib.
- Chronic bleeding from the tumor is not a contraindication to starting imatinib.
- Mutational analysis is part of a complete assessment of GIST.
- In the adjuvant setting, an increased frequency of surveillance after imatinib discontinuation due to the higher risk of tumor recurrence over the next 6–18 months should be considered.
- In patients treated with neoadjuvant imatinib, imatinib can be safely stopped the day before surgery and restarted when resuming p.o. intake. Sunitinib should be stopped at least 1–2 weeks before surgery due to the higher complication rate as compared to imatinib.
- Neoadjuvant imatinib may be associated with initial pseudoprogression. Evaluation of an early triple-phase CT scan by a surgical oncologist with experience in GIST treatment is essential.
- The appearance of new cystic lesion(s) in the liver after starting imatinib likely represents liver metastasis responding to the drug.
- When operating on metastatic patients, the preoperative CT scan often underestimates the tumor burden.
- Follow-up schedule should be personalized based on the individual risk of tumor recurrence/progression and the patient's life circumstances.

References

1. Fletcher CDM, Bridge JA, Hogendoorn PCW, Mertens F. WHO classification of tumours of soft tissue and bone. Lyon: International Agency for Research on Cancer; 2013.
2. von Mehren M, Joensuu H. Gastrointestinal stromal tumors. J Clin Oncol. 2018;36(2):136–43.
3. Soreide K, Sandvik OM, Soreide JA, Giljaca V, Jureckova A, Bulusu VR. Global epidemiology of gastrointestinal stromal tumours (GIST): a systematic review of population-based cohort studies. Cancer Epidemiol. 2016;40:39–46.
4. Blackstein ME, Blay JY, Corless C, Driman DK, Riddell R, Soulieres D, et al. Gastrointestinal stromal tumours: consensus statement on diagnosis and treatment. Can J Gastroenterol. 2006;20(3):157–63.
5. Miettinen M, Lasota J. Gastrointestinal stromal tumors: pathology and prognosis at different sites. Semin Diagn Pathol. 2006;23(2):70–83.
6. Kawanowa K, Sakuma Y, Sakurai S, Hishima T, Iwasaki Y, Saito K, et al. High incidence of microscopic gastrointestinal stromal tumors in the stomach. Hum Pathol. 2006;37(12):1527–35.
7. Hirota S, Isozaki K, Moriyama Y, Hashimoto K, Nishida T, Ishiguro S, et al. Gain-of-function mutations of c-kit in human gastrointestinal stromal tumors. Science. 1998;279(5350):577–80.
8. Heinrich MC, Corless CL, Duensing A, McGreevey L, Chen CJ, Joseph N, et al. PDGFRA activating mutations in gastrointestinal stromal tumors. Science. 2003;299(5607):708–10.
9. Niinuma T, Suzuki H, Sugai T. Molecular characterization and pathogenesis of gastrointestinal stromal tumor. Transl Gastroenterol Hepatol. 2018;3:2.
10. Charville GW, Longacre TA. Surgical pathology of gastrointestinal stromal tumors: practical implications of morphologic and molecular heterogeneity for precision medicine. Adv Anat Pathol. 2017;24(6):336–53.
11. Miettinen M, Wang ZF, Lasota J. DOG1 antibody in the differential diagnosis of gastrointestinal stromal tumors: a study of 1840 cases. Am J Surg Pathol. 2009;33(9):1401–8.
12. Kindblom LG, Remotti HE, Aldenborg F, Meis-Kindblom JM. Gastrointestinal pacemaker cell tumor (GIPACT): gastrointestinal stromal tumors show phenotypic characteristics of the interstitial cells of Cajal. Am J Pathol. 1998;152(5):1259–69.
13. American Joint Committee on Cancer 2017. AJCC cancer staging manual. 8th ed. Chicago: Springer; 2017.
14. Fletcher CD, Berman JJ, Corless C, Gorstein F, Lasota J, Longley BJ, et al. Diagnosis of gastrointestinal stromal tumors: a consensus approach. Hum Pathol. 2002;33(5):459–65.
15. Joensuu H. Risk stratification of patients diagnosed with gastrointestinal stromal tumor. Hum Pathol. 2008;39(10):1411–9.
16. Cancer Protocol Templates – College of American Pathologists. Available at: https://www.cap.org/protocols-and-guidelines/cancer-reporting-tools/cancer-protocol-templates. Accessed 4 May 2019.
17. Joensuu H, Vehtari A, Riihimaki J, Nishida T, Steigen SE, Brabec P, et al. Risk of recurrence of gastrointestinal stromal tumour after surgery: an analysis of pooled population-based cohorts. Lancet Oncol. 2012;13(3):265–74.
18. Pantaleo MA, Nannini M, Corless CL, Heinrich MC. Quadruple wild-type (WT) GIST: defining the subset of GIST that lacks abnormalities of KIT, PDGFRA, SDH, or RAS signaling pathways. Cancer Med. 2015;4(1):101–3.
19. Martin J, Poveda A, Llombart-Bosch A, Ramos R, Lopez-Guerrero JA, Garcia del Muro J, et al. Deletions affecting codons 557-558 of the c-KIT gene indicate a poor prognosis in patients with completely resected gastrointestinal stromal tumors: a study by the Spanish Group for Sarcoma Research (GEIS). J Clin Oncol. 2005;23(25):6190–8.
20. Patrikidou A, Le Cesne A. Key messages from the BFR14 trial of the French Sarcoma Group. Future Oncol. 2017;13(3):273–84.
21. DeMatteo RP, Ballman KV, Antonescu CR, Corless C, Kolesnikova V, von Mehren M, et al. Long-term results of adjuvant imatinib mesylate in localized, high-risk, primary gastrointestinal stromal tumor: ACOSOG Z9000 (Alliance) intergroup phase 2 trial. Ann Surg. 2013;258(3):422–9.

22. Joensuu H, Rutkowski P, Nishida T, Steigen SE, Brabec P, Plank L, et al. KIT and PDGFRA mutations and the risk of GI stromal tumor recurrence. J Clin Oncol. 2015;33(6):634–42.
23. Gill AJ, Chou A, Vilain R, Clarkson A, Lui M, Jin R, et al. Immunohistochemistry for SDHB divides gastrointestinal stromal tumors (GISTs) into 2 distinct types. Am J Surg Pathol. 2010;34(5):636–44.
24. Nannini M, Biasco G, Astolfi A, Pantaleo MA. An overview on molecular biology of KIT/PDGFRA wild type (WT) gastrointestinal stromal tumours (GIST). J Med Genet. 2013;50(10):653–61.
25. Miettinen M, Killian JK, Wang ZF, Lasota J, Lau C, Jones L, et al. Immunohistochemical loss of succinate dehydrogenase subunit A (SDHA) in gastrointestinal stromal tumors (GISTs) signals SDHA germline mutation. Am J Surg Pathol. 2013;37(2):234–40.
26. Pasini B, McWhinney SR, Bei T, Matyakhina L, Stergiopoulos S, Muchow M, et al. Clinical and molecular genetics of patients with the Carney-Stratakis syndrome and germline mutations of the genes coding for the succinate dehydrogenase subunits SDHB, SDHC, and SDHD. Eur J Hum Genet. 2008;16(1):79–88.
27. Wada R, Arai H, Kure S, Peng WX, Naito Z. "Wild type" GIST: clinicopathological features and clinical practice. Pathol Int. 2016;66(8):431–7.
28. Chetty R, Serra S. Molecular and morphological correlation in gastrointestinal stromal tumours (GISTs): an update and primer. J Clin Pathol. 2016;69(9):754–60.
29. Mussi C, Schildhaus HU, Gronchi A, Wardelmann E, Hohenberger P. Therapeutic consequences from molecular biology for gastrointestinal stromal tumor patients affected by neurofibromatosis type 1. Clin Cancer Res. 2008;14(14):4550–5.
30. Zoller ME, Rembeck B, Oden A, Samuelsson M, Angervall L. Malignant and benign tumors in patients with neurofibromatosis type 1 in a defined Swedish population. Cancer. 1997;79(11):2125–31.
31. Forde PM, Cochran RL, Boikos SA, Zabransky DJ, Beaver JA, Meyer CF, et al. Familial GI stromal tumor with loss of heterozygosity and amplification of mutant KIT. J Clin Oncol. 2016;34(3):e13–6.
32. Ricci R. Syndromic gastrointestinal stromal tumors. Hered Cancer Clin Pract. 2016;14:15; eCollection 2016.
33. Agaram NP, Wong GC, Guo T, Maki RG, Singer S, Dematteo RP, et al. Novel V600E BRAF mutations in imatinib-naive and imatinib-resistant gastrointestinal stromal tumors. Genes Chromosomes Cancer. 2008;47(10):853–9.
34. Boikos SA, Pappo AS, Killian JK, LaQuaglia MP, Weldon CB, George S, et al. Molecular subtypes of KIT/PDGFRA wild-type gastrointestinal stromal tumors: a report from the National Institutes of Health Gastrointestinal Stromal Tumor Clinic. JAMA Oncol. 2016;2(7):922–8.
35. National Comprehensive Cancer Network. Clinical practice guidelines: soft tissue sarcoma (2.2019). Available at: https://www.nccn.org/professionals/physician_gls/pdf/sarcoma.pdf. Accessed 29 Apr 2019.
36. Casali PG, Abecassis N, Aro HT, Bauer S, Biagini R, Bielack S, et al. Gastrointestinal stromal tumours: ESMO-EURACAN Clinical Practice Guidelines for diagnosis, treatment and follow-up. Ann Oncol. 2018;29(Supplement_4):iv267.
37. Joensuu H, Hohenberger P. Management of small gastrointestinal stromal tumours – Authors' reply. Lancet. 2013;382(9906):1701–2.
38. Kobara H, Mori H, Rafiq K, Fujihara S, Nishiyama N, Chiyo T, et al. Analysis of the amount of tissue sample necessary for mitotic count and Ki-67 index in gastrointestinal stromal tumor sampling. Oncol Rep. 2015;33(1):215–22.
39. Na HK, Lee JH, Park YS, Ahn JY, Choi KS, Kim DH, et al. Yields and utility of endoscopic ultrasonography-guided 19-gauge Trucut biopsy versus 22-gauge fine needle aspiration for diagnosing gastric subepithelial tumors. Clin Endosc. 2015;48(2):152–7.
40. Shin SY, Lee SJ, Jun JH, Park JK, Seo HI, Han KH, et al. Mucosal incision and forceps biopsy for reliable tissue sampling of gastric subepithelial tumors. Clin Endosc. 2017;50(1):64–8.
41. Uesato M, Tamachi T, Hanari N, Muto Y, Kagaya A, Urahama R, et al. Drill needle aspiration biopsy for submucosal tumors in an experimental study. Gastric Cancer. 2017;20(3):475–80.

42. Joo MK, Park JJ, Kim H, Koh JS, Lee BJ, Chun HJ, et al. Endoscopic versus surgical resection of GI stromal tumors in the upper GI tract. Gastrointest Endosc. 2016;83(2):318–26.
43. Eriksson M, Reichardt P, Sundby Hall K, Schutte J, Cameron S, Hohenberger P, et al. Needle biopsy through the abdominal wall for the diagnosis of gastrointestinal stromal tumour - Does it increase the risk for tumour cell seeding and recurrence? Eur J Cancer. 2016;59:128–33.
44. Holmebakk T, Bjerkehagen B, Boye K, Bruland O, Stoldt S, Sundby HK. Definition and clinical significance of tumour rupture in gastrointestinal stromal tumours of the small intestine. Br J Surg. 2016;103(6):684–91.
45. Nishimura J, Nakajima K, Omori T, Takahashi T, Nishitani A, Ito T, et al. Surgical strategy for gastric gastrointestinal stromal tumors: laparoscopic vs. open resection. Surg Endosc. 2007;21(6):875–8.
46. Zhi X, Jiang B, Yu J, Roe OD, Qin J, Ni Q, et al. Prognostic role of microscopically positive margins for primary gastrointestinal stromal tumors: a systematic review and meta-analysis. Sci Rep. 2016;6:21541.
47. Rutkowski P, Nowecki ZI, Michej W, Debiec-Rychter M, Wozniak A, Limon J, et al. Risk criteria and prognostic factors for predicting recurrences after resection of primary gastrointestinal stromal tumor. Ann Surg Oncol. 2007;14(7):2018–27.
48. Andtbacka RH, Ng CS, Scaife CL, Cormier JN, Hunt KK, Pisters PW, et al. Surgical resection of gastrointestinal stromal tumors after treatment with imatinib. Ann Surg Oncol. 2007;14(1):14–24.
49. Sjolund K, Andersson A, Nilsson E, Nilsson O, Ahlman H, Nilsson B. Downsizing treatment with tyrosine kinase inhibitors in patients with advanced gastrointestinal stromal tumors improved resectability. World J Surg. 2010;34(9):2090–7.
50. Mei L, Du W, Idowu M, von Mehren M, Boikos SA. Advances and challenges on management of gastrointestinal stromal tumors. Front Oncol. 2018;8:135.
51. Du CY, Zhou Y, Song C, Wang YP, Jie ZG, He YL, et al. Is there a role of surgery in patients with recurrent or metastatic gastrointestinal stromal tumours responding to imatinib: a prospective randomised trial in China. Eur J Cancer. 2014;50(10):1772–8.
52. Raut CP, Posner M, Desai J, Morgan JA, George S, Zahrieh D, et al. Surgical management of advanced gastrointestinal stromal tumors after treatment with targeted systemic therapy using kinase inhibitors. J Clin Oncol. 2006;24(15):2325–31.
53. Fairweather M, Balachandran VP, Li GZ, Bertagnolli MM, Antonescu C, Tap W, et al. Cytoreductive surgery for metastatic gastrointestinal stromal tumors treated with tyrosine kinase inhibitors: a 2-institutional analysis. Ann Surg. 2018;268(2):296–302.
54. Raut CP, Wang Q, Manola J, Morgan JA, George S, Wagner AJ, et al. Cytoreductive surgery in patients with metastatic gastrointestinal stromal tumor treated with sunitinib malate. Ann Surg Oncol. 2010;17(2):407–15.
55. Fero KE, Coe TM, Fanta PT, Tang CM, Murphy JD, Sicklick JK. Surgical management of adolescents and young adults with gastrointestinal stromal tumors: a US population-based analysis. JAMA Surg. 2017;152(5):443–51.
56. Eisenberg BL, Harris J, Blanke CD, Demetri GD, Heinrich MC, Watson JC, et al. Phase II trial of neoadjuvant/adjuvant imatinib mesylate (IM) for advanced primary and metastatic/recurrent operable gastrointestinal stromal tumor (GIST): early results of RTOG 0132/ACRIN 6665. J Surg Oncol. 2009;99(1):42–7.
57. Wang D, Zhang Q, Blanke CD, Demetri GD, Heinrich MC, Watson JC, et al. Phase II trial of neoadjuvant/adjuvant imatinib mesylate for advanced primary and metastatic/recurrent operable gastrointestinal stromal tumors: long-term follow-up results of Radiation Therapy Oncology Group 0132. Ann Surg Oncol. 2012;19(4):1074–80.
58. Dematteo RP, Ballman KV, Antonescu CR, Maki RG, Pisters PW, Demetri GD, et al. Adjuvant imatinib mesylate after resection of localised, primary gastrointestinal stromal tumour: a randomised, double-blind, placebo-controlled trial. Lancet. 2009;373(9669):1097–104.
59. Joensuu H, Eriksson M, Sundby Hall K, Reichardt A, Hartmann JT, Pink D, et al. Adjuvant imatinib for high-risk GI stromal tumor: analysis of a randomized trial. J Clin Oncol. 2016;34(3):244–50.

60. Casali PG, Le Cesne A, Poveda Velasco A, Kotasek D, Rutkowski P, Hohenberger P, et al. Time to definitive failure to the first tyrosine kinase inhibitor in localized GI stromal tumors treated with imatinib as an adjuvant: a European Organisation for Research and Treatment of Cancer Soft Tissue and Bone Sarcoma Group Intergroup Randomized Trial in Collaboration with the Australasian Gastro-Intestinal Trials Group, UNICANCER, French Sarcoma Group, Italian Sarcoma Group, and Spanish Group for Research on Sarcomas. J Clin Oncol. 2015;33(36):4276–83.
61. Raut CP, Espat NJ, Maki RG, Araujo DM, Trent J, Williams TF, et al. Efficacy and tolerability of 5-year adjuvant imatinib treatment for patients with resected intermediate- or high-risk primary gastrointestinal stromal tumor: the PERSIST-5 clinical trial. JAMA Oncol. 2018;4(12):e184060.
62. Demetri GD, von Mehren M, Blanke CD, Van den Abbeele AD, Eisenberg B, Roberts PJ, et al. Efficacy and safety of imatinib mesylate in advanced gastrointestinal stromal tumors. N Engl J Med. 2002;347(7):472–80.
63. Blanke CD, Demetri GD, von Mehren M, Heinrich MC, Eisenberg B, Fletcher JA, et al. Long-term results from a randomized phase II trial of standard- versus higher-dose imatinib mesylate for patients with unresectable or metastatic gastrointestinal stromal tumors expressing KIT. J Clin Oncol. 2008;26(4):620–5.
64. Verweij J, Casali PG, Zalcberg J, LeCesne A, Reichardt P, Blay JY, et al. Progression-free survival in gastrointestinal stromal tumours with high-dose imatinib: randomised trial. Lancet. 2004;364(9440):1127–34.
65. Casali PG, Zalcberg J, Le Cesne A, Reichardt P, Blay JY, Lindner LH, et al. Ten-year progression-free and overall survival in patients with unresectable or metastatic GI stromal Tumors: long-term analysis of the European Organisation for Research and Treatment of Cancer, Italian Sarcoma Group, and Australasian Gastrointestinal Trials Group Intergroup Phase III Randomized Trial on Imatinib at two dose levels. J Clin Oncol. 2017;35(15):1713–20.
66. Blanke CD, Rankin C, Demetri GD, Ryan CW, von Mehren M, Benjamin RS, et al. Phase III randomized, intergroup trial assessing imatinib mesylate at two dose levels in patients with unresectable or metastatic gastrointestinal stromal tumors expressing the kit receptor tyrosine kinase: S0033. J Clin Oncol. 2008;26(4):626–32.
67. Blay JY, Le Cesne A, Ray-Coquard I, Bui B, Duffaud F, Delbaldo C, et al. Prospective multicentric randomized phase III study of imatinib in patients with advanced gastrointestinal stromal tumors comparing interruption versus continuation of treatment beyond 1 year: the French Sarcoma Group. J Clin Oncol. 2007;25(9):1107–13.
68. Le Cesne A, Ray-Coquard I, Bui BN, Adenis A, Rios M, Bertucci F, et al. Discontinuation of imatinib in patients with advanced gastrointestinal stromal tumours after 3 years of treatment: an open-label multicentre randomised phase 3 trial. Lancet Oncol. 2010;11(10):942–9.
69. Kang YK, Ryu MH, Yoo C, Ryoo BY, Kim HJ, Lee JJ, et al. Resumption of imatinib to control metastatic or unresectable gastrointestinal stromal tumours after failure of imatinib and sunitinib (RIGHT): a randomised, placebo-controlled, phase 3 trial. Lancet Oncol. 2013;14(12):1175–82.
70. Demetri GD, van Oosterom AT, Garrett CR, Blackstein ME, Shah MH, Verweij J, et al. Efficacy and safety of sunitinib in patients with advanced gastrointestinal stromal tumour after failure of imatinib: a randomised controlled trial. Lancet. 2006;368(9544):1329–38.
71. Demetri GD, Reichardt P, Kang YK, Blay JY, Rutkowski P, Gelderblom H, et al. Efficacy and safety of regorafenib for advanced gastrointestinal stromal tumours after failure of imatinib and sunitinib (GRID): an international, multicentre, randomised, placebo-controlled, phase 3 trial. Lancet. 2013;381(9863):295–302.
72. Joensuu H, Eriksson M, Collan J, Balk MH, Leyvraz S, Montemurro M. Radiotherapy for GIST progressing during or after tyrosine kinase inhibitor therapy: a prospective study. Radiother Oncol. 2015;116(2):233–8.
73. Gatto L, Nannini M, Saponara M, Di Scioscio V, Beltramo G, Frezza GP, et al. Radiotherapy in the management of gist: state of the art and new potential scenarios. Clin Sarcoma Res. 2017;7:1; eCollection 2017.

Geriatric Surgical Oncology

13

Tyler R. Chesney, Naser AlQurini, and Shabbir M. H. Alibhai

Introduction

Older adults are the fastest growing cohort requiring surgery and have the greatest incidence of cancer [1–3]. The median age at cancer diagnosis is nearing 70 years, and by 2030 nearly 70% of incident cancers will be in older adults [4–6]. For older adults, cancer care decision-making has inherent complexities due to altered risk-benefit profiles, underlying health status, remaining life expectancy, and heterogeneity in patient values and goals [7–9]. Older adults often place higher importance on outcomes such as long-term functional independence, quality of life, and avoidance of prolonged recovery [10–13]. Recommendations applicable to geriatric surgical oncology emphasize preoperative discussions regarding personal goals and preferences, while incorporating counseling about older adult-specific outcomes such as postoperative delirium, functional decline, loss of independence, and long-term care admissions [14–21]. However, age alone does not adequately describe the diversity in health status of older adults with cancer [22, 23]. Focused consideration

T. R. Chesney
Department of Surgery, University of Toronto, Toronto, ON, Canada

N. AlQurini
Division of Geriatric Medicine, Department of Medicine, University of Toronto, Toronto, ON, Canada

Department of Medicine, University of Toronto, Toronto, ON, Canada
e-mail: naser.alqurini@uhn.ca

S. M. H. Alibhai (✉)
Division of Geriatric Medicine, Department of Medicine, University of Toronto, Toronto, ON, Canada

Institute of Health Policy, Management, and Evaluation, University of Toronto, Toronto, ON, Canada

Department of Medicine, University Health Network, Toronto, ON, Canada
e-mail: shabbir.alibhai@uhn.ca

F. C. Wright et al. (eds.), *Surgical Oncology Manual*,
https://doi.org/10.1007/978-3-030-48363-0_13

Table 13.1 Approach to older adults with cancer when surgery is a treatment option [25–28]

Confirm diagnosis and clinically stage cancer
Assess for vulnerability using a geriatric screening tool with defined measurement properties
Refer for CGA if abnormal geriatric screening or other age-related concern
Assess risk of surgery using surgical risk tool with defined measurement properties
Estimate underlying life expectancy using a prognostic tool with defined measurement properties
Describe treatment options in light of above assessments including options for preoperative optimization based on CGA and prehabilitation
Elicit goals and values from patient to make treatment recommendation
The following sections provide further detail on aspects of this approach

on patient assessment, patient-centered decision-making, and perioperative care for older adults tailored to individual needs will optimize disease control and quality of life [24]. This chapter acts as an overview to guide the integration of geriatric principles into the overall surgical care of older adults with cancer (Table 13.1); it does not provide cancer-type specific considerations or treatment recommendations.

Terminology

- *Geriatric Oncology*: The practice of geriatric oncology incorporates geriatric principles into the care of older adults with cancer. This includes tailored assessments, decision-making, and treatment options including addressing geriatric syndromes. A *geriatric oncologist* may have a background in geriatric medicine, medical oncology, radiation oncology, or surgical oncology along with expertise in the care of older adults with cancer. All clinicians caring for older adults with cancer can apply these principles to practice and seek expert consultation when needed.
- *Older Adult*: To avoid negative stereotypes and discriminative connotation, the preferred term for referring to individuals aged 65 and older is "older adult" and including a specific age range as relevant [1]. The diversity in physiologic, functional, and social health among older adults must be recognized [29, 30].
- *Comprehensive Geriatric Assessment (CGA)*: A CGA includes assessment by a trained assessor in all four cardinal domains: physical health (comorbidities, medications, nutritional status), functional status (basic and instrumental activities of daily living), psychological status (cognitive and emotional), and socioeconomic factors (living situation, financial resources) [31, 32]. Typically, CGA includes a multidisciplinary team with geriatric expertise using structured and validated instruments in each domain sufficient for diagnosis and management. Importantly, CGA also includes implementation and monitoring of a treatment plan for identified deficits.
- *Geriatric Screening*: In contrast to CGA, geriatric screening involves the use of abbreviated evaluations not requiring advanced geriatric training [31]. Many geriatric screening tools have been developed with varying degrees of

methodological rigor and investigation of measurement properties [33–37]. While many studies have aimed to assess the prognostic and predictive value of individual geriatric screening tools, geriatric screening is best used to identify older adults who would benefit from CGA [31–33, 35].

- *Geriatric Syndromes*: Geriatric syndromes are multifactorial health conditions that are common in older adults and manifested by multiple interacting contributing factors [38]. Examples include delirium, dementia, falls, frailty, sarcopenia, pressure ulcers, malnutrition, and incontinence.
- *Frailty*: Frailty is a state of vulnerability to stressors associated with a multisystem decline in physiologic reserve and function and increased risk of adverse health outcomes [39–43]. Frailty is operationalized both as a *cumulative deficit model* reflecting coaction of intrinsic and extrinsic factors and as a *phenotype model* reflecting multidimensional biological changes [39, 40]. Many tools now exist to screen for frailty to predict adverse outcomes, and an abnormal screen prompts a comprehensive assessment for treatment planning [44, 45].
- *Sarcopenia*: Sarcopenia includes loss of skeletal muscle mass, strength, and physical performance [46–49]. Some definitions use muscle mass alone, but incorporating a measure of strength or performance is recommended [46–48, 50–52]. Examples of measurements include cross-sectional imaging (skeletal muscle index, total psoas index, total psoas volume, total psoas area), bioimpedance analysis, dual X-ray absorptiometry, grip strength, physical performance batteries, and timed walking tests. Depending on the definition, prevalence of sarcopenia in surgical oncology patients ranges from 12% to 78%, but when a measure of strength or performance is included, prevalence ranges from 12% to 21% [52]. In surgical oncology, sarcopenia is associated with reduced overall survival and increased complications; this association is greater when a measure of strength or performance is included [51, 52].

Frailty for Surgeons

Frailty is associated with increased risk of falls, disability, hospitalization, functional dependence, chemotherapy intolerance, and poorer postoperative outcomes including overall complications, postoperative mortality, readmission, need for institutional care, and overall survival [42, 53–60]. Frailty is present in 10–20% of the general older adult population and up to 40% of older adults with cancer [57, 61, 62].

Several definitions exist. Those without frailty are described as fit, well, or robust. Some definitions use a range from very fit to very severely frail, some use a dichotomous definition of fit versus frail, and some have a middle category between fit and frail labeled as pre-frail or vulnerable [40, 42, 57]. Over 70 tools exist to measure frailty, many without validation [42, 63]. Broadly these are use for screening using either single or short assessments or comprehensive assessment [45]. Others have been designed for research purposes using administrative data. A CGA can identify frailty based on the number of identified deficits and has the advantage of identifying deficits amenable to intervention [57]. Gold-standard frailty measurements include the Rockwood Frailty Index assessing accumulation of deficits across 30–70 items and the Fried Frailty Phenotype of weight loss, low activity, weak grip strength, slow gait speed, and exhaustion [64–66].

Given the association of frailty with poorer postoperative, functional, and oncologic outcomes, surgeons should routinely include a geriatric screening tool when assessing older adults with cancer and use the screening results to prompt referral for CGA [63, 67–70].

Assessing Older Adults Before Cancer Surgery

Traditional metrics of risks such as ASA physical status (American Society of Anesthesiologists), ECOG performance status (Eastern Cooperative Oncology Group), Karnofsky performance status, and clinical judgment alone miss important modifiable deficits and underestimate treatment intolerance, complications, impairments in function, and mortality [53, 71–77]. Older adult-specific assessments should be used [21]. An approach that uses brief geriatric screening tools to select older adults who should be referred for CGA is a practicable approach for surgeons [28, 33, 34, 78]. There are several goals of preoperative assessment outlined in Table 13.2.

Geriatric Screening Tools

Many screening tools have been developed to identify vulnerable older adults who are most likely to benefit from referral for CGA [31–36, 42]. These tools offer feasibility over CGA, but each has incumbent tradeoffs in comprehensiveness. These screening tools vary in the domains assessed, method of administration, time to complete, and test properties [28, 33, 34]. Surgeons should select a tool based on resources available, and familiarity or recommendations of local geriatric services. At minimum, surgeons caring for older adults with cancer should select one screening tool to use routinely. This can be done by the surgeon or trained delegate (e.g., residents, physician assistants, and nurses) and some are self-administered by

Table 13.2 Goals of preoperative assessment [18, 19, 28, 32]

Provide estimates of postoperative outcomes and competing causes of death and poor outcomes to aid decision-making and preparedness planning
Identify areas of vulnerability that may be optimized, including candidates for prehabilitation
Tailor treatment choices and supportive care
Anticipate postoperative needs
Plan for early rehabilitation
Delirium prevention and monitoring strategies
Proactive discharge planning including caregiver preparation and home care needs

patients. Older adults with an abnormal screening test score can then be referred to local multidisciplinary geriatric service for CGA and recommendations [63, 67–70].

Geriatric screening tools to identify vulnerability or frailty (an abnormal score should prompt CGA)

- Two commonly used geriatric screening tools that are sensitive for abnormalities in CGA and for postoperative outcomes in older adults with cancer are VES-13 (Vulnerable Elders Survey-13) (Table 13.3) and the G8 (Table 13.4.) [34, 79–81]. Both can be done in <5 minutes. VES-13 can be self-administered and G8 is administered by a healthcare professional. G8 has better sensitivity but worse specificity than VES-13 [34]. The G8 has been optimized in a single prospective cohort study to a shortened 6-item G6 tool with improved performance on internal validation, but it is yet to undergo external validation [82].
- Other available tools include GFI (Groningen Frailty Indicator), FRAIL Scale, SAOP2 (Senior Adult Oncology Program 2), Abbreviated CGA, TRST (Triage Risk Screening Tool), Clinical Frailty Scale, Edmonton Frail Scale, and PRISMA-7.

Other than frailty, if resources are available, additional single domain assessment tools that often are included as part of a CGA can be used (Table 13.5). Components that are most associated with postoperative outcomes and offer targets for interventions are functional status, cognition, depression, nutritional status, and comorbidities [86–88].

Table 13.3 Vulnerable Elders Survey-13 (VES-13) [42, 79]

Category		Points
Age (years)	<75	0
	75–85	1
	≥85	3
Self-rated health	Good, very good, or excellent	0
	Fair or poor	1
Physical disability	Difficulty with any of the following Stooping, crouching, or kneeling Lifting or carrying objects as heavy as 10 lbs Reaching or extending arms above shoulder level Writing, handing, or grasping small objects Walking a quarter mile (400 m) Doing heavy housework	0 (0 items) 1 (1 item) 2 (≥2 items)
Functional disability	Need assistance because of health/physical condition for any of the following: Shopping for personal items Managing money Walking across the room (cane or walker okay) Doing light housework Bathing or showering	0 (0 items) 4 (≥1 item)
A score of ≥3 is abnormal (frail)		

Table 13.4. G8 Tool [80]

Item	Answers	Points
Has food intake declined over the past 3 months due to loss of appetite, digestive problems, chewing, or swallowing difficulties?	Severe decrease in food intake	0
	Moderate decrease in food intake	1
	No decrease in food intake	2
Weight loss during the last 3 months	Weight loss >3 kg	0
	Does not know	1
	Weight loss between 1 and 3 kg	2
	No weight loss	3
Mobility	Bed or chair bound	0
	Able to get out of bed/chair but does not go out	1
	Goes out	2
Neuropsychological problems	Severe dementia or depression	0
	Mild dementia or depression	1
	No psychological problems	2
Body mass index (BMI, kg/m^2)	<19	0
	19 to <21	1
	21 to <23	2
	≥23	3
Takes >3 medications per day	Yes	0
	No	1
In comparison to other people of the same age, how does patient consider their health status?	Not as good	0
	Does not know	0.5
	As good	1
	Better	2
Age	>85	0
	80–85	1
	<80	2
A score of ≤14 is abnormal (frail)		

A mobile app for frailty screening (Essential Frailty Toolset) has been developed to assess patients undergoing aortic valve replacement [89]. The Essential Frailty Toolset has not been assessed in general surgery or oncology patients, but it is a simple four-item tool and is free to download (frailtytool.com).

Table 13.5 Single domain tools to consider if resources are available

Tool	Domains evaluated	Abnormal score	Time to complete	Comments
Timed Up and Go (TUG) [83]	Rise from chair, walk 3 m (10 ft), and return to sitting in chair	>12 s to complete	<1 minute	Simple test; requires timer and walking space Associated with major postoperative complications
Falls [84]	Ask patient about falls in the past 6 months	Report of any fall in the past 6 months	<1 minute	One-third patients had reported a fall when asked Strongly associated with postoperative complication and institutional discharge Sensitivity for frailty unreported
Mini-Cog [85]	Cognitive screening tool 3-word recall (scored 0–3) Clock drawing with all numbers and time set to 10 past 11 (scored 0 or 2)	≤3	≤3 minutes	Short screen for cognitive impairment Associated with postoperative complications, institutional discharge, and death at 6 months Poor performance with limited education
Nutrition	BMI Weight loss MNA-SF	BMI < 21 <80% of ideal weight or weight loss (>5% in 1 month or 10% in 6 months)	1–3 minutes	Associated with increased complications, hospital stay, and mortality [18]

BMI body mass index, *MNA-SF* mini nutritional assessment short form

Comprehensive Geriatric Assessment

CGA (Table 13.6) reveals unrecognized health issues, predicts postoperative outcomes, and can influence oncologic and non-oncologic treatment decisions [105–107]. In hospitalized patients, CGA has been associated with decreased mortality and functional decline at 3, 6, and 12 months.

CGA is recommended by multiple clinical oncology societies for those aged 70–75 years or older and those who are younger with age-related health concerns [18, 20, 32, 90, 108, 109]. If resources do not allow this, then geriatric screening tests can be used to select older adults for CGA [63, 67–70]. For CGA, any of various models and combinations of tools that assess the cardinal domains are acceptable [31, 32, 90]. Some geriatric oncology centers have developed electronic assessments [110, 111]. The Preoperative Assessment of Cancer in the Elderly (PACE) is a battery

Table 13.6 Comprehensive geriatric assessment [32, 90]

<table>
<tr><th>Domain</th><th>Example tools</th><th>Impact</th><th>Treatment options [90]</th></tr>
<tr><td>Functional independence</td><td>ADL (Katz index)
IADL (Lawton scale)</td><td rowspan="3">Impairs independent living
Adverse health-related outcomes
Treatment complications
Increased risk of death
Falls typically multifactorial
Consider impact of chemotherapy-associated neuropathy [91]</td><td rowspan="3">Home care assistance
Prehabilitation, anticipate postoperative rehabilitation
Physical therapy
Exercise program/ falls prevention program
Occupational therapy
Home safety evaluation
Medication review for falls</td></tr>
<tr><td>Physical performance [92, 93]</td><td>Grip strength
Gait speed
Timed Up and Go (TUG)
Short Physical Performance Battery (SPPB)</td></tr>
<tr><td>Falls [94]</td><td>Prior falls history
Location and circumstance</td></tr>
<tr><td>Comorbidity [95]</td><td>Charlson Comorbidity Index (CCI)
Cumulative Illness Rating Scale-Geriatric (CIRS-G)</td><td>Perioperative considerations
Severe comorbidity may be more life-limiting than cancer diagnosis</td><td>Optimize medical management</td></tr>
<tr><td>Nutrition [96]</td><td>Mini Nutritional Assessment (MNA)
Unintentional weight loss
Serum albumin
BMI</td><td>Treatment complications
Increased mortality
Increased hospital stay
Poor adjuvant chemotherapy tolerance</td><td>Dietician
Specific dietary recommendations
Oral care
Social work, home care, occupational therapy</td></tr>
<tr><td>Polypharmacy [97]</td><td>STOPP/START Criteria [98]
Beers Criteria [99]
Medication Appropriateness Index (MAI)</td><td>Drug interactions
Adverse events
Altered renal or liver function
Medication appropriateness</td><td>ACS-AGS guidelines for perioperative medication management [21]
Pharmacist medication review
Geriatrician management</td></tr>
<tr><td>Social support</td><td>Living situation
Power of Attorney
Availability of caregiver(s)
Social isolation
Financial status</td><td>Impaired treatment tolerability
Prolonged and difficult recovery
Difficulty with discharge planning</td><td>Social work
Transportation assistance
Home care assistance
Caregiver support
Spiritual care</td></tr>
</table>

Table 13.6 (continued)

Domain	Example tools	Impact	Treatment options [90]
Cognition (MCI, dementia, and delirium)	Mini-Cog (screening test) Montreal Cognitive Assessment (MoCA) Mini-Mental State Exam (MMSE) Rowland Universal Dementia Assessment Scale (RUDAS) [100] Confusion Assessment Method (CAM) for delirium	Capacity for informed consent Ability to follow complex treatment instructions Risk factor for postoperative delirium	Delirium prevention strategies [101, 102] Involve caregiver Involve SDM if capacity for informed consent is lacking Evaluate home supports Review medication appropriateness
Psychological status (depression, anxiety, distress) [103, 104]	Geriatric Depression Scale (GDS) Patient Health Questionnaire (PHQ-9) Distress Thermometer (DT)	Poor QoL Caregiver burden Functional decline	Geriatrician or PCP treatment Psycho-oncology Social work/ counseling Geriatric psychiatry
Other geriatric syndromes	Urinary incontinence	Social withdrawal and dermatitis Increased infections Increased health care costs	Lifestyle and pharmacotherapy
	Pressure ulcers	Physical restriction and social isolation Increased infections Increased health care costs	Multidisciplinary wound care team
	Osteoporosis	Falls and fracture risk	Geriatrician or PCP treatment
	Sarcopenia	Disability, hospitalization, and death	Dietician and nutritional recommendations Exercise program

CGA should be conducted by a team with geriatric expertise
Specific tools used are not standard but should include assessment in all four cardinal domains of physical health, functional status, psychological status, and socioeconomic factors and include management plans for identified deficits [31, 32].
Individual tools can be used alone or in shorter batteries for screening

ACS-AGS American College of Surgeons and American Geriatrics Society, *ADL* activities of daily living, *CGA* comprehensive geriatric assessment, *IADL* instrumental activities of daily living, *MCI* mild cognitive impairment, *PCP* primary care provider, *SDM* substitute decision-maker

investigated in older adults having cancer surgery [60]. Treatment strategies exist for deficits identified on CGA; however, specific guidance on how oncologic treatments should be altered based on CGA is not yet available.

Estimating Surgical Risk

Frailty, abnormal geriatric screening tests, and CGA are associated with surgical outcomes; however, several prognostic models have been developed aiming to give individual estimates of postoperative outcomes [35]. Few meet high-quality methodological standards for development and validation in older adults and older adults with cancer [88, 112–115]. The American College of Surgeons (ACS) Surgical Risk Calculator is a commonly used prognostic model that has undergone sound development, validation, and recalibration to improve test performance (Table 13.7) [116, 117].

Estimating Life Expectancy

Estimating an older adult's underlying life expectancy can assist with contextualizing treatment choices for cancer control by relating life expectancy with the risk of cancer-related morbidity, recurrence, and death. Discussing overall prognosis is helpful in supporting patients make choices about their healthcare and may strengthen the physician-patient relationship [118, 119]. Clinician predictions of life expectancy are often inaccurate, and prognosis calculators are helpful (Table 13.8) [7, 123–125]. An easy-to-use web-interface with life expectancy calculators informed by a systematic review of prognostic indices is available (ePrognosis) [7, 126]. Project Big Life also developed and validated a newer population-based life expectancy calculator with an easy-to-use web-interface [122, 127].

Table 13.7 Prediction model to estimate surgical risk

ACS Surgical Risk Calculator (riskcalculator.facs.org/RiskCalculator)	Web-based calculator Presents risk referenced against average patient Printable patient-friendly report	Outcomes of most interest Serious complication Death Return to OR Discharge to institution (short-term only)

Table 13.8 Free web-based life expectancy calculators

ePrognosis (eprognosis.ucsf.edu/calculators/#/)	Multiple calculators available Informed by systematic review [7] Lee Schonberg Index is most relevant [120, 121] Estimates 5-, 10-, and 14-year mortality Prints or emails patient-friendly report
Project Big Life (www.projectbiglife.ca/)	Canadian population-based prediction model [122] Patient-friendly online results display

Communication and Patient-Centered Decision-Making

Results of geriatric screening, CGA, life expectancy, and surgical risk estimates allow more informed patient-centered decision-making [26, 68]. There are no high-level clinical trial data to guide specific oncologic treatment modifications, but treatment recommendations should incorporate multidisciplinary recommendations in a shared decision-making model that integrates the patient's preferences and values [18, 20, 24, 28, 42, 68, 87].

For a fit older adult, standard treatments are appropriate. Based on patient preferences, tailored options can be considered (e.g., watch and wait, local excision, no surgical axillary staging, omission of radiotherapy after breast conserving surgery).

For a vulnerable or frail older adult – or when life expectancy is short enough that cancer control is a lesser priority due to low likelihood of cancer-related morbidity or mortality – management options include prehabilitation, less-invasive or organ-sparing treatment, or a palliative/non-curative symptom management approach.

Inadequate assessment and communication pitfalls can lead to nonbeneficial interventions with unintended consequences and unwanted burdens [26, 128, 129]. Uncertainty can lead to pressures for more aggressive treatments, and well-informed patients may choose differently [130–132]. Poor quality of the decision-making conversation, lack of shared decision-making, and unexpected poor postoperative quality of life all contribute to regret [133].

If surgery is chosen, it is important to discuss goals and preferences. Surgeons may discuss surgery with a "fix-it" model, convey risk as "big surgery", and insist on "surgical buy-in" to aggressive interventions in the case of major complications, and patients focus on logistical concerns [134–136]. However, an approach that narratively describes the types of patient-centered outcomes that are reasonably possible conveys more meaningful information [137]. Simply asking what a patient "wants" can lead to unattainable expectations or unexpected excessive burden [128, 138–140]. Explore and understand the types of patient-reported outcomes that would be unacceptable to the patient and the relative importance of longevity-based or comfort-based care if major complications occur, particularly a prolonged trajectory of accumulating complications [141, 142]. Question prompt lists are being investigated to facilitate discussing choices, expectations if everything goes well, and what happens if things go wrong [143].

Preparing for Surgery

What Is Prehabilitation?

Prehabilitation is a coordinated process aimed at improving the capacity of a patient to withstand an upcoming stressor like surgery. For patients with frailty, interventions that have been tested include physical activity, protein or other nutritional supplementation, psychosocial interventions, medication management, pharmacotherapy, and multifaceted interventions [68, 144]. Currently available evidence for prehabilitation, particularly in oncology, is mixed and inconclusive [145–149]. Multifaceted prehabilitation guided by CGA is likely to be most effective, with high yield for programs incorporating supervised combined nutrition and exercise interventions in individuals at increased risk of functional decline or with functional deficits at baseline.

Nutrition

Malnutrition is a common finding in older adults with cancer, particularly gastrointestinal cancers and when symptoms like anorexia, early satiety, nausea, and vomiting are present [96]. Malnutrition is associated with postoperative complications, mortality, and decreased survival [96, 150].

There are many tools to screen for malnutrition, or it may be identified on CGA. Screen with BMI (≤21), unintentional weight loss (>5% in 1 month or 10% in 6 months), serum albumin (<35 g/L), or MNA-SF (Mini Nutritional Assessment-Short Form) [96, 151]. If a patient screens positive for malnutrition, refer to a dietician if available and for CGA for suggested interventions (Table 13.9). Additionally, follow standard ERAS pathways with preoperative carbohydrate load, short liquid fast, and early postoperative diet [17].

Caring for Older Adults After Surgery

The American College of Surgeons and American Geriatrics Society provide detailed recommendations for older adults undergoing surgery (these are not specific to oncology) [17, 21]. Largely, older adults should be cared for similarly to younger adults, including ERAS pathways, with added attention to proactive early

Table 13.9 Suggested interventions for malnutrition (best done with dietician involvement) [96, 152]

Nutritional counseling	Individualized Focus on protein intake; recommend minimum of 20-35 g protein/meal and at least 1 g/kg/day Oral nutrition supplements typically low in protein; use protein-rich preparations Whey protein isolates or whole milk powder contain high-quality proteins
Pharmacologic	Anti-emetics Pain control Branched-chain amino acids (leucine) promote protein synthesis in older adults (renal impairment is contraindication) Omega-3 fatty acids (fish oil) may improve appetite and body weight (2 g/day) Insufficient evidence for cannabinoids Corticosteroids considered to increase appetite (<1–3 weeks, usually not used due to numerous side effects)
Physical activity	Daily aerobic and strength training; can stimulate appetite and anabolism

Table 13.10 Postoperative considerations requiring added attention in older adults [17, 24, 68]

Proactive early mobilization [153]	Remove barriers (crowding furniture) and restraints (proactive removal of Foley and nasogastric tube, saline lock intravenous) Up to chair at meal times even if not eating; active range-of-motion exercises if in bed; head-of-bed at 30 ° if aspiration risk Encourage ambulation; walking aids as needed Physiotherapy as needed
Delirium prevention [101, 102]	Avoid physical restraints, orient to surroundings (lighting, clock, date), family members present, sleep hygiene (limit nighttime interruptions, early waking, and napping during daytime), hearing and visual aids Optimal pain control, but limit opioids as much as possible Avoid inappropriate medications Screening with Confusion Assessment Method (CAM); is a work-up of suspected delirium for reversible causes, and prevent complications Antipsychotics (risperidone, olanzapine, quetiapine, or ziprasidone) at the lowest effective dose for shortest possible duration considered if behavioral measures have failed and severely agitated, distressed, or threatening substantial harm to self, others, or both
Avoid inappropriate medications	Beers or STOPP-START criteria [99] Avoid benzodiazepines (e.g., lorazepam), anticholinergics (e.g., dimenhydrinate), and antihistamines (e.g., diphenhydramine) Limit opioids as much as possible

mobilization, avoidance of inappropriate medications (Beers criteria), delirium prevention, and discharge planning including caregiver education, home care planning, rehabilitation planning (Table 13.10) [17, 24, 68].

For vulnerable patients who undergo surgery, although largely studied in emergency and orthopedic surgical populations, a proactive geriatric co-management strategy may provide some benefit [70, 154–156]. While all routine postoperative management applies to older adults, older adults are at increased risk for the hazards of hospitalization including delirium, malnutrition, pressure ulcers, falls, restraint use, functional decline, and adverse drug effects [24, 157]. Postoperative geriatrics teams can assist with management of medications and chronic medical conditions; prevention, recognition, and treatment of common postoperative complications including delirium; and discharge planning and caregiver education for post-hospital care [17, 24, 70].

Toronto Pearls

- In general, age is not the primary consideration to guide decision-making for cancer treatment, and older adults have unique vulnerabilities that require assessment beyond the traditional preoperative evaluation.
- Many resources exist that can be adapted to local clinical environments (Table 13.11).
- Surgeons, or a delegate, should employ a screening tool to guide referral for CGA when planning cancer treatments.

Table 13.11 List of key guidelines and geriatric oncology resources [27, 28]

Guideline or resource	Contents
International Society of Geriatric Oncology (SIOG) (www.siog.org/content/comprehensive-geriatric-assessment-cga-older-patient-cancer)	Guidelines Screening Tools (Geriatric 8, Triage Risk Screening Tool, Vulnerable Elderly Survey-13) Geriatric Assessment Tools
Cancer-Type Specific Guidelines	SIOG breast cancer guideline [158] SIOG rectal cancer guideline [87] SIOG colorectal cancer guideline [159]
ACS-AGS preoperative and perioperative guidelines [17, 21]	Detailed recommendations for older adults undergoing surgery not specific to oncology
AGS Postoperative Delirium [101, 102]	Detailed recommendations for prevention, screening, diagnosis, work-up, and management
American Society of Clinical Oncology (ASCO) Geriatric Oncology (www.asco.org/practice-guidelines/cancer-care-initiatives/geriatric-oncology)	Compilation of geriatric oncology resources, tools, updates, and research
Cancer & Aging Research Group (CARG) Tools http://www.mycarg.org/SelectQuestionnaire	Online Chemo-Toxicity Calculator Online Geriatric Assessment Tool in multiple languages
Senior Adult Oncology Program (SOAP) Tools, Moffitt Cancer Center (moffitt.org/for-healthcare-providers/clinical-programs-and-services/senior-adult-oncology-program/senior-adult-oncology-program-tools)	Chemotherapy Risk Assessment Scale for High-Age Patients (CRASH) CalculatorCumulative Illness Rating Scale-Geriatric (CIRS-G) Calculator SAOP2 Screening Questionnaire
ConsultGeri, The Hartford Institute for Geriatric Nursing (consultgeri.org/tools/try-this-series)	Geriatric assessment tools with video tutorials

ACS-AGS American College of Surgeons and American Geriatrics Society

- Surgeons should identify local resources available to assist in caring for older adults with cancer as these will vary.
- Results of screening and CGA as needed, risk of surgery estimation, and life expectancy estimation should be combined with patient preferences in a shared decision-making model to guide treatment choices and perioperative planning.

This systematic multidomain and holistic approach to provide assessment and intervention in the perioperative settings optimizes life prolongation, geriatric syndrome prevention, subjective well-being improvement, and functional status.

References

1. Lundebjerg NE, Trucil DE, Hammond EC, Applegate WB. When it comes to older adults, language matters: Journal of the American Geriatrics Society adopts modified American Medical Association style. J Am Geriatr Soc. 2017;65:1386–8.

2. Balducci L, Ershler WB. Cancer and ageing: a nexus at several levels. Nat Rev Cancer. 2005;5:655.
3. Etzioni DA, Liu JH, Maggard MA, Ko CY. The aging population and its impact on the surgery workforce. Ann Surg. 2003;238:170.
4. Ries LAG, Reichman ME, Lewis DR, Hankey BF, Edwards BK. Cancer survival and incidence from the Surveillance, Epidemiology, and End Results (SEER) program. Oncologist. 2003;8:541–52.
5. Edwards BK, Howe HL, Ries LAG, Thun MJ, Rosenberg HM, Yancik R, Wingo PA, Jemal A, Feigal EG. Annual report to the nation on the status of cancer, 1973–1999, featuring implications of age and aging on US cancer burden. Cancer. 2002;94:2766–92.
6. Smith BD, Smith GL, Hurria A, Hortobagyi GN, Buchholz TA. Future of cancer incidence in the United States: burdens upon an aging, changing nation. J Clin Oncol. 2009;27:2758–65.
7. Yourman LC, Lee SJ, Schonberg MA, Widera EW, Smith AK. Prognostic indices for older adults: a systematic review. JAMA. 2012;307:182–92.
8. Hutchins LF, Unger JM, Crowley JJ, Coltman CA Jr, Albain KS. Underrepresentation of patients 65 years of age or older in cancer-treatment trials. N Engl J Med. 1999;341:2061–7.
9. Talarico L, Chen G, Pazdur R. Enrollment of elderly patients in clinical trials for cancer drug registration: a 7-year experience by the US Food and Drug Administration. J Clin Oncol. 2004;22:4626–31.
10. Fried TR, Van Ness PH, Byers AL, Towle VR, O'Leary JR, Dubin JA. Changes in preferences for life-sustaining treatment among older persons with advanced illness. J Gen Intern Med. 2007;22:495–501.
11. Barnato AE, Herndon MB, Anthony DL, Gallagher PM, Skinner JS, Bynum JPW, Fisher ES. Are regional variations in end-of-life care intensity explained by patient preferences?: a study of the US Medicare Population. Med Care. 2007;45:386.
12. Teno JM, Fisher ES, Hamel MB, Coppola K, Dawson NV. Medical care inconsistent with patients' treatment goals: association with 1-year Medicare resource use and survival. J Am Geriatr Soc. 2002;50:496–500.
13. Nabozny MJ, Kruser JM, Steffens NM, Brasel KJ, Campbell TC, Gaines ME, Schwarze ML. Constructing high-stakes surgical decisions: it's better to die trying. Ann Surg. 2016;263:64.
14. Hurria A, Mohile SG, Dale W. Research priorities in geriatric oncology: addressing the needs of an aging population. J Natl Compr Cancer Netw. 2012;10:286–8.
15. Dall TM, Gallo PD, Chakrabarti R, West T, Semilla AP, Storm MV. An aging population and growing disease burden will require alarge and specialized health care workforce by 2025. Health Aff. 2013;32:2013–20.
16. Section for Enhancing Geriatric Understanding and Expertise Among Surgical and Medical Specialists (SEGUE) AGS. Retooling for an aging America: building the Healthcare Workforce: a white paper regarding implementation of recommendation 4.2 of this Institute of Medicine Report of April 14, 2008, that "All licensure, certification and maintenance of certification for healthcare professionals should include demonstration of competence in care of older adults as a criterion". J Am Geriatr Soc. 2011;59:1537–9.
17. Mohanty S, Rosenthal RA, Russell MM, Neuman MD, Ko CY, Esnaola NF. Optimal perioperative management of the geriatric patient: a best practices guideline from the American College of Surgeons NSQIP and the American Geriatrics Society. J Am Coll Surg. 2016;222:930–47.
18. National Comprehensive Cancer Network older adult oncology (version 2.2018). https://www.nccn.org/professionals/physician_gls/pdf/senior.pdf. Accessed 19 Oct 2018.
19. Kristjansson SR, Spies C, Veering BTH, Silverstein JH, Vigano AAL, Mercadante S, Jack S, Zaniboni A, Schmidt M, Watt HL. Perioperative care of the elderly oncology patient: a report from the SIOG task force on the perioperative care of older patients with cancer. J Geriatr Oncol. 2012;3:147–62.
20. Aapro M, Schrijvers D. ESMO handbook of cancer in the senior patient. 2nd ed. London: ESMO; 2015.

21. Chow WB, Rosenthal RA, Merkow RP, Ko CY, Esnaola NF. Optimal preoperative assessment of the geriatric surgical patient: a best practices guideline from the American College of Surgeons National Surgical Quality Improvement Program and the American Geriatrics Society. J Am Coll Surg. 2012;215:453–66.
22. Lowsky DJ, Olshansky SJ, Bhattacharya J, Goldman DP. Heterogeneity in healthy aging. J Gerontol A Biol Sci Med Sci. 2013;69:640–9.
23. Wildiers H, Mauer M, Pallis A, Hurria A, Mohile SG, Luciani A, Curigliano G, Extermann M, Lichtman SM, Ballman K. End points and trial design in geriatric oncology research: a joint European organisation for research and treatment of cancer–Alliance for Clinical Trials in Oncology–International Society Of Geriatric Oncology position article. J Clin Oncol. 2013;31:3711–8.
24. Shahrokni A, Kim SJ, Bosl GJ, Korc-Grodzicki B. How we care for an older patient with cancer. J Oncol Pract. 2017;13:95–102.
25. Shapiro GR. Introduction: decision making with older cancer patients. Cancer J. 2017;23:199–200.
26. Chesney TR, Schwarze ML. Patient-centered surgical decision making. In: Rosenthal R, Zenilman M, Katlic M, editors. Principles and practice of geriatric surgery. 3rd ed. Cham: Springer; 2017. p. 1–13.
27. Soto-Perez-de-Celis E, Li D, Yuan Y, Lau YM, Hurria A. Functional versus chronological age: geriatric assessments to guide decision making in older patients with cancer. Lancet Oncol. 2018;19:e305–16.
28. Loh KP, Soto-Perez-de-Celis E, Hsu T, de Glas NA, Battisti NML, Baldini C, Rodrigues M, Lichtman SM, Wildiers H. What every oncologist should know about geriatric assessment for older patients with cancer: Young International Society of Geriatric Oncology position paper. J Oncol Pract. 2018;14:85–94.
29. Ghignone F, Van Leeuwen BL, Montroni I, Huisman MG, Somasundar P, Cheung KL, Audisio RA, Ugolini G. The assessment and management of older cancer patients: a SIOG surgical task force survey on surgeons' attitudes. Eur J Surg Oncol. 2016;42:297–302.
30. Chesney TR, Pang G, Ahmed N. Caring for older surgical patients: contemporary attitudes, knowledge, practices, and needs of general surgeons and residents. Ann Surg. 2017;268:77. https://doi.org/10.1097/SLA.0000000000002363.
31. Puts MTE, Alibhai SMH. Fighting back against the dilution of the comprehensive geriatric assessment. J Geriatr Oncol. 2018;9:3–5.
32. Wildiers H, Heeren P, Puts M, Topinkova E, Janssen-Heijnen MLG, Extermann M, Falandry C, Artz A, Brain E, Colloca G. International Society of Geriatric Oncology consensus on geriatric assessment in older patients with cancer. J Clin Oncol. 2014;32:2595–603.
33. Decoster L, Van Puyvelde K, Mohile S, Wedding U, Basso U, Colloca G, Rostoft S, Overcash J, Wildiers H, Steer C. Screening tools for multidimensional health problems warranting a geriatric assessment in older cancer patients: an update on SIOG recommendations. Ann Oncol. 2014;26:288–300.
34. Hamaker ME, Jonker JM, de Rooij SE, Vos AG, Smorenburg CH, van Munster BC. Frailty screening methods for predicting outcome of a comprehensive geriatric assessment in elderly patients with cancer: a systematic review. Lancet Oncol. 2012;13:e437–44.
35. Eamer G, Al-Amoodi M, Holroyd-Leduc J, Rolfson DB, Warkentin L, Khadaroo RG. Review of risk assessment tools to predict morbidity and mortality in elderly surgical patients brief title: review of surgical risk assessment tools. Am J Surg. 2018;216:585–94.
36. Watt J, Tricco AC, Talbot-Hamon C, Rios P, Grudniewicz A, Wong C, Sinclair D, Straus SE. Identifying older adults at risk of harm following elective surgery: a systematic review and meta-analysis. BMC Med. 2018;16:2.
37. Mokkink LB, Terwee CB, Patrick DL, Alonso J, Stratford PW, Knol DL, Bouter LM, de Vet HCW. The COSMIN study reached international consensus on taxonomy, terminology, and definitions of measurement properties for health-related patient-reported outcomes. J Clin Epidemiol. 2010;63:737–45.

38. Inouye SK, Studenski S, Tinetti ME, Kuchel GA. Geriatric syndromes: clinical, research, and policy implications of a core geriatric concept: (See Editorial Comments by Dr. William Hazzard on pp 794–796). J Am Geriatr Soc. 2007;55:780–91.
39. Clegg A, Young J, Iliffe S, Rikkert MO, Rockwood K. Frailty in elderly people. Lancet. 2013;381:752–62.
40. Robinson TN, Walston JD, Brummel NE, Deiner S, Brown CH, Kennedy M, Hurria A. Frailty for surgeons: review of a National Institute on Aging Conference on Frailty for Specialists. J Am Coll Surg. 2015;221:1083–92.
41. Anaya DA, Johanning J, Spector SA, Katlic MR, Perrino AC, Feinleib J, Rosenthal RA. Summary of the panel session at the 38th Annual Surgical Symposium of the Association of VA Surgeons: what is the big deal about frailty? JAMA Surg. 2014;149:1191–7.
42. Ethun CG, Bilen MA, Jani AB, Maithel SK, Ogan K, Master VA. Frailty and cancer: implications for oncology surgery, medical oncology, and radiation oncology. CA Cancer J Clin. 2017;67:362–77.
43. Morley JE, Vellas B, Van Kan GA, Anker SD, Bauer JM, Bernabei R, Cesari M, Chumlea WC, Doehner W, Evans J. Frailty consensus: a call to action. J Am Med Dir Assoc. 2013;14:392–7.
44. Buta BJ, Walston JD, Godino JG, Park M, Kalyani RR, Xue Q-L, Bandeen-Roche K, Varadhan R. Frailty assessment instruments: systematic characterization of the uses and contexts of highly-cited instruments. Ageing Res Rev. 2016;26:53–61.
45. Rockwood K, Theou O, Mitnitski A. What are frailty instruments for? Age Ageing. 2015;44:545–7.
46. Cruz-Jentoft AJ, Baeyens JP, Bauer JM, Boirie Y, Cederholm T, Landi F, Martin FC, Michel J-P, Rolland Y, Schneider SM. Sarcopenia: European consensus on definition and diagnosis report of the European Working Group on Sarcopenia in older people. Age Ageing. 2010;39:412–23.
47. Fielding RA, Vellas B, Evans WJ, Bhasin S, Morley JE, Newman AB, van Kan GA, Andrieu S, Bauer J, Breuille D. Sarcopenia: an undiagnosed condition in older adults. Current consensus definition: prevalence, etiology, and consequences. International working group on sarcopenia. J Am Med Dir Assoc. 2011;12:249–56.
48. Studenski SA, Peters KW, Alley DE, Cawthon PM, McLean RR, Harris TB, Ferrucci L, Guralnik JM, Fragala MS, Kenny AM. The FNIH sarcopenia project: rationale, study description, conference recommendations, and final estimates. J Gerontol A Biol Sci Med Sci. 2014;69:547–58.
49. Muscaritoli M, Anker SD, Argiles J, Aversa Z, Bauer JM, Biolo G, Boirie Y, Bosaeus I, Cederholm T, Costelli P. Consensus definition of sarcopenia, cachexia and pre-cachexia: joint document elaborated by Special Interest Groups (SIG) "cachexia-anorexia in chronic wasting diseases" and "nutrition in geriatrics". Clin Nutr. 2010;29:154–9.
50. Clynes MA, Edwards MH, Buehring B, Dennison EM, Binkley N, Cooper C. Definitions of sarcopenia: associations with previous falls and fracture in a population sample. Calcif Tissue Int. 2015;97:445–52.
51. Levolger S, Van Vugt JLA, De Bruin RWF, IJzermans JNM. Systematic review of sarcopenia in patients operated on for gastrointestinal and hepatopancreatobiliary malignancies. Br J Surg. 2015;102:1448–58.
52. Simonsen C, de Heer P, Bjerre ED, Suetta C, Hojman P, Pedersen BK, Svendsen LB, Christensen JF. Sarcopenia and postoperative complication risk in gastrointestinal surgical oncology: a Meta-analysis. Ann Surg. 2018;268:58–69.
53. Makary MA, Segev DL, Pronovost PJ, Syin D, Bandeen-Roche K, Patel P, Takenaga R, Devgan L, Holzmueller CG, Tian J. Frailty as a predictor of surgical outcomes in older patients. J Am Coll Surg. 2010;210:901–8.
54. Shamliyan T, Talley KMC, Ramakrishnan R, Kane RL. Association of frailty with survival: a systematic literature review. Ageing Res Rev. 2013;12:719–36.
55. Pawlik TM, Gleisner AL, Bauer TW, Adams RB, Reddy SK, Clary BM, Martin RC, Scoggins CR, Tanabe KK, Michaelson JS. Liver-directed surgery for metastatic squamous cell carcinoma to the liver: results of a multi-center analysis. Ann Surg Oncol. 2007;14:2807–16.

56. Tan K-Y, Kawamura YJ, Tokomitsu A, Tang T. Assessment for frailty is useful for predicting morbidity in elderly patients undergoing colorectal cancer resection whose comorbidities are already optimized. Am J Surg. 2012;204:139–43.
57. Handforth C, Clegg A, Young C, Simpkins S, Seymour MT, Selby PJ, Young J. The prevalence and outcomes of frailty in older cancer patients: a systematic review. Ann Oncol. 2014;26:1091–101.
58. Li Y, Pederson JL, Churchill TA, Wagg AS, Holroyd-Leduc JM, Alagiakrishnan K, Padwal RS, Khadaroo RG. Impact of frailty on outcomes after discharge in older surgical patients: a prospective cohort study. Can Med Assoc J. 2018;190:E184–90.
59. Hewitt J, Long S, Carter B, Bach S, McCarthy K, Clegg A. The prevalence of frailty and its association with clinical outcomes in general surgery: a systematic review and meta-analysis. Age Ageing. 2018;47:793–800.
60. Audisio RA. Shall we operate? Preoperative assessment in elderly cancer patients (PACE) can help A SIOG surgical task force prospective study. Crit Rev Oncol Hematol. 2008;48:16–31.
61. Collard RM, Boter H, Schoevers RA, Voshaar RCO. Prevalence of frailty in community-dwelling older persons: a systematic review. J Am Geriatr Soc. 2012;60:1487–92.
62. Song X, Mitnitski A, Rockwood K. Prevalence and 10-year outcomes of frailty in older adults in relation to deficit accumulation. J Am Geriatr Soc. 2010;58:681–7.
63. Huisingh-Scheetz M, Walston J. How should older adults with cancer be evaluated for frailty? J Geriatr Oncol. 2017;8:8–15.
64. Mitnitski AB, Mogilner AJ, Rockwood K. Accumulation of deficits as a proxy measure of aging. Sci World J. 2001;1:323–36.
65. Rockwood K, Song X, MacKnight C, Bergman H, Hogan DB, McDowell I, Mitnitski A. A global clinical measure of fitness and frailty in elderly people. Can Med Assoc J. 2005;173:489–95.
66. Fried LP, Tangen CM, Walston J, Newman AB, Hirsch C, Gottdiener J, Seeman T, Tracy R, Kop WJ, Burke G. Frailty in older adults: evidence for a phenotype. J Gerontol A Biol Sci Med Sci. 2001;56:M146–57.
67. Hall DE, Arya S, Schmid KK, Carlson MA, Lavedan P, Bailey TL, Purviance G, Bockman T, Lynch TG, Johanning JM. Association of a frailty screening initiative with postoperative survival at 30, 180, and 365 days. JAMA Surg. 2017;152:233–40.
68. Alvarez-Nebreda ML, Bentov N, Urman RD, Setia S, Huang JC-S, Pfeifer K, Bennett K, Ong TD, Richman D, Gollapudi D. Recommendations for preoperative management of frailty from the Society for Perioperative Assessment and Quality Improvement (SPAQI). J Clin Anesth. 2018;47:33–42.
69. Magnuson A, Canin B, van Londen GJ, Edwards B, Bakalarski P, Parker I. Incorporating geriatric medicine providers into the care of the older adult with cancer. Curr Oncol Rep. 2016;18:65.
70. McDonald SR, Heflin MT, Whitson HE, Dalton TO, Lidsky ME, Liu P, Poer CM, Sloane R, Thacker JK, White HK. Association of integrated care coordination with postsurgical outcomes in high-risk older adults: the Perioperative Optimization of Senior Health (POSH) initiative. JAMA Surg. 2018;153:454–62.
71. Robinson TN, Eiseman B, Wallace JI, Church SD, McFann KK, Pfister SM, Sharp TJ, Moss M. Redefining geriatric preoperative assessment using frailty, disability and co-morbidity. Ann Surg. 2009;250:449–55.
72. Kristjansson SR, Nesbakken A, Jordhøy MS, Skovlund E, Audisio RA, Johannessen H-O, Bakka A, Wyller TB. Comprehensive geriatric assessment can predict complications in elderly patients after elective surgery for colorectal cancer: a prospective observational cohort study. Crit Rev Oncol Hematol. 2010;76:208–17.
73. Jolly TA, Deal AM, Nyrop KA, Williams GR, Pergolotti M, Wood WA, Alston SM, Gordon B-BE, Dixon SA, Moore SG. Geriatric assessment-identified deficits in older cancer patients with normal performance status. Oncologist. 2015;20:379–85.

74. Kirkhus L, Benth JŠ, Rostoft S, Grønberg BH, Hjermstad MJ, Selbæk G, Wyller TB, Harneshaug M, Jordhøy MS. Geriatric assessment is superior to oncologists' clinical judgement in identifying frailty. Br J Cancer. 2017;117:470.
75. Revenig LM, Canter DJ, Henderson MA, Ogan K, Kooby DA, Maithel SK, Liu Y, Kim S, Master VA. Preoperative quantification of perceptions of surgical frailty. J Surg Res. 2015;193:583–9.
76. Hoffmann TC, Del Mar C. Clinicians' expectations of the benefits and harms of treatments, screening, and tests: a systematic review. JAMA Intern Med. 2017;177:407–19.
77. Sacks GD, Dawes AJ, Ettner SL, Brook RH, Fox CR, Maggard-Gibbons M, Ko CY, Russell MM. Surgeon perception of risk and benefit in the decision to operate. Ann Surg. 2016;264:896–903.
78. Korc-Grodzicki B, Holmes HM, Shahrokni A. Geriatric assessment for oncologists. Cancer Biol Med. 2015;12:261.
79. Saliba D, Elliott M, Rubenstein LZ, Solomon DH, Young RT, Kamberg CJ, Roth RNC, MacLean CH, Shekelle PG, Sloss EM. The Vulnerable Elders Survey: a tool for identifying vulnerable older people in the community. J Am Geriatr Soc. 2001;49:1691–9.
80. Bellera CA, Rainfray M, Mathoulin-Pelissier S, Mertens C, Delva F, Fonck M, Soubeyran PL. Screening older cancer patients: first evaluation of the G-8 geriatric screening tool. Ann Oncol. 2012;23:2166–72.
81. Yokom DW, Alibhai SMH, Sattar S, Krzyzanowska MK. Puts MTE (2018) Geriatric oncology screening tools for CGA-based interventions: results from a phase II study of geriatric assessment and management for older adults with cancer. J Geriatr Oncol. 2018;9(6):683–6.
82. Martinez-Tapia C, Canoui-Poitrine F, Bastuji-Garin S, Soubeyran P, Mathoulin-Pelissier S, Tournigand C, Paillaud E, Laurent M, Audureau E. Optimizing the G8 screening tool for older patients with cancer: diagnostic performance and validation of a six-item version. Oncologist. 2016;21:188–95.
83. Huisman MG, Van Leeuwen BL, Ugolini G, Montroni I, Spiliotis J, Stabilini C, de'Liguori Carino N, Farinella E, de Bock GH, Audisio RA. "Timed up & go": a screening tool for predicting 30-day morbidity in onco-geriatric surgical patients? a multicenter cohort study. PLoS One. 2014;9:e0086863.
84. Jones TS, Dunn CL, Wu DS, Cleveland JC, Kile D, Robinson TN. Relationship between asking an older adult about falls and surgical outcomes. JAMA Surg. 2013;148:1132–8.
85. Robinson TN, Wu DS, Pointer LF, Dunn CL, Moss M. Preoperative cognitive dysfunction is related to adverse postoperative outcomes in the elderly. J Am Coll Surg. 2012;215:12–7.
86. Feng MA, McMillan DT, Crowell K, Muss H, Nielsen ME, Smith AB. Geriatric assessment in surgical oncology: a systematic review. J Surg Res. 2015;193:265–72.
87. Montroni I, Ugolini G, Saur NM, Spinelli A, Rostoft S, Millan M, Wolthuis A, Daniels IR, Hompes R, Penna MM. Personalized management of elderly patients with rectal cancer: expert recommendations of the European Society of Surgical Oncology, European Society of Coloproctology, International Society of Geriatric Oncology, and American College of Surgeons Commission. Eur J Surg Oncol. 2018;44:1685–702.
88. Katlic MR, Coleman J, Khan K, Wozniak SE, Abraham JH. Sinai abbreviated geriatric evaluation: development and validation of a practical test. Ann Surg. 2019;269:177–83.
89. Afilalo J, Lauck S, Kim DH, Lefèvre T, Piazza N, Lachapelle K, Martucci G, Lamy A, Labinaz M, Peterson MD. Frailty in older adults undergoing aortic valve replacement: the FRAILTY-AVR study. J Am Coll Cardiol. 2017;70:689–700.
90. Mohile SG, Velarde C, Hurria A, Magnuson A, Lowenstein L, Pandya C, O'Donovan A, Gorawara-Bhat R, Dale W. Geriatric assessment-guided care processes for older adults: a Delphi consensus of geriatric oncology experts. J Natl Compr Cancer Netw. 2015;13:1120–30.
91. Gewandter JS, Fan L, Magnuson A, Mustian K, Peppone L, Heckler C, Hopkins J, Tejani M, Morrow GR, Mohile SG. Falls and functional impairments in cancer survivors with chemotherapy-induced peripheral neuropathy (CIPN): a University of Rochester CCOP study. Support Care Cancer. 2013;21:2059–66.

92. Cesari M, Kritchevsky SB, Newman AB, Simonsick EM, Harris TB, Penninx BW, Brach JS, Tylavsky FA, Satterfield S, Bauer DC. Added value of physical performance measures in predicting adverse health-related events: results from the Health, Aging and Body Composition Study. J Am Geriatr Soc. 2009;57:251–9.
93. Studenski S, Perera S, Patel K, Rosano C, Faulkner K, Inzitari M, Brach J, Chandler J, Cawthon P, Connor EB. Gait speed and survival in older adults. JAMA. 2011;305:50–8.
94. Wildes TM, Dua P, Fowler SA, Miller JP, Carpenter CR, Avidan MS, Stark S. Systematic review of falls in older adults with cancer. J Geriatr Oncol. 2015;6:70–83.
95. Williams GR, Mackenzie A, Magnuson A, Olin R, Chapman A, Mohile S, Allore H, Somerfield MR, Targia V, Extermann M. Comorbidity in older adults with cancer. J Geriatr Oncol. 2016;7:249–57.
96. Mislang AR, Di Donato S, Hubbard J, Krishna L, Mottino G, Bozzetti F, Biganzoli L. Nutritional management of older adults with gastrointestinal cancers: an International Society of Geriatric Oncology (SIOG) review paper. J Geriatr Oncol. 2018;9:382–92.
97. Prithviraj GK, Koroukian S, Margevicius S, Berger NA, Bagai R, Owusu C. Patient characteristics associated with polypharmacy and inappropriate prescribing of medications among older adults with cancer. J Geriatr Oncol. 2012;3:228–37.
98. Gallagher P, Ryan C, Byrne S, Kennedy J, O'Mahony D. STOPP (screening tool of older person's prescriptions) and START (screening tool to alert doctors to right treatment). Consensus validation. Int J Clin Pharmacol Ther. 2008;46:72–83.
99. Panel AGS, BCUE, Fick DM, Semla TP, Beizer J, Brandt N, Dombrowski R, CE DB, Eisenberg W, Epplin JJ, Flanagan N, et al. American Geriatrics Society 2015 updated beers criteria for potentially inappropriate medication use in older adults. J Am Geriatr Soc. 2015;63:2227–46.
100. Storey JE, Rowland JTJ, Conforti DA, Dickson HG. The Rowland universal dementia assessment scale (RUDAS): a multicultural cognitive assessment scale. Int Psychogeriatr. 2004;16:13–31.
101. Samuel M. Postoperative delirium in older adults: best practice statement from the American Geriatrics Society. J Am Coll Surg. 2015;220:136.
102. Oh ES, Fong TG, Hshieh TT, Inouye SK. Delirium in older persons: advances in diagnosis and treatment. JAMA. 2017;318:1161–74.
103. Weiss Wiesel TR, Nelson CJ, Tew WP, Hardt M, Mohile SG, Owusu C, Klepin HD, Gross CP, Gajra A, Lichtman SM. The relationship between age, anxiety, and depression in older adults with cancer. Psycho-Oncology. 2015;24:712–7.
104. Canoui-Poitrine F, Reinald N, Laurent M, Guery E, Caillet P, David J, Tournigand C, Lagrange J, Bastuji-Garin S, Lemogne C. Geriatric assessment findings independently associated with clinical depression in 1092 older patients with cancer: the ELCAPA Cohort Study. Psycho-Oncology. 2016;25:104–11.
105. Caillet P, Laurent M, Bastuji-Garin S, Liuu E, Culine S, Lagrange J-L, Canoui-Poitrine F, Paillaud E. Optimal management of elderly cancer patients: usefulness of the Comprehensive Geriatric Assessment. Clin Interv Aging. 2014;9:1645.
106. Hamaker ME, Te Molder M, Thielen N, van Munster BC, Schiphorst AH, van Huis LH. The effect of a geriatric evaluation on treatment decisions and outcome for older cancer patients – a systematic review. J Geriatr Oncol. 2018;9:430–40.
107. Kim K, Park K-H, Koo K-H, Han H-S, Kim C-H. Comprehensive geriatric assessment can predict postoperative morbidity and mortality in elderly patients undergoing elective surgery. Arch Gerontol Geriatr. 2013;56:507–12.
108. Pallis AG, Ring A, Fortpied C, Penninckx B, Van Nes MC, Wedding U, Vonminckwitz G, Johnson CD, Wyld L, Timmer-Bonte A. EORTC workshop on clinical trial methodology in older individuals with a diagnosis of solid tumors. Ann Oncol. 2011;22:1922–6.
109. Pallis AG, Fortpied C, Wedding U, Van Nes MC, Penninckx B, Ring A, Lacombe D, Monfardini S, Scalliet P, Wildiers H. EORTC elderly task force position paper: approach to the older cancer patient. Eur J Cancer. 2010;46:1502–13.

110. Shahrokni A, Tin A, Downey RJ, Strong V, Mahmoudzadeh S, Boparai MK, McMillan S, Vickers A, Korc-Grodzicki B. Electronic rapid fitness assessment: a novel tool for preoperative evaluation of the geriatric oncology patient. J Natl Compr Cancer Netw. 2017;15:172–9.
111. Hurria A, Akiba C, Kim J, Mitani D, Loscalzo M, Katheria V, Koczywas M, Pal S, Chung V, Forman S. Reliability, validity, and feasibility of a computer-based geriatric assessment for older adults with cancer. J Oncol Pract. 2016;12:e1025–34.
112. Moons KGM, Altman DG, Reitsma JB, Ioannidis JPA, Macaskill P, Steyerberg EW, Vickers AJ, Ransohoff DF, Collins GS. Transparent reporting of a multivariable prediction model for Individual Prognosis or Diagnosis (TRIPOD): explanation and elaboration. Ann Intern Med. 2015;162:W1–W73.
113. Buettner S, Wagner D, Kim Y, Margonis GA, Makary MA, Wilson A, Sasaki K, Amini N, Gani F, Pawlik TM. Inclusion of sarcopenia outperforms the modified frailty index in predicting 1-year mortality among 1,326 patients undergoing gastrointestinal surgery for a malignant indication. J Am Coll Surg. 2016;222:397–407.
114. Olufajo OA, Reznor G, Lipsitz SR, Cooper ZR, Haider AH, Salim A, Rangel EL. Preoperative assessment of surgical risk: creation of a scoring tool to estimate 1-year mortality after emergency abdominal surgery in the elderly patient. Am J Surg. 2017;213:771–7.
115. Min L, Hall K, Finlayson E, Englesbe M, Palazzolo W, Chan C-L, Hou H, Miller A, Diehl KM. Estimating risk of postsurgical general and geriatric complications using the VESPA preoperative tool. JAMA Surg. 2017;152:1126–33.
116. Selby D, Cascella A, Gardiner K, Do R, Moravan V, Myers J, Chow E. A single set of numerical cutpoints to define moderate and severe symptoms for the Edmonton Symptom Assessment System. J Pain Symptom Manag. 2010;39:241–9.
117. Sherman SK, Poli EC, Kapadia MR, Turaga KK. Estimating surgical risk for patients with severe comorbidities. JAMA Surg. 2018;153:778–80.
118. Fenton JJ, Duberstein PR, Kravitz RL, Xing G, Tancredi DJ, Fiscella K, Mohile S, Epstein RM. Impact of prognostic discussions on the patient-physician relationship: prospective cohort study. J Clin Oncol. 2017;36:225–30.
119. Smith AK, Williams BA, Lo B. Discussing overall prognosis with the very elderly. N Engl J Med. 2011;365:2149.
120. Lee SJ, Boscardin WJ, Kirby KA, Covinsky KE. Individualizing life expectancy estimates for older adults using the Gompertz Law of Human Mortality. PLoS One. 2014;9:e108540.
121. Schonberg MA, Li V, Marcantonio ER, Davis RB, McCarthy EP. Predicting mortality up to 14 years among community-dwelling adults aged 65 and older. J Am Geriatr Soc. 2017;65:1310–5.
122. Manuel DG, Perez R, Sanmartin C, Taljaard M, Hennessy D, Wilson K, Tanuseputro P, Manson H, Bennett C, Tuna M. Measuring burden of unhealthy behaviours using a multivariable predictive approach: life expectancy lost in Canada attributable to smoking, alcohol, physical inactivity, and diet. PLoS Med. 2016;13:e1002082.
123. Cheon S, Agarwal A, Popovic M, Milakovic M, Lam M, Fu W, DiGiovanni J, Lam H, Lechner B, Pulenzas N. The accuracy of clinicians' predictions of survival in advanced cancer: a review. Ann Palliat Med. 2015;5:22–9.
124. Lamont EB, Christakis NA. Complexities in prognostication in advanced cancer: to help them live their lives the way they want to. JAMA. 2003;290:98–104.
125. Downar J, Goldman R, Pinto R, Englesakis M, Adhikari NKJ. The "surprise question" for predicting death in seriously ill patients: a systematic review and meta-analysis. Can Med Assoc J. 2017;189:E484–93.
126. Lee S, Smith A, Widera E, Yourman L, Schonberg M, Ahalt C. ePrognosis. https://eprognosis.ucsf.edu/index.php. Accessed 6 Jan 2018.
127. Manuel DG, Perez R, Sanmartin C, Taljaard M, Hennessy D, Wilson K, Tanuseputro P, Manson H, Bennett C, Tuna M. Project big life. https://www.projectbiglife.ca/. Accessed 6 Jan 2018.

128. Cooper Z, Courtwright A, Karlage A, Gawande A, Block S. Pitfalls in communication that lead to nonbeneficial emergency surgery in elderly patients with serious illness: description of the problem and elements of a solution. Ann Surg. 2014;260:949–57.
129. Kwok AC, Semel ME, Lipsitz SR, Bader AM, Barnato AE, Gawande AA, Jha AK. The intensity and variation of surgical care at the end of life: a retrospective cohort study. Lancet. 2011;378:1408–13.
130. Morris RS, Ruck JM, Conca-Cheng AM, Smith TJ, Carver TW, Johnston FM. Shared decision-making in acute surgical illness: the surgeon's perspective. J Am Coll Surg. 2018;226:784–95.
131. Raiten JM, Neuman MD. " If I had only known"--on choice and uncertainty in the ICU. N Engl J Med. 2012;367:1779–81.
132. Fried TR, Bradley EH, O'leary J. Prognosis communication in serious illness: perceptions of older patients, caregivers, and clinicians. J Am Geriatr Soc. 2003;51:1398–403.
133. Wilson A, Ronnekleiv-Kelly SM, Pawlik TM. Regret in surgical decision making: a systematic review of patient and physician perspectives. World J Surg. 2017;41:1454–65.
134. Kruser JM, Pecanac KE, Brasel KJ, Cooper Z, Steffens N, McKneally M, Schwarze ML. "And I think that we can fix it": mental models used in high-risk surgical decision making. Ann Surg. 2015;261:678–84.
135. Pecanac KE, Kehler JM, Brasel KJ, Cooper Z, Steffens NM, McKneally MF, Schwarze ML. "It's big surgery": preoperative expressions of risk, responsibility and commitment to treatment after high-risk operations. Ann Surg. 2014;259:458–63.
136. Nabozny MJ, Kruser JM, Steffens NM, Pecanac KE, Brasel KJ, Chittenden EH, Cooper Z, McKneally MF, Schwarze ML. Patient-reported limitations to surgical buy-in: a qualitative study of patients facing high-risk surgery. Ann Surg. 2017;265:97–102.
137. Taylor LJ, Nabozny MJ, Steffens NM, Tucholka JL, Brasel KJ, Johnson SK, Zelenski A, Rathouz PJ, Zhao Q, Kwekkeboom KL. A framework to improve surgeon communication in high-stakes surgical decisions: best case/worst case. JAMA Surg. 2017;152:531–8.
138. Schwarze ML, Campbell TC, Cunningham TV, White DB, Arnold RM. You can't get what you want: innovation for end-of-life communication in the intensive care unit. Am J Respir Crit Care Med. 2016;193:14–6.
139. Quill TE, Holloway R. Time-limited trials near the end of life. JAMA. 2011;306:1483–4.
140. Cooper Z, Koritsanszky LA, Cauley CE, Frydman JL, Bernacki RE, Mosenthal AC, Gawande AA, Block SD. Recommendations for best communication practices to facilitate goal-concordant care for seriously ill older patients with emergency surgical conditions. Ann Surg. 2016;263:1–6.
141. Case SM, Fried TR, O'Leary J. How to ask: older adults' preferred tools in health outcome prioritization. Patient Educ Couns. 2013;91:29–36.
142. van Summeren JJGT, Haaijer-Ruskamp FM, Schuling J. Eliciting preferences of multimorbid elderly adults in family practice using an outcome prioritization tool. J Am Geriatr Soc. 2016;64:e143–8.
143. Taylor LJ, Rathouz PJ, Berlin A, Brasel KJ, Mosenthal AC, Finlayson E, Cooper Z, Steffens NM, Jacobson N, Buffington A. Navigating high-risk surgery: protocol for a multisite, stepped wedge, cluster-randomised trial of a question prompt list intervention to empower older adults to ask questions that inform treatment decisions. BMJ Open. 2017;7:e014002.
144. Ismail H, Cormie P, Burbury K, Waterland J, Denehy L, Riedel B. Prehabilitation prior to major cancer surgery: training for surgery to optimize physiologic reserve to reduce postoperative complications. Curr Anesthesiol Rep. 2018;8:1–11.
145. Barberan-Garcia A, Ubré M, Roca J, Lacy AM, Burgos F, Risco R, Momblán D, Balust J, Blanco I, Martínez-Pallí G. Personalised prehabilitation in high-risk patients undergoing elective major abdominal surgery: a randomized blinded controlled trial. Ann Surg. 2018;267:50–6.

146. Luther A, Gabriel J, Watson RP, Francis NK. The impact of total body prehabilitation on post-operative outcomes after major abdominal surgery: a systematic review. World J Surg. 2018;42:1–11.
147. Gillis C, Buhler K, Bresee L, Carli F, Gramlich L, Culos-Reed N, Sajobi TT, Fenton TR. Effects of nutritional prehabilitation, with and without exercise, on outcomes of patients who undergo colorectal surgery: a systematic review and meta-analysis. Gastroenterology. 2018;155:391–410.
148. Stephensen D, Hashem F, Corbett K, Bates A, George M, Hobbs RP, Hopkins M, Hutchins I, Lowery DP, Pellatt-Higgins T. Effects of preoperative and postoperative resistance exercise interventions on recovery of physical function in patients undergoing abdominal surgery for cancer: a systematic review of randomised controlled trials. BMJ Open Sport Exerc Med. 2018;4:e000331.
149. Vermillion SA, James A, Dorrell RD, Brubaker P, Mihalko SL, Hill AR, Clark CJ. Preoperative exercise therapy for gastrointestinal cancer patients: a systematic review. Syst Rev. 2018;7:103.
150. Huisman MG, Veronese G, Audisio RA, Ugolini G, Montroni I, de Bock GH, van Leeuwen BL, Vigano A, Gilbert L, Spiliotis J. Poor nutritional status is associated with other geriatric domain impairments and adverse postoperative outcomes in onco-geriatric surgical patients–a multicentre cohort study. Eur J Surg Oncol. 2016;42:1009–17.
151. Rubenstein LZ, Harker JO, Salvà A, Guigoz Y, Vellas B. Screening for undernutrition in geriatric practice: developing the short-form mini-nutritional assessment (MNA-SF). J Gerontol A Biol Sci Med Sci. 2001;56:M366–72.
152. Vigano A, Kasvis P, Di Tomasso J, Gillis C, Kilgour R, Carli F. Pearls of optimizing nutrition and physical performance of older adults undergoing cancer therapy. J Geriatr Oncol. 2017;8:428–36.
153. Moore JE, Mascarenhas A, Marquez C, Almaawiy U, Chan W-H, D'Souza J, Liu B, Straus SE. Mapping barriers and intervention activities to behaviour change theory for Mobilization of Vulnerable Elders in Ontario (MOVE ON), a multi-site implementation intervention in acute care hospitals. Implement Sci. 2014;9:160.
154. Van Grootven B, Flamaing J, Dierckx de Casterlé B, Dubois C, Fagard K, Herregods M-C, Hornikx M, Laenen A, Meuris B, Rex S. Effectiveness of in-hospital geriatric co-management: a systematic review and meta-analysis. Age Ageing. 2017;46:903–10.
155. Walke LM, Rosenthal RA, Trentalange M, Perkal MF, Maiaroto M, Jeffery SM, Marottoli RA. Restructuring care for older adults undergoing surgery: preliminary data from the Co-Management of Older Operative Patients En Route Across Treatment Environments (CO-OPERATE) model of care. J Am Geriatr Soc. 2014;62:2185–90.
156. Shipway D, Koizia L, Winterkorn N, Fertleman M, Ziprin P, Moorthy K. Embedded geriatric surgical liaison is associated with reduced inpatient length of stay in older patients admitted for gastrointestinal surgery. Futur Hosp J. 2018;5:108–16.
157. Creditor MC. Hazards of hospitalization of the elderly. Ann Intern Med. 1993;118:219–23.
158. Biganzoli L, Wildiers H, Oakman C, Marotti L, Loibl S, Kunkler I, Reed M, Ciatto S, Voogd AC, Brain E. Management of elderly patients with breast cancer: updated recommendations of the International Society of Geriatric Oncology (SIOG) and European Society of Breast Cancer Specialists (EUSOMA). Lancet Oncol. 2012;13:e148–60.
159. Papamichael D, Audisio RA, Glimelius B, De Gramont A, Glynne-Jones R, Haller D, Köhne C-H, Rostoft S, Lemmens V, Mitry E. Treatment of colorectal cancer in older patients: International Society of Geriatric Oncology (SIOG) consensus recommendations 2013. Ann Oncol. 2014;26:463–76.

Hepatocellular Carcinoma

14

Blayne Amir Sayed, Shiva Jayaraman, Calvin H. L. Law, Alice C. Wei, Paul D. Greig, and Gonzalo Sapisochin

Introduction

Hepatocellular carcinoma (HCC) is the sixth most common cancer in the world and the third leading cause of cancer death [1]. Worldwide in 2018, there were over 840,000 new cases diagnosed and over 780,000 deaths attributable to primary liver cancer [2]. Over 80% of HCC occurs in Asia and sub-Saharan secondary to hepatitis B virus (HBV) and aflatoxin B1 exposure [1].

Annually in the United States, more than 42,000 new cases are diagnosed and 31,000 deaths attributed to primary liver cancer [3]. In Canada in 2017, there were an estimated 2500 new cases and 1200 deaths from HCC [4]. It is the 18th most common cancer in Canada with an expected 5-year survival of 19% (Table 14.1). Overall the incidence of HCC is increasing in North America, partially due to the increase in patients with hepatitis C virus (HCV) and nonalcoholic steatohepatitis (NASH). The incidence of HCV-related liver disease is expected to plateau in the near future, but it appears that despite viral eradication, cirrhotic patients have a life-long risk for HCC, and with the increased incidence of other causes of liver disease, HCC rates may remain static or even continue to increase.

The management of HCC depends on the stage of the tumor and the underlying liver function (Tables 14.2, 14.4, and 14.5). Disease-free survival is significantly

B. A. Sayed · P. D. Greig · G. Sapisochin (✉)
Abdominal Organ Transplant and Hepatopancreatobiliary Surgery, Department of Surgery, University of Toronto, Toronto, ON, Canada
e-mail: blayne.sayed@uhn.ca; paul.greig@uhn.ca; gonzalo.sapisochin@uhn.ca

S. Jayaraman · C. H. L. Law
Department of Surgery, University of Toronto, Toronto, ON, Canada
e-mail: jayars@stjoe.on.ca; Calvin.Law@sunnybrook.ca

A. C. Wei
Department of Surgery, Memorial Sloan Kettering Cancer Center, New York, NY, USA
e-mail: weia@mskcc.org

F. C. Wright et al. (eds.), *Surgical Oncology Manual*,
https://doi.org/10.1007/978-3-030-48363-0_14

Table 14.1 Prognosis

Presentation	Prognosis [5] 5-Year overall survival (OS)
Solitary tumor, no vascular involvement (resection)	60–70%
Multiple tumors, none > 5 cm	35–40%
Lymph node or major vascular involvement	15%
Distant metastatic disease	0%

less than the overall survival because of the high incidence of recurrence or "de novo" tumors due to the underlying cirrhotic tissue, which is the main risk factor for developing HCC. Even for resectable solitary tumors with no vascular invasion, the 5-year recurrence rate is around 70%.

Special Notes

- Staging of HCC is complex: both the extent of the tumor and the underlying liver function have to be considered. The most commonly used clinical staging system worldwide is the BCLC (Table 14.3).
- The most commonly used pathological staging system is the AJCC.
- For transplantation, the Milan criteria are the most commonly used transplant criteria. Patients within criteria are allocated exception points for priority on the waiting list. Other staging systems are center-specific, but not widely used. The criteria used in Ontario appear in section "Liver Transplantation."

Special Notes

- HCC diagnosis is based on dynamic imaging techniques showing contrast enhancement on the arterial phase and "washout" in the venous phase.
- *Considerations for Surgical Resection*:
  – Cirrhotic patient must be Child's A (well-preserved liver function).
  – To reduce the risk of postoperative liver failure, the target volume of the future liver remnant (FLR) should be >25–30% in non-cirrhotic livers and >40% in cirrhotic livers.
  – For marginal or small FLRs, portal vein embolization (PVE) or transarterial radioembolization can be considered to induce preoperative hypertrophy and increase FLR volume.
  – The radiological response to embolization may be a proxy of the hepatic regenerative capacity.
  – Some centers routinely utilize lobar transarterial radioembolization (Y90) instead of PVE, which is theorized to provide an (a) equivalent lobectomy effect as surgical resection and/or (b) preoperative PVE for appropriate patients with bilobar disease. This is not established by randomized data.

Table 14.2 Management of solitary HCC

Workup	Treatment	Follow-up
If < 1 cm:	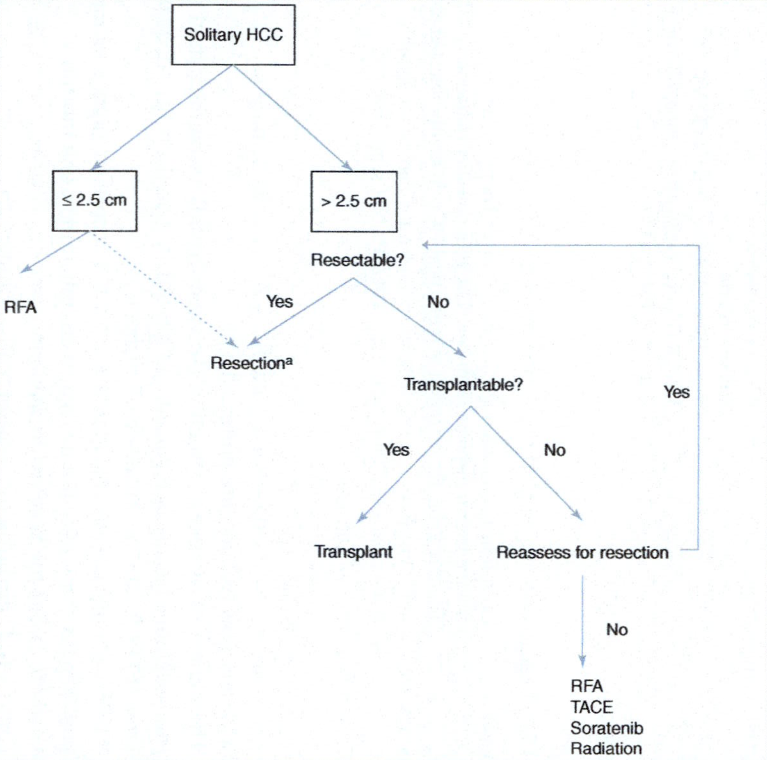	Every 3–6 months for the first 5 years: AFP CT chest/abdomen
Difficult to fully characterize lesions <1 cm		Treat recurrences accordingly
Recommend 3-month follow-up		After 5 years, return to routine surveillance for HCC in high-risk patients (q6 monthly US + AFP)
If > 1 cm:		
Labs: AFP Hepatitis panel Bilirubin, transaminases, ALP, PT or INR, TB		
Imaging: CT chest, abdomen, pelvis Liver MRI or triphasic CT		
Biopsy in case of indeterminate lesion both at CT and MRI		

AFP α-feto protein, *RFA* radiofrequency ablation, *MWA* microwave ablation, *TACE* transarterial chemoembolization, *US* ultrasound
[a]Consider liver resection depending on liver function and tumor location

Table 14.3 Staging systems [6]

Clinical (preoperative)	*Barcelona Clinic for Liver Cancer (BCLC)* Okuda International HPB Association (IHPBA) Cancer of the Liver Italian Program Score (CLIP) American Study of Liver Tumor Group Chinese University Prognostic Index (CUPI)
Pathological staging system (postoperative)	*American Joint Committee on Cancer (AJCC), 7th Ed* Japanese Integrated Score (JIP) Tokyo Score
Transplant staging system	*Milan Criteria*[a] UCSF Criteria[a] Total Tumor Volume Criteria (TTV)[a] UNOS (United Network of Organ Sharing) TNM Extended Toronto Criteria

[a]For priority on the waitlist

Table 14.4 Management of multifocal HCC/advanced stage

Multifocal	Liver transplant evaluation (see Sect. "Liver Transplantation") If not a liver transplant candidate, TACE or consider radiation There is a role for resection in multifocal HCC in highly selected patients
Advanced stage	In Child's B, C cirrhotic patients, radiotherapy may be an option If not candidates for radiotherapy, consider best supportive care

TACE transarterial chemoembolization

  - There are no well-established guidelines for resection margins. In general, wide margins (>2 cm) are preferred. [7]
  - The choice of anatomic resection (segment-based) vs parenchymal sparing (non-segment-based) is nuanced and should be based on (a) adequate margins, (b) FLR, and (c) presence of cirrhosis.
  - ALPSS should not be considered for HCC because of higher incidence of post-hepatectomy liver failure, major complications, and mortality.
- *Contraindications for Surgical Resection*:
  - Child's B, C cirrhosis (non-preserved liver function)
  - Portal hypertension: portosystemic varices, splenomegaly, thrombocytopenia (platelet count <100/mm [8])
  - Major vascular invasion: main portal venous branches or hepatic veins
  - Extrahepatic disease
- *For large (>5 cm) or multi-focal tumors*:
  - Size and number are not contraindications to surgery.
  - If not a resection candidate, consider transplant evaluation (Tables 14.4 and 14.5). If the tumor(s) exceed guidelines for transplantation, consider attempt at downstaging with other treatment options such as ablation, TACE, Y90, sorafenib, or radiotherapy.

Table 14.5 Liver transplantation

Criteria	Management
Ontario criteria	Minimum for listing: Absence of vascular invasion and extrahepatic spread *and* (a) One HCC nodule greater than or equal to 2 cm *or* (b) Multiple nodules greater than or equal to 1 cm *or* (c) Multiple biopsy proven nodules of any size *or* (d) Any size recurrent/persistent HCC nodule(s) after therapy with the intent to cure The following tumors are eligible for MELD Exception points: Milan criteria *or* UCSF criteria *or* TTV <145 cm^3 and AFP <1000 If otherwise a suitable transplant candidate, list for liver transplant and start locoregional therapy (TACE or ablation (RFA or MWA) or radiation), "bridging therapy" while waiting Tumors that exceed these criteria may become eligible if successfully "downstaged" and stable for a minimum of 3 months
Toronto extended criteria	For tumors beyond the Ontario criteria: If the tumor is well or moderately differentiated and aFP < 1000 and otherwise a suitable transplant candidate, the patient may be eligible for live donor liver transplant
	For all tumor patients, consider live donor liver transplant if a suitable live donor available

TACE transarterial chemoembolization, *TTV* total tumor volume, *RFA* radiofrequency ablation, *MWA* microwave ablation

- "Salvage" transplantation (i.e., transplantation following previous ablation or resection for HCC) is effective: outcomes following transplantation are comparable for patients successfully downstaged into transplant criteria vs those within criteria initially.

Special Notes

- Milan criteria: one tumor up to 5 cm or three tumors up to 3 cm, with no major vascular invasion, no metastases
- UCSF criteria: one tumor up to 6.5 cm or three tumors up to 4.5 cm with total tumor diameter <8 cm with no major vascular invasion, no metastases
- *Toronto Extended Criteria*: no size or number restrictions. Well- or moderately differentiated tumors on biopsy, no constitutional symptoms, no major vascular invasion, no metastases. AFP ≤1000 [9]

Landmark Publications

Radiofrequency Ablation (Table 14.6)

- Utilized for destination therapy vs resection for solitary lesions ≤2.5 cm
- Also used for locoregional control to bridge to transplantation

Table 14.6 RFA

HCC	Study	Methods	Results
≤2 cm	Multicenter Livraghi et al. [7]	Prospective, RFA <2 cm	Local recurrence: 0.9% 5-year survival 68.5% (resection candidates)
≤3 cm	Meta-analysis Mulier et al. [10]	Meta-analysis	Local recurrence 14%
3–5 cm	Meta-analysis Mulier et al. [10]	Meta-analysis	Local recurrence 25%
≤5 cm	RCT Chen et al. [11]	RFA vs. resection for <5 cm	No difference in overall survival or recurrence between RFA and resection
Early	Meta-analysis, Zhou et al. [12]	Meta-analysis of RFA vs. liver resection	Liver resection was superior to RFA, specially in HCC >3 cm
Early	Meta-analysis, Wang et al. [13]	Meta-analysis of RCT and non-RCT of RFA vs. liver resection	Similar overall survival but higher recurrence rate with RFA

HCC hepatocellular carcinoma, *RCT* randomized controlled trial, *RFA* radiofrequency ablation

Transarterial Chemoembolization (TACE) (Table 14.7)

- Doxorubicin mixed with lipiodol (targeting agent) administered via subsegmental hepatic artery followed by embolization
- Doxorubicin delivered by drug-eluting microspheres may have lower toxicity and higher efficacy and be suitable for Child's A and B patients.

Transarterial Radioembolization (Y90) (Table 14.8)

- Yttrium-90 (Y90) glass microspheres administered at 120-Gy dose via segmental
- or subsegmental hepatic artery
- The efficacy of Y90 and the correct comparative therapy are still in question:
- There is no phase III RCT evidence supporting Y90 vs sorafenib
- There is phase II RCT data supporting Y90 vs TACE

Surgical Resection (Table 14.9)

- Even for resectable solitary tumors with no vascular invasion, the 5-year recurrence rate is around 70%.
- Cirrhotic patients must have well-preserved liver function, no portal hypertension, and a sufficient FLR.

Table 14.7 TACE

Clinical scenario	Study	Methods	Results
Unresectable HCC	Llovet et al. [14]	RCT TACE vs. symptomatic treatment	TACE improved OS compared with symptomatic treatment TACE: OS: 1 year = 82% and 2 year = 63% Control: OS: 1 year = 63% and 2 year = 27%
	Hong Kong Lo et al. [15] [10]	RCT TACE vs. symptomatic treatment	TACE improved OS TACE: 1-year OS = 57%, 2-year OS = 31%, and 3-year OS = 26% Control: 1-year OS = 32%, 2-year OS = 11%, and 3-year OS = 3%

HCC hepatocellular carcinoma, *RCT* randomized controlled trial, *RFA* radiofrequency ablation, *OS* overall survival

Table 14.8 Y90

Clinical scenario	Study	Methods	Results
Unresectable HCC, Child's A	*SIRveNIB* Chow et al. [16]	RCT, phase III Y90 ($N = 182$) vs. sorafenib ($N = 178$)	Primary endpoint OS No benefit associated with Y90 MOS less with Y90 vs sorafenib: 8.8 vs 10.0 months
Unresectable HCC, Child's A or B	*SARAH* Vilgrain et al. [17]	RC, phase III Y90 ($N = 237$) vs. sorafenib ($N = 222$)	Primary endpoint OS No benefit associated with Y90 MOS less with Y90 vs sorafenib: 8.0 vs 19.9 months
All stage HCC, Child's A or B	Salem et al. [18]	RCT, phase II Y90 ($N = 24$) vs. TACE ($N = 21$)	Y90 improved median TTP vs TACE: >26 vs 6.8 months

OS overall survival, *RCT* randomized controlled trial, *TACE* transarterial chemoembolization, *TTP* time to progression, *Y90* transarterial radioembolization

Table 14.9 Resection

HCC	Study	Methods	Results
>10 cm	Liau et al. [19]	Prospective cohort	Long-term survival similar after resection for select patients with HCC >10 cm vs. <10 cm
Multifocal HCC	Kim et al. [20]	Retrospective study	High recurrence rate but long-term survival if aggressive treatment of recurrence
Small HCC	Roayaie et al. [21]	Retrospective study	5-year overall survival 70%, 5-year recurrence rate 68%
Margins 2 cm vs. 1 cm	Shi et al. [22]	RCT	Long-term survival better with wide (2 cm) margin than narrow (<1 cm) margin (e.g., 5-year survival 74.9% vs. 70.9%)

HCC hepatocellular carcinoma, *RCT* randomized controlled trial

Table 14.10 Transplantation

Study	Methods	Results
Milan criteria Mazzaferro et al. [23]	Retrospective $N = 48$ patients	4-year survival of 75%
UCSF criteria Yao et al. [24]	Retrospective $N = 70$ patients	1-year survival (OS) of 90% 5-year survival of 75%
Toronto criteria Sapisochin et al. [9]	Retrospective $N = 605$ patients Two cohorts	Cohort 1: M vs M+: 5-year survival 72% vs 70% Cohort 2: M vs M+: 5-year survival 78% vs 68% Combined: M vs M+: 5-year survival 76% vs 68%; 10-year survival 60% vs 50%

OS overall survival, *DFS* disease-free survival, *M* within Milan criteria, *M+* outside Milan criteria, *UCSF* University of California, San Francisco

Transplantation (Table 14.10)

- For multifocal tumors in setting of cirrhosis, transplant offers only curative therapy.
- 5- and 10-year survival may exceed 75% and 60%, respectively, depending on indication and biology.

Systemic Therapy (Table 14.11)

- Sorafenib is the standard for unresectable HCC in patients with preserved liver function.
- Levatinib has recently demonstrated to be non-inferior to sorafenib, and several studies have provided evidence for new second-line treatments.
- Although the use of checkpoint inhibitors is highly anticipated, there is no RCT evidence demonstrating utility of these agents.

Table 14.11 Systemic therapy

Study	Methods	Results
SHARP trial [25]	RCT, phase III Primary treatment for advanced HCC in Child's A cirrhotics *N* = 299 sorafenib, 303 placebo	Primary endpoint OS Sorafenib vs placebo extends MOS by 2.8 months (10.7 vs 7.9)
Kudo et al. [26]	RCT, phase III Primary treatment for advanced HCC in Child's A cirrhotics *N* = 478 levatinib, 476 sorafenib	Primary endpoint OS Levatinib vs sorafenib extends MOS by 1.3 months (13.6 vs 12.3 months)
RESORCE trial [27]	RCT, phase III Second-line treatment, progression on sorafenib for advanced HCC in Child's A cirrhotics *N* = 379 regorafenib, 194 placebo	Primary endpoint OS Regorafenib vs placebo extends MOS by 2.8 months (10.6 vs 7.8)
CELESTIAL trial [28]	RCT, phase III Second-line treatment, progression on sorafenib for advanced HCC in Child's A cirrhotics *N* = 467 cabozantinib, 237 placebo	Primary endpoint OS Cabozantinib vs placebo extends MOS by 2.2 months (10.2 vs 8.0)
REACH-2 trial [29]	RCT, phase III Second-line treatment, progression on sorafenib for advanced HCC in Child's A cirrhotics, AFP > 400 *N* = 197 ramucirumab, 95 placebo	Primary endpoint OS Ramucirumab vs placebo extends MOS by 1.2 months (8.5 vs 7.3)

MOS median overall survival, *OS* overall survival, *RCT* randomized controlled trial

Guidelines and Consensus Documents

1. American Association for the Study of Liver Diseases (AASLD) Guidelines [30]
2. European Association for the Study of Liver Guidelines [31]
3. Consensus conference on liver transplantation for HCC [32]

Referral to Medical Oncology/HCC-Focused Hepatology

1. Patients who are candidates for TACE (Child's A, B, no contraindications for angiography)
2. Patients who are candidates for sorafenib, levatinib, or other systemic therapies (Child's A, advanced HCC)

Referral to Radiation Oncology

HCC not amenable to TACE or other ablation.

Referral to Multidisciplinary Cancer Conference

All HCC patients are discussed at the Multidisciplinary Cancer Conference (MCC) due to the multidisciplinary nature of their management.

University of Toronto Pearls

- When considering resection, if there is any doubt about FLR, perform portal vein embolization (PVE). We do not routinely use Y90.
- *Definitive* treatment of solitary lesions <2.5 cm: liver resection if appropriate, ablation if not a surgical candidate or thought to be a better approach.
- For single lesions, ablation is preferable to TACE if it meets the size criteria.
- Consider resection in patients with single HCC who are not transplant candidates.
- Patients with very large (>10 cm) tumors may be amenable for liver resection.
- For patients with multifocal disease outside of Ontario/Milan criteria: Regardless of tumor size and volume, utilize Extended Toronto Criteria to consider if liver transplantation is appropiate.

References

1. Forner A, Reig M, Bruix J. Hepatocellular carcinomas. Lancet. 2018;391:1301–14.
2. Globocan. Liver cancer worldwide: Globocan 2018 Report. 2018;876:2018–2019.
3. Cancer facts and figures. 2019. Available at: www.cancer.org.
4. Canadian Cancer Statistics. Canadian Cancer Society's Steering Committee on Cancer Statistics. 2018.
5. Vauthey JN, et al. Simplified staging for hepatocellular carcinoma. J Clin Oncol. 2002;20:1527–36.
6. Burkhart RA, Pawlik TM. Staging and prognostic models for hepatocellular carcinoma and intrahepatic cholangiocarcinoma. Cancer Control. 2017;24:1–11.

7. Livraghi T, et al. Sustained complete response and complications rates after radiofrequency ablation of very early hepatocellular carcinoma in cirrhosis: is resection still the treatment of choice? Hepatology. 2008;47:82–9.
8. Maithel SK, et al. Importance of low preoperative platelet count in selecting patients for resection of hepatocellular carcinoma: a multi-institutional analysis. J Am Coll Surg. 2011;212:638–48.
9. Sapisochin G, et al. The extended Toronto criteria for liver transplantation in patients with hepatocellular carcinoma: a prospective validation study. Hepatology. 2016;64:2077–88.
10. Mulier S, et al. Local recurrence after hepatic radiofrequency coagulation. Ann Surg. 2005;242:158–71.
11. Chen M-S, et al. A prospective randomized trial comparing percutaneous local ablative therapy and partial hepatectomy for small hepatocellular carcinoma. Ann Surg. 2006;243:321–8.
12. Zhou Y, et al. Meta-analysis of radiofrequency ablation versus hepatic resection for small hepatocellular carcinoma. BMC Gastroenterol. 2010;10:78.
13. Wang Y, et al. Radiofrequency ablation versus hepatic resection for small hepatocellular carcinomas: a meta-analysis of randomized and nonrandomized controlled trials. PLoS One. 2014;9:e84484.
14. Llovet JM, et al. Arterial embolisation or chemoembolisation versus symptomatic treatment in patients with unresectable hepatocellular carcinoma: a randomised controlled trial. Lancet. 2002;359:1734–9.
15. Lo CM, et al. Randomized controlled trial of transarterial Lipiodol chemoembolization for unresectable hepatocellular carcinoma. Hepatology. 2002;35:1164–71.
16. Yoong BK, et al. SIRveNIB: selective internal radiation therapy versus Sorafenib in Asia-Pacific patients with hepatocellular carcinoma. J Clin Oncol. 2018;36:1913–21.
17. Vilgrain V, et al. Efficacy and safety of selective internal radiotherapy with yttrium-90 resin microspheres compared with sorafenib in locally advanced and inoperable hepatocellular carcinoma (SARAH): an open-label randomised controlled phase 3 trial. Lancet Oncol. 2017;18:1624–36.
18. Salem R, et al. Y90 radioembolization significantly prolongs time to progression compared with chemoembolization in patients with hepatocellular carcinoma. Gastroenterology. 2016;151:1155–1163.e2.
19. Liau K-H, et al. Outcome of partial hepatectomy for large (> 10 cm) hepatocellular carcinoma. Cancer. 2005;104:1948–55.
20. Kim PTW, et al. Outcomes after hepatic resection and subsequent multimodal treatment of recurrence for multifocal hepatocellular carcinoma. Br J Surg. 2013;100:1516–22.
21. Roayaie S, et al. Resection of hepatocellular cancer ≤2 cm: results from two Western centers. Hepatology. 2013;57:1426–35.
22. Shi M, et al. Partial hepatectomy with wide versus narrow resection margin for solitary hepatocellular carcinoma: a prospective randomized trial. Ann Surg. 2007;245:36–43.
23. Mazzaferro V, et al. Liver transplantation for the treatment of small hepatocellular carcinomas in patients with cirrhosis. N Engl J Med. 1996;334:693–9.
24. Yao FY, et al. Liver transplantation for hepatocellular carcinoma: expansion of the tumor size limits does not adversely impact survival. Hepatology. 2001;33:1394–403.
25. Llovet JM, et al. Sorafenib in advanced hepatocellular carcinoma. N Engl J Med. 2008;359:378–90.
26. Kudo M, et al. Lenvatinib versus sorafenib in first-line treatment of patients with unresectable hepatocellular carcinoma: a randomised phase 3 non-inferiority trial. Lancet. 2018;391:1163–73.
27. Bruix J, et al. Regorafenib for patients with hepatocellular carcinoma who progressed on sorafenib treatment (RESORCE): a randomised, double-blind, placebo-controlled, phase 3 trial. Lancet. 2017;389:56–66.
28. Cicin I, et al. Cabozantinib in patients with advanced and progressing hepatocellular carcinoma. N Engl J Med. 2018;379:54–63.

29. Zhu AX, et al. Ramucirumab after sorafenib in patients with advanced hepatocellular carcinoma and increased α-fetoprotein concentrations (REACH-2): a randomised, double-blind, placebo-controlled, phase 3 trial. Lancet Oncol. 2019;20:282–96.
30. Bruix J, Sherman M, American Association for the Study of Liver Diseases. Management of hepatocellular carcinoma: an update. Hepatology. 2011;53:1020–2.
31. Galle PR, et al. EASL clinical practice guidelines: management of hepatocellular carcinoma. J Hepatol. 2018;69:182–236.
32. Clavien P-A, et al. Recommendations for liver transplantation for hepatocellular scarcinoma: an international consensus conference report. Lancet Oncol. 2012;13:e11–22.

Malignancy of Unknown Primary 15

Jessica Bogach, Christine Elser, and Savtaj S. Brar

Introduction

A malignancy or cancer of unknown primary (CUP) is a histologically proven metastatic malignancy where a site of origin cannot be identified, despite comprehensive workup. Generally, cancer of unknown primary is divided into five main categories [1]:

- Adenocarcinoma
- Squamous cell carcinoma
- Carcinoma not otherwise specified (NOS) or poorly differentiated carcinoma
- Neuroendocrine tumor
- Poorly differentiated malignant neoplasm (may include melanoma, sarcoma, lymphoma, germ cell tumor, thyroid cancer)

J. Bogach
General Surgical Oncology, University of Toronto, Toronto, ON, Canada
e-mail: Jessica.Bogach@one-mail.on.ca

C. Elser
Department of Medical Oncology, Princess Margaret Cancer Centre, Toronto, ON, Canada

Deparment of Medical Oncology, University of Toronto, Toronto, ON, Canada
e-mail: christine.elser@uhn.ca

S. S. Brar (✉)
Department of Surgery, University of Toronto, Toronto, ON, Canada
e-mail: savtaj.brar@sinaihealth.ca

F. C. Wright et al. (eds.), *Surgical Oncology Manual*,
https://doi.org/10.1007/978-3-030-48363-0_15

Table 15.1 Histology-based survival outcomes [3]

Histology	Proportion of CUPs (%)	Median survival (months)	12-month survival (%)
Adenocarcinoma	60	2	15
Squamous cell carcinoma	5	15	53
Carcinoma NOS/poorly differentiated carcinoma	29	2	15
Neuroendocrine	1	11	48

Epidemiology

Cancer of unknown primary makes up 3–5% of all malignancies; however, the incidence is decreasing [2, 3]. In 20–50% of patients, the primary tumor is never identified, even after the completion of postmortem evaluation [4]. When a primary is identified, the most common sites are lung (27%) and pancreas (24%), followed by other hepatobiliary sites (8%) and kidney (8%) [5].

Unknown primaries are slightly more common in females (52% of CUPs); however, squamous cell carcinomas with unknown primary sites are more commonly diagnosed in men (67% are male) [3]. In general, prognosis is poor, with median survival of 3–9 months [6]. Histologic diagnosis will impact the survival, with longer survival seen in neuroendocrine tumors and squamous cell carcinomas, while shorter survival is seen in adenocarcinoma and carcinoma not otherwise specified (NOS) (Table 15.1).

Diagnostic Workup

Although the majority of patients have poor outcomes, the goal of investigations is to try and identify the primary tumor site, to identify favorable subgroups that may benefit from directed therapy, and avoid unnecessary investigations or delays [7]. At any point in the workup, if the site of the primary is identified, the treatment algorithm (Table 15.2) should be redirected to that tumor type.

Pathologic Assessment

When obtaining tissue for diagnosis, core biopsies are preferred over fine-needle aspirated (FNA) biopsies to allow pathologic assessment [1]. The exception is in head and neck nodes where FNA is acceptable [8]. It is critical to give the pathologist the full clinical picture and inform them of investigations to date to guide testing including immunohistochemistry (IHC). IHC can predict a primary site in 35–40% [1].

Initial stains that help determine the cell line of origin are listed here [9, 10]:

Epithelial: PanKeratin, CAM5.2, AE1, AE3
Squamous cell carcinoma: CK5/6, p63/p40

Table 15.2 Basic workup, special test, and invasive procedures required to assess the site of primary tumor

Basic workup[a]	Special tests	Invasive procedures
Indicated in all patients with CUP	Should be guided by pathology and clinical presentation	Not recommended for initial workup Should be guided by pathology and clinical presentation
Complete history and physical exam: include complete skin exam including the perineum, scalp, head and neck, breast and pelvic exam Review any prior biopsies, prior regressing lesions CBC, chemistry CT chest, abdomen, and Pelvis Urine cytology, urinalysis Mammogram (female) *Core biopsy with pathology review and appropriate immunohistochemistry (IHC)*	Breast MRI and ultrasound – in a female with isolated axillary nodes and negative mammogram PET CT – SCC metastases in the neck, can also be considered in a single metastasis to rule out other occult disease [7] Bone scan if bone metastases Gynecology oncology consult if female with pelvic disease Serum tumor markers[b]	Gastroscopy and colonoscopy if liver metastases, or symptoms CT enteroclysis or capsule endoscopy if small bowel primary is suspected Cystoscopy: for retroperitoneal nodes and suspicious urine cytology Triple endoscopy for isolated neck nodes (laryngoscopy, esophagoscopy, nasopharyngoscopy)

[a]Primary only considered "unknown" if basic workup fails to identify primary site
[b]Tumor marker ordering should not be empiric but suggested by clinical picture. Consider AFP, PSA, beta-hCG, chromogranin A, CEA, Ca125, CA 19-9, thyroglobulin

Table 15.3 Common epithelial tumor sites based on staining patterns of CK7 and CK20 [9]

CK7+/CK20+	*CK7-/CK20+*
Upper gastrointestinal adenocarcinoma Pancreatic ductal adenocarcinoma Urothelial	Colorectal Merkel cell
CK7+/CK20-	*CK7-/CK20-*
Breast Ovarian Pulmonary adenocarcinoma Endometrial and endocervical adenocarcinoma Thyroid Salivary gland adenocarcinoma	Prostate Hepatocellular Renal cell Adrenal cortical Squamous cell Carcinoma (including lung)

Melanoma: S100, SOX10
Lymphoma: LCA, CD20, CD3
Germ cell tumor: OCT 3/4, SALL4
Mesothelial: WT1, calretinin, mesothelin, D2-40
Sarcoma: vimentin, actin, desmin S100, c-kit

If an epithelial marker is determined, CK7 and CK20 status help determine the site of origin (Table 15.3). Further stains can help assess for a primary site (Table 15.4).

Table 15.4 Common tumor-specific antibodies [11]

Carcinoma	Antibody	Sensitivity	Specificity	Other cancers
Breast	GATA3 GCDFP-15	+++ +	++ ++	TCC, salivary, skin Salivary, sweat gl.
CRC	CDX2	+++	+++	Gastric, pancreas
Lung-adeno	TTF-1	+++	+++	Thyroid, NE
GYN	PAX8	++++	++	Thyroid, RCC
Serous Ovarian	WT1	++++	+++	Mesothelioma
RCC	PAX8	++	++	GYN, thyroid
TCC, squamous	P63 p40	++++ ++++	++++ ++++	Thymoma, salivary, NE, trophoblastic
Prostate	PSA	++++	++++	
Thyroid	Tg	+++	++++	

Adapted from Kandalaft and Gown [11]
TCC transitional cell carcinoma, *NE* neuroendocrine, *RCC* renal cell carcinoma, *GYN* gynecologic malignancy

Molecular Testing

When the basic workup, targeted investigations, and IHC are still unable to localize the likely site of the primary, molecular profiling may be attempted. Gene expression profiling (GEP) has been used to identify gene expression patterns of tumor subtypes and helps to identify the primary site. There are many commercial tests available. Studies have compared GEP with site-specific therapy to empiric treatment [12, 13]. A randomized prospective study found that identifying the tissue of origin has not led to improved survival; however, it may allow better prognostication for patients by identifying tumor types that are more likely to respond to treatment [13]. Given that they have not shown improved survival, guidelines are not recommending the use of these tests as the standard of care [14]. Next-generation sequencing may be able to identify targetable mutations; however, similar to gene expression profiling, the impact on outcomes has not been defined and it is not routinely recommended [14].

When there is a suspected tissue of origin based on pathology or pattern of disease, molecular tests may be useful in directing treatment. For example, a patient with a likely diagnosis of lung cancer should have EGFR, ALK, and ROS1 mutation testing. Similarly, KRAS and MSI testing should be performed for colorectal cancer. PDL1 testing should be considered for lung, urothelial, and renal cell cancers.

Special Considerations in Workup

Neck Mass

A mass in the neck is a common presentation for a head and neck primary and has a unique workup.

Following CT scans of the head and neck, FDG-PET scan should be obtained in order to identify a primary site. If there is no primary identified, fiberoptic examination of the nasopharynx, oropharynx, hypopharynx, and larynx should be performed as an examination under anesthesia [15]. If histology is squamous cell, Human Papilloma Virus (HPV) and Epstein Barr Virus (EBV) testing should be performed on the biopsy. HPV positivity is often correlated with a tonsil or base of tongue primary [16]. Selective biopsies should be taken depending on the nodal location. Deep tonsillar biopsies or ipsilateral tonsillectomy should be performed at the time of examination under anesthesia as the base of tongue and tonsils will harbor the majority of primary tumors [8, 17, 18].

Adenocarcinoma in the neck should trigger an evaluation for a thyroid primary with thyroglobulin and calcitonin levels. Nodes in levels IV and V should be a signal of a possible infraclavicular primary tumor.

If no primary is identified, treatment is determined by histology and location of the metastatic nodes.

Neuroendocrine Tumors (NET)

Forty to fifty percent of patients with NETs will present with metastatic disease, often in lymph nodes and the liver, and rarely in the bone. In 13% of patients presenting with metastatic disease, the primary tumor location is unknown. The most common site of the primary in these cases will be the small intestine or the lung [19]. Many other tumor types can have neuroendocrine differentiation and should be considered in the differential when pathology suggests neuroendocrine features (Table 15.5). IHC suggestive of a neuroendocrine tumor includes epithelial stains, synaptophysin, chromogranin, and CD56 [1].

Identifying the primary site is important for definitive management, particularly when the metastatic disease is resectable. Radiologic evaluation may include CT chest, abdomen and pelvis, capsule endoscopy, functional imaging (Octreotide Scan or ^{68}Ga-DOTATOC PET-CT) and upper and lower endoscopy [19, 20]. It is important to distinguish the primary site if possible as some systemic treatment decisions are dictated by the site of the primary tumor [19]

Pathologic grade (determined by Ki67 and mitoses) can guide a management plan.

Table 15.5 Tumors that have neuroendocrine differentiation

Indolent	Aggressive
Well-differentiated neuroendocrine tumor	Small-cell and large-cell neuroendocrine lung cancers
Well-differentiated pancreatic NET	High-grade NET
Medullary thyroid cancer	Extra-pulmonary small-cell carcinoma
Paraganglioma	Merkel cell carcinoma
Pheochromocytoma	Neuroblastoma

Table 15.6 Favorable and unfavorable presentations of CUP [1, 21–24]

Favorable presentation	Unfavorable presentation
Adenocarcinoma in a female with axillary lymph node disease	Adenocarcinoma
Female with peritoneal papillary adenocarcinoma	More than two metastatic sites
Squamous cell carcinoma nodes in the neck or inguinal region	Liver metastases
Poorly differentiated carcinoma in a young male with mediastinal or retroperitoneal (midline) disease (features of germ cell tumors)	Poor performance status (ECOG > 2)
Colorectal cancer IHC profile (CDX2+, CK20+, CK7−)	Elevated LDH
Neuroendocrine features	Low albumin
Isolated resectable metastasis	Non-papillary peritoneal adenocarcinoma
Men with skeletal-only metastases	

Management of CUP

Commonly, patients with CUP are classified as having a favorable or unfavorable presentation (Table 15.6). Patients with favorable presentations make up to 15–20% of patients with CUP and they tend to present with good performance status and clinical features that suggest a specific tumor subtype that has appropriate treatment. Treatment in these patients can often offer reasonable oncologic outcomes. The remaining 80–85% of patients present with unfavorable features and tend to have poor prognosis [21].

Approach to Patients with Favorable Subtypes

Recognition of favorable subtypes is essential as many patients in this category can be approached with curative intent. The following is a list of favorable presentations and how they are approached:

Isolated or single site of metastasis

- Consideration should be given to surgical resection if technically possible. Definitive radiation can be considered if applicable.
- Consideration can be given to PET scan to consider other occult disease prior to surgical resection.
- If it is a retroperitoneal mass, evaluate whether histology is consistent with germ cell tumor [14].
  - If it is a non-germ cell histology, surgical excision can be considered.

Female with papillary adenocarcinoma in the peritoneal cavity

- Should be treated like a stage III ovarian cancer. Cytoreduction followed by platinum-based systemic chemotherapy can achieve complete response and prolonged disease-free intervals in some patients [23]
- If serous histology, BRCA testing should be performed.

Axillary mass in a female

- With negative mammogram, MRI, and ultrasound and pathology suggestive of a breast primary, it can be approached as stage II or III breast cancer [14]. The absence of a radiologically evident primary in the breast does not rule out the breast as the primary site.
  - Prognosis is similar to stage II/III breast cancer.
- Hormone receptor (ER, PR) and HER2 status should be evaluated.
- The breast can be treated with mastectomy or whole breast irradiation.
- Management of the axilla should follow principles of management for breast cancer presenting with clinical node involvement.
- In a male presenting with axillary adenocarcinoma, axillary dissection is recommended.

Young males (<40) with mediastinal or retroperitoneal poorly differentiated carcinoma

- Can be approached as germ cell tumors.
- Serum AFP, beta-hCG, and testicular ultrasound should be ordered [21].
- Treatment often consists of systemic therapy (etoposide, cisplatin ± bleomycin) [25].

Inguinal adenopathy [14]

- If squamous cell carcinoma:
  - Investigations should be directed at a pelvic or anal primary
  - Nodal dissection followed by radiation can be performed for patients with no primary identified
- If adenocarcinoma is isolated to a single lymph node basin:
  - Can be treated with therapeutic nodal dissection ± adjuvant radiation

Isolated liver metastases

- If no primary is identified, and patient is fit, resection should be considered if technically feasible
  - Pathology should be assessed for possible intra-hepatic cholangiocarcinoma

Colorectal cancer IHC profile

- Investigated with upper and lower endoscopy [21]
- Managed as a stage IV colon cancer with systemic therapy and consideration of resection in appropriate patients

Male with skeletal metastases

- Serum PSA should be ordered
- Even without evidence of prostate disease, a trial of hormonal therapy and bisphosphonates can be considered [21]

Neck mass

- Squamous cell carcinoma: can be definitively treated with neck dissection, radiation therapy, or chemoradiation. In patients that undergo neck dissection, consideration for adjuvant radiation should be given [15].
- Adenocarcinoma: If no thyroid primary is identified, nodes in levels I-III can be treated with neck dissection with parotidectomy followed by radiation.

Neuroendocrine features

- Both low-grade and high-grade neuroendocrine tumors are considered favorable.
- Low-grade tumors tend to be indolent and may be amenable to surgery or to somatostatin analogues.
- High-grade tumors, often called "small cell" neuroendocrine carcinomas, can show good responses to systemic chemotherapy [1, 26].

Approach to Patients with Unfavorable Prognosis CUP

It is essential to identify favorable presentations such as patients benefit from specific, multidisciplinary treatment approaches. Patients who present with unfavorable prognosis CUP typically receive empiric systemic therapy [1].

When deciding on the optimal systemic therapy regimen, clinical presentation, pathology including IHC, and molecular tests all need to be considered. If a putative primary is suggested, then the patient should be treated accordingly.

Patients with CUP tend to have disease that is not very responsive to chemotherapy. Some of the poor outcomes are thought to be related to chromosomal instability in CUP tumors, which results in atypical behavior and chemoresistance [27]. Despite poor outcomes, in those with adequate performance status, chemotherapy should be considered.

When choosing chemotherapy regimens, drugs that are often selected are those that are included in multiple common regimens, such as taxanes and platinum-based drugs, with hopes of broad efficacy. In phase II studies and small randomized studies, no single superior chemotherapy regimen has been identified, and response rates are generally in the range of 10–65%. A meta-analysis by Golfinopoulos et al. [28] could not identify a single regimen to recommend. This analysis attempted to formally exclude favorable prognosis subtypes when possible; however, the heterogeneity in this population makes it difficult to study. Based on current evidence, recommended regimens should include a platinum, a taxane, or both [14]. Commonly used regimens include carboplatinum/paclitaxel, gemcitabine/cisplatinum, carboplatinum/paclitaxel/etoposide, and cisplatinum/paclitaxel/5-FU (used for SCC) [14].

Landmark Trials

- As CUP patients are heterogeneous and often have advanced disease or poor performance status, prospective studies are challenging to perform. Current practice guidelines are based on multiple small trials; no landmark trials exist in this field [14].

Referral to Multidisciplinary Case Conference

- All patients without an identified primary tumor should be reviewed in a multidisciplinary case conference before considering surgical excision.

Referral to Medical Oncology

- All patients with unknown primary tumors should be seen by medical oncologists.

Referral to Radiation Oncology

- Adjuvant therapy after therapeutic lymph node dissection
- Definitive management of some squamous cell carcinomas
- Palliative treatment of symptomatic metastases

References

1. Greco FA, Hainsworth JD. Cancer of unknown primary site. In: DeVita VT, editor. Cancer: principles and practice of oncology. 8th ed. Philadelphia: Lippincott Williams & Wilkins; 2015.
2. Pavlidis N, Pentheroudakis G. Cancer of unknown primary site. Lancet. 2012;379(9824):1428–35.
3. Urban D, Rao A, Bressel M, Lawrence YR, Mileshkin L. Cancer of unknown primary: a population-based analysis of temporal change and socioeconomic disparities. Br J Cancer. 2013;109(5):1318–24.
4. Blaszyk H, Hartmann A, Bjornsson J. Cancer of unknown primary: clinicopathologic correlations. APMIS. 2003;111(12):1089–94.
5. Pentheroudakis G, Golfinopoulos V, Pavlidis N. Switching benchmarks in cancer of unknown primary: from autopsy to microarray. Eur J Cancer. 2007;43(14):2026–36.
6. Pavlidis N, Briasoulis E, Hainsworth J, Greco FA. Diagnostic and therapeutic management of cancer of an unknown primary. Eur J Cancer. 2003;39(14):1990–2005.
7. Fizazi K, Greco FA, Pavlidis N, Daugaard G, Oien K, Pentheroudakis G, et al. Cancers of unknown primary site: ESMO Clinical Practice Guidelines for diagnosis, treatment and follow-up. Ann Oncol. 2015;26(Suppl 5):v133–8.
8. Network NCC. Head and neck cancers. Version 1 2019. NCCN; 2019.
9. Conner JR, Hornick JL. Metastatic carcinoma of unknown primary: diagnostic approach using immunohistochemistry. Adv Anat Pathol. 2015;22(3):149–67.

10. Oien KA, Dennis JL. Diagnostic work-up of carcinoma of unknown primary: from immunohistochemistry to molecular profiling. Ann Oncol. 2012;23(Suppl 10):x271–7.
11. Kandalaft PL, Gown AM. Practical applications in immunohistochemistry: carcinomas of unknown primary site. Arch Pathol Lab Med. 2016;140(6):508–23.
12. Hayashi H, Kurata T, Takiguchi Y, Arai M, Takeda K, Akiyoshi K, et al. Randomized phase II trial comparing site-specific treatment based on gene expression profiling with carboplatin and paclitaxel for patients with cancer of unknown primary site. J Clin Oncol. 2019;37(7):570–9.
13. Hainsworth JD, Rubin MS, Spigel DR, Boccia RV, Raby S, Quinn R, et al. Molecular gene expression profiling to predict the tissue of origin and direct site-specific therapy in patients with carcinoma of unknown primary site: a prospective trial of the Sarah Cannon research institute. J Clin Oncol. 2013;31(2):217–23.
14. Network NCC. NCCN guidelines: occult primary. NCCN; 2019.
15. Network NCC. NCCN practical guidelines in oncology: head and neck cancers. 2018.
16. Begum S, Gillison ML, Nicol TL, Westra WH. Detection of human papillomavirus-16 in fine-needle aspirates to determine tumor origin in patients with metastatic squamous cell carcinoma of the head and neck. Clin Cancer Res. 2007;13(4):1186–91.
17. Lapeyre M, Malissard L, Peiffert D, Hoffstetter S, Toussaint B, Renier S, et al. Cervical lymph node metastasis from an unknown primary: is a tonsillectomy necessary? Int J Radiat Oncol Biol Phys. 1997;39(2):291–6.
18. Mendenhall WM, Mancuso AA, Amdur RJ, Stringer SP, Villaret DB, Cassisi NJ. Squamous cell carcinoma metastatic to the neck from an unknown head and neck primary site. Am J Otolaryngol. 2001;22(4):261–7.
19. Pavel M, O'Toole D, Costa F, Capdevila J, Gross D, Kianmanesh R, et al. ENETS consensus guidelines update for the Management of Distant Metastatic Disease of intestinal, pancreatic, bronchial neuroendocrine neoplasms (NEN) and NEN of unknown primary site. Neuroendocrinology. 2016;103(2):172–85.
20. Menda Y, O'Dorisio TM, Howe JR, Schultz M, Dillon JS, Dick D, et al. Localization of unknown primary site with 68Ga-DOTATOC PET/CT in patients with metastatic neuroendocrine tumor. J Nucl Med. 2017;58(7):1054–7.
21. Collado Martín R, García Palomo A, de la Cruz ML, Borrega García P, Barón Duarte FJ. Clinical guideline SEOM: cancer of unknown primary site. Clin Transl Oncol. 2014;16(12):1091–7.
22. Culine S, Kramar A, Saghatchian M, Bugat R, Lesimple T, Lortholary A, et al. Development and validation of a prognostic model to predict the length of survival in patients with carcinomas of an unknown primary site. J Clin Oncol. 2002;20(24):4679–83.
23. Pavlidis N. Forty years experience of treating cancer of unknown primary. Acta Oncol. 2007;46(5):592–601.
24. Varadhachary GR, Raber MN, Matamoros A, Abbruzzese JL. Carcinoma of unknown primary with a colon-cancer profile-changing paradigm and emerging definitions. Lancet Oncol. 2008;9(6):596–9.
25. Network NCC. Testicular cancer. 2019.
26. Hainsworth JD, Johnson DH, Greco FA. Poorly differentiated neuroendocrine carcinoma of unknown primary site. A newly recognized clinicopathologic entity. Ann Intern Med. 1988;109(5):364–71.
27. Vikeså J, Møller AK, Kaczkowski B, Borup R, Winther O, Henao R, et al. Cancers of unknown primary origin (CUP) are characterized by chromosomal instability (CIN) compared to metastasis of know origin. BMC Cancer. 2015;15:151.
28. Golfinopoulos V, Pentheroudakis G, Salanti G, Nearchou AD, Ioannidis JP, Pavlidis N. Comparative survival with diverse chemotherapy regimens for cancer of unknown primary site: multiple-treatments meta-analysis. Cancer Treat Rev. 2009;35(7):570–3.

Melanoma

16

Andrea M. Covelli, Hyeyoun (Elise) Min,
David R. McCready, Nicole J. Look Hong, Joan E. Lipa,
Teresa M. Petrella, and Frances C. Wright

Hyeyoun (Elise) Min contributed to the technical part of this chapter.

Introduction

Melanoma is the seventh most common diagnosed malignancy across Canada [1]. Melanoma represents less than 5% of all incident skin cancers but accounts for the most attributable deaths from skin cancer. In 2017, of all new cancers diagnosed, 3.9% in males and 3.1% in females were melanoma. Overall there were an estimated 7322 new cases, and 1240 deaths from melanoma in 2017. The incidence rates of melanoma continue to increase by approximately 2% per year for both men and women and the mortality rate by 1% per year for men and 0.3% for women [1].

A. M. Covelli
General Surgical Oncology Fellowship, University of Toronto, Toronto, ON, Canada
e-mail: Andrea.covelli@utoronto.ca

H. (E.) Min
Division of Plastic & Reconstructive Surgery, Sunnybrook University of Toronto, Toronto, ON, Canada

D. R. McCready · N. J. Look Hong · F. C. Wright (✉)
Department of Surgery, University of Toronto, Toronto, ON, Canada
e-mail: David.McCready@uhn.ca; Nicole.LookHong@sunnybrook.ca; frances.wright@sunnybrook.ca

J. E. Lipa
Department of Surgery, Division of Plastics and Reconstructive Surgery, University of Toronto, Toronto, ON, Canada

Department of Medical Oncology and Hematology, University of Toronto, Toronto, ON, Canada
e-mail: Joan.Lipa@sunnybrook.ca

T. M. Petrella
Department of Medical Oncology, University of Toronto, Toronto, ON, Canada
e-mail: Teresa.Petrella@sunnybrook.ca

F. C. Wright et al. (eds.), *Surgical Oncology Manual*,
https://doi.org/10.1007/978-3-030-48363-0_16

Similar trends in increasing incidence have been reported in the United States, United Kingdom, Sweden, and Norway [2]. Melanoma is the fourth most common cancer in adolescents and adults ages 15–49 [1].

Exposure to ultraviolet radiation through exposure to sunlight, tanning beds, and sun lamps are a major risk factor for melanoma. Other risk factors include having a fair complexion, the number and type of moles, personal and family history of skin cancer, a weakened immune system, and a history of severe blistering sunburn [3].

Historically, melanoma has been divided into four main subtypes: superficial spreading melanoma (SSM), lentigo maligna melanoma (LMM), nodular melanoma (NM), and acral lentiginous melanoma (ALM) based on histopathological features of the intra-dermal component of the tumour adjacent to a dermal invasive component [4]. SSM is the most common subtype in European descent accounting for approximately 60% of cutaneous melanoma. They occur in younger patients (median age 5th decade) and arise in areas of intense intermittent sun exposure such as trunk and lower limbs [4–6]. SSM presents as a flat irregularly shaped macule with variation in colour (brown, black, pink, blue) and atypical reticular pattern on dermatoscopy [6, 7]. SSM subtype is the largest contributor to the increasing incidence of melanoma [8].

Lentigo Maligna Melanoma presents similarly to SSM, a large variegated macule with irregular edges. LMM tends to occur later in life (median 8th decade) and in chronically sun-exposed areas (head and neck, forearms). It is estimated to be 5–15% of all diagnosed melanomas but up to 25% of those diagnosed on head and neck [9, 10]. On histology there is evidence of severely sun-damaged skin with lentiginous proliferation of atypical melanocytes [4]. The 'ABCD' (asymmetry, border irregularity, colour variegation, diameter 6 mm) melanoma warning signs are hallmarks of SSM and LMM [11].

In contrast, NM and ALM do not fall into the 'ABCD' presentation. Nodular melanomas tend to occur in older patients (median age 7th decade), any location, and present as a rapidly expanding nodule often detected as changing lesions by patients. NMs account for 10–30% of diagnosed melanomas [8, 12]. Despite this, approximately half of all cutaneous melanomas >2 mm in depth are NMs, reflecting their increased vertical growth rate and resultant more advanced stage on presentation [12, 13]. In comparison with SSM, NM are more often ulcerated, have a higher mitotic index, and more frequently have an NRAS mutation [12, 14]. ALM appears as a pigmented lesion on non-sun–exposed extremities, specifically the palms of hands, soles of feet, and at the base of nail beds. The relative proportion of ALM varies across ethnicities. In white populations of European descent, ALM is reported to be 1–7% of all cutaneous melanomas; however, in Asian populations, ALM ranges from 18% to 47% and nearly 40% in African populations [15–17]. ALM has demonstrated lower overall 5 year and 10 year survival rates compared to other cutaneous melanomas of equivalent stage; however, given the rarity of the subtype and paucity of prospective data, it is unclear if this observation has been due solely to delay in diagnosis and later stages of presentation [15, 16].

Desmoplastic melanoma (DM) is a rare variant (<4%) of cutaneous melanoma and is most commonly located on the head and neck. Neurotropism and absence of BRAF mutation are common features of DM. Clinically it can be confused for lentigo maligna or more often be amelanotic. On histology it can often appear as an amelanocytic spindle with abundant collagen formation and is thought to be a

Table 16.1 Clinical presentation and prognosis

Presentation	Prognosis 5-Year overall survival (OS) [21]
Localized disease (82–85%)	82–99%
Regional metastasis (10–13%)	32–93%
Distant metastasis (2–5%)	20–30%[a]

[a]In the setting of checkpoint inhibitors and targeted therapy, 5 year OS for stage IV disease has increased from a historical 5 year OS of approx. 6%

sarcomatoid melanoma. There are two histological variants of DM, pure and mixed. In pure DM (pDM) the lesion is predominately desmoplastic and fibrosis is seen throughout. In mixed DM (mDM) fibrosis is limited and more cellularity is seen throughout the lesion. DM has higher rates of local recurrence compared to other melanoma histological subytpes [4, 18]. Additionally, pDM demonstrates higher rates of local recurrence, less frequent lymph node involvement, and overall better prognosis than mDM [18, 19]. In contrast, the rate of lymph node involvement and overall prognosis in mDM is similar to other melanoma histological subytpes [20]. Other uncommon melanoma subtypes include nevoid melanoma, (histologically resembles a nevus) and spitzoid melanoma (resembling a spitz nevus) [4].

Clinically melanoma can present a localized disease, with involved regional lymph node basins (regional metastatic disease), or with distant metastasis. Overall prognosis is reflective of extent of disease (Table 16.1).

Staging

The American Joint Committee on Cancer (AJCC) 8th edition is the current recommended melanoma staging system. In the 8th edition of the AJCC staging system, T1 thin melanomas (previously <1 mm) have been subcategorized into T1a <0.8 mm without ulceration and T1b <0.8 mm with ulceration, or 0.8–1 mm with or without ulceration [21, 22]. A significant decrease in 10 year melanoma-specific survival (MSS) was demonstrated for melanomas >0.8 mm with localized disease alone compared to melanomas <0.8 mm (73% vs. 86% $p < 0.01$) [23].

AJCC 8th edition no longer differentiates between satellite and in-transit lesions as 2 cm from the previous excision was an arbitrary cut-off.

While the extent of lymph node positivity is the greatest prognostic factor for MSS in the non-metastatic population, more accurate prognostic estimates are obtained by including tumour thickness [24]. This is reflected in the AJCC 8th edition which has expanded Stage III subcategories to reflect tumour thickness in addition to ulceration and the extent of nodal and/or in-transit disease [22, 24].

The AJCC 8th staging system has also re-categorized central nervous system (CNS) metastatic disease as M1d irrespective of other sites of disease. This reflects both the poorer prognosis of CNS metastasis compared to other sites of metastasis as well as the stratification in systemic therapy studies [22, 24]. Additionally, elevated lactate dehydrogenase (LDH) is no longer classified as M1c. LDH level is now combined with metastatic site such that each Ma-d has a subcategory designation (0 to indicate normal LDH and 1 for an elevated LDH).

Management

Primary Localized Melanoma

Notes: 5 mm margin is generally adequate particularly for MIS that is non-lentigo maligna (LM) type [28]. The borders of LM can be less distinct and have higher rates of incomplete excision [29]. In a large prospective study, 86% of MIS were completely excised with 6 mm margins, whereas 99% were completely excised with 9 mm margins [30]. Surgery is commonly performed to the depth of the deep subcutaneous fascia because occult invasive melanoma (generally less than 0.5 mm) has been reported in up to a third of MIS [31] (Table 16.2).

Special Notes

- Thin melanomas <1 mm in depth, discuss the option of SLNB to patients with any of the following features:
    - Between 0.8 and 1 mm (T1b)
    - Ulceration
    - Microsatellitosis
    - Clark IV/V
    - Higher mitotic count (>3)
- Once considered potential 'high-risk' features in thin melanomas, newer studies suggest that lymphovascular invasion, tumour regression >50%, vertical growth rate, and absence of tumour infiltrating lymphocytes are not independent risk factors for lymph node positivity. The presence of one of these criteria in isolation cannot be interpreted as a clear indication for SLNB [32–34].
- While most thin melanomas have <4.5% likelihood of a positive sentinel lymph node, the likelihood increases to 8.8% for melanomas 0.75–1 mm. Consideration for SLNB should therefore be given to patients based on Breslow thickness of >0.75 mm alone (rounded to 0.8 mm in AJCC 8th edition, T1b) [21, 32, 35–37] (Table 16.3).
- Ulceration is an independent prognostic factor for both melanoma-specific survival (MSS) and sentinel lymph node positivity. While ulceration in thin melano-

Table 16.2 Management of melanoma in situ

Workup	Wide local excision (margins) [25]	Lymph node assessment	Follow-up (F/U) [26, 27]
History and physical exam No labs No radiologic studies	5 mm clinical margin with the aim of achieving histological negative margins increase to 10 mm clinical margin if necessary	SLNB is not indicated	Clinically: Instruct patients on skin examinations (patient education) Refer to dermatologist One clinical visit per year with dermatologist (or more frequently as clinically indicated based on skin exam)

SLNB sentinel lymph node biopsy

Table 16.3 Management of melanoma ≤1 mm (Breslow depth)

Workup	Wide local excision (margins) [25]	Lymph node assessment	Follow-up (F/U) [26, 27]
History and physical exam Clinical assessment of regional lymph nodes and in-transit lesions No labs No radiologic studies	1 cm clinical margin Including skin and subcutaneous tissue to the fascia (but not the fascia)	SLNB is not indicated in most cases <0.8 mm SLNB should be considered and discussed for melanoma 0.8–1 mm and <0.8 mm with ulceration	Follow-up is dependent on clinical stage based on the results of sentinel lymph node biopsy Stage IA Clinically: Instruct patients on skin examinations (patient education) Refer to dermatologist Every 6–12 months for first 3 years, and then annually with a dermatologist no oncologist follow-up is necessary No labs No imaging

SLNB sentinel lymph node biopsy

mas is seen predominately in those >0.8 mm, the presence of ulceration is an independent risk factor for sentinel lymph node positivity even in melanomas <0.75 mm [37–39]. For melanomas <0.8 mm with ulceration, consideration should be given to SLNB [35] (Table 16.3).

- While mitotic rate was previously felt to be an independent prognostic factor for sentinel lymph node positivity in thin melanomas, recent data suggests that the impact of mitotic rate >1 mm is interdependent with Breslow thickness and depth >0.75 mm is a stronger predictor than mitotic rate [38, 40].
- There is limited evidence to inform follow-up frequency and imaging.
- For subungual melanomas, the appropriate surgical management is a functional amputation (proximal to closest joint or ray amputation).

Special Notes

- There have been no prospective randomized studies to date which compare 1 cm and 2 cm margins for intermediate thickness 1–2 mm melanoma. WHO Melanoma Group RCT 1 versus 3 cm for <2 mm melanoma demonstrated no difference in MSS but increased local recurrence with 1 cm excision [41]. A recent meta-analysis (although combines various tumour thickness) suggests that a narrow margin (1–2 cm) results in significantly worse local recurrence and MSS [42] compared to a wider margin (3–5 cm). This is the only publication that has demonstrated better survival with a wider margin of excision (Tables 16.4 and 16.10).
- RCTs for melanoma >2 mm have compared 1 versus 3 cm margins and 2 versus 4 cm margins. There was no significant difference in overall survival (OS) or local recurrence when comparing 2–4 cm margins [43, 44]. There was no difference in OS, but there was a significantly improved MSS in patients who had 3 cm margins compared to 1 cm margins [45] (Table 16.10).

Table 16.4 Management of melanoma 1.1–4 mm (Breslow depth)

Workup	Wide local excision (margins) [25]	Lymph node assessment	Follow-up (F/U) [26, 27]
History and physical exam Clinical assessment of regional lymph nodes and in-transit lesions No labs No routine radiologic studies Further imaging only as clinically indicated	1–2 mm melanoma: 1–2 cm clinical margin, 2 cm if feasible without compromising cosmetic or functional outcome or requiring reconstructive surgery 2–4 mm melanoma: 2 cm clinical margin Margins may be modified to accommodate functional or anatomic considerations Consultation with plastic surgery if primary closure is compromised (i.e., lower arm/lower leg/ high on the back) No need to remove fascia	offer SLNB	Follow-up is dependent on clinical stage based on the results of sentinel lymph node biopsy Clinically: Instruct patients on skin examinations (patient education) Refer to dermatologist Stage IB/IIA: Every 6–12 months for 3 years and then annually with a dermatologist No oncologist follow-up is necessary No labs No imaging Stage IIB: Every 6 months with an oncologist (medical and/or surgical) for first 3 years, then annually Every 6–12 months with a dermatologist No labs No imaging Stages III–IV (see Tables 16.5 and 16.7)

SLNB sentinel lymph node biopsy

- The updated available Level I evidence is insufficient to determine optimal excision margins for melanoma [46]. Recommendations are based on consensus/ guidelines.
- MelMarT-II (NCT 03860883) is an actively recruiting prospective trial randomizing patients 1–2 mm with ulceration and >2 mm with or without ulceration (pT2b-T4b AJCC 8th ed.) to 1 versus 2 cm resection to determine differences in disease-free survival (DFS) with narrow margins.
- May consider wider margins with desmoplastic melanoma (DM). Local recurrence rate (LRR) is higher than other cutaneous melanomas, 6.7–56% [47]. The increased LRR is believed to be due to both microscopic residual disease and neurotropism (seen 17–78%) [18, 47]. For pure DM lesions <2 mm resected with 1 cm margins cumulative index mortality was 25.2% higher than lesions <2 mm resected with 2 cm margins [48]. While there is no data specifically for DM, <1 mm current recommendations for excision all DM is 2 cm when feasible [18].
- Margins are determined from the edge of the clinically visible lesion or the incision excision/biopsy scar. Adequate margins are assessed clinically. Re-excision is recommended with involved margins.

Table 16.5 Management of melanoma>4 mm (Breslow depth)

Workup	Wide local excision (margins) [25]	Lymph node assessment	Follow-up (F/U) [26, 27]

History and physical exam
Clinical assessment of regional lymph nodes and in-transit lesions
No labs
Imaging:
  CT or MRI of brain[a]
AND
  CT chest, abdomen and pelvis
OR
  PET/CT ± MRI brain[a]
	2 cm clinical margin
	Margins may be modified to accommodate functional or anatomic considerations
	Consultation with plastic surgery if necessary if primary closure is compromised
		Discuss and offer SLNB	Follow-up is dependent on clinical stage based on the results of sentinel lymph node biopsy
			Clinically:
			  Instruct patients on skin examinations (patient education)
			  Refer to dermatologist
			Stage IIB/C:
			  Every 6 months with an oncologist for first 3 years, then annually
			  Every 6–12 months with a dermatologist
			No labs
			No routine imaging
			Refer to medical oncology for consideration of adjuvant clinical trial in Stage 2b/c
			Stages III–IV (see Tables 16.5 and 16.7)

SLNB sentinel lymph node biopsy
[a]Depending on institutional preference or availability

- Based on limited data, it is recommended that the depth of excision should extend to the level of the fascia, but the fascia itself does not require excision except in the case of documented clinical or radiologic invasion [28, 49] (Table 16.4).

Special Notes

- There is very limited data with no evidence about improved outcomes with standard metastatic workup at the time of initial workup for patients with thick melanomas (>4 mm) and no evidence of nodal or in-transit disease. Imaging at initial presentation is left to the discretion of individual physicians (Table 16.5).
- Controversy exists regarding the clinical value of sentinel lymph node assessment for thick melanoma as T4 melanomas have higher risk of systemic metastases at initial diagnosis. However, for thick melanomas without distant metastases, SLNB remains useful for staging (and directing adjuvant treatment), prognostication, and locoregional control [35, 50, 51]. Thick melanomas have a 42% risk of node positivity at 10 years, and SLN status still represents the most important survival prognostic factor [50]. SLNB confers a 10-year disease-free survival benefit for intermediate and thick melanomas [50].
- There is a lack of valid prospective studies of the efficacy of routine follow-up.
- No study has demonstrated an improvement in survival due to routine imaging surveillance. However, melanoma-specific survival for Stage IIB are lower than that of Stage IIIA and Stage IIC mirror that of IIIB suggesting that imaging as part of surveillance for high-risk Stage II patients might be warranted. The utility and implementation of routine imaging for surveillance in high-risk Stage II patients remain to be determined (Table 16.5).

- Surveillance imaging is currently left to the discretion of individual physicians. Some centres complete surveillance CT scans annually in the high-risk population while recognizing the current lack of data to support this.

Regionally Metastatic Melanoma

Special Notes

- The rate of successful SLNB is 98.1% with an overall false-negative rate of 12.5%. In high-volume centres with >50 cases, a false-negative rate of 5% (local recurrence rate 5%) is achieved [60, 61]. We recommend performing SLNB with preoperative lymphoscintigraphy and using both blue dye and radioactive dye [62]. Approximately 15–20% of patients with a positive sentinel lymph node will have melanoma metastases identified in completion lymphadenectomy [50, 61]. Table 16.7 desrcibes the rationale for sentinel lymph node biopsy.
- Based on retrospective data and the results of the MSLT-1 trial, there was controversy around the role of CLND after positive SLN alone. MSLT-1 demonstrated an improvement in disease-free survival in both intermediate and thick melanomas, but this translated into an improved MSS only for intermediate thickness melanomas when comparing SLNB positive with CLND to those patients who present with clinically palpable disease. This effect was not demonstrated for thick melanomas [50] (Table 16.11).
- Given that the SLN is the only positive node (i.e. no further positive lymph nodes identified on CLND) in 80–85% of patients, and the limited population in which CLND may confer survival benefit (MSLT-1), numerous patients undergoing routine CLND solely for SLNB positivity may be exposed to unnecessary morbidity [63, 64]. This was the basis for 2 RCTs prospectively examining the benefit of CLND after positive SLNB versus close observation, with CLND only in the setting of subsequently identified clinical or radiographic disease [52–54]. These RCTs demonstrated no difference in OS, MSS, or distant metastatic-free survival. MSLT-2 noted a higher disease free survival in the CLND group rather than observation group, but this did not translate into improved OS nor MSS, as patients underwent CLND at the time of lymph node disease progression [52] (Tables 16.6 and 16.11).
- Patients excluded from these RCTs included: concomitant microsatellitosis, immunosuppression of the patient, extracapsular spread/extension (MSLT-2 only), more than two involved nodal basins (MSLT-2 only), and disease >2 mm within the SLN (DeCOG-SLT only). Additionally, 66% positive SLNBs in both studies had <1.01 mm of lymph node disease [52, 54]. CLND, rather than close observation, can be considered for patients with the above features following discussion with the patient and MCC (Tables 16.6 and 16.11).
- In MSLT-2 subset analyses, no patients were seen to benefit from routine CLND including those with higher volume disease in the lymph nodes and higher number of nodes involved. Site of primary melanoma also did not affect outcome.

Table 16.6 Management of regional metastatic melanoma

Clinical scenario	Workup	Treatment approach	Follow-up
Sentinel lymph node biopsy (SLNB) positive [35, 52–54]	Mutational analysis Metastatic work-up with: CT head or MRI of brain AND CT chest, abdomen, and pelvis (C/A/P) OR PET/CT ± MRI brain	Completion lymphadenectomy (CLND) is no longer offered routinely to all patients based on the results of MSLT-2 and deCOG-SLT Rather than CLND: clinical exam + ultrasound (U/S) monitoring of SLNB positive lymph node basins q 4–6 months for the first 2 years. then q6 months for 3 years Discussion and consideration of CLND for those patients: who are unable to go onto close surveillance and/or did not meet inclusion criteria for MSLT-2 and deCOG-SLT Refer to medical oncology for assessment of adjuvant therapy	Clinically: Instruct patients on skin examinations (patient education) Stage III: Every 3–6 months with an oncologist for first 3 years, then every 6 months for 2 years, then annually Every 6–12 months with a dermatologist U/S of SLNB positive basins q4–6 months for first 2 years then q 6 months for 3 years Consider imaging: CT C/A/P q 6–12 months or as clinically indicated CT/ MRI brain as clinically indicated -no role for routine bone scan No routine labs
Clinically Positive Lymph Nodes[a] [35, 52–54]	FNA or lymph node biopsy Mutational analysis Imaging: CT or MRI of brain AND CT chest, abdomen, and pelvis OR PET/CT ± MRI brain	Therapeutic lymphadenectomy, or completion lymphadenectomy if previous SLNB, of involved basin(s) Consideration of neoadjuvant therapy to enable resection and potentially improve survival Refer to medical oncology for assessment of neoadjuvant or adjuvant therapy Consider consultation with radiation oncology for adjuvant therapy to nodal basin and/or for unresectable disease	
Local recurrence, in-transit or satellite lesions[b] [27, 55, 56–59]	Excisional/incisional biopsy or FNA Mutational analysis Imaging: CT or MRI of brain AND CT chest, abdomen, and pelvis OR PET/CT ± MRI brain	*Local recurrence* Surgical excision with negative margins *One to four in-transit/satellite lesion*: Surgical excision with clear margins Refer to medical oncology for assessment of adjuvant therapy *Multiple lesions* (no consensus): Local surgical therapy options Resection if feasible Amputation (very rarely necessary) Intralesional therapy with IL-2, interferon-α, BCG, VP10/Rose Bengal ORR 69–87% and CR rates for IL-2 range from 32% to 69%. CR correlated with improved PFS and OS. Addition of topical therapies to IL-2 has increased the CR to 60–100% T-VEC[c]: viral vaccine talimogene laherparepvec. Phase 3 RTC T-VEC vs.G-CSF. 15% with TVEC in injected lesions, 8% in uninjected (bystander) and 3% in visceral lesions. Median OS response improved with T-VEC (23.3 months vs. 18.9) Topical therapy with imiquimod or diphencyprone cream (DPCP). OR 60–100% and CR rates 40–100% have been reported with imiquimod. OR 13–46% and CR rates 40–80% have been reported with DPCP Radiation therapy for unresectable disease has demonstrated up to 66% CR and 100% ORR for subcutaneous metastasis Regional therapy options Heated isolated limb perfusion (HILP)/infusion (ILI) with melphalan ± TNF-α. Possible improvement in DFS and OS with complete response. Higher CR and ORR with HILP than ILI (26–69% CR and 67–95% ORR with HILP a 25–38% CR and 45–77% ORR with ILI). Similar 5 year OS rates 49% with HILP and 46% with ILI. Increased toxicity with HILP Combination of systemic therapy with intralesional treatments are ongoing in clinical trials	

(continued)

Table 16.6 (continued)

SLNB sentinel lymph node biopsy, *FNA* fine-needle aspiration, *CLND* completion lymphadenectomy, *ILI* isolated limb infusion, *HILP* heated isolated limb perfusion, *BCG* Bacille Calmette-Guérin, *OS* overall survival, *CR* complete response, *ORR* overall response rate (complete + partial response)

[a]Clinically palpable lymph nodes should be managed as described even in the setting of no obvious primary melanoma

[b]Local recurrence is thought to represent persistent disease and presents at the margin of the WLE scar, therefore recommendation is for re-excision to negative margins. Satellite (within 2 cm of the WLE scar)/ in-transit metastases (> 2 cm from the WLE excision) represent intralymphatic spread of melanoma and can present as cutaneous or subcutaneous masses between the WLE scar and the regional lymph node basin

[c]T-VEC is currently unavailable in Canada outside of a clinical trial

Table 16.7 Rationale for sentinel lymph node biopsy

Accurate staging Allows a more directed treatment planning (ex. adjuvant therapy) and rational follow-up strategy [52]	
Prognostic factor The 5-year overall survival for patients with nodal micrometastases (<2 mm) is 67% and with nodal macrometastases 43% [82]	
Better locoregional control Among patients with intermediate thickness melanomas, MSS is improved when regional metastasis was identified via SLNB rather than clinical presentation (62.1% vs. 41.5%) [50, 83]	
Decreased complication rates Complication rates of SLNB vs. lymphadenectomy: 4.6% vs. 23.2% [62] Lymphedema rate for axillary SLNB vs. complete lymphadenectomy: 1.7% and 9%, respectively [52, 62] Lymphedema rate for groin SLNB vs. complete lymphadenectomy: 1.7% and 26%, respectively [52, 62]	
Potential survival benefit SLNB has been associated an increase in DFS for both intermediate and thick melanomas [50] SLNB has been associated with an increase in MSS for patients with an intermediate thickness melanoma that have metastases in their lymph nodes	
Impact in adjuvant therapy Accurate nodal staging information is important in order to offer patients adjuvant targeted therapy or checkpoint immunotherapy and/or enrolment in clinical trials	
Tumour thickness likelihood of positive SN [84]	
<0.75 mm[a]	1–3.6%
0.76–1.5 mm	7–9.8%
1.5–4.0 mm	20.9–24.6%
>4.0 mm	31.4–39.7%

[a]Without evidence of ulceration

- As the role for CLND in the setting of positive SLNB has decreased, most lymphadenectomies in the groin will be performed either as a CLND for clinically/ radiographically diagnosed disease or therapeutic lymph node dissection (TLND; i.e. clinically identified lymph node involvement without previous SLNB). In the pre-MSLT-2/de-COG setting of CLND for only positive SLNB (without evidence of further disease), lymphadenectomy was limited to the superficial inguinal LN basin and deep (iliac/obturator) dissection was reserved for clinically palpable disease or radiographic pelvic node involvement [65] (Tables 16.6 and 16.11).

- In the setting of CLND (for clinically palpable)/TLND, the rates of deep (iliac and/or obturator) LN involvement are approximately 30–35% [66, 67]. In the setting of palpable lymphadenopathy or recurrent disease after SLNB, both a superficial and deep groin dissection is currently offered at our centre.
- It is not known whether in the setting of radiographically detected involvement of the superficial compartment (while on surveillance for a resected positive sentinel lymph node) one can safely omit the deep dissection. This is currently under investigation in a multi-centre RCT EAGLE-FM (NCT02166788).
- Completion/therapeutic lymphadenectomy in the axilla usually requires levels 1, 2, and 3 dissection with selective transection of pectoralis minor [68, 69]. In the setting of clinically diagnosed disease, rates of level 3 lymph node involvement are 18–31% and 100% when presenting with bulky disease (defined by a large fixed axillary mass or matted nodes presenting in all three levels) [70, 71].
- Neoadjuvant therapies in the context of unresectable/borderline resectable regional disease are being studied. Phase II trials using both targeted therapies (dual BRAF and MEK inhibitors) as well as checkpoint inhibitors (CTLA-4 and PD-1 inhibitors) in the neoadjuvant setting have demonstrated complete pathological responses between 25% and 58% with higher rates of near-complete and partial pathological responses. This has translated into an improved event-free survival and absolute overall survival of 18–23% [72–75]. Currently there are multiple ongoing studies to determine the comparative utility of neoadjuvant versus adjuvant therapies for clinically/marginally resectable disease, the optimal duration of neoadjuvant therapy, as well as the optimal therapeutic regime (Table 16.12).
- Intralesional interleukin-2 (IL-2) for the treatment of in-transit melanoma has an overall response rate of 82%, with complete clinical response in 51–69% of patients and complete pathologic response rate of 32% [57]. When complete clinical response is achieved, an increase in 5-year overall survival can be obtained, compared to partial responders (80% vs. 33%, respectively) [76, 77]. However, this increase in survival might not necessarily represent a direct effect of intra-tumoral IL-2 and could be biased by selection of cases with less aggressive disease [78]. Unlike systemic IL-2, intralesional IL-2 is well tolerated with much less toxicity. 58–100% complete pathologic response has been demonstrated when IL-2 injections are combined with topic imiquimod and retenoids [79–81] (Table 16.6).

Adjuvant Therapy

Recent studies have demonstrated the utility of adjuvant checkpoint inhibitors or targeted therapy in the setting of lymph node positivity (either following detection of microscopic disease on SLN biopsy or after resection of clinically involved lymph nodes). For those patients with a BRAF V600E/K mutation,dual targeted therapy (dabrafenib + trametinib) has demonstrated an improved 4-year recurrence-free survival, decreased relapse rate, improved distant metastasis-free survival (compared to placebo), and an estimated 4-year cure rate of 54% (vs. 37% with placebo) [85, 86] (Table 16.12). In patients both with and without a BRAF mutation, immune checkpoint inhibitors have also demonstrated an improvement in recurrence free survival and overall survival (for ipilimumab). Ipilimumab (a CTL4-A inhibitor) demonstrated an improved 5 year recurrence-free survival (40.8%), distant metastasis-free survival, and overall survival (65.4%) compared to placebo (54.4%) [87] (Table 16.12). Nivolumab (a PD-1 Inhibitor) has demonstrated an improved 18 month recurrence-free survival in comparison to ipilimumab (70.5% vs. 60.8%); however, overall survival has not yet been reported [88] (Table 16.12). Pembrolizumab (a PD-1 Inhibitor) has also demonstrated an improved 18 month recurrence-free survival (71.4%) compared with placebo (53.2%); however, OS has also not been reported [89] (Table 16.12).

Patients with Stage IIB/IIIC and high-risk stage IIIA should routinely be considered for adjuvant immunotherapy. It is unclear whether the benefits outweigh the potential toxicities of immunotherapy for Stage IIIA patients with a low burden of disease (1 SLN positive with <1 mm and no evidence of ulceration) as these patients were excluded from the stage III RCTs [27]. Table 16.8 presents a comparison of the current adjuvant therapies.

There is limited data around the role for radiation therapy (RT) in the setting of effective adjuvant immunotherapies. Prior to the advent of effective immunotherapy, adjuvant RT to the site of primary WLE was considered in desmoplastic melanoma with high-risk features (>4 mm, extensive neurotropism/perineural

Table 16.8 Comparison of adjuvant therapies

	Nivolumab vs. Ipilimumab (Checkmate 238) [88]	Dabrafenib + Trametinib vs. placebo (Combi-AD) [86]	Pembrolizumab vs. placebo (Keynote 054) [89]	Ipilimumab vs. placebo (EORTC 18071) [87]
Patients	IIIb/c, IV (no brain mets)	IIIa (>1 mm), IIIb, IIIc	IIIa (>1 mm), IIIb, IIIc (no intransits)	IIIa (>1 mm), IIIb, IIIc (no intransits)
Duration of Therapy	1 year	1 year	1 year	1 year
RFS	1 year 70% vs. 60% HR 0.65	4 year 54% vs. 38% HR 0.57	1 year 75% vs. 61% HR 0.57	5 year 40% vs. 30% HR 0.75
DMFS	HR 0.73	HR 0.53	N/A	5 year 48% vs. 38%
OS	N/A	3 year 86% vs. 77% HR 0.57	N/A	5 year 65% vs. 54%

invasion, and narrow resection margins, located on head and neck) [27, 90]. Adjuvant RT to the lymph node basins has been demonstrated to reduced nodal recurrence (but not relapse-free or overall survival) in patients at high risk of nodal recurrence including gross/macroscopic extranodal extension, ≥1 positive parotid LN, ≥2 cervical LNs, ≥3 axillary or ilioinguinal LNs [27, 91]. Adjuvant RT is also associated with a higher rate of lymphedema especially for patients receiving inguinal radiation. In the current era of adjuvant therapy, the role RT as an adjuvant treatment is unclear.

Distant Metastatic Melanoma

Special Notes

- Most common causes of death with metastatic melanoma are respiratory failure and intracranial metastases.
- No head-to-head trials have been conducted on the use of targeted therapy compared to immunotherapy in BRAF mutated patients. The use and sequencing of targeted and/or immunotherapies in the metastatic setting is dependent on multiple factors including the extent of disease, rapidity of growth, location of disease (CNS involvement), symptoms, tolerability of potential adverse events, and drug funding (Tables 16.8 and 16.13).
- Similarly, the utility of surgical resection in the setting of metastatic disease in the era of immunotherapy is dependent on the extent of disease, responsiveness of disease to targeted/immunotherapy, location of disease, and patient symptoms (Tables 16.9 and 16.13).
- A phase II trial of complete resection for stage IV melanoma (SWOG, S9430 trial) reported a 4-year OS of 31% with median survival of 21 months [93]. 5-Year survival of 40% has also been reported for complete metastasectomy when tumour-free margins are obtained [110]. Prior to the advent of immunotherapy when resection of melanoma metastases ± systemic therapy was compared to systemic medical therapy alone, median survival was 15.8 versus 6.9 months and surgical treatment conferred a 4-year survival of 20.8% versus 7.0%. Distant disease-free interval of more than 12 months, M1a, and lower number of organ sites of metastases were associated with improved survival [96].
- In the era of immunotherapy while the number of metastatectomies does not appear to have increased, the nature of the metastatectomies has increased from predominately resection of in-transit disease to predominately intra-abdominal surgery. There was a significant increase in potentially curative surgery for residual oligometastatic disease [95]. Optimal sequencing of metastasectomy with targeted and immunotherapies remains unclear (Table 16.9).

Table 16.9 Management of distant metastatic disease

Workup	Surgical approach [92–95]	Systemic therapy
Labs: Serum LDH CBC, lytes, BUN, Cr, LFTs, TSH Mutational Analysis/ BRAF and next-generation sequencing testing Imaging: CT or MRI of brain CT chest, abdomen, and pelvis PET/CT scan to identify otherwise occult metastatic disease if considering surgical intervention	Role of metastasectomy has evolved in the setting of systemic targeted and checkpoint immunotherapies Consider mastectomy as an adjunct after initiation of systemic therapy. Evolving evidence for resection of residual or active oligometastatic disease (<3 sites) after treatment with immunotherapy or targeted therapy as 'curative intent' surgery. Increased resection of intra-abdominal disease for non-palliation purposes. Prior to advent of effective systemic immunotherapy, complete resection of highly selected patients with oligometastatic disease resulted in 20–30% 5 year OS including: [92–94, 96] Pulmonary metastases –most common site of solid organ metastasis Symptomatic or isolated GI (4% of stage IV) metastases Subcutaneous metastases Distant lymph node basins Liver, adrenal, and pancreas Symptomatic brain metastases (surgery, stereotactic radiosurgery, or whole-brain radiation) Palliation of symptoms (bleeding, bowel obstruction, neurologic sequelae) 75–90% can obtain symptom relief	Targeted therapies dependent on mutational status (BRAF, KIT, MEK, NRAS genes) [3] V600E/K BRAF mutation positive (43–50% of cases) Combination-targeted therapy (BRAF inhibitor + MEK inhibitor) has demonstrated improved sustained long-term response (OS, PFS,) compared to monotherapy [97–100] BRAF inhibitor (vemurafenib, dabrafenib, encorafenib) + MEK inhibitor (trametinib, cobimetinib, binimetinib) rapid tumour response, but common progression of disease within 12 months of treatment NRAS is mutated in approximately 15–30% of melanomas. There is limited data around targeted therapy for NRAS mutated melanoma. Binimetinib (MEK inhibitor) has demonstrated a mild improvement in progression-free survival in stage IV disease [101] BRAF and NRAS mutations are mutually exclusive (occurring together <0.5%) KIT mutations occur in 2–8% of all cutaneous melanomas: more common in acral (25%) and mucosal (22%) melanoma tyrosine kinase inhibitors demonstrate approx. 20% response rate in the metastatic setting [102–104] Checkpoint inhibitors Ipilimumab (CTLA-4 Inhibitor): Slow but durable response in 20% of patients [105] Anti-PD1: Pembrolizumab and Nivolumab Pembrolizumab: 5 year OS in Stage IV is 34%, (41% when used as 1st line) [106] Nivolumab: 3 year OS 51.2% when used 1st line [107] Combined immunotherapy (Ipilimumab + Nivolumab) – 3 year OS was 58% in the Nivo + Ipi, Treatment-related adverse events grade 3/4 occurred in 59% with combination verses 21–28% with single agent immunotherapy [108, 109] Systemic chemotherapy (dacarbazine, temozolomide, carbo/taxol and abraxane): used after progression on checkpoint inhibitors ± targeted immunotherapy. Limited clinical response rate. Consider clinical trial whenever available and appropriate

LFT liver function test, *PET* positron emission tomography, *OS* overall survival, *PFS* progression-free survival

Table 16.10 Wide local excision-margins

Melanoma (Breslow thickness)	Study	Methods	Results
In situ (MIS) No RCTs	Kunishigie et al. [30]	Prospective case series 1982–2008 $N = 1120$ MIS All moh's microsurgery (3 mm margin + additional 3 mm) If positive margin additional 3 mm resected	All patients have a minimum of 6 mm margins 86% had negative margins with 6 mm increased to 97% with 9 mm margins Local recurrence with negative margins 0.3% at 3 years 0.8% at 5 years
	Akhtar et al. [29]	Retrospective case series 2001–2009 $N = 192$ MIS (75 lentigo maligna - LM) All excised ≥2006 had 5 mm margins (58%)	29.3% of LM were incompletely excised on initial excision 7/75 left incompletely excised with recurrence rate of 29% 2 (1%) recurred of completely excised, also LM margins 0.8 and 1.4 mm
<1 mm	French Cooperative Surgical Trial [111]	$N = 337$ (melanoma < 2.1 mm) RCT Excision margins: 2 cm vs. 5 cm Excluded acral lentiginous Median F/U: 16 years	No difference in OS (87% vs. 86%) Time to recurrence was 37.6–43 months 10-year disease-free survival was 85% with 2-cm margin and 83% with 5-cm margin. LRR 5.6%
	Swedish Cooperative Surgical Trial [112]	$N = 989$ (melanoma 0.8–2.0 mm) RCT Excision margins: 2 cm vs. 5 cm Median F/U: 11 years	No difference in 10 year OS (79% vs. 76%) 5-year recurrence-free survival was 81% with 2 cm and 83% with 5 cm (no difference). LR: <1% overall
	WHO Melanoma Program Trial [113] [41]	$N = 612$ (melanoma ≤ 2 mm) RCT Excision margins: 1 cm vs. ≥3 cm (3–5 cm) Median F/U: 15 years	No difference in OS 8 year OS 89.6% 1 cm vs. 90.3% ≥ 3 cm and 12 year OS were 85.1% and 87.2% respectively Differences (not significant) in LR narrow And wide excision (2.6% 1 cm excision vs.0.1%, ≥ 3 cm

(continued)

Table 16.10 (continued)

Melanoma (Breslow thickness)	Study	Methods	Results
1–4 mm French, Swedish and WHO trials plus:	Intergroup Melanoma Surgical Trial [44, 114]	*N* = 740 (melanoma 1.0–4.0 mm) RCT Excision margins: 2 cm vs. 4 cm on trunk and proximal extremity Median F/U: 10 years	No difference in 10 year OS 70% with 2 cm vs. 77% with 4 cm No difference is LR with 2 cm vs. 4 cm margins whether the comparisons were made as first relapse 0.4% vs. 0.9%) or anytime (2.1% vs. 2.6%)
	British Cooperative Group Trial [45, 115]	*N* = 675 (melanoma 2.0–4.0 mm) RCT excision margins: 1 cm vs. 3 cm Median F/U: 8.8 years	No difference in OS Melanoma-specific survival improved with 3 cm margins compared to 1 cm margins HR 1.24 Cumulative incidence of death due to melanoma at 8.8 years was 47.9% with 1 cm and 38.1% with 3 cm margins Lower LR with 3 cm margins ($p = 0.05$)
	Swedish Melanoma Study Group + Danish Melanoma Group [43]	*N* = 936 (melanoma ≥2 mm) RCT 1:1 Excision margins: 2 cm vs. 4 cm (50% >3 cm) Median F/U: 6.7 years (11.8 in Swedish cohort)	No difference in OS at 5 years (65% vs. 65%) or 10 years No difference in MSS at 5 years Difference (non-significant $p = 0.06$) in local recurrence 1 cm (4.3%) vs. 3 cm (1.9%)
>4 mm	British Cooperative Group Trial [45, 115]	*N* = 225 (melanoma > 4 mm) Excision margins: 3 cm vs. 1 cm Median F/U: 8.8 years	No difference in OS (as above)

F/U follow-up, *RCT* randomized controlled trials, *WLE* wide local excision, *OS* overall survival, *NS* not significant, *LRR* locoregional recurrence, LR local recurrence (within/adjacent to the scar). *CLND* completion lymphadenectomy – previous SLNB, *DFS* disease-free survival, *TLND* therapeutic lymphadenectomy – palpable or radiographic disease without previous SLNB, *SLN* sentinel lymph node

Table 16.11 Sentinel lymph node biopsy and completion lymphadenectomy

Study	Methods	Results
Multicenter Selective Lymphadenectomy Trial (MSLT-1) [50]	Phase III Multicentre RCT $N = 1347$ (melanoma 1.2–3.5 mm), 314 with thick melanoma Groups: WLE + SLNB (with CLND if SLNB positive, observation if SLNB negative) vs. WLE and observation alone (with TLND when clinically nodal relapse) Median F/U: 10 years	5-year DFS 78% vs. 73% ($p = 0.009$) 10-year DFS SLNB vs. observation for intermediate thickness: 71.3% vs. 64.7% ($p = 0.01$) and for thick melanoma: 50.7% vs. 40.5% ($p = 0.03$) No significant difference in 10-year melanoma-specific survival in intermediate-thickness melanoma (81.4% in SLNB group vs. 78.3% in observation group, $p = 0.18$) and in thick melanoma (58.9% vs. 64.4%, $p = 0.56$) Subgroup analysis in positive sentinel node patients: Better 10-year MSS in those who were SLN+ and had CLND vs. those who had TLND (62.1% vs. 41.5%, $p = 0.006$) Node-negative patients have 10-year OS of 85.1% vs. 62.1% for those with node-positive disease ($p < 0.001$) In multivariable analysis, sentinel node status is the strongest predictor of disease recurrence and death from melanoma
Multicenter Selective Lymphadenectomy Trial (MSLT-2) [52]	Phase III multicentre RCT $N = 1939$ Intermediate and thick melanomas (≥1.2 mm) with positive SLNB (all underwent WLE and SLNB) 1:1 Randomization to either: Completion lymph node dissection Close observation with clinical exam and ultrasound and completion dissection with additional nodal disease	Median f/u 43 months 3 year MSS did not differ between the CLND group and the nodal observation group (86% vs. 86%) Sub-group analysis did not identify any group with improved MSS with CLND vs. observation 3 year DFS higher with CLND (68%) vs. observation (63%) 2nd to decreased nodal recurrence at 3 years (92% with CLND vs. 77% with observation) No difference in distant metastasis-free survival Median thickness in both groups 2.1 mm, 69–72% had only one SLN positive, median size of metastasis in SLN 0.61–0.67 mm, approx. 65% had ≤1 mm of disease in SLN
De-COG SLT [53, 54]	Phase III multicentre RCT $N = 438$ (trial closed early 2nd to limited accrual) Intermediate and thick melanomas (≥1 mm) with positive SLNB (all underwent WLE and SLNB) 1:1 Randomization to either: completion lymph node dissection close observation with clinical exam and ultrasound and completion dissection with additional nodal disease	Median f/u 72 months No difference in Distant metastasis-free survival (DMFS) at 3 years 77% with observation and 74.9% with CLND, or 5 years 68% with observation and 65% with CLND No difference in OS at 3 years (81.7% observation and 81.2% CLND) or 5 years No difference in recurrence free survival (RcFS) at 3 years (67.4% observation vs. 66.8% CLND) and 5 years Median thickness in both groups 2.4 mm, 91–93% had only one SLN positive, approx. 65% had ≤1 mm of disease in SLN

RCT randomized controlled trial, *WLE* wide local excision, *OS* overall survival, *LR* locoregional recurrence, *NS* not significant, *CLND* completion lymphadenectomy – immediate, *TLND* therapeutic lymphadenectomy – delayed, *SLN* sentinel lymph node, *DFS* disease-free survival, RcFS recurrence-free survival, *DMFS* distant-metastasis-free survival

Table 16.12 Adjuvant systemic therapy

Drug	Study	Methods	Results
Dual targeted therapy: Dabrafenib (BRAF inhibitor) + Trametinib (MEK inhibitor)	Hauschild et al., Long et al. [85, 86] *N* = 870	Phase 3 RCT (COMBI-AD) Resected Stage III (IIIA only if >1 mm of disease in ≥1 lymph node), BRAF V600E/K mutated All patients had completion lymphadenectomy prior to trial enrollment RCT 1:1 adjuvant Dabrafenib + Trametinib 12 months vs. placebo Post-hoc subgroup analysis (AJCC 7th vs. AJCC 8th staging) to assess for RcFS (recurrence + death)	3- and 4-year RcFS rates 59% and 54% dabrafenib (Dab) plus trametinib (Tram) vs. 40% and 38% placebo Dab + Tram median recurrence not reached at 44 months, vs. 16.6 placebo Relapse rates 40% Dab + Tram vs. 59% placebo DMS with Dab + Tram HR 0.53 3-year OS 86% with combination vs. 77% with placebo (not significant) Estimated 54% Dab + Tram vs. 37% placebo will never recur (estimated cure rate) RcFS improved across all stages (both 7th and 8th staging) with Dab-Tram
Checkpoint inhibitors:			
Ipilimumab (CTLA-4 inhibitor)	Eggermont et al. [87] *N* = 951	Phase 3 RCT (EORTC 18071) Resected Stage III (IIIA only if >1 mm of disease in ≥1 lymph node) All patients had completion lymphadenectomy prior to trial enrollment RCT 1:1 ipilimumab (Ipi) 10 mg/kg q 3 weeks * 4 cycles then q3 months for up to 3 years vs. placebo	5-year RcFS rates 40.8% Ipi vs. 30.3% placebo Ipi improved RcFS in both micro- and macrometastasis Overall survival was significantly longer with Ipi 5 year OS was 65.4% Ipi vs. 54.4% placebo 5 year DMS 48.3% Ipi vs. 38.9 placebo (HR 0.76)
Pembrolizumab (PD-1 inhibitor)	Eggermont et al. [89] *N* = 1014	Phase 3 RCT (Keynote 054) Stage III patients stratification via Stage IIIA (only if >1 mm of disease in ≥1 lymph node) /IIIB/IIIC (<4 lymph nodes) and IIIC(>4 nodes) All patients had completion lymphadenectomy prior to trial enrollment 1:1 Pembrolizumab (Anti-PD-1) 200 mg q 3 weeks *18 weeks (1 year) vs. placebo	Median f/u 15 months 12-month RcFS was 75.4% with pembrolizumab (Pembro) and 61.0% with placebo (HR 0.57) 18-month RcFS significantly higher with pembro vs. placebo 71.4% vs. 53.2%, Benefit of Pembro was similar across stages IIIA, IIIB, IIIC, and microscopic and macroscopic nodal ds Adverse events grades 3 to 5 with pembro were 14.7% vs. 3.4% with placebo

Nivolumab (PD-1 Inhibitor)	Weber et al. *N* = 906 [88]	Phase 3 RCT (Checkmate 238) Stage IIIB, IIIC or resected Stage IV (including brain metastasis) All patients had completion lymphadenectomy prior to trial enrollment 1:1 Nivolumab (Nivo) 3 mg/kg q 2 weeks for 1 year or Ipilimumab (Ipi) 10 mg/kg q 2 weeks * 4 dose then q 12 weeks for 1 year total	18 month median f/u, median recurrence-free survival not reached in patients with stage III or stage IV disease, irrespective of disease stage more benefit with nivo than ipi 12-month RcFS 70.5% with Nivo vs. 60.8% with Ipi, 18-month RcFS were 66.4% and 52.7%, respectively Grade 3/4 adverse events were 14.4% with Nivo and 45.9% with Ipi
Neoadjuvant trials			
Dual targeted therapy: Dabrafenib (BRAF inhibitor) + Trametinib (MEK Inhibitor)	Amaria et al. *N* = 21 [72]	Phase 2 randomized trial Stage IIIB/C or Stage IV resectable oligometastases 1:2: upfront surgery vs. Dab + Tram 8 weeks pre-op and 44 weeks post-op Only one patient in the surgery arm received adjuvant treatment with a 5 drug combination regime	DFS at 18.6 months 71% dual therapy vs. 0% with surgery alone Median event-free survival 19.7 months dual therapy vs. 2.9 months surgery alone Trial stopped early due to longer than expected event-free survival with Dab + Tram 58% complete response and 17% partial response
Dual Checkpoint Inhibition: Ipilimumab (CTLA-4 Inhibitor) + Nivolumab (PD-1 Inhibitor)	Blank et al., Rozeman et al. [74, 75] *N* = 20 Ipilimumab 3 mg/kg + Nivolumab 1 mg/kg	Phase 2 randomized trial (OpACIN) Palpable stage 3 1:1: Ipi + Nivo either 4 cycles after surgery or 2 cycles pre-op, 2 cycles post-op 90% of patients developed grade 3 or 4 adverse events Based on A/Es neo-OpACIN being undertaken to identify optimal dosing	78% with >50% necrosis on pathology (7/9) (3 with <10% viable tumour and 3 with pCR) 31 month f.u 0/7 patients with path response developed recurrent disease Neoadjuvant arm: 30 month recurrence-free survival 80%, OS 90% Adjuvant arm: 30 month recurrence-free survival 60%, OS 67%
	Amaria et al. [73] *N* = 23 Nivolumab 3 mg/kg vs Ipilimumab 3 mg/kg + Nivolumab 1 mg/kg	Phase 2 randomized trial Stage IIIB/C or Stage IV resectable oligometastases 1:1 Nivo alone 4 cycles q2 weeks pre-op, VS. Nivo + Ipi 3 cycles q3 weeks pre-op post-op both arms Nivo alone 3 mg/kg q2 weeks Trial stopped early bc of disease progression events in Nivo only arm and high rate of A/Es in the combo arm	2 pts in Nivo arm progressed and were unresectable pCR 25% in Nivo alone, 45% in Nivo + Ipi PFS at 15 months 82% in combo vs. 58% Nivo alone OS at 22 months 100% in combo vs. 76% in Nivo alone PFS and OS not significant (? 2nd to small sample size) Improved PFS and OS in patients who achieved pCR vs. those who did not

Table 16.13 Systemic therapy for metastatic disease

Drug	Study	Methods	Results
Targeted immunotherapy:			
Dabrafenib (BRAF inhibitor) + Trametinib (MEK inhibitor)	Long, G. et al. [116] *N* = 423	Phase 3 RCT (Combi-D) BRAF V600E/K mutation unresectable stage III or IV 1:1 Dabrafenib + Trametinib vs. Dabrafenib alone No prior systemic tx for Stage IV disease, excluded untreated brain metastasis	3-year PFS was 22% with combination therapy versus 12% with monotherapy 3-year OS was 44% vs. 32%, respectively Greatest 3 year OS benefit in pts with baseline LDH ≤ ULN and <3 organ sites with metastasis 62% vs. 25%
	Robert, C. et al. [99, 117] *N* = 704	Phase 3 RCT (Combi-V) BRAF V600E/K mutation unresectable stage III or IV 1:1 Dabrafenib + Trametinib vs. Vemurafenib alone No prior systemic tx for Stage IV disease, excluded untreated brain metastasis	3-y PFS, 25% with combination therapy vs. 11% with monotherapy 3-year OS, 45% vs. 32% respectively Greatest 3 year OS benefit in pts with baseline LDH ≤ ULN and <3 organ sites with metastasis 70% vs. 46%
Vemurafenib (BRAF inhibitor) + Cobimetinib (MEK inhibitor)	Ascierto et al. [97] *N* = 495	Phase 3 RCT (CoBRIM) BRAF V600E/K mutation, unresectable stage III or IV RCT 1:1 Vemurafenib + Cobimetinib vs. Vemurafenib alone No prior systemic tx for Stage IV disease, excluded untreated brain metastasis	Median progression-free survival was 12.3 months for combined therapy vs. 7.2 months for monotherapy Median overall survival was 22.3 months versus 17.4 months respectively
Encorafenib (BRAF Inhibitor) + Binimetinib (MEK Inhibitor)	Dummer et al. [98] *N* = 577	Phase 3 RCT (Columbus Trial) BRAF V600E/K mutation, unresectable stage III or IV 1:1:1 Encorafenib + Binimetinib vs. Encorafenib alone vs. Vemurafenib alone No prior systemic tx for Stage IV disease, excluded untreated brain metastasis	median progression-free survival was 14·9 months with combination therapy vs. 9.6 months with encorafenib alone vs. 7·3 months with vemurafenib alone median follow-up 16.6 months, median OS not yet reached
Checkpoint inhibitors:			
Ipilimumab (CTLA-4 Inhibitor)	Robert C et al. [118] *N* = 502	Phase 3 RCT tx naive unresectable stage III or IV Ipilimumab 10 mg/kg + dacarbazine vs. dacarbazine + placebo	OS significantly longer in Ipi + D vs. D + placebo—11.2 vs. 9.1 months with higher survival rates at: 1 year 47% vs. 36%, 2 year 28% vs. 18%, and 3 year 20.8% vs. 12.2%

Table 16.13 (continued)

Drug	Study	Methods	Results
	Hodi et al. [119] $N = 676$	Phase 3 RCT previously treated unresectable stage III or IV, HLA-A*0201 positive 3:1:1 ipilimumab 3 mg/kg + gp100, vs. ipilimumab 3 mg/kg vs. gp100	median overall survival was 10 months among patients receiving ipilimumab ± gp100 vs. 6 months with gp100 alone progression-free survival was highest in the ipi alone group 57.7% at 12 weeks (vs. 49% with combination and 49% with gp100 alone Ipi alone group had best ORR 10.9%
	Schadendorf et al. [105]	Patient level OS-analysis, 1861 patients unresectable stage III or IV, previously treated (1257) or treatment naive (604) 2 trials, (10 prospective and 2 retrospective including 2 phase III trials) comparisons of ipilimumab with controls (3 mg/kg in 52%, 10 mg/kg in 40% of patients)	median OS was 11.4 months 3 year OS rates were 22% for all patients 26% for treatment-naive patients, and 20% for previously treated patients
Nivolumab (PD-1 inhibitor)			
	Weber et al. [120] $N = 631$	Phase 3 RCT (Checkmate 037) Unresectable stage III or IV progressed on ipilimumab ± BRAF/MEK inhibitor 2:1 nivolumab 3 mg/kg q2 week vs. cytotoxic chemotherapy (ICC) (dacarbazine/paclitaxel)	ORR 31. 7%, in the nivolumab group vs. 10. 6%, in the ICC group Median duration of response had not yet been reached at 8.4 months with nivolumab vs. 3·5 months with ICC
	Ascierto et al. [107] Robert et al. [121] $N = 418$	Phase 3 RCT (Checkmate 066) unresectable stage III or IV, treatment naive BRAF wt 1:1 nivolumab 3 mg/kg q2 week vs. dacarbazine q3 week	3-year OS 51.2% with nivolumab vs. 21.6% with Dacarbazine median OS was 37.5 vs. 11.2 months Complete and partial responses were 19.0% and 23.8% with Nivo

(continued)

Table 16.13 (continued)

Drug	Study	Methods	Results
Pembrolizumab (PD-1 inhibitor)	Robert et al. [122] *N* = 173	Phase 1 trial (Keynote-001) unresectable stage III or IV progressed on ipilimumab Pembrolizumab 2 mg/kg q3 week vs. 10 mg/kg q3 week	ORR 26% at 8 months f/u in both groups A/E rate was the same in both groups
	Hamid et al. [106], Robert el al [123]. *N* = 655	Phase 1b trial, (Keynote-001) unresectable stage III or IV Pembro 2 mg/kg q3week vs. 10 mg/kg q3 week vs. 10 mg/kg q2 week 151 treatment naive, 496 had previous systemic treatment (excluding PD-1 inhibitors)	5 year OS 34% in all patients and 41% in treatment (tx)-naive patients Median OS was 23.8 months in all patients and 38.6 months in tx naïve patients 16.0% achieved CR at median 12 months, 2 year sustained DFS 90% and sustained CR 88% at 30 months
	Schacter et al. [124] Robert et al. [125] *N* = 834	Phase 3 RCT (Keynote-006) unresectable stage III or IV 1:1:1 Pembrolizumab 10 mg/kg q 2 weeks vs. Pembrolizumab 10 mg/kg q 3 week vs. Ipilimumab 3 mg/kg Prior systemic tx for Stage IV disease (excluding PD-1 and CTLA-4 inhibitors)	ORR 36% in pembro group vs. 13% in ipi group median OS not reached in pembro at 23 months, median OS with ipi 16 months 2 year OS was 55% in the pembro arms vs. 43% in ipi arm
Combination therapy:	Hodi et al., Wolchok et al. [108, 109] *N* = 94	Phase 3 RCT (Checkmate-067) tx naive unresectable stage III or IV 1:1:1 Nivolumab 1 mg/kg + Ipilimumab 3 mg/kg q 3 weeks * 4 doses then Nivolumab alone 3 mg/kg q 2 weeks vs. Nivolumab alone 3 mg/kg q 2 weeks vs. Ipilimumab alone 3 mg/kg q 3 weeks * 4 doses	median OS was not reached at 48months in the Nivo + Ipi group vs. 36.9 months with Nivo vs. 19.9 months with Ipi 3 year OS was 58% in the Nivo + Ipi group vs. 52% in the Nivo group vs. 34% in the Ipi group Treatment-related adverse events grade 3/4 occurred in 59% with combination, 21% with Nivo alone and 28% with Ipi alone

RCT randomized controlled trial, *PFS* progression-free survival, *OS* overall survival, *D* dacarbazine, *RFS* relapse-free survival, *DFS* disease-free survival, *IFN* interferon, *Ipi* ipilimumab, *Nivo* nivolumab, *Pembro* pembrolizumab, *RcFS* recurrence-free survival

Landmark Trials

Systemic Therapy

Referring to Medical Oncology (Patients with High-Risk Melanoma)

1. Primary melanoma with Breslow thickness >4 mm
2. Node-positive melanoma (palpable and sentinel node positive)
3. In-transit or satellite lesions
4. Metastatic disease
5. Recurrent disease
6. Unknown primary melanoma

Patients with metastatic melanoma should be referred for clinical trials whenever possible. Metastatic melanoma of the unknown primary site is diagnosed in approximately 2–9% of all melanoma cases. It is usually diagnosed if metastatic melanoma is confirmed clinically and pathologically, and if no cutaneous, uveal, or mucosal melanoma primary can be found. Data suggests that unknown primary melanoma can be accurately staged using the AJCC staging system and have equal survival stage per stage [126].

Referring to Radiation Oncology [90, 91]

1. Unresectable or gross residual nodal disease
2. Extracapsular nodal extension
3. ≥1 parotid, ≥2 cervical, ≥2 axillary, ≥3 inguinal palpable lymph nodes involved
4. Cervical lymph node ≥2 cm, axillary and inguinal lymph node ≥3 cm
5. Metastatic disease – if symptomatic from focal disease; treatment of brain metastases with stereotactic radiosurgery
6. Pure desmoplastic melanoma with narrow margins, locally recurrent or extensive neurotropism
7. Multiple local recurrences at the primary site (after resection), positive margins around primary site from microsatellites
8. In transit/satellite disease unsuitable for surgery, intralesional, or topical therapies or systemic therapy

Referring to Multidisciplinary Cancer Conference (MCC)

1. Bulky nodal disease
2. New metastatic disease
3. In-transit or locoregional recurrence

4. Any consideration of non-standard multimodal therapy
5. Consideration of available clinical trials

Technical Aspects of Melanoma Defect Reconstruction

There are various coverage options following melanoma excision. The decision-making process for selection of the best coverage method is dependent on the following factors: defect location, size, adjacent skin laxity, history of radiation or need for adjuvant treatment, and the patient's medical comorbidities. In general, the simplest closure method is used that will provide optimal function and cosmesis.

Generally, a full-thickness circular tissue defect, going down to fascia, periosteum, or paratenon, is present after a melanoma excision. The commonly used coverage options are listed below with a brief description of their appropriate use and important perioperative care.

Primary Closure

Primary closure is the simplest closure available and is recommended whenever possible. It requires adequate laxity in the surrounding tissue and can be used in any part of the body. It is also easily done in a clinic setting with the use of local anesthetics.

As for technical tips, a preoperative elliptical excision marking allows a linear closure without a dog-ear formation that would otherwise result from closing a circular defect. It may be necessary to undermine both sides of the skin flaps at the pre-fascial level to allow adequate advancement. It is recommended to suture the incision in a layered fashion to approximate the superficial fascia where present, the deep dermis, and finally the skin closure.

Skin Graft

When primary closure is not possible, skin graft may be useful in areas where there is a lack of adjacent skin laxity. A skin graft is a fast procedure, but it takes longer to heal, requires postoperative wound care, and has worse aesthetics than flap coverage. Furthermore, a skin graft should not be used in a previously irradiated tissue or in an area that will likely receive adjuvant radiation.

There are two types of skin grafts: (1) full thickness skin graft (FTSG) that consists of epidermis and the full thickness of dermis and (2) split thickness skin graft (STSG) that consists of epidermis and a partial thickness of dermis.

The FTSG may be useful across a joint as it does not undergo significant secondary contraction like STSG. However, it is important to remember that an FTSG has a limitation to the size that can be harvested since the donor site requires a primary closure (i.e. groin, supraclavicular region, etc.), and an FTSG takes less readily than the STSG. Intraoperatively, it is pie-crusted using a scalpel to prevent hematoma or seroma formation under the graft, and it is sutured to the defect skin edges with gut sutures.

The STSG is useful in a larger surface area over any soft tissue (muscle, fascia, fat), periosteum, perichondrium, paratenon, and medullary bone. Frequently harvested using a dermatome from any healthy skin (i.e. commonly thighs), the common thickness used is 0.012″ and STSGs may be used as a pie-crusted sheet graft or meshed to enlarge the surface area and improve its ability to conform to irregular contours. The STSG may be sutured or stapled to the recipient site, and the donor site undergoes secondary healing over the course of approximately 2 weeks.

Postoperative care is necessary to allow adequate graft healing. This may be achieved using a bolster dressing using a Reston foam or a VAC dressing, which is necessary for approximately 5 days postop to provide compression, avoid shear, and avoid fluid accumulation under the graft. After removal of the initial dressings, daily non-adherent dressing changes are required for approximately 2 weeks afterwards until the skin graft has fully healed. Patients may require splints during the immediate postoperative graft healing period if skin grafts are placed in extremities and do not have a VAC dressing on in order to prevent tendon or muscle movement below the graft.

Local Flaps [1]

Local flaps may be a better option over skin grafts when the coverage requires better tissue colour and contour match and durability. Local flaps consist of skin, subcutaneous tissue, and superficial fascia, where the tissues in the immediate vicinity of the primary defect are raised and transferred to the defect size. There are a variety of local flaps, and the commonly used types in melanoma defect coverage include advancement, transposition, rotation, and keystone flaps. It is important to note that after a local flap is performed, it may interfere with accuracy of sentinel lymph node mapping and make re-excision more challenging.

Advancement Flap

Advancement flap as shown in Fig. 16.1 is a unidirectional linear advancement of tissue. There are many varieties of this flap. The single advancement flap, which demonstrates the general principle of this flap design, is demonstrated below. The flap is designed by making parallel incisions along a tangent to the defect at the depth of the defect. Tension may be reduced by undermining both opposing wound edges and by utilizing Burrow's triangle excisions.

Transposition Flap

An example of a transposition flap is the classic rhomboid flap as shown in Fig. 16.2. A defect is shaped into a rhombus shape with angles of 60 and 120 degrees. The flap is designed as an extension of the short axis of the rhomboid in the region of the maximal adjacent skin laxity. The flap is lifted and transposed into the defect as the tension vector changes by 90 degrees, and the donor site is closed primarily.

Fig. 16.1 Single advancement flap

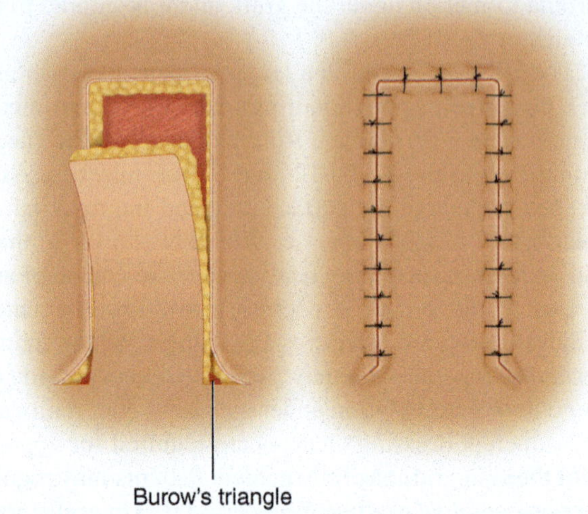

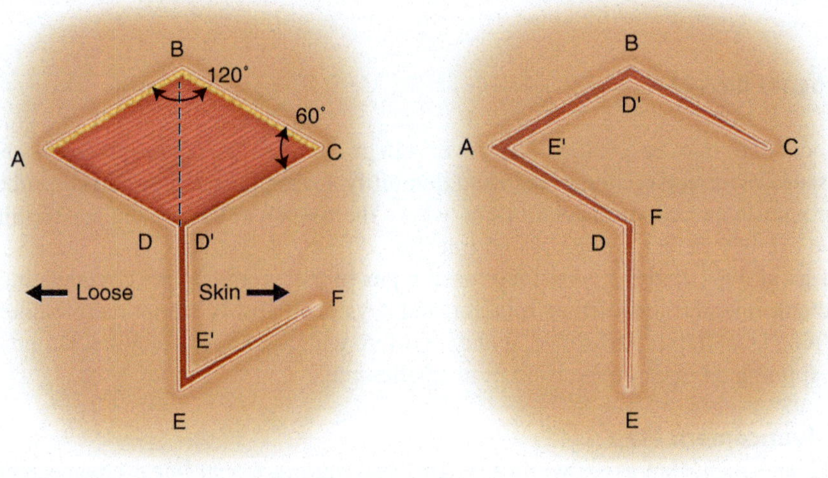

Fig. 16.2 Rhomboid flap

Rotation Flap

Rotation flaps repair defects that cannot be closed along a single tension vector by an advancement flap as shown in Fig. 16.3. It is designed by extending an arc from beyond the base of the defect (of approximately 5–6 times the base of the triangulated defect), with a pivot point about 2 times in length of the triangulated defect. The rotation results in a secondary defect along the arc of rotation, which is often closed by re-distribution of the elevated flap over this defect and the defect form the

Fig. 16.3 Rotation flap

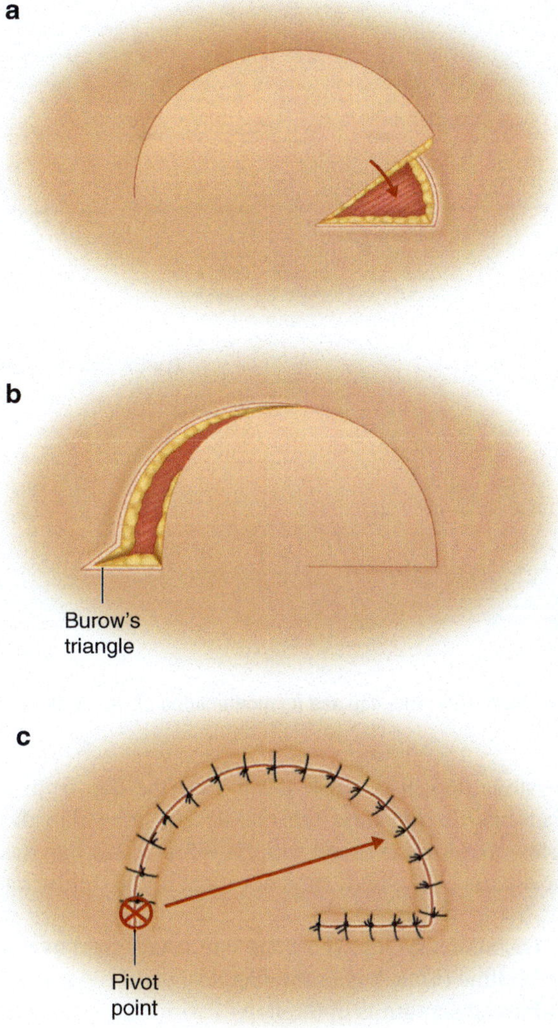

melanoma excision. Alternatively, a Burrow's triangle allows a closure without a dog ear and by eliminating the secondary defect. A Burrow's triangle may also be used to relax the line of maximal tension of the flap, to avoid ischemic compromise to the flap.

Keystone Flap

Keystone flap as shown in Fig. 16.4 is a fasciocutaneous flap based on muscular perforators that can be considered in most parts of the body, and is particularly useful in back, chest, abdomen, and longitudinally oriented leg or arm defects. It requires having intact fascia with intact perforators supplying it. When designing a

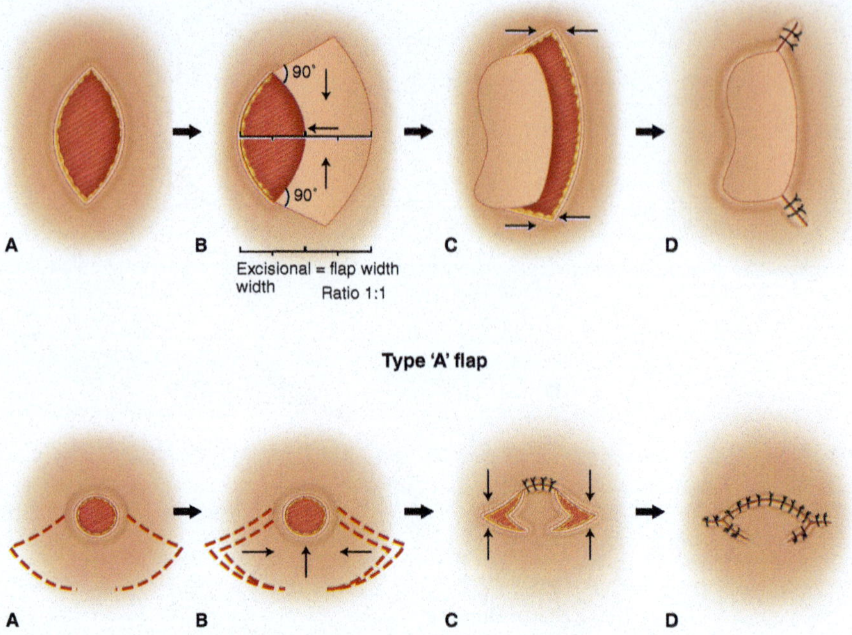

Fig. 16.4 Keystone flap and its modification (Type 'A' flap) [2]

keystone flap, it is important to take the flap from area of maximal laxity. Below diagrams demonstrate the classic keystone flap design and a modification of it below to optimize blood supply. While it is a flap design that may be considered in most parts of the body, it is not ideal in the following situations:

- Distal medial leg where the flap is designed over the bone
- Midline of back is in the flap design
- Fascial septum is in the flap
- Skin has been elevated off the fascia perforators already (i.e. if an advancement flap has been attempted and didn't reach)

Regional Flaps

Regional flaps, which are tissue with its own blood supply, are used for larger defects. They are useful in irradiated defects or defects that may have exposed critical structures, such as major vessels, nerves, bones and/or tendons; for example, in a larger defect with exposed axillary vessels, a pectoralis muscle flap or a latissimus dorsi flap may be indicated. Free flaps, which are distant transfers of tissue with its own blood supply using microsurgical techniques, are less commonly performed in melanoma and non-melanoma coverage situations. In situations where regional flaps would be needed or when local flap options are not straightforward, early plastic surgery consultation is recommended to allow operative planning and coordinated surgery.

Toronto Pearls

- Groin dissection flaps should preserve Scarpa's fascia with the flap.
- Saphenous vein preservation during groin dissection could be considered.
- Level 3 axillary dissection should be completed in the presence of palpable axillary disease.
- Superficial and deep groin dissection should be completed in the presence of palpable disease.
- If patient does not undergo completion lymphadenectomy after a positive SLNB, perform ultrasound monitoring of the axilla and/or groin every 4–6 months for 3 years and then yearly to 5 years.
- Pembrolizumab is the preferred adjuvant therapy in non-BRAF mutated patients (2nd to q3 week drug dosing) over nivolumab.
- Consider radiation for multiple local recurrences at the site of primary disease following re-excision.
- Currently we do not have access to VP10, T-VEC, or interferon-α as injectable treatment for in-transit disease.
- Our centre routinely uses IL-2 intra-tumoral injection and aldara and retinoid creams (triple therapy) in the management of multiple in-transit metastases as first-line treatment after surgery.
- Topical immunotherapy (diphencyprone – DPCP) or systemic immunotherapy is 2nd line after triple therapy for ongoing in-transit disease.
- Radiation is rarely used for in-transit disease.

References

1. Society CC. Canadian Cancer Statistics 2019. 2019. https://www.cancer.ca/~/media/cancer.ca/CW/cancer%20information/cancer%20101/Canadian%20cancer%20statistics/Canadian-Cancer-Statistics-2019-EN.pdf?la=en.
2. Olsen CM, Green AC, Pandeya N, Whiteman DC. Trends in melanoma incidence rates in eight susceptible populations through 2015. J Invest Dermatol. 2019;139:1392.
3. Leonardi GC, Falzone L, Salemi R, et al. Cutaneous melanoma: from pathogenesis to therapy (review). Int J Oncol. 2018;52(4):1071–80.
4. Scolyer RA, Long GV, Thompson JF. Evolving concepts in melanoma classification and their relevance to multidisciplinary melanoma patient care. Mol Oncol. 2011;5(2):124–36.
5. Duncan L. The classification of cutaneous melanoma. Hematol Oncol Clin North Am. 2009;23:501–13.
6. Singh P, Kim HJ, Schwartz RA. Superficial spreading melanoma: an analysis of 97 702 cases using the SEER database. Melanoma Res. 2016;26(4):395–400.

7. Ferrari Júnior NM, Muller H, Ribeiro M, Maia M, Sanches Júnior JA. Cutaneous melanoma: descriptive epidemiological study. Sao Paulo Med J. 2008;126:41–7.
8. Shaikh WR, Xiong M, Weinstock MA. The contribution of nodular subtype to melanoma mortality in the United States, 1978 to 2007. Arch Dermatol. 2012;148(1):30–6.
9. Kvaskoff M, Siskind V, Green AC. Risk factors for lentigo maligna melanoma compared with superficial spreading melanoma: a case-control study in Australia. Arch Dermatol. 2012;148(2):164–70.
10. Greveling K, Wakkee M, Nijsten T, van den Bos RR, Hollestein LM. Epidemiology of lentigo maligna and lentigo maligna melanoma in the Netherlands, 1989–2013. J Invest Dermatol. 2016;136(10):1955–60.
11. Rigel DS, Russak J, Friedman R. The evolution of melanoma diagnosis: 25 years beyond the ABCDs. CA Cancer J Clin. 2010;60(5):301–16.
12. Warycha MA, Christos PJ, Mazumdar M, et al. Changes in the presentation of nodular and superficial spreading melanomas over 35 years. Cancer. 2008;113(12):3341–8.
13. Demierre MF, Chung C, Miller DR, Geller AC. Early detection of thick melanomas in the United States: beware of the nodular subtype. Arch Dermatol. 2005;141:745–50.
14. Lee JH, Choi JW, Kim YS. Frequencies of BRAF and NRAS mutations are different in histological types and sites of origin of cutaneous melanoma: a meta-analysis. Br J Dermatol. 2011;164(4):776–84.
15. Teramoto Y, Keim U, Gesierich A, et al. Acral lentiginous melanoma: a skin cancer with unfavourable prognostic features. A study of the German central malignant melanoma registry (CMMR) in 2050 patients. Br J Dermatol. 2018;178(2):443–51.
16. Bradford PT, Goldstein AM, McMaster ML, Tucker MA. Acral lentiginous melanoma: incidence and survival patterns in the United States, 1986–2005. Arch Dermatol. 2009;145(4):427–34.
17. Cress RD, Holly EA. Incidence of cutaneous melanoma among non-Hispanic whites, Hispanics, Asians, and blacks: an analysis of California cancer registry data, 1988–93. Cancer Causes Control. 1997;8:246–52.
18. Chen LL, Jaimes N, Barker CA, Busam KJ, Marghoob AA. Desmoplastic melanoma: a review. J Am Acad Dermatol. 2013;68(5):825–33.
19. Murali R, Shaw HM, Lai K, et al. Prognostic factors in cutaneous desmoplastic melanoma: a study of 252 patients. Cancer. 2010;116(17):4130–8.
20. Hawkins WG, Busam KJ, Ben-Porat L, et al. Desmoplastic melanoma: a pathologically and clinically distinct form of cutaneous melanoma. Ann Surg Oncol. 2005;12(3):207–13.
21. Gershenwald JE, Scolyer RA. Melanoma staging: American joint committee on cancer (AJCC) 8th edition and beyond. Ann Surg Oncol. 2018;25:2105–10.
22. Gershenwald JE, Scolyer RA, Hess KR, et al. Chapter 47 melanoma of the skin. In: American Joint of Committee on cancer manual. 8th ed. New York: Springer International Publishing; 2017.
23. Lo SN, Scolyer RA, Thompson JF. Long-term survival of patients with thin (T1) cutaneous melanomas: a breslow thickness cut point of 0.8 mm separates higher-risk and lower-risk tumors. Ann Surg Oncol. 2018;25(4):894–902.
24. Gershenwald JE, Scolyer RA, Hess KR, et al. Melanoma staging: evidence-based changes in the American Joint Committee on Cancer eighth edition cancer staging manual. CA Cancer J Clin. 2017;67:472–92.
25. Wright F, Souter LH, Kellet S, Easson A, Murray C, et. al. Primary excision margins and sentinel lymph node biopsy in cutaneous melanoma. 2017;Guideline 8–2. Current Oncology. 2019;26(4):e541–550.
26. Rajagopal S, Souter LH, Baetz T, et al. Follow-up of Patients with Cutaneous Melanoma who were Treated with Curative Intent. In: Ontario CC, editor. https://www.cancercareontario.ca/en/guidelines-advice/types-of-cancer/317762019.
27. Coit DG, Thompson JA, Albertini MR, Barker C, Carson WE, et al. NCCN guidelines version 2.2019 cutaneous melanoma. J Natl Compr Canc Netw. 2019;17:367–402.
28. Swetter SM, Tsao H, Bichakjian CK, et al. Guidelines of care for the management of primary cutaneous melanoma. J Am Acad Dermatol. 2019;80(1):208–50.

29. Akhtar S, Bhat W, Magdum A, Stanley PR. Surgical excision margins for melanoma in situ. J Plast Reconstr Aesthet Surg. 2014;67(3):320–3.
30. Kunishige JH, Brodland DG, Zitelli JA. Surgical margins for melanoma in situ. J Am Acad Dermatol. 2012;66(3):438–44.
31. Bax MJ, Johnson TM, Harms PW, et al. Detection of occult invasion in melanoma in situ. JAMA Dermatol. 2016;152(11):1201–8.
32. Cordeiro E, Gervais MK, Shah PS, Look Hong NJ, Wright FC. Sentinel lymph node biopsy in thin cutaneous melanoma: a systematic review and meta-analysis. Ann Surg Oncol. 2016;23(13):4178–88.
33. Andtbacka RH, Gershenwald JE. Role of sentinel lymph node biopsy in patients with thin melanoma. J Natl Compr Canc Netw. 2009;7(3):308–17.
34. McClain SE, Shada AL, Barry M, Patterson JW, Slingluff CL Jr. Outcome of sentinel lymph node biopsy and prognostic implications of regression in thin malignant melanoma. Melanoma Res. 2012;22(4):302–9.
35. Wong SL, Faries MB, Kennedy EB, Agarwala SS, et al. Sentinel lymph node biopsy and management of regional lymph nodes in melanoma: American Society of Clinical Oncology and Society of Surgical Oncology clinical practice guideline update. J Clin Oncol. 2018;36(4):399–413.
36. Faries M, Wanek L, Elashoff D, Wright BE, Morton DL. Predictors of occult nodal metastasis in patients with thin melanoma. Arch Surg. 2010;145:137–42.
37. Maurichi A, Miceli R, Camerini T, et al. Prediction of survival in patients with thin melanoma: results from a multi-institution study. J Clin Oncol. 2014;32(23):2479–85.
38. Han D, Zager JS, Shyr Y, et al. Clinicopathologic predictors of sentinel lymph node metastasis in thin melanoma. J Clin Oncol. 2013;31(35):4387–93.
39. Kupferman ME, Kubik MW, Bradford CR, et al. The role of sentinel lymph node biopsy for thin cutaneous melanomas of the head and neck. Am J Otolaryngol. 2014;35(2):226–32.
40. Wat H, Senthilselvan A, Salopek TG. A retrospective, multicenter analysis of the predictive value of mitotic rate for sentinel lymph node (SLN) positivity in thin melanomas. J Am Acad Dermatol. 2016;74(1):94–101.
41. Cascinelli N. Margin of resection in the management of primary melanoma. Semin Surg Oncol. 1998;14(4):272–5.
42. Wheatley K, Wilson JS, Gaunt P, Marsden JR. Surgical excision margins in primary cutaneous melanoma: a meta-analysis and Bayesian probability evaluation. Cancer Treat Rev. 2016;42:73–81.
43. Gillgren P, Drzewiecki KT, Niin M, et al. 2-cm versus 4-cm surgical excision margins for primary cutaneous melanoma thicker than 2 mm: a randomised, multicentre trial. Lancet. 2011;378(9803):1635–42.
44. Balch CM, Soong SJ, Smith T, et al. Long-term results of a prospective surgical trial comparing 2 cm vs. 4 cm excision margins for 740 patients with 1–4 mm melanomas. Ann Surg Oncol. 2001;8(2):101–8.
45. Hayes AJ, Maynard L, Coombes G, et al. Wide versus narrow excision margins for high-risk, primary cutaneous melanomas: long-term follow-up of survival in a randomised trial. Lancet Oncol. 2016;17:184–92.
46. Sladden MJ, Balch C, Barzilai DA, Berg D, Freiman A, et al. Surgical excision margins for primary cutaneous melanoma. Cochrane Database Syst Rev. 2009;(4):Art. No.: CD004835. https://doi.org/10.1002/14651858.CD004835.pub2.
47. Lens MB, Newton-Bishop JA, Boon AP. Desmoplastic malignant melanoma: a systematic review. Br J Dermatol. 2005;152(4):673–8.
48. Maurichi A, Miceli R, Camerini T, et al. Pure desmoplastic melanoma: a melanoma with distinctive clinical behavior. Ann Surg. 2010;252(6):1052–7.
49. Grotz TE, Markovic SN, Erickson LA, et al. Mayo Clinic consensus recommendations for the depth of excision in primary cutaneous melanoma. Mayo Clin Proc. 2011;86(6):522–8.
50. Morton DL, Thompson JF, Cochran AJ, et al. Final trial report of sentinel-node biopsy versus nodal observation in melanoma. N Engl J Med. 2014;370(7):599–609.

51. Ribero S, Osella-Abate S, Sanlorenzo M, et al. Sentinel lymph node biopsy in thick-melanoma patients (N=350): what is its prognostic role? Ann Surg Oncol. 2015;22:1967–73.
52. Faries MB, Thompson JF, Cochran AJ, et al. Completion dissection or observation for sentinel-node metastasis in melanoma. N Engl J Med. 2017;376(23):2211–22.
53. Leiter U, Stadler R, Mauch C, et al. Complete lymph node dissection versus no dissection in patients with sentinel lymph node biopsy positive melanoma (DeCOG-SLT): a multicentre, randomised, phase 3 trial. Lancet Oncol. 2016;17(6):757–67.
54. Leiter U, Stadler R, Mauch C, et al. Final analysis of DECOG-SLT trial: survival outcomes of complete lymph node dissection in melanoma patients with positive sentinel node. (Abstract). J Clin Oncol. 2018;36(15):9501.
55. Squires MH, Delman KA. Current treatment of locoregional recurrence of melanoma. Curr Oncol Rep. 2013;15(5):465–72.
56. Read T, Lonne M, Sparks DS, et al. A systematic review and meta-analysis of locoregional treatments for in-transit melanoma. J Surg Oncol. 2019;119:887–96.
57. Hassan S, Petrella TM, Zhang T, et al. Pathologic complete response to intralesional interleukin-2 therapy associated with improved survival in melanoma patients with in-transit disease. Ann Surg Oncol. 2015;22(6):1950–8.
58. Andtbacka RHI, Ross M, Puzanov I, et al. Patterns of clinical response with talimogene laherparepvec (T-VEC) in patients with melanoma treated in the OPTiM phase III clinical trial. Ann Surg Oncol. 2016;23:4169–77.
59. Barker CA, Lee NY. Radiation therapy for cutaneous melanoma. Dermatol Clin. 2012;30(3):525–33.
60. Morton DL, Cochran AJ, Thompson JF, et al. Sentinel node biopsy for early-stage melanoma. Trans Meet Am Surg Assoc. 2005;123:10–20.
61. Valsecchi ME, Silbermins D, de Rosa N, Wong SL, Lyman GH. Lymphatic mapping and sentinel lymph node biopsy in patients with melanoma: a meta-analysis. J Clin Oncol. 2011;29(11):1479–87.
62. McMasters KM, Noyes RD, Reintgen DS, et al. Lessons learned from the sunbelt melanoma trial. J Surg Oncol. 2004;86(4):212–23.
63. van der Ploeg AP, van Akkooi AC, Verhoef C, Eggermont AM. Completion lymph node dissection after a positive sentinel node: no longer a must? Curr Opin Oncol. 2013;25(2):152–9.
64. Wong SL, Morton DL, Thompson JF, et al. Melanoma patients with positive sentinel nodes who did not undergo completion lymphadenectomy: a multi-institutional study. Ann Surg Oncol. 2006;13(6):809–16.
65. Mack LA, McKinnon JG. Controversies in the management of metastatic melanoma to regional lymphatic basins. J Surg Oncol. 2004;86(4):189–99.
66. Faut M, Kruijff S, Hoekstra HJ, van Ginkel RJ, Been LB, van Leeuwen BL. Pelvic lymph node dissection in metastatic melanoma to the groin should not be abandoned yet. Eur J Surg Oncol. 2018;44(11):1779–85.
67. Oude Ophuis CM, van Akkooi AC, Hoekstra HJ, et al. Risk factors for positive deep pelvic nodal involvement in patients with palpable groin melanoma metastases: can the extent of surgery be safely minimized?: a retrospective, multicenter cohort study. Ann Surg Oncol. 2015;22(Suppl 3):S1172–80.
68. Mohan N, Brar S, Rich JT, Wright F, Higgins K. The use of pectoralis major flaps during axillary dissection for bulky axillary lymphadenopathy. Open Access Surg. 2013;6:33.
69. Hadjiminas DJ, Zacharioudakis KE. Direct transpectoral approach for level III axillary lymph node clearance. Ann R Coll Surg Engl. 2014;96(6):481–2.
70. Nessim C, Law C, McConnell Y, Shachar S, McKinnon G, Wright F. How often do level III nodes bear melanoma metastases and does it affect patient outcomes? Ann Surg Oncol. 2013;20(6):2056–64.
71. Gentile D, Covarelli P, Picciotto F, et al. Axillary lymph node metastases of melanoma: management of third-level nodes. In Vivo. 2016;30:141–6.

72. Amaria RN, Prieto PA, Tetzlaff MT, et al. Neoadjuvant plus adjuvant dabrafenib and trametinib versus standard of care in patients with high-risk, surgically resectable melanoma: a single-centre, open-label, randomised, phase 2 trial. Lancet Oncol. 2018;19(2):181–93.
73. Amaria RN, Reddy SM, Tawbi HA, et al. Neoadjuvant immune checkpoint blockade in high-risk resectable melanoma. Nat Med. 2018;24(11):1649–54.
74. Blank CU, Rozeman EA, Fanchi LF, et al. Neoadjuvant versus adjuvant ipilimumab plus nivolumab in macroscopic stage III melanoma. Nat Med. 2018;24(11):1655–61.
75. Rozeman EA, Sikorska K, van de Wiel B, et al. 30 months relapse-free survival, overall survival, and long-term toxicity update of (neo)adjuvant ipilimumab (ipi) 1 nivolumab (nivo) in macroscopic stage III melanoma (OPACIN trial) (abstract). Ann Oncol. 2018;29(Suppl_10):42.
76. Weide B, Derhovanessian E, Pflugfelder A, et al. High response rate after intratumoral treatment with interleukin-2: results from a phase 2 study in 51 patients with metastasized melanoma. Cancer. 2010;116(17):4139–46.
77. Boyd KU, Wehrli BM, Temple CL. Intra-lesional interleukin-2 for the treatment of in-transit melanoma. J Surg Oncol. 2011;104(7):711–7.
78. Temple-Oberle CF, Byers BA, Hurdle V, Fyfe A, McKinnon JG. Intra-lesional interleukin-2 therapy for in transit melanoma. J Surg Oncol. 2014;109(4):327–31.
79. Shi VY, Tran K, Patel F, et al. 100% complete response rate in patients with cutaneous metastatic melanoma treated with intralesional interleukin (IL)-2, imiquimod, and topical retinoid combination therapy: results of a case series. J Am Acad Dermatol. 2015;73(4):645–54.
80. Garcia MS, Ono Y, Martinez SR, et al. Complete regression of subcutaneous and cutaneous metastatic melanoma with high-dose intralesional interleukin 2 in combination with topical imiquimod and retinoid cream. Melanoma Res. 2011;21(3):235–43.
81. Nadler A, Look-Hong N, Alavi N, Abadir W, Wirght FC. Local therapies for in-transit melanoma: an evidence-based algorithm. University of Toronto. J Surg Oncol. 2019.
82. Balch CM, Gershenwald JE, Soong SJ, et al. Multivariate analysis of prognostic factors among 2,313 patients with stage III melanoma: comparison of nodal micrometastases versus macrometastases. J Clin Oncol. 2010;28(14):2452–9.
83. Kachare SD, Brinkley J, Wong JH, Vohra NA, Zervos EE, Fitzgerald TL. The influence of sentinel lymph node biopsy on survival for intermediate-thickness melanoma. Ann Surg Oncol. 2014;21(11):3377–85.
84. Lens MB, Daews M, Newton-Bishop A, Goodacre T. Tumour thickness as a predictor of occult lymph node metastases in patients with stage I and stage II melanoma undergoing sentinel lymph node biopsy. Br J Surg. 2002;89:1223–7.
85. Hauschild A, Dummer R, Schadendorf D, et al. Longer follow-up confirms relapse-free survival benefit with adjuvant Dabrafenib plus Trametinib in patients with resected BRAF V600–mutant stage III melanoma. J Clin Oncol. 2018;36(35):3441–9.
86. Long GV, Hauschild A, Santinami M, et al. Adjuvant Dabrafenib plus Trametinib in stage III BRAF-mutated melanoma. N Engl J Med. 2017;377(19):1813–23.
87. Eggermont AMM, Chiarion-Sileni V, Grob J-J, et al. Prolonged survival in stage III melanoma with ipilimumab adjuvant therapy. NEJM. 2016;375(19):1845–55.
88. Weber J, Mandala M, Del Vecchio M, Gogas HJ, et al. Adjuvant nivolumab versus ipilimumab in resected stage III or IV melanoma. N Engl J Med. 2017;377(19):1824–35.
89. Eggermont AMM, Blank CU, Mandala M, et al. Adjuvant pembrolizumab verses placebo in resected stage III melanoma. NEJM. 2018;378(19):1789–801.
90. Strom T, Caudell JJ, Han D, et al. Radiotherapy influences local control in patients with desmoplastic melanoma. Cancer. 2014;120(9):1369–78.
91. Henderson MA, Burmeister BH, Ainslie J, et al. Adjuvant lymph-node field radiotherapy versus observation only in patients with melanoma at high risk of further lymph-node field relapse after lymphadenectomy (ANZMTG 01.02/TROG 02.01): 6-year follow-up of a phase 3, randomised controlled trial. Lancet Oncol. 2015;16(9):1049–60.
92. Bello DM. Indications for the surgical resection of stage IV disease. J Surg Oncol. 2019;119(2):249–61.

93. Sosman JA, Moon J, Tuthill RJ, et al. A phase 2 trial of complete resection for stage IV melanoma: results of Southwest Oncology Group Clinical Trial S9430. Cancer. 2011;117(20):4740–06.
94. Faries MB, Mozzillo N, Kashani-Sabet M, et al. Long-term survival after complete surgical resection and adjuvant immunotherapy for distant melanoma metastases. Ann Surg Oncol. 2017;24(13):3991–4000.
95. Smith MJF, Smith HG, Joshi K, et al. The impact of effective systemic therapies on surgery for stage IV melanoma. Eur J Cancer. 2018;103:24–31.
96. Howard JH, Thompson JF, Mozzillo N, et al. Metastasectomy for distant metastatic melanoma: analysis of data from the first Multicenter Selective Lymphadenectomy Trial (MSLT-I). Ann Surg Oncol. 2012;19(8):2547–55.
97. Ascierto PA, McArthur GA, Dréno B, et al. Cobimetinib combined with vemurafenib in advanced BRAFV600-mutant melanoma (coBRIM): updated efficacy results from a randomised, double-blind, phase 3 trial. Lancet Oncol. 2016;17(9):1248–60.
98. Dummer R, Ascierto PA, Gogas HJ, et al. Encorafenib plus binimetinib versus vemurafenib or encorafenib in patients with BRAF -mutant melanoma (COLUMBUS): a multicentre, open-label, randomised phase 3 trial. Lancet Oncol. 2018;19(5):603–15.
99. Robert C, Karaszewska B, Schachter J, et al. Three-year estimate of overall survival in COMBI-v, a randomized phase 3 study evaluating first-line dabrafenib (D) + trametinib (T) in patients (pts) with unresectable or metastatic BRAF V600E/K–mutant cutaneous melanoma. Ann Oncol. 2016;27(suppl_6).
100. Long GV, Stroyakovskiy D, Gogas H, et al. Combined BRAF and MEK inhibition versus BRAF inhibition alone in melanoma. N Engl J Med. 2014;371(20):1877–88.
101. Dummer R, Schadendorf D, Ascierto PA, et al. Binimetinib versus dacarbazine in patients with advanced NRAS -mutant melanoma (NEMO): a multicentre, open-label, randomised, phase 3 trial. Lancet Oncol. 2017;18(4):435–45.
102. Tzen C-Y, Wu Y-H, Tzen C-Y. Characterization of KIT mutation in melanoma. Dermatol Sin. 2014;32(1):7–12.
103. Hodi FS, Corless CL, Giobbie-Hurder A, et al. Imatinib for melanomas harboring mutationally activated or amplified KIT arising on mucosal, acral, and chronically sun-damaged skin. J Clin Oncol. 2013;31(26):3182–90.
104. Carvajal RD, Antonescu CR, Wolchok JD, Chapman PB, Roman R-A, Teitcher J. KIT as a therapeutic target in metastatic melanoma. JAMA. 2011;305(22):2327–34.
105. Schadendorf D, Hodi FS, Robert C, et al. Pooled analysis of long-term survival data from phase II and phase III trials of ipilimumab in unresectable or metastatic melanoma. J Clin Oncol. 2015;33(17):1889–94.
106. Hamid O, Robert C, Daud A, et al. Five-year survival outcomes for patients with advanced melanoma treated with pembrolizumab in KEYNOTE-001. Ann Oncol. 2019;30:582–8.
107. Ascierto PA, Long GV, Robert C, et al. Survival outcomes in patients with previously untreated BRAF wild-type advanced melanoma treated with nivolumab therapy: three-year follow-up of a randomized phase 3 trial. JAMA Oncol. 2019;5:187–94.
108. Hodi FS, Chiarion-Sileni V, Gonzalez R, et al. Nivolumab plus ipilimumab or nivolumab alone versus ipilimumab alone in advanced melanoma (CheckMate 067): 4-year outcomes of a multicentre, randomised, phase 3 trial. Lancet Oncol. 2018;19(11):1480–92.
109. Wolchok JD, Chiarion-Sileni V, Gonzalez R, et al. Overall survival with combined nivolumab and ipilimumab in advanced melanoma. N Engl J Med. 2017;377(14):1345–56.
110. Ollila DW. Complete metastasectomy in patients with stage IV metastatic melanoma. Lancet Oncol. 2006;7(11):919–24.
111. Khayat D, Rixe O, Martin G, et al. Surgical margins in cutaneous melanoma (2 cm versus 5 cm for lesions measuring less than 2.1-mm thick). Cancer. 2003;97(8):1941–6.
112. Cohn-Cedermark G, Rutqvist LE, Andersson R, et al. Long term results of a randomized study by the Swedish Melanoma Study Group on 2-cm versus 5-cm resection margins for patients with cutaneous melanoma with a tumour thickness of 0.8–2.0 mm. Cancer. 2000;89:1495–501.

113. Veronesi U, Cascinelli N. Narrow excision (1-cm margin): a safe procedure for thin cutaneous melanoma. Arch Surg. 1991;125:438–41.
114. Balch CM, Urist MM, Karakousis CP, et al. Efficacy of 2-cm surgical margins for intermediate-thickness melanomas (1 to 4 mm). Results of a multi-institutional randomized surgical trial. Ann Surg. 1993;218:262.
115. Thomas JM, Newton-Bishop J, A'Hern R, et al. Excision margins in high-risk malignant melanoma. N Engl J Med. 2004;350:757–66.
116. Long GV, Flaherty KT, Stroyakovskiy D, et al. Dabrafenib plus trametinib versus dabrafenib monotherapy in patients with metastatic BRAF V600E/K-mutant melanoma: long-term survival and safety analysis of a phase 3 study. Ann Oncol. 2017;28(7):1631–9.
117. Robert C, Karaszewska B, Schachter J, et al. Improved overall survival in melanoma with combined dabrafenib and trametinib. N Engl J Med. 2015;372(1):30–9.
118. Robert C, Thomas L, Bondarenko I, et al. Ipilimumab plus dacarbazine for previously untreated metastatic melanoma. N Engl J Med. 2011;364(26):2517–26.
119. Hodi FS, O'Day SJ, McDermott DF, et al. Improved survival with ipilimumab in patients with metastatic melanoma. N Engl J Med. 2010;363:711–23.
120. Weber JS, D'Angelo SP, Minor D, et al. Nivolumab versus chemotherapy in patients with advanced melanoma who progressed after anti-CTLA-4 treatment (CheckMate 037): a randomised, controlled, open-label, phase 3 trial. Lancet Oncol. 2015;16(4):375–84.
121. Robert C, Long GV, Brady B, et al. Nivolumab in previously untreated melanoma without BRAF mutation. N Engl J Med. 2015;372(4):320–30.
122. Robert C, Ribas A, Wolchok JD, et al. Anti-programmed-death-receptor-1 treatment with pembrolizumab in ipilimumab-refractory advanced melanoma: a randomised dose-comparison cohort of a phase 1 trial. Lancet. 2014;384(9948):1109–17.
123. Robert C, Ribas A, Hamid O, et al. Durable complete response after discontinuation of pembrolizumab in patients with metastatic melanoma. JCO. 2018;36(17):1668–74.
124. Schachter J, Ribas A, Long GV, et al. Pembrolizumab versus ipilimumab for advanced melanoma: final overall survival results of a multicentre, randomised, open-label phase 3 study (KEYNOTE-006). Lancet. 2017;390(10105):1853–62.
125. Robert C, Schachter J, Long GV, et al. Pembrolizumab versus ipilimumab in advanced melanoma. N Engl J Med. 2015;372(26):2521–32.
126. Pfeil AF, Leiter U, Buettner PG, et al. Melanoma of unknown primary is correctly classified by the AJCC melanoma classification from 2009. Melanoma Res. 2011;21(3):228–34.

Technical Aspects of Melanoma Defect Reconstruction – References

Bhat SP. Keystone flaps in coloured skin: flap technology for the masses? Indian J Plast Surg. 2013;46:36–47.

Budd ME, Hovsepian R, Basseri B, Evans GRD. Chapter 8 flaps. In: Guyuron B, Eriksson E, Persing J, editors. Plastic surgery: indications and practice. UK: Elsevier; 2009. p. 70–3.

Merkel Cell Carcinoma

17

Andrea M. Covelli, Anthony M. Joshua, Joan E. Lipa,
Marcus O. Butler, Laura Snell, Alexander Sun,
and Frances C. Wright

Introduction

Merkel cell carcinomas (MCCs) are rare cutaneous neuroendocrine neoplasms that are clinically aggressive due to a relatively high local, regional, and distant metastatic recurrence potential [1]. These tumours are thought to be more aggressive

A. M. Covelli (✉)
General Surgical Oncology, University of Toronto, Toronto, ON, Canada
e-mail: Andrea.covelli@utoronto.ca

A. M. Joshua
Kinghorn Cancer Centre, St Vincents Hospital, Sydney, NSW, Australia
e-mail: Anthony.joshua@svha.org.au

J. E. Lipa
Department of Medical Oncology and Hematology, University of Toronto, Toronto, ON, Canada

Department of Surgery, Division of Plastics and Reconstructive Surgery, University of Toronto, Toronto, ON, Canada
e-mail: Joan.Lipa@sunnybrook.ca

M. O. Butler
Department of Medical Oncology and Hematology, University of Toronto, Toronto, ON, Canada

Department of Medicine, University of Toronto, Toronto, ON, Canada
e-mail: Marcus.Butler@uhn.ca

L. Snell · F. C. Wright
Department of Surgery, Division of Surgical Oncology, University of Toronto, Toronto, ON, Canada
e-mail: Laura.Snell@sunnybrook.ca; frances.wright@sunnybrook.ca

A. Sun
Department of Radiation Oncology, University of Toronto, Toronto, ON, Canada
e-mail: Alex.Sun@rmp.uhn.on.ca

F. C. Wright et al. (eds.), *Surgical Oncology Manual*,
https://doi.org/10.1007/978-3-030-48363-0_17

than melanoma and are associated with an overall historical 5-year survival rate between 13.5% and 56% depending on stage at time of initial presentation [2–4]. They are found most commonly in Caucasian (94%), elderly patients, with the average age at presentation being 72 years [5–9]. The most common sites of involvement include the head and neck (46–48%), followed by the extremities (35–38%), and trunk (11–17%) [5, 7]. Risk factors include extensive sun exposure, immunosuppression, and/or infection with the polyomavirus [7, 10–12]. It is estimated that 60-80% of MCC in the Northern Hemisphere are related to the polyomavirus [13, 14].

MCCs usually present as non-tender (86%), rapidly growing (63%), painless, red to violaceous intradermal papules (56%), or large nodules [1, 10]. MCC can also be flesh toned and the overlying epidermis is usually preserved [1]. A common clinical presentation is an elderly Caucasian man with a rapidly growing, otherwise asymptomatic, nodule in a sun-exposed area, often with other signs of background sun exposure [1, 5, 7, 15]. Given their relatively non-specific clinical presentation, diagnosis is often delayed leading to advanced disease at the time of diagnosis. Approximately half of all MCC are considered to be benign lesions on visual inspection alone [10]. The "AEIOU" acronym can be used to assist with diagnosis: A—asymptomatic, E—expanding, I—immunosuppressed, O—older than age >50 years, and U—ultraviolet-exposed fair skin [1, 10]. Ultimately, diagnosis is established by excisional or punch biopsy demonstrating the characteristic "small, round, blue cells" with large prominent nuclei [16].

Three histological subtypes of Merkel cell include: (i) small-cell variant which is poorly differentiated and indistinguishable from bronchial small-cell carcinoma on histology alone, (ii) intermediate variant, which is the most common, and (iii) trabecular variant, which is the most well-differentiated and also the most uncommon; it is often only seen as a component of a mixed variant with the other two histologic subtypes [14, 16]. While the utility of differentiating the variants remains unclear, it is thought that the trabecular variant is least aggressive whereas the small-cell variant the most aggressive.

Immunohistochemical analysis has been instrumental in identifying markers characteristic of MCC, facilitating its differentiation from other "small round, blue cell tumours" commonly seen with bronchial small-cell carcinoma, poorly differentiated neuroendocrine tumours, lymphoma, and small-cell melanoma. Cytokeratin-20 (CK-20 and neuron-specific enolase (NSE) are highly specific for MCC. CK-20 staining is positive in 89–100% of MCCs. In contrast, thyroid transcription factor-1 (TTF-1) and CK-7 stain positive in bronchial small cell but are generally absent in MCC [1, 16]. Small-cell melanoma stains positive for S-100 and HBM-45 but negative for CK-20 differentiating it from MCC [16].

The American Joint Committee on Cancer AJCC eighth edition is the current recommended staging system for MCCs. Clinically and pathologically node negative patients (Stage I and Stage II) demonstrate improved overall survival (OS) with smaller MCCs at the time of presentation. In Stage I patients (i.e. <2 cm), the 5-year OS is 45.0%, whereas in Stage IIA (>2 cm), 5-year OS is 30.9%, and MCC with local invasion into the fascia, muscle, cartilage, or bone (Stage IIB) 5-year OS is

Table 17.1 Clinical presentation and prognosis

Presentation [3, 17]	Prognosis [8] 5-Year overall survival (OS)
Localized disease (65–66%)	51
Regional metastasis (27–28%)	35%
Distant metastasis (7–8%)	14%

27.3% [17]. Prognostically overall survival is also related to nodal involvement. 5-year OS is highest in patients who are clinically and pathologically node negative (50.6%) (Table 17.1). Those who are discovered to be node-positive on pathological examination (micrometastasis identified within a sentinel lymph node) demonstrate a 5-year OS 39.7% which decreases to 26.8% in patients with clinically discovered regional lymph node involvement at the time of diagnosis [17] (Table 17.1).

Management

Wide Local Excision

Wide local excision (WLE) is considered the cornerstone of treatment for localized MCC (Table 17.2). While no trials have demonstrated, the absolute size of margin required to reduce local recurrence current recommendations are 1–2 cm down to the fascia or pericranium, irrespective of size of the MCC [2, 19] (Table 17.2). The intent behind wide local excision is not to achieve wide negative margins on the primary lesion itself, but rather to remove microscopic satellite disease [19].

40-50% of MCC occur in the head and neck region.WLE with 1–2 cm is attempted whenever possible; however, when WLE would preclude appropriate functional and/or cosmetic outcomes, Mohs micrographic surgery can be considered. There has been no prospective data comparing the outcomes of Mohs micrographic surgery to WLE ≥1 cm. Retrospective studies have demonstrated that when microscopically negative margins are achieved, Mohs' microsurgery did not confer worse recurrence nor overall survival compared to WLE for stage I and II disease [20, 21].

Sentinel Lymph Node Biopsy

The single most important prognostic characteristic of clinically localized MCC is the presence or absence of occult nodal metastases [2, 9, 17]. The incidence of sentinel node metastases in MCC ranges anywhere between 14 and 47%, and approximately 30% of clinically node-negative patients will harbour micrometastatic disease [2, 3, 17, 24] . While an increase in size of the primary MCC has been

Table 17.2 Management of localized Merkel cell carcinoma [2, 18, 19]

Workup	Surgical excision (margins)	Lymph node assessment	Adjuvant therapy	Follow-up
History and physical examination Complete skin and lymph node examination Biopsy (H + E, IHC) No labs Imaging studies at physician discretion	Wide local excision (WLE) (1–2 cm margins) to investing fascia Mohs micrographic surgical excision with negative margins and then re-excision (0.5–1.0 cm margins)[a]	Offer and discuss SLNB—Ideally done at time of definitive resection	Refer to radiation oncology for consideration of adjuvant RTX to the primary site No role for systemic chemotherapy in the adjuvant or neoadjuvant setting Adjuvant immuno-therapy is being investigated in clinical trials	History and physical exam every 3–6 months for 3 years including full skin exam and assessment of lymph node basins and then every 6–12 months thereafter

H + E hematoxylin and eosin staining, *IHC* immunohistochemistry, *SLNB* sentinel lymph node biopsy, *RTX* radiation therapy

[a]Mohs surgery is not routinely recommended but can be considered in cosmetically sensitive areas when 1–2 cm margins are not feasible or would result in significant morbidity

associated with an increase in occult lymph node metastasis, sentinel lymph node (SLN) positivity has been demonstrated up to 14% in MCCs <1 cm [9, 17]. Overall, however, SLN positivity has been associated with (a) primary tumour size (25% for tumours ≤2 cm vs. 45% for tumours >2 cm) and (b) the presence of lymphovascular invasion (55% for tumours with lymphovascular invasion vs. 4% for tumours with no evidence of lymphovascular invasion) [9, 25].

Undergoing SLNB may offer local therapeutic benefit as there has been decreased regional nodal recurrence compared to patients who underwent observation alone [2, 26]. In addition, patients with a positive sentinel lymph node appear to be at significantly higher risk of distant metastasis and death from MCC and thus may benefit from additional treatment [2, 18, 24, 26–28]. False negative rates with sentinel lymph node biopsy (SLNB) have been reported to range from 0 to 57% with recent patient-level systematic review reporting ~15% [24]. False negative rates are likely secondary to lymphatic dysfunction and/or the relatively high number of MCCs on the head and neck leading to multiplicity of lymph node basins compared to other sites.

Current recommendations following a positive SLN include completion lymph node dissection and/or radiation therapy [19] (Table 17.3). While there have been no clinical trials comparing local-regional treatments (completion lymph node dissection (CLND) alone, nodal irradiation (NRT) alone, and CLND plus nodal radiation) following a positive SLN, large series single institute studies have not demonstrated a difference in recurrence *or survival outcomes* between local-regional treatment options [29, 30] (Table 17.3). Patients undergoing NRT tend to be older with more medical comorbidities whereas those who undergo both CLND + NRT tend to be

Table 17.3 Management of regional metastatic Merkel cell carcinoma [19, 22, 23]

Clinical scenario	Workup[a]	Surgical approach
SLNB positive	Imaging: CT chest, abdomen, and pelvis PET-CT[a] MRI[b]	Completion lymphadenectomy (CLND) should be offered and discussed Level I–III axillary lymph node dissection Superficial and deep groin dissection Refer to radiation oncology for consideration of treatment to primary site and nodal basin. There may be a role for radiation to the nodal basin instead of CLND in some patients Refer to medical oncology for assessment of adjuvant therapy clinical trial
Clinically positive lymph nodes	FNA or core biopsy Imaging: CT chest, abdomen, and pelvis PET-CT[a] MRI[b]	Therapeutic lymphadenectomy should be offered and discussed Refer to radiation oncology for assessment of adjuvant therapy Refer to medical oncology for assessment of adjuvant therapy clinical trial

SLNB sentinel lymph node biopsy, *FNA* fine-needle aspiration, *CLND* completion lymphadenectomy

[a]PET-CT is gaining importance and may be preferred in some instances

[b]MRI can be used if PET-CT is unavailable

younger with a higher SLN disease burden. No study has demonstrated a significant difference in local-regional recurrence (LRR) in the lymph node basin irrespective of treatment modality. Overall LRR alone occurred in less than 10% of patients across all treatment modalities [25, 29].

While there has been no demonstrated difference in local-regional or distant recurrence or disease-specific survival, CLND offers the advantage over radiation therapy of identifying non-sentinel lymph node positive disease. Non-sentinel lymph node positivity is demonstrated in approximately 32% of patients who undergo CLND and confers a worse prognosis than positive sentinel lymph nodes alone (5 year Merkel cell-specific survival 51% vs. 90% and 5 year disease-free survival 33% vs. 64% after controlling for number of involved lymph nodes) [30].

Metastatic Merkel Cell Carcinoma

Adjuvant Therapy for Merkel Cell Carcinoma

Indications for Post-Operative Radiation Therapy [19]

- Radiation to the primary site*
  - Primary tumour >1 cm in diameter
  - Salvage operation for recurrent disease

  - Positive margins that cannot be surgically re-excised
- Radiation to the nodal basin
  - Absence of surgical assessment of lymph node basin
  - Positive sentinel node without completion of node dissection/ alternative to CLND (Table 17.5)
  - Bulky nodal disease with multiple (4+ axillary and 10+ inguinal) lymph node metastases
  - Extracapsular spread

*can consider omitting adjuvant RT in MCC <1 cm, with negative margins and negative SLN [19, 26].

Table 17.4 Management of distant metastatic Merkel cell carcinoma [19]

Workup	Surgical approach	Systemic therapy
Imaging: CT chest, abdomen, and pelvis PET-CT MRI No specific labs	May be considered for patients with oligometastasis after multidisciplinary tumour board consultation [31] For palliation of symptoms such as bleeding, pain, intestinal obstruction, or perforation of intestinal metastases	Refer to radiation and medical oncology for assessment of combination therapy ± clinical trial enrollment Single-agent immunotherapy: Avelumab Multi-agent chemotherapy: Carboplatin/etoposide Cisplatin/etoposide Cyclophosphamide/doxorubicin/vincristine

Notes: Immunotherapy has recently demonstrated promise for metastatic disease both as a first-line agent and a second-line agent after progression on chemotherapy. There is no data currently combining immunotherapy with radiation therapy. Combining chemotherapy and radiation therapy may provide better palliation of advanced locoregional disease compared to chemotherapy alone

Table 17.5 Radiation therapy for Merkel cell carcinoma

Study	Treatment	Conclusions	Comment
Mojica P et al. [32]	Surgery ± adjuvant RT to the primary site $N = 1187$	OS was significantly increased with adjuvant RT vs. surgery alone	SEER registry data; no information on RFS or DSS RT-treated patients significantly younger than surgery-alone patients
Jouary T et al. [33]	Surgery + RT to the primary site and regional nodal basin vs. surgery + observation $N = 83$	Adjuvant RT associated with improvement in regional recurrence compared to observation (0% vs. 16.7%); no improvement in OS	RCT of patients with stage I disease Prematurely closed due to a drop in recruitment with the advent of SLNB

Table 17.5 (continued)

Study	Treatment	Conclusions	Comment
Bhatia S et al. [34]	Surgery ± adjuvant RT or RT alone (RT alone only 5% of study cohort) to the primary site and regional nodal basin *N* = 6908	Adjuvant RT had significantly improved overall survival compared to surgery alone for localized disease stages I & II but not with nodal involvement (stage III) Relative risk reduction 29% and 23% in stage I/II	Retrospective cohort NCDB registry, no information on DSS Unable to assess RT fields (i.e. local site +/− lymph node basins) which may be key in stage III
Chen et al. [20]	Head and neck MCC surgery ± adjuvant RT or ChemoRT (only 13% of study cohort) to the primary site and regional nodal basin *N* = 4815	Adjuvant RT provided a survival benefit over surgery alone (HR 0.80 [95% CI, 0.70-0.92])	Retrospective cohort NCDB Registry (1998–2011), no information on DSS
Hasan et al. [35]	Surgery ± adjuvant RT/ adjuvant chemoRT to the primary site and regional nodal basin *N* = 4475	Adjuvant RT had significantly improved overall survival compared to surgery alone Reduced recurrence rate (38% surgery alone vs. 23% surgery + RT) and improved 3-year overall survival was 55% with surgery alone and (78%) with surgery + RT	Systematic review of 34 studies All studies were primary Merkel that underwent WLE and either observation or adjuvant therapy RT included both the primary site and lymph node basin
Perez et al. [29]	Surgery (completion lymph node dissection) or RT alone (nodal basin irradiation), or surgery+RT after positive SLN *N* = 71 (CLND = 11, RT alone = 40, CLND + RT = 20)	No difference in DSS or distant metastasis or regional recurrence between groups Regional failure <10% in all treatment arms	Single institute retrospective database (1998–2005) Median f/u 22.3 months Higher burden of nodal disease in combination group, lowest in CLND Limited number of patients in the CLND group
Lee et al. [30]	Surgery (completion lymph node dissection) or RT (nodal basin irradiation) after positive SLN *N* = 163 (CLND = 137, RT = 26)	No difference in DSS, DFS, or regional recurrence between treatments Decreased DSS, DFS, distant recurrence in patients with positive non-SLNs vs. positive SLNs alone	Single institute prospective database (2006–2017) Median f/u 1.9 years Limited number of patients in the RT alone group

RT radiation therapy, *OS* overall survival, *DFS* disease-free survival, *DSS* disease-specific survival, *RFS* recurrence-free survival, *RCT* randomized controlled trial, *CLND* completion lymph node dissection, *SLN* sentinel lymph node

Systemic Therapy for Merkel Cell Carcinoma

While MCC is a chemosensitive disease, there is no evidence supporting the use of chemotherapy as an adjuvant to resected high-risk MCC (stage III) [19, 36, 37]. Similarly, there is limited data around the utility of adjuvant chemotherapy in the setting of resectable local-regional recurrent disease [19, 34]. The use of immunotherapy in the adjuvant setting is currently being investigated.

Despite sparse literature on chemotherapeutic options for MCC, until recently chemotherapy was used at most institutions with or without or radiation therapy for stage IV (distant metastatic disease) [19, 38] (Table 17.4). While MCC does appear to be chemosensitive the response duration is short and patients often experience significant toxicities [14, 39]. Additionally, it is unclear from retrospective studies whether there is a significant survival benefit with palliative chemotherapy particularly given the associated toxicities [4, 14, 34].

Recent emerging data has demonstrated the benefit of immunotherapy in unresectable stage III and Stage IV disease. Both PD-1 (pembrolizumab and nivolumab) and PDL-1 (avelumab) inhibitors have demonstrated high response rates and appear to be much more durable compared to chemotherapy. Pembrolizumab as first-line therapy demonstrated an overall response rate (ORR) of 56% with 2-year progression-free survival of 48% [40, 41]. Avelumab as a first-line agent has demonstrated an objective response rate of 62.1% and when used as second-line treatment an overall response rate (ORR) of 33% with duration >1 year in over 74% of responders [42–44]. Given these findings, immunotherapy is now considered the preferred treatment for metastatic disease [19] (Table 17.4). Enrollment in clinical trials is encouraged whenever available and appropriate, particularly as approval for immunotherapy is not yet widely available.

Referring to Medical Oncology

- All patients with histologically confirmed MCCs, other than those with localized, non-nodal disease should be referred to medical oncology to (1) evaluate the risk of tumour recurrence and (2) to establish the role of systemic therapy. If any doubt exists regarding patient risk stratification, referral to medical oncology is warranted.

Referring to Radiation Oncology

- All patients with histologically confirmed MCCs should be referred to radiation oncology for consideration of adjuvant, neoadjuvant, or primary therapy.

Referring to Multidisciplinary Cancer Conference (MCC)

- All patients with a diagnosis of MCC should be discussed to confirm pathologic diagnosis, and evaluate the indications for adjuvant or therapy.

Toronto Pearls

- The multidisciplinary management of MCCs is the cornerstone of evidence-based treatment.

References

1. Senchenkov A, Moran SL. Merkel cell carcinoma: diagnosis, management, and outcomes. Plast Reconstr Surg. 2013;131(5):771e–8e.
2. Allen PJ, Bowne WB, Jaques DP, Brennan MF, Busam K, Coit DG. Merkel cell carcinoma: prognosis and treatment of patients from a single institution. J Clin Oncol. 2005;23(10):2300–9.
3. Lemos BD, Storer BE, Iyer JG, et al. Pathologic nodal evaluation improves prognostic accuracy in Merkel cell carcinoma: analysis of 5823 cases as the basis of the first consensus staging system. J Am Acad Dermatol. 2010;63(5):751–61.
4. Bichakjian CK, Lowe L, Lao CD, et al. Merkel cell carcinoma: critical review with guidelines for multidisciplinary management. Cancer. 2007;110(1):1–12.
5. Albores-Saavedra J, Batich K, Chable-Montero F, Sagy N, Schwartz AM, Henson DE. Merkel cell carcinoma demographics, morphology, and survival based on 3870 cases: a population based study. J Cutan Pathol. 2010;37(1):20–7.
6. Miller RW, Rabkin CS. Merkel cell and melanoma: etiological similarities and differences. Cancer Epidemiol Biomark Prev. 1999;8:153–8.
7. Agelli M, Clegg LX. Epidemiology of primary Merkel cell carcinoma in the United States. J Am Acad Dermatol. 2003;49:832–41.
8. Bichakjian CK, Nghiem P, Johnson T, Wright CL, Sober AJ. Merkel cell carcinoma. In: American joint of committee on cancer manual. 8th ed; 2017.
9. Iyer JG, Storer BE, Paulson KG, et al. Relationships among primary tumor size, number of involved nodes, and survival for 8044 cases of Merkel cell carcinoma. J Am Acad Dermatol. 2014;70(4):637–43.
10. Heath M, Jaimes N, Lemos B, et al. Clinical characteristics of Merkel cell carcinoma at diagnosis in 195 patients: the AEIOU features. J Am Acad Dermatol. 2008;58(3):375–81.
11. Clarke CA, Robbins HA, Tatalovich Z, et al. Risk of merkel cell carcinoma after solid organ transplantation. J Natl Cancer Inst. 2015;107(2):dju382.
12. Engels EA, Frisch M, Goedert JJ, Biggar RJ, Miller RW. Merkel cell carcinoma and HIV infection. Lancet. 2002;359(9305):497–8.
13. Feng H, Shuda M, Chang Y, Moore PS. Clonal intergration of a polymavirus in human Merkel cell carcinoma. Science. 2008;319(5866):1096–100.
14. Schadendorf D, Lebbe C, Zur Hausen A, et al. Merkel cell carcinoma: epidemiology, prognosis, therapy and unmet medical needs. Eur J Cancer. 2017;71:53–69.
15. Fitzgerald TL, Dennis S, Kachare SD, Vohra NA, Wong JH, Zervos EE. Dramatic increase in the incidence and mortality from Merkle cell carcinaoma in the United States. Am Surg. 2015;81:802–6.

16. Jaeger T, Ring J, Andres C. Histological, immunohistological and clinical features of Merkel cell carcinoma in correlation to Merkel cell polyomavirus status. J Skin Cancer. 2012;2012:983421–5.
17. Harms KL, Healy MA, Nghiem P, et al. Analysis of prognostic factors from 9387 Merkel cell carcinoma cases forms the basis for the new 8th edition AJCC staging system. Ann Surg Oncol. 2016;23(11):3564–71.
18. Medina-Franco H, Urist MM, Fiveash J, Heslin MJ, Bland KI, Beenken SW. Multimodality treatment of Merkel cell carcinoma: case series and literature review of 1024 cases. Ann Surg Oncol. 2000;8(3):204–8.
19. Schmults CD, Blitzblau R, Aasi SZ, Alam M, Andersen JS, Bordeaux J, Bowen GM, Chen P-L. Merkel cell carcinoma. In: National comprehensive cancer network guidelines. National Comprehensive Cancer Network: Fort Washington; 2019.
20. Chen MM, Roman SA, Sosa JA, Judson BL. The role of adjuvant therapy in the management of head and neck merkel cell carcinoma: an analysis of 4815 patients. JAMA Otolaryngol Head Neck Surg. 2015;141(2):137–41.
21. Singh B, Qureshi MM, Truong MT, Sahni D. Demographics and outcomes of stage I and II Merkel cell carcinoma treated with Mohs micrographic surgery compared with wide local excision in the National Cancer Database. J Am Acad Dermatol. 2018;79(1):126–34.. e123
22. Siva S, Byrne K, Seel M, et al. 18F-FDG PET provides high-impact and powerful prognostic stratification in the staging of Merkel cell carcinoma: a 15-year institutional experience. J Nucl Med. 2013;54(8):1223–9.
23. Hawryluk EB, O'Regan KN, Sheehy N, et al. Positron emission tomography/computed tomography imaging in Merkel cell carcinoma: a study of 270 scans in 97 patients at the Dana-Farber/Brigham and Women's Cancer center. J Am Acad Dermatol. 2013;68(4):592–9.
24. Gunaratne DA, Howle JR, Veness MJ. Sentinel lymph node biopsy in Merkel cell carcinoma: a 15-year institutional experience and statistical analysis of 721 reported cases. Br J Dermatol. 2016;174(2):273–81.
25. Fields RC, Busam KJ, Chou JF, et al. Recurrence and survival in patients undergoing sentinel lymph node biopsy for merkel cell carcinoma: analysis of 153 patients from a single institution. Ann Surg Oncol. 2011;18(9):2529–37.
26. Gupta SG, Wang LC, Penas PF, Gellenthin M, Lee SJ, Nghiem P. Sentinel lymph node biopsy for evaluation and treatment of patients with Merkel cell carcinoma: the Dana-Farber experience and meta-analysis of the literature. Arch Dermatol. 2006;142:685–90.
27. Kachare SD, Wong JH, Vohra NA, Zervos EE, Fitzgerald TL. Sentinel lymph node biopsy is associated with improved survival in Merkel cell carcinoma. Ann Surg Oncol. 2014;21(5):1624–30.
28. Mehrany K, Otley CC, Weenig RH, Philips PK, Roenigk RK, Nguyen TH. A meta-analysis of the prognostic significance of sentinel lymph node status in Merkle cell carcinoma. Dermatol Surg. 2002;2002(28):2.
29. Perez MC, Oliver DE, Weitman ES, et al. Management of sentinel lymph node metastasis in Merkel cell carcinoma: completion lymphadenectomy, radiation, or both? Ann Surg Oncol. 2019;26(2):379–85.
30. Lee JS, Durham AB, Bichakjian CK, et al. Completion lymph node dissection or radiation therapy for sentinel node metastasis in Merkel cell carcinoma. Ann Surg Oncol. 2019;26(2):386–94.
31. Gonzalez RJ, Padhya TA, Cherpelis BS, et al. The surgical management of primary and metastatic Merkel cell carcinoma. Curr Probl Cancer. 2010;34(1):77–96.
32. Mojica P, Smith D, Ellenhorn JD. Adjuvant radiation therapy is associated with improved survival in Merkel cell carcinoma of the skin. J Clin Oncol. 2007;25(9):1043–7.
33. Jouary T, Leyral C, Dreno B, et al. Adjuvant prophylactic regional radiotherapy versus observation in stage I Merkel cell carcinoma: a multicentric prospective randomized study. Ann Oncol. 2012;23(4):1074–80.

34. Bhatia S, Storer BE, Iyer JG, et al. Adjuvant radiation therapy and chemotherapy in Merkel cell carcinoma: survival analyses of 6908 cases from the national cancer data base. J Natl Cancer Inst. 2016;108(9):djw042.
35. Hasan S, Liu L, Triplet J, Li Z, Mansur D. The role of post-operative radiation and chemoradiation in Merkel cell carcinoma: a systematic review of the literature. Fronteir Oncology. 2013;3:276.
36. Fields RC, Busam KJ, Chou JF, et al. Recurrence after complete resection and selective use of adjuvant therapy for stage I through III Merkel cell carcinoma. Cancer. 2012;118(13):3311–20.
37. Poulsen MG, Rischin D, Porter I, Walpole E, Harvey J, Hamilton C, Keller J, Tripcony L. Does chemotherapy improve survival in high-risk stage I and II Merkel cell carcinoma of the skin? International Journal of Radiation Oncology. 2006;64(1):114–9.
38. Desch L, Kunstfeld R. Merkel cell carcinoma: chemotherapy and emerging new therapeutic options. J Skin Cancer. 2013;2013:327150.
39. Voog EB, Biron P, Martin JP, Blay JY. Chemotherapy for patients with locally advanced or metastatic Merkel cell carcinoma. Cancer. 1999;85(12):2589–95.
40. Nghiem P, Bhaita S, Lipson EJ, Sharfman WH, Kudchadkar RR, Brohl AS, Friedlander PA, Daud A. Durable tumor regression and overall survival in patients with advanced Merkel cell carcinoma receiving pembrolizumab as first-line therapy. J Clin Oncol. 2019;37(9):693–702.
41. Nghiem PT, Bhatia S, Lipson EJ, Kudchadkar RR, Miller NJ. PD-1 blockade with pembrolizumab in advanced Merkel-cell carcinoma. N Engl J Med. 2016;374(26):2542–52.
42. Kaufman HL, Russell J, Hamid O, et al. Avelumab in patients with chemotherapy-refractory metastatic Merkel cell carcinoma: a multicentre, single-group, open-label, phase 2 trial. Lancet Oncol. 2016;17(10):1374–85.
43. Kaufman HL, Russell JS, Hamid O, et al. Updated efficacy of avelumab in patients with previously treated metastatic Merkel cell carcinoma after >/=1 year of follow-up: JAVELIN Merkel 200, a phase 2 clinical trial. J Immunother Cancer. 2018;6(1):7.
44. D'Angelo SP, Russell J, Lebbe C, et al. Efficacy and safety of first-line avelumab treatment in patients with stage IV metastatic Merkel cell carcinoma: a preplanned interim analysis of a clinical trial. JAMA Oncol. 2018;4(9):e180077.

Neuroendocrine Tumors (Gastroenteropancreatic)

18

Mohammadali Khorasani, Calvin H. L. Law, Sten Myrehaug, Simron Singh, Angela Assal, Eugene Hsieh, Moises Cukier, and Julie Hallet

Introduction

An increasing incidence (per 100,000 population per year) has been reported in multiple recent population-based studies throughout the world. In the USA, the prevalence of neuroendocrine tumors (NETs) is 3.5 per 100,000 [1]. In Ontario, Canada, the incidence of NETs went from 2.48 (1994) to 5.86 (2009) [2]. This increase is likely explained by better detection, diagnosis, and classification [2]. Combined with prolonged survival, this explains that NETs are now more prevalent than esophageal, gastric, and pancreatic carcinoma combined [2–4]. Distribution and survival of various NETs are summarized in Table 18.1.

M. Khorasani
General Surgical Oncology, University of Toronto, Toronto, ON, Canada
e-mail: mohammadali.khorasani@alumni.ubc.ca

C. H. L. Law · J. Hallet (✉)
Department of Surgery, University of Toronto, Toronto, ON, Canada
e-mail: Calvin.Law@sunnybrook.ca; julie.hallet@sunnybrook.ca

S. Myrehaug
Department of Radiation Oncology, University of Toronto, Toronto, ON, Canada
e-mail: sten.myrehaug@sunnybrook.ca

S. Singh · A. Assal
Department of Medicine, University of Toronto, Toronto, ON, Canada
e-mail: simron.singh@sunnybrook.ca; angela.assal@sunnybrook.ca

E. Hsieh
Department of Pathology, University of Toronto, Toronto, ON, Canada
e-mail: eugene.hsieh@sunnybrook.ca

M. Cukier
Department of Surgical Oncology, National Cancer Institute, Panama City, Panama

F. C. Wright et al. (eds.), *Surgical Oncology Manual*,
https://doi.org/10.1007/978-3-030-48363-0_18

Table 18.1 Distribution, presentation, and survival of neuroendocrine tumors [2]

Site	Proportion of all NETs (%)	Metastases at presentation (%)	Metachronous metastases (%)	10-year overall survival (%)
Stomach	5.0	10.6	23	49.7
Small intestine	18.1	34	42.3	51.2
Colon[a]	12.9	22.6	37.6	48.3
Rectum	12.3	3.3	13.3	84.0
Pancreas	9.4	23.4	57.8	30.2
Broncho-pulmonary	25.0	14.3	33.9	49.7
Others	17.3	28.8	50.7	23.1

[a]This group includes appendiceal NET

For the purpose of this chapter, we focus on well-differentiated gastroenteropancreatic (GEP) NETs. Primary pulmonary, thyroid, or thymic NETs and gynecological and poorly differentiated NETs are beyond the scope of this chapter.

Pathological Classification and Grading

- If the histology is suggestive of NET, confirmation of GEP-NET requires immunohistochemistry (IHC) for low molecular keratin and chromogranin, as well as synaptophysin (optional). The neuroendocrine granules contained in the cells stain strongly for chromogranin and most often synaptophysin [5, 6].
- The histological grading system of NETs is determined by both the proliferation index (using the Ki-67 labeling index or the mitotic index) and differentiation. It is most commonly classified according to the World Health Organization (WHO) and UICC/AJCC, which is endorsed by the European Neuroendocrine Tumor Society (ENETS) and the North American Neuroendocrine Tumor Society (NANETS) [7]. This grading system is independent of tumor stage.
- Ki-67 labeling index requires automated or manual counting of 1000 cells. The grade is assigned based on the region with most intensive labeling ("hotspot") [6].
- The most recent WHO grading classification of NETs was updated in 2017 [3] and is summarized in Table 18.2. It includes a new distinction between poorly-differentiated G3 (G3 neuroendocrine *cancers*) and well-differentiated G3. NENs (G3 neuroendocrine *tumors*) recognizes different biology, response to treatment, and prognosis, and was initially developed for pancreatic tumors [30].
- In case of metastatic disease without identified primary tumor, additional IHC can support identification of the primary tumor site (see Table 18.3) [6].

Table 18.2 Derived from 2017 World Health Organization neuroendocrine neoplasm classification [8]

	Differentiation		Criteria
Grade 1 (G1)	Well differentiated (called neuroendocrine tumor)		<2 mitosis/10 HPF <3% Ki-67 index
Grade 2 (G2)	Well differentiated (called neuroendocrine tumor)		3–20% Ki-67 index 2–20 mitosis/10 HPF
Grade 3 (G3)	**Well differentiated** (neuroendocrine tumor)		>20 mitosis/10 HPF >30% Ki-67 index
	Poorly differentiated (neuroendocrine cancer)	Small cells Large cells	>20 mitosis/10 HPF >30% Ki-67 index
Mixed neuroendocrine non-neuroendocrine neoplasms **(MiNEN)**		Combination of neuroendocrine histology with another histology, each accounting for ≥30% of the specimen	Grade is assigned based on grading of the most aggressive histological component

GEP gastroentropancreatic, *NET* neuroendocrine tumor, *GI* gastrointestinal, *Panc* pancreatic, *HPF* high power field

Table 18.3 IHC differential diagnosis of suspected NET

IHC stains	Primary tumor site	Confirmation IHC stains
TTF-1	Thyroid (medullary thyroid carcinoma) Broncho-pulmonary	CEA and calcitonin + in thyroid NET
CDX-2	Small intestine Pancreas	Serotonin + in small intestine. Pancreatic hormones + in pancreas
ISL-1 PDX-1	Pancreas	Pancreatic hormones +
PSAP	Rectum	
Tyrosine hydroxylase (and keratin negative)	Pheochromocytoma Paraganglioma	

Adapted from [6]

Staging

Two TNM staging systems are currently available, the American Joint Committee on Cancer/Union for International Cancer Control (AJCC/UICC) and ENETS [9, 10]. Staging systems are specific to each primary tumor site. The College of American Pathologists (CAP) has based their protocol on the AJCC classification. Neither staging system includes patient-level variables or information on associated endocrinopathy.

- Given the variability in staging systems, it is essential that pathology reports clearly identify the system that was used to classify, grade, and stage the tumor.
- Survival for GEP-NETs is dictated by (1) grade and (2) primary tumor localization, and (3) metastases [1, 2].
- Minimal dataset for pathology reporting of NET include: anatomic site of primary tumor, presence of multicentric disease, immunohistochemistry (IHC) for chromogranin and synaptophysin, grade (proliferation rate assessed by Ki-67 and mitotic rate), presence of other non-neuroendocrine components, lymph node metastases, and their characteristics [11].

Workup

The workup of NETs can be divided into the following:

1. *Primary tumor site and extent of disease*
   (a) Primary tumor site:
   - Cross-sectional imaging:
   - CT C/A/P for pancreas and lungs
   - CT-enterogram for small intestine
   - MRI for pancreas if further assessment required after CT
   - Upper and lower gastrointestinal endoscopy for stomach, colon, and rectum
   - Endoscopic ultrasound for pancreas if further assessment and tissue diagnosis require

   (b) Extent disease
   - Cross-sectional imaging with arterial and venous phases – NETs are typically hypervascular hyperenhancing tumors that require an arterial phase for identification. Liver metastases can be isointense to the normal parenchyma on venous phase and thus overlooked.
   - CT scan C/A/P
   - MRI liver if further assessment of liver metastases required for surgery-Functional imaging (see below)
2. *Grading*
   (a) Tissue diagnosis for histological grade classification
   (b) Functional imaging for biology behavior classification (see below)
3. *Endocrinopathy* (hormonal status)
   (a) Clinical evaluation for functional syndromes
   (b) Biochemical assessment, based on primary tumor site (see below)
   (c) Echo if serotonin secretion

Primary Tumor and Extent of Disease

Imaging and Endoscopy

Initial investigations in the workup of NETs are summarized in Table 18.4.

Table 18.4 Initial workup for NETs

Tumor site	Endoscopy	CT chest	CT triphasic abdo-pelvis	CT enterogram	Biochemical markers	Other
Stomach	Gastroscopy	X	X		Gastrin (off PPI)	Biopsy of antrum to document the presence of atrophic gastritis
Small intestine	Colonoscopy	X	X	X	24 h-u5HIAA	
Appendix	Colonoscopy	X		X	24 h-u5HIAA	Role of video capsule is limited due to risk of obstruction and small luminal size of small intestine NETs
Colon	Colonoscopy	X	X		24 h-u5HIAA	
Rectum	Colonoscopy	X	X		Targeted by symptoms (see below)	If >2 cm or high risk signs[a]: local staging with ERUS or MRI pelvis
Pancreas		X	X		Targeted by symptoms (see below)	MRI pancreas if additional information required after CT scan
Metastases with unknown primary	Gastroscopy Colonoscopy	X	X	X	24 h-u-5HIAA Targeted by symptoms (see below)	MRI pancreas if other investigations negative

[a]High risk sign for rectum NET: ulceration, umbilication, hyperaemia, semi-pedunculated

Special Notes

- CT-enterogram is an important imaging modality to identify primary small bowel NET and synchronous tumors. It should be performed and interpreted in specialized centers, as sensitivity and specificity of the test is related to expertise and volume.
- Over 50% of small bowel NETs are multifocal. Identification of multiple sites of intestinal NETs is important in planning therapy. CT-enterogram is therefore useful for workup of small intestine NETs.
- Unknown primary has been reported in up to 46% of NETs diagnosed initially by identification of distant metastases. Detailed preoperative workup can identify the primary tumor in the majority of those cases. With preoperative workup, 10% of metastatic NETs may not have a primary tumor identified. Surgical exploration, including staging laparoscopy, can identify the primary tumor in half of those cases. It is indicated if identification of the primary tumor will alter surgical or medical management [12, 13].
- MRI of the liver can further define the extent of metastatic disease. It is most useful for: (1) identification of occult metastases when suspected based on endocrinopathy or other clinical signs and (2) detailing number and localization of metastases in planning for maximal surgical cytoreduction.
- The risk of synchronous or metachronous neoplasia in patients with GEP-NETs is 20–25% in contemporary studies [14–16]. It has been suggested that this association could be related to higher detection rate of NET in patients with other cancers as a result of surveillance strategies.

Functional/Somatostatin Receptor-Based Imaging Techniques

- Given many well-differentiated NETs express somatostatin receptors, radiolabeled somatostatin analog can be utilized to produce functional images. The most commonly used somatostatin receptor analog imaging (SRI) techniques are indium-111 pentetreotide scan (OctreoScan) and somatostatin receptor positron emission tomography (SSTR-PET, e.g., 68-Ga DOTATATE PET/CT).
- With improvement in cross-sectional imaging and introduction of new functional imaging modalities (such as SSTR-PET), the role of Octreoscan is limited. SSTR-PET should replace Octreoscan [17].
- Use of SSTR-PET can be useful in the following situations [17]:
  - Staging after initial histologic diagnosis of NET, if the identification of additional disease sites will change management
  - Evaluation of a mass suggestive of NET but not amenable to endoscopic or percutaneous biopsy
  - Staging prior to planned surgery, if the identification of additional disease sites will change the indication or extent of surgery

- Evaluation of unknown primary (after completing other workup)
- Evaluation of patients with biochemical evidence of NET without evidence on conventional imaging, or re-staging of patients with biochemical or clinical evidence of progression without progression on conventional imaging
- New indeterminate lesion on conventional imaging with unclear etiology and not amenable to biopsy

- The avidity of NETs on functional imaging can help assess the tumor biology:
  - As the grade of NENs increases, their somatostatin receptor expression decreases, making grade 3 well-differentiated NETs less likely to be avid on SSTR-PET than their grade counterparts [18].
  - Grade 3 and/or poorly differentiated NENs are more likely to be avid on FDG-PET [18–20].

Grading

- Histology confirmation and grading is necessary for classification and therapeutic decision-making.
- Fine needle aspiration (FNA) can obtain adequate cells for establishing the diagnosis of NENs via performing specific staining and/or IHC.
- Morphological assessment can also be performed on the FNA samples to try to distinguish poorly-differentiated NEC from well-differentiated NETs [5].
- Larger amount of material through core biopsies are usually required for more accurate grading assessment and calculation of mitotic rate or Ki-67 index as analysis on the FNA can underestimate the grade [5, 21, 22].
- IHC profile can be used to identify the primary tumor site and orient workup for patients with distant metastases with unknown primary (see section "Pathological Classification and Grading")

Endocrinopathy

Tumor site		Hormone	Clinical syndrome	Diagnosis
Stomach	Type I	None		
	Type II	Gastrin		
	Type III	Serotonin Histamine	Atypical carcinoid syndrome	Elevated 24-hour u5HIAA Elevated 24-hour urinary N-methyl histamine
	Type IV	Rare		
Small intestine		Serotonin	Carcinoid syndrome	Elevated 24-hour u5HIAA

Tumor site		Hormone	Clinical syndrome	Diagnosis
Pancreas	Insulinoma	Insulin	Whipple's triad: Documented hypoglycemia (BG <3.0 mmol/L) associated with symptoms of hypoglycemia (confusion, sweating, weakness, unconsciousness), and immediate relief with administration of glucose Weight gain	Inappropriately elevated insulin (>20 pmol/L) and C-peptide (>200 pmol/L) when hypoglycemic (<3.0) 48–72 hours supervised fasting test: glucose, insulin, c-peptide, pro-insulin, beta-hydroxybutyrate, sulfonylurea screen, drawn at the time of hypoglycemia(<3.0 mmol/L) Can also assess response to glucagon
	Gastrinoma	Gastrin	Zollinger-Ellison syndrome (ZES): Multiple ulcers Diarrhea (may resolve with PPI)	Elevated fasting serum gastrin (off PPI for 1 week, can use H2 blockers during this period) Usually >200 pg/mL If >1000 pg/mL: diagnostic of ZES unless hypochlorhydria present If <1000 pg/mL: confirm with secretin or calcium simulated gastrin or acidic gastric acid Gastroscopy: Gastric pH <2 (perform off PPI to avoid false negatives) Document peptic ulcer disease
	Glucagonoma	Glucagon	"Sweet" syndrome: 4Ds: Dermatosis (necrolytic migratory erythema) Depression Deep venous thrombosis Diabetes: 40–90% will have glucose intolerance Weight loss	Fasting serum glucagon >500 pg/ml (normal≤50) (check with a blood glucose to rule out a physiologic response to hypoglycemia)
	VIPoma	Vasoactive intestinal peptide (VIP)	Verner-Morrison syndrome: Watery, secretory diarrhea (>700 ml/day) Hypokalemia Hypochlorhydria Hypercalcemia	Elevated serum VIP
	Somatostatinoma	Somatostatin	Secretory diarrhea that persists with fasting Possible steatorrhea (secondary to somatostatin inhibition of digestive enzymes) Cholelithiasis Diabetes Hypochlorhydria	Elevated fasting serum somatostatin
Colon		Serotonin	Carcinoid syndrome	Elevated 24-hour u5HIAA
Rectum		Very rare Histamine		Elevated 24-hour urinary N-methyl histamine

u5HIAA urinary 5-hydroxyindoleacetic acid [23, 24]

Biochemical Testing for Endocrinopathy

- *24-Hour urinary 5-HIAA (U5-HIAA):* 5-Hydroxyindoleacetic acid is an end product of serotonin metabolism and may be elevated in well-differentiated NETs that produce serotonin, most commonly in midgut primary NETs versus rarely in foregut, hindgut, or pancreatic NETs [25].
  - Its levels can be falsely elevated by a variety of foods and medications, which should be avoided when possible before testing [25].
  - In patients with elevated U5-HIAA at diagnosis, this marker can be followed as a marker after treatment [21].
  - All patients with symptoms suggestive of carcinoid syndrome should have U5-HIAA levels checked as the marker to confirm serotonin excess [6] and to monitor effective serotonin inhibition after treatment.
- *Functional pancreatic NETs hormones:* 10% of pancreatic NETs are functional.
  - Routine testing for hypersecretion of pancreatic hormones is not recommended. Biochemical testing should be performed in the presence of clinical signs and symptoms suggestive of a pancreatic endocrine syndrome [6, 21].
  - Hormones should be checked at a fasting state, as secretion is stimulated postprandially
  - Hormone testing needs to be interpreted in the context of the clinical situation. An elevated value is not always pathologic, if it is an appropriate physiologic response.

Carcinoid Syndrome

- *Constellation of symptoms including secretary diarrhea, dry flushing (no sweating), and/or bronchospasm, as a result of excess serotonin in the systemic circulation* [6, 26].
- *Most common primary tumor sites* [6, 26].:
  - *Small intestine*
  - *Colon*
  - *Pancreatic: rarely*
  - *Rectal: rarely*
- *As serotonin is inactivated in the liver, carcinoid syndrome usually occurs in the context of liver metastasis or when the portal circulation is bypassed if there is disease in sites not drained by the portal system (such as retroperitoneum)* [6, 27].
- *20–30% of patients with liver metastases will present clinical carcinoid syndrome* [27].
- *Fibrosis: desmoplastic reaction and fibrosis can develop as a complication of serotonin excess, with or without clinical manifestations of carcinoid syndrome* [28].
  - *Mesenteric and retroperitoneal fibrosis: 50% of patients with midgut NETs and can lead to:*

Intestinal obstruction
Mesenteric angina or ischemia
Mesenteric venous ischemia
Ureteral obstruction

- *Cardiac valvulopathy: 40% of patients with carcinoid syndrome and is due to fibrosis in the right-heart leading to:*
  Pulmonic insufficiency in 50%
  Tricuspid insufficiency in 90%
  Left ventricular dysfunction, if the left heart exposed to serotonin (e.g., lung secretion of serotonin), in 10%
- *All patients with elevated 24 h-u5HIAA should have an echocardiogram to rule out carcinoid heart disease upon diagnosis, and yearly thereafter for follow-up.*

• *Biochemical workup: 24-hour urinary 5-HIAA acid*
  - *24-Hour urinary collection.*
  - *Diet restrictions with a low-amine diet should be followed in days prior and during the collection to ensure accuracy.*

• *Diagnosis:*
  - *Carcinoid syndrome symptoms with elevated 24 h-u5HIAA.*
  - *Patients may have endocrinopathy and functional tumors with hypersecretion of serotonin (elevated 24 h-u5HIAA) without reporting typical symptoms.*

Other Biochemical Markers

• *Serum chromogranin A (CgA)*: It is a protein that is stored in neuroendocrine tissue. Elevated serum CgA levels can be associated with functional or nonfunctional well-differentiated GEP NETs [29].
  - CgA is nonspecific and can be falsely elevated by different medications, foods, and medical conditions [29, 30].
  - CgA alone should not be used for diagnosis of NETs, but with caution, its levels can be used as one of the tools in assessing disease progression, response to treatment, or as a sign of disease recurrence in surveillance [21, 29].
  - CgA level changes should not be used alone as the reason to modify treatment [21, 25].

Management of Gastroenteropancreatic NETs with Locoregional Disease

Goals of Therapy

Incidental Finding

When an NET is identified incidentally, the management should be tailored to the risk of nodal and distant metastases, the morbidity of therapy, and the acceptability/feasibility of monitoring. Clinical observation can be indicated.

Curative Intent

When the disease is localized (local or locoregional), curative intent management can be undertaken. The risk of recurrence is however high, and recurrence can occur over a prolonged period of time [31]. See section below for details regarding recommended surveillance protocols.

Noncurative Intent

Patients with NETs have prolonged survival even with active metastatic disease and can experience complications and deteriorating quality of life from hormonal hypersecretion. It can be considered a "chronic cancer [1].

With metastatic disease, curative intent management is unlikely. Half of liver metastases are not detectable on preoperative imaging and measure <2 mm [32].

Considering the unique characteristics of NETs, the goals of therapy are:

1. Control of tumor burden
2. Control of endocrinopathy/hormonal hypersecretion
3. Prevention of locoregional complications from primary tumor site

Gastric NETs

Characteristics, workup, and management of gastric NET subtypes are summarized in Table 18.5.

Duodenal NETs

Characteristics, workup, and management of duodenal NETs are summarized in Table 18.6.

Special Notes

- Although liver metastases are rare in duodenal NETs, lymph node dissection (LND) is advised if imaging suggests lymph node involvement.
- Duodenal/ampullary NETs are classified separately from jejunal in the eighth edition of AJCC TNM staging (2017)
- Ampullary NETs appear to have a higher nodal metastasis rate even in smaller than 2 cm lesions [38, 39] and may need to be treated more aggressively even when small [36].

Ileal/Jejunal NETs

Characteristics, workup, and management of small bowel NETs are summarized in Table 18.7.

Table 18.5 Characteristics and management of locoregional gastric NETs [21, 33–35]

Type	I	II	III	IV
Frequency	75%	4%	20%	1%
Associated conditions	Atrophic gastritis Pernicious anemia (50%)	ZES MEN-1	Sporadic Atypical carcinoid syndrome	Sporadic
Size and number	<1 cm Multifocal	<2 cm Multifocal	>2 cm Solitary	4-5 cm Solitary
Grade	G1-G2	G1-G2	G3	G3 Poorly differentiated Small cells
Gastrin (off PPI)	Elevated	Elevated	Normal	Normal
Gastric pH (off PPI)	Elevated	Low	Normal	Normal
Nodal metastases	<2%	30%	70%	>75%
Distant metastases	<2%	10–30%	25–75%	50–100%
5-year OS	100%	90%	50%	<10%
Workup	Gastroscopy with biopsy of polyps and *antrum* Fasting serum gastrin (off PPI[a])			
	CT chest-abdo-pelvis	CT chest-abdo-pelvis MRI pancreas +/– EUS Genetics (MEN-1)	CT chest-abdo-pelvis U5HIAA	CT chest-abdo-pelvis
Management	Monitoring: gastroscopy q 1–2 years Lesion ≥1 cm on monitoring: Endoscopic resection Surgical wedge resection if endoscopic not feasible Anemia refractory to medical management: can consider antrectomy (very rare indication)	Management of the gastrinoma	Locoregional: gastrectomy with LND Metastatic: systemic therapy (regimen based on Ki67 and differentiation)	Systemic therapy: cytotoxic chemotherapy (cisplatin-etoposide)

PPI proton pump inhibitors, *ZES* Zollinger–Ellison syndrome, *MEN-1* multiple endocrine neoplasia type 1, *OS* overall survival. *EUS* endoscopic ultrasound

[a]PPI should be stopped at least 7 days prior to measuring serum gastrin

Table 18.6 Characteristics and management of locoregional duodenal NET [2, 36, 37]

Types		**5 types**: Sporadic or gastrinoma occurring in the setting of MEN-1/ZES (most common) Somatostatinomas occurring near ampulla, associated with NF-1 (~18%) Gangliocytic paraganglioma Nonfunctional NET containing serotonin, gastrin, or calcitonin positive cells Neuroendocrine carcinoma
Associated conditions		MEN-1/ZES (40%) NF-1
Nodal metastases		40% Increases with grade, larger tumor size, and higher grade
Distant metastases		Rare
Workup	Lab	24 h u5HIAA Serum gastrin (off PPI) or somatostatin if suggestive clinical manifestations
	Endoscopy	Gastro-duodenoscopy with biopsy: localization and grading
	Imaging	CT chest-abdo-pelvis EUS (define depth of invasion)[a] Consider SSTR-PET if identification of additional disease will alter management
Management	<2 cm Confined to mucosa or submucosa No nodal disease on imaging REF	Endoscopic resection If endoscopic not feasible: Wedge duodenal resection Transduodenal resection if D2/periampullary
	≥2 cm Or when endoscopic criteria not met	Segmental resection with LND Avoid aggressive resection with pancreaticoduodenectomy by performing transduodenal or segmental duodenal resection with LND if possible
	Metastases	Limited role for resection of primary tumor and liver cytoreduction (exception: functional tumors, for palliation of endocrinopathy) See section below on metastatic disease

U5HIAA urinary 5-hydroxyindoleacetic acid, *ZES* Zollinger–Ellison syndrome, *MEN-1* multiple endocrine neoplasia type 1, *NF-1* neurofibromatosis type 1, *LND* lymph node dissection
[a]Gastrinomas can be submucosal, making detection difficult on upper GI endoscopy/EUS

Table 18.7 Characteristics and management of locoregional ileal/jejunal NETs [2, 36, 40]

Nodal metastases		70%
Distant metastases		76%
Workup	Labs	24 h u5HIAA
	Endoscopy	Colonoscopy to rule out synchronous neoplasm
	Imaging	CT chest-abdo-pelvis CT-enterogram, to assess the number and localization of multifocal primary tumors Consider SSTR-PET if identification of additional disease will alter management
Management	Localized (no lymphadenopathy on imaging)	Segmental resection with LND[a]
	Locoregional (mesenteric lymphadenopathy on imaging)	Segmental resection with LND Avoid aggressive extensive small bowel resection to achieve resection of mesenteric mass[a]
	Distant metastases	See section below on metastatic disease

U5HIAA urinary 5-hydroxyindoleacetic, *LND* lymph node dissection
[a]See special notes below

Special Notes

- Consider resection of primary and lymph nodes even if clearly metastatic, for locoregional control, symptom management, and possibly survival benefit [40–42].
- Inspect and palpate the entire small bowel looking for additional tumors:
  - Multifocal tumors are most often located within 100 cm of the ileocecal valve.
  - Tumors are rarely located in the first 100 cm from angle of Treitz [43].
- After initial resection performed in an emergency setting (e.g., for small bowel obstruction), re-image with CT scan to rule out residual/unresected mesenteric nodal disease. Consider resection of residual/unresected mesenteric nodal disease to prevent complications from mesenteric fibrosis.
- Cross-sectional imaging should be used to carefully assess the relationship of mesenteric bulky nodal disease to the superior mesenteric artery/vein in the assessment of resectability. Desmoplasia/fibrosis can make resection of bulky nodal disease more challenging. Mesenteric lymph node metastases are divided into four stages [44]:
  - Stage 1: close to the edge of small bowel NET
  - Stage 2: involve the distal branches of the mesenteric arteries
  - Stage 3: extend proximally on the SMA, without encasement
  - Stage 4: cephalad regional disease, including retropancreatic/retroperitoneal nodal disease, and encasement of the SMA/SMV
- Resection of bulky mesenteric nodal disease may result in ischemia of more length of small bowel than required to clear the primary disease, determining the needed extent of small bowel resection.
  - Avoid extensive small bowel resection.
  - Favor mesenteric-sparing small bowel resection, with "peeling-off" of nodal mass from mesenteric vessels, to limit the length of small bowel resected.

  - If mesenteric nodal disease initially deemed unresectable (e.g., due to proximal localization on superior mesenteric artery), consider referral to specialized center.
- Stage 1–3, and selected stage 4 nodal disease can be resected [40]:
  - Stage 1 and 2: as part of segmental small bowel resection
  - Stage 3: segmental small bowel resection, and separate resection of the proximal nodes along the vessels (incision of the peritoneum and dissection off the vessels up to the root of the mesentery)
  - Stage 4: typically deemed unresectable, depending on localization can be resected in specialized centers.
- Consider sparing the ileocecal valve to reduce the functional impacts of diarrhea (due to post-enterectomy syndrome or carcinoid syndrome).
- Consider cholecystectomy at the time of surgery to avoid subsequent issues with gallstone disease from potential for long-term use of somatostatin analogs and/or ischemic cholecystitis from potential embolization for liver metastases.

Colonic NETs

Characteristics, workup, and management of colonic NETs are summarized in Table 18.8.

Appendiceal NETs

Characteristics, workup, and management of appendiceal NETs are summarized in Table 18.9.

Table 18.8 Characteristics and management of locoregional colonic NETs

Distant metastases [2]		60%
Workup	Labs	24 h u5HIAA
	Endoscopy	Colonoscopy
	Imaging	CT chest-abdo-pelvis Consider SSTR-PET if identification of additional disease will alter management
Management [45]	<2 cm Limited to mucosa or submucosa No lymphadenopathy on imaging	Endoscopic resection with tattoo of resection site [45]
	≥2 cm Or when endoscopic criteria not met	Segmental colectomy with LND – same oncological principles as for colonic adenocarcinoma
	Distant metastases	Limited role for resection of primary tumor and liver cytoreduction (exception: functional tumors, for palliation of endocrinopathy) See section below on metastatic disease

U5HIAA urinary 5-hydroxyindoleacetic, *LND* lymph node dissection

Table 18.9 Characteristics and management of locoregional appendiceal NETs [46]

Workup	Labs	24 h u5HIAA
	Endoscopy	Colonoscopy to rule out synchronous neoplasm
	Imaging	CT chest-abdo-pelvis Consider SSTR-PET if identification of additional disease will alter management
Management	<1 cm No lymphadenopathy on imaging	Appendectomy If incidental finding post-appendectomy: R0 resection: no additional surgery R1 resection: completion surgery, consider partial cecectomy to achieve negative margin
	1–2 cm No lymphadenopathy on imaging	Appendectomy If incidental finding post-appendectomy: No high-risk feature: no additional surgery High-risk feature (G2 or invasion mesoappendix >3 mm): completion right hemicolectomy
	1–2 cm Lymphadenopathy on imaging	Right hemicolectomy If incidental finding post-appendectomy: completion right hemicolectomy
	>2 cm	Right hemicolectomy If incidental finding post-appendectomy: completion right hemicolectomy
	Distant metastases	Same principles as for small bowel NETs

u5HIAA urinary 5-Hydroxyindoleacetic Acid

Special Notes

- Management of appendiceal well-differentiated NETs that are 1–2 cm is controversial.
  - Survival for appendiceal NET is excellent, regardless of whether patients undergo appendectomy or right hemicolectomy [46].
  - The role of right hemicolectomy is to achieve a larger LND, and there is a higher rate of microscopic nodal metastases with right hemicolectomy [46–49].
  - There is no established survival benefit from right hemicolectomy in this subset of patients [46–49].
  - Right hemicolectomy carries a risk of short- (anastomotic leak) and long-term morbidity (functional diarrhea).
  - The risk of nodal metastases is increased if: lymphadenopathy identified on imaging, tumor >1 cm, invasion of mesoappendix >3 mm, and tumor localization at the base of the appendix [46].
  - Therefore, decisions should be personalized for each patient, balancing risks associated with right hemicolectomy and LND against chance of residual disease/recurrence. It is recommended that management of these patients be discussed at multidisciplinary rounds.
- Appendiceal NENs with mixed histology should be treated according to their most aggressive histological component.

Rectal NETs

Characteristics, workup, and management of rectal NETs are summarized in Table 18.10.

Special Notes

- Complete endoscopic excision of incidental well-differentiated rectal NETs that are less than 1 cm may be adequate [21, 53, 54].
- In case of indeterminate margins following endoscopic resection, two options are possible for G1 tumors[48]:
  - Clinical monitoring with sigmoidoscopy and pelvis MRI q 1–2 years for prolonged period time due to long interval to recurrence with indolent biology
  - Completion transanal excision of the scar to clear any residual disease and achieve R0 resection.
  - Patients with complete excision (R0) of T1 rectal NETs do not require further surveillance and can be discharged

Table 18.10 Characteristics and management of locoregional rectal NETs [46, 50–52]

Nodal metastases	T1 (<2 cm invading submucosa)	1%
	T2 (>2 cm invading submucosa, or any size beyond muscularis propria)	26%
	T3/4 (any size invading beyond sub-serosa)	53%
Distant metastases	T1	< 1%
	T2	25%
	T3/4	67%
Workup	Labs	Hormonal testing if clinical manifestation suggestive of endocrinopathy (rare)
	Endoscopy	Colonoscopy with tattoo of site ERUS if need to confirm depth on invasion
	Imaging	CT chest-abdo-pelvis MRI pelvis if need to stage pelvis Consider SSTR-PET if identification of additional disease will alter management
Management	<1 cm No lymphadenopathy on imaging	
	T1	Endoscopic resection Or Transanal excision[a]
	≥T2 Locoregional lymphadenopathy	Total mesorectal excision – same oncological principles as for rectal adenocarcinoma

[a]See special note below

- In case of indeterminate margins following endoscopic resection for G2 tumors: consider transanal excision of the scar/residual disease to ensure complete excision [45].
- Transanal minimally invasive surgery (TAMIS) facilitates transanal excision for rectal NETs with low morbidity [52].
- Management of rectal NETs should be individualized, and discussion at MCC is recommended.

Pancreatic NETs (pNETs)

10% of all pNETs are functional [55].

- Functionality is primarily determined based on clinical symptoms due to excess hormones.
- Biochemical testing is not indicated routinely.
- Biochemical testing is indicated in the presence of symptoms suspicious of endocrinopathy. Screening and confirmatory testing are required to meet all criteria and establish an endocrine diagnosis (See above section Endocrinopathy).
- Note: Endocrinopathy is not defined by positive stains on IHC.

Characteristics, workup, and management of pancreatic NETs subtypes are summarized in Table 18.11.

Special Notes

- *Small nonfunctional PNETs* (<2 cm):
  - *Typical imaging characteristics*: Isodense on noncontrast phase, avidly hyperenhancing on arterial phase, and hyperenhancing on venous phase, homogeneous lesion with smooth contours that does not distort the pancreatic parenchyma. The differential diagnosis is: metastatic renal cell carcinoma or melanoma (associated with history of those malignancies), or solid serous cystadenoma and splenule (benign lesions) [59, 60].
  - *EUS-biopsy* is indicated if there is doubt about diagnosis on imaging. EUS biopsy is limited in accuracy to grade small PNETs due to small tumor size and intratumoral heterogeneity.
  - *Observation is recommended* in small nonfunctional PNETs with no evidence of nodal metastases on imaging. Retrospective analyses indicates growth 0.1 mm/year, favorable long-term survival, no progression to metastatic or unresectable disease, rare need for surgery during follow-up (majority due to patient preference) [61–63].
  - *Monitoring regimen:* [60, 64]

    Cross-sectional imaging at 6 months initially to demonstrate stability

    Thereafter: cross-sectional imaging every 1–2 years

    If the lesion is visible on ultrasound, this modality can also be used for monitoring

Table 18.11 Characteristics and management of locoregional pancreatic NETs [23, 55–58]

		Non-functional		Insulinoma	Gastrinoma	Glucagonoma Somatostatinoma	VIPoma
		<2 cm	>2 cm				
Nodal metastases		6%	30%				
Distant metastases		Rare	60%	10%	60%	80%	80%
Associated conditions – MEN-1		25%		5%	25%	15%	6%
Workup	Labs	As indicated by clinical signs and symptoms		See above section on endocrinopathy work-up			
	Endoscopy	EUS: Localization of small tumors Identification of relationship with pancreatic duct Biopsy (FNA or FNB) for histology diagnosis and grading Note: for small PNET <2 cm, biopsy is not required for observation, as small size limits accuracy of biopsy for histology and grading					
	Imaging	CT chest-abdo-pelvis MRI pancreas Consider SSTR-PET if identification of additional disease will alter management					
Management – surgical		Monitoring[a]: if no clinical lymphadenopathy (imaging)	Surgical resection with LND	Surgical resection: for symptoms, local resection favored[a] Intraoperative ultrasound Blind distal pancreatectomy is not indicated[a]	Hypergastrinemia: PPIs [17] Surgical resection with LND: for symptoms and curative intent to prevent distant metastases	Surgical resection with LND	Surgical resection with LND
Medical management of endocrinopathy		NA		Diet changes (snacks, frequent smaller meals with complex carbs, fat, and protein) Diazoxide Somatostatin analogs Verapamil Afinitor (for side effect of hyperglycemia) Last resort: steroids	Somatostatin analogs High dose PPIs H2 blockers	Somatostatin analogs (glucagonoma only) Management of diabetes Pancreatic enzymes (somatostatinoma)	Somatostatin analogs Volume and electrolyte replacement

LND lymph node dissection
[a]See special notes below

- *Pancreatic sparing resections* (enucleation, central pancreatectomy) can be considered in selected patients with small lesions
  - They have higher rate of postoperative pancreatic fistula but lower rates of long-term endocrine and exocrine insufficiency [65].
  - To consider for insulinoma and gastrinoma without evidence of nodal disease
  - When deciding between observation versus enucleation versus formal resection, location of tumor (head vs. tail), the associated surgical morbidity with surgical resection, patients' wishes, and their comorbidities all need to be taken into account.
  - Ideal candidates are tumors <2 cm in the head (enucleation) or neck (central pancreatectomy) of the pancreas.
- *LND* for PNETs is not associated with better progression-free or overall survival [66]
  - LND is performed for accurate nodal staging.
  - Nodal metastases identified on imaging should be resected, especially for functional tumors.
- *Insulinoma* [64, 67–69]
  - It is an indolent disease – only 5–15% are potentially malignant.
  - Surgery is undertaken mostly to control and prevent complications from the endocrinopathy.
  - 80–90% are isolated and < 2 cm.
  - Endocrine cure is 95–100% with resection, with 10-year recurrence of 6%.
  - If the primary PNET cannot be localized on imaging:

    There is no indication for blind resection of the tail of the pancreas, as the risk is the same throughout the gland.

    Laparoscopic intraoperative ultrasound can be considered in expert centers, as part of the imaging workup.

    The role of formal surgical exploration is limited, considering the low risk of malignancy, the need for extensive mobilization of the pancreas, 10% of lesions are nonvisible and nonpalpable, and the ability to manage symptoms medically.
  - Patients can be effectively managed medically with somatostatin analogs and diazoxide.
  - Benign insulinomas (no nodal or distant metastases) do not require long-term follow-up. Routine surveillance has not been shown to reduce the incidence of relapsing insulinomas [7].
- *Gastrinoma* [70–75]
  - It is an aggressive disease – 60% are malignant and metastases are frequent.
  - MEN-1 patients with gastrinoma have better overall survival than patients with sporadic gastrinoma.
  - Endocrine cure is 50% immediately after resection and 40% at 10 years.
  - If the PNET is localized:

    Surgery is indicated.

    LND is important to improve endocrine cure.

- If the PNET is not localized on imaging:

  Surgical exploration with duodenotomy is extremely rarely needed in contemporary practice.

  Nonlocalized tumors are most often located in the duodenum, small, with lower gastrin levels, and associated with longer overall survival.

  Results of surgical exploration with duodenotomy rely on data from patients treated prior to the introduction of new imaging techniques (1980 to 2000).

  Long-term endocrine cure with exploration is 46% at 10 years.

  Medical therapy with PPI can effectively control hyperacidity and symptoms for up to 20 years.

- *Other rare functional PNETs*: While there are no large series reported, consensus statements and expert opinions are to resect locoregional tumors [64, 68, 76].
- *Local ablation* can be used for symptomatic patients with functional PNETs but not medically fit for surgery. Options include pancreatic radiofrequency ablation, alcohol ablation, or stereotactic ablative radiotherapy (SABR) [78, 79].
- *Aggressive locoregional resection for functional PNETs:* Debulking procedures for locally advanced functional PNETs can be used in selected patients, with the goal to control endocrine symptoms. This has to be discussed in multidisciplinary teams and balance patients' wishes, comorbidities, technical feasibility and risks of the surgical procedure, alternative options for therapy, and response to medical management of the endocrinopathy.

Special cases: PNETs as part of hereditary syndromes [23, 57, 58, 77, 80].

- *MEN-1:*
  - 80–100% will develop non-functioning pNETs.

    54% gastrinomas (>80% duodenal): majority are multifocal

    18% insulinoma

    <5% glucagonoma, somatostatinoma, VIPoma
  - Prognosis:

    0–13% of those pNETs will grow and cause symptoms [14].

    The majority have good prognosis without surgery [13].
  - Surgery:

    Usually not indicated due to low rate of symptoms and growth, good prognosis, and multifocality requiring extensive procedures that may not clear all the disease.

    Indication for surgery: Nonfunctioning PNET >2 cm.
  - If MEN-1 is suspected when working up a PNET: Measure serum calcium and parathormone, as 95% of MEN-1 will have hyperparathyroidism.
  - Associated conditions: Parathyroid adenoma, pituitary adenoma, adrenal tumors, thymic and bronchial NETs.
- *VHL:* [80]
  - Two-thirds will develop pNET.
  - 98% are nonfunctioning PNETs.

- 10–20% develop pheochromocytoma or rare extra-adrenal paragangliomas. Check serum or urine metanephrines, normetanephrines prior to any surgery.
- Prognosis: The natural history of those pNETs is variable, but they are less aggressive than sporadic PNETs.
- Surgery:
  Usually not indicated
  Indications for surgery: >3 cm and with either (1) mutation in exon 3 of the VHL gene or (2) doubling time > 500 days.

Metastatic

Workup and management recommendations for metastatic NETs are summarized in Table 18.12.

Special Notes

- Compared to other cancers, the indolent nature of NET liver metastases and the pattern of growth by pushing rather than infiltrating within the parenchyma makes surgical debulking possible [40].
- NET liver metastases can be divided in *three types:* [81]
  - Type 1: single metastasis
  - Type 2: isolated bulky metastases with smaller bilobar lesions
  - Type 3: disseminated bilobar metastases with no normal liver
- *Benefits of liver debulking:*
  - Reduce tumor burden for symptom control: Endocrine control achieved in 96%
  - Potentially improve efficacy of antiproliferative effects of long-acting somatostatin analogs, by reducing tumor burden.
  - Delay the need for other lines for medical therapy.
- *R0 resection is not achievable for metastatic NETs*
  - Recurrence is expected (>90%) [82, 83].
  - There is no survival benefit in attempting R0 resection.
  - Avoid anatomic or extensive resection with the goal of achieving R0 resection, to preserve function.
- *Goal of liver debulking:* Cytoreduction of 70% of liver metastases. It yields the same results as traditional goal of 90% [84, 85].
- *Contraindications for liver debulking* [40]:
  - Poor performance status
  - Significant liver replacement (>50–70%)
- *Indications and benefits of liver debulking are for small intestinal primary NETs.*
  - For other primaries, the benefits of liver debulking are controversial.
  - Liver debulking can be considered for other *functional* NETs, when benefits of symptom controls are a goal of therapy.
  - *For PNETs:* Liver resection and debulking and extrahepatic metastasectomy are controversial. PNETs have a worse prognosis than small intestinal NETs, are rarely functional, and have fewer long-term local complications. Retrospective series are limited to small samples from single institutions [86].

Table 18.12 Characteristics and management of metastatic GEP-NET

Workup	Labs	24 h-u5hIAA Other depending on primary tumor site and targeted by clinical signs and symptoms (see prior sections)
	Imaging	CT chest-abdo-pelvis MRI liver Consider SSTR-PET if identification of additional disease will alter management
	Endoscopy	Depending on primary tumor site (see prior sections)
	Other	Echocardiogram if elevated u5HIAA
Surgical management	Resectable (debulking possible)	*Liver*: Consider liver debulking to achieve >70% cytoreduction* Use parenchymal-preserving technique and avoid anatomic resections Consider concomitant intraoperative ablation to increase proportion of cytoreduction Combine with medical management *Extrahepatic*: Consider debulking for reduction of tumor burden, local or endocrine symptoms in selected patients with G1 NET, and good performance status[a]
	Unresectable (debulking not possible)	Liver embolization (TAE, TACE, RFA)* Liver ablation (RFA, SABR) Combine with medical management Liver transplantation in selected patients
Medical management (see below for more details)		Long-acting somatostatin analogs Targeted therapy (Afinitor, Sunitinib) Peptide receptor radionuclide therapy (PRRT) Cytotoxic chemotherapy: capecitabine-temozolomide
Resection of primary tumor site if unresectable metastases[a]	Small intestine	Consider
	Pancreas	In highly selected patients
	Colon	Not usually
	Rectum	Not usually

TAE transarterial embolization, *TACE* transarterial chemoembolization, *RFA* radiofrequency ablation, *SABR* stereotactic ablative radiotherapy
[a]See special notes

Resection of metastatic disease for PNETs should be individualized depending on tumor burden, grade, response to prior therapies, and patient age and comorbidities.

Functional PNETs: Consider resection if necessary for symptom control.

Nonfunctional PNETs: No routine resection of metastases – highly selected cases in specialized NETs centers.

- *Technical considerations:*
  - Consider cholecystectomy at the time of surgery for any patient-potential long-term use of somatostatin analogs or eventual need for liver embolization.
  - Liver resection: Parenchymal sparing procedures (PSP) are recommended, including enucleation, wedge resection, and intraoperative ablation [40].
    PSP preserves functional liver parenchyma which ensures patients remain candidates for future procedures upon progression or recurrence (such as repeat surgery, liver embolization, ablation).
    Avoid anatomic resection and/or portal vein embolization in preparation for extensive anatomic resection.
- Liver debulking can be *combined* with:
  - Postoperative ablative therapies (HAE/TACE).
  - Medical therapy with long-acting somatostatin analogs.
  - Limited evidence is currently available on the benefits of multimodal therapy with PRRT.
- *Extrahepatic NETs metastases* [87]:
  - They are not a contraindication to liver debulking, but the burden of extrahepatic disease and morbidity associated with resection should be carefully considered.
  - Cytoreduction of extrahepatic disease can be considered in selected patients with good performance status, G1 tumors, and small bowel NETs primaries.
    Goals of improving symptoms and endocrinopathy, improving local symptoms, reducing tumor burden, and delaying the need for additional lines of medical therapy
    Endocrine response in 70% after surgery
    Favorable long-term outcomes: 77% 5-year overall survival and 51% 5-year progression-free survival
- *Resection of primary tumor in case of unresectable metastases:*
  - Primary PNETs have a different risk profile than small intestinal NETs. Local complications are less common and can be managed nonoperatively (radiation therapy for bleeding and stents for obstruction). Resection of the primary carries higher morbidity and mortality (whipple or distal pancreatectomy).
  - Emerging retrospective studies have suggested a benefit for resection of primary PNETs in the setting of unresectable metastases. Overall survival of resected patients was superior than for patients who were offered resection but declined it [88].
  - Resection of primary PNET with unresectable metastases can be considered in carefully selected cases (lower Ki67, lower liver tumor burden <25%, located in body/tail of pancreas) [88, 89].

Medical Management in NETs

Systemic Therapy: Adjuvant Therapy

There is no evidence for adjuvant therapy following resection of locoregional G1-G2 GEP-NETs.

Systemic Therapy: Somatostatin Analogs

- Somatostatin analogs play two roles in medical management of NETs: (1) symptom control and (2) antiproliferative effect.
- Antiproliferative effect (prolonged progression-free survival) of long-acting forms has been demonstrated in randomized controlled trials for well-differentiated enteric and pancreatic NETs (PROMID trial, CLARINET trial).
- Long-acting agents are the backbone of systemic therapy for NETs and can be used alone or in combination with surgery in case of residual disease, for recurrent disease, or metastatic disease.

Systemic Therapy: Chemotherapy

- Well-differentiated NETs are traditionally resistant to chemotherapy agents, due to slow proliferation. In certain cases such as bulky/progressive disease that is not responding to other treatments, cytotoxic chemotherapy can be considered [60, 90]. However, advances in alternative treatment options such as peptide receptor radionuclide therapy (PRRT) continues to diminish the role of cytotoxic chemotherapy in well-differentiated NETs.
  - Capecitabine–temozolomide can be used for well-differentiated NETs:
    - Benefit in overall and progression-free survival in advanced PNETs in ECOG-ACRIN E2211 randomized trial [91]
    - Activity reported in small phase 2 trials for all NETs liver metastases [92].
  - FOLFOX can be used in selected cases of well-differentiated NETs; some activity has been demonstrated in small phase 2 trials [93].
- For advanced/metastatic high grade (G3) NETs or poorly-differentiated NECs, chemotherapy is the mainstay of treatment. Platinum-based chemotherapy (cisplatin–etoposide) is the regimen of choice [94].

Systemic Therapy: Biologic Agents

- Indicated for metastatic or progressing GI and pancreatic NETs.
- PNETs: Everolimus and Sutent have been associated with improved progression-free survival and overall survival [95–98].
- GI NETs: In a phase 3 randomized placebo-controlled trial (RADIANT-4), everolimus showed improved PFS and better disease control over placebo in advanced non-functional well-differentiated GINET, while maintaining the overall quality of life in these patients [98, 99].

Systemic Therapy: Peptide Receptor Radionuclide Therapy (PRRT)

- For patients with well-differentiated NETs, which are somatostatin receptor positive, PRRT can be utilized as a treatment option.

- Currently, the use is mostly limited to advanced progressive/metastatic well-differentiated NETs that do not respond to long-acting somatostatin analog.
- A phase 3 randomized controlled trial (NETTER-1) of PRRT showed improved PFS, with suggested improved OS at interim analysis when using ^{177}Lu-Dotatate compared to escalation of dose of Octreotide LAR in patients with inoperable somatostatin receptor positive well-differentiated GINET, whose disease was progressing on standard dose of Octreotide LAR [100]. In addition, time to deterioration of quality of life was significantly higher in the ^{177}Lu-Dotatate group [101]. PNETs were not included in this trial.
- The possible applications of PRRT in treatment of advanced somatostatin receptor positive NETs is evolving.

Perioperative Management

Elevated u5HIAA and/or Carcinoid Syndrome

- *Carcinoid heart disease*: Preoperative echocardiogram to rule out carcinoid heart disease prior to general anesthetic:
  - If carcinoid heart disease is identified: refer to cardiology for assessment regarding medical management and valve replacement.
  - If valve replacement is indicated, abdominal surgery should be delayed. In patients with very elevated u5HIAA who need better endocrine control prior to cardiac surgery, alternative nonoperative options can be used, including somatostatin analogs and liver embolization.
  - If valve replacement is not indicated, abdominal surgery can proceed when the patient is deemed optimized by cardiology.
- *Carcinoid crisis*: Physiological stress and tumor manipulation during surgery under general anesthetic can trigger acute release of serotonin leading to carcinoid crisis:
  - Plan for perioperative octreotide administration to control serotonin secretion in patients with elevated u5HIAA [102].
  - If an infusion of octreotide is initiated during surgery: continue for 24 hours and discontinue if patient is hemodynamically stable.
  - Intraoperative crisis occurs in up to one-third of the patients.
  - Other products have also been implicated in carcinoid crisis: bradykinin, kallikrein, and histamine, but are not targeted by perioperative octreotide preparation.

Table 18.13 provides an example of guidelines used for perioperative management of patients with carcinoid syndrome.

Table 18.13 Perioperative clinical preparation for NETs with elevated u5HIAA

Clinical scenario	Preparation
Patients well controlled on long-acting somatostatin analog (20 mg–30 mg IM)	Additional dose of long-acting somatostatin analog 2–3 weeks prior to procedure Supplementary dose of octreotide 250 µg–500 µg SC 1–2 h before procedure Carcinoid crisis with hypotension: Fluid resuscitation Intraoperative octreotide 500 µg–1000 µg IV q5 min, may require infusion 50 µg–200 µg/h Patients who have required supplemental doses intraoperatively should have 50 µg–200 µg/h infusion for 4–24 h postoperatively
Patients poorly controlled on long-acting somatostatin analog	Additional dose of octreotide LAR 60 mg 2–3 weeks prior to procedure Supplementary dose of octreotide IR 500 µg–1000 µg SC 1–2 h before procedure Infusion of 100 µg–250 µg/h starting 1 h before procedure, continue 12–24 h after surgery, wean as tolerated
Patients not on therapy or for emergency surgery	500 µg–1000 µg SC 1–2 h before procedure Consider postoperative infusion 100 µg–250 µg/h

Adapted from: Belo S, Department of Anesthesia. Protocol for Perioperative Management of Patients with Carcinoid Syndrome. Sunnybrook Heath Sciences Centre. University of Toronto. 2011

Functional PNETs [68, 103]

- Carcinoid syndrome is rare with PNET (<50 cases reported).
- *For functional PNETs: the endocrine syndrome should be optimized prior to surgery.*
- *Insulinoma:*
  - Diazoxide: control of hypoglycemia (50–60%)
  - Somatostatin analogs: control insulin hypersecretion (35–50%)
- *Gastrinoma*:
  - PPI: management of hyperacidity and ulcer disease
- Somatostatin analogs: control insulin hypersecretion*Glucagonoma*:
  - Somatostatin analogs: minimize the catabolic state
  - Doppler ultrasound: rule out DVT
  - Management of electrolytes disturbances
  - Management of hyperglycemia
- *VIPoma*:
  - Somatostatin analogs: control diarrhea
  - Management of electrolytes disturbances

Follow-Up

- There is no level-1 evidence regarding the benefits or ideal regimen for surveillance and follow-up of NETs.
- Recommendations for resected primary NETs have been released by the Commonwealth Neuroendocrine Tumors Society (CommNETS) following a

RAND-UCLA appropriateness methods study. These recommendations take into consideration the high rate but slow pace of recurrence in GEP-NETs [31].
- Cumulative incidence of recurrence 48.5% at 10 years.
- Median time to recurrence is 8.7 years for small intestine NET and 7.2 years for PNETs.
- Low and decreasing risk of recurrence after 10 years post-resection.
- Thoracic imaging is not recommended.
- CT scan is the modality of choice. The role of ultrasound and MRI to detect recurrence is not well established, but they can be considered as alternative when it is desirable to avoid CT scan.

• Monitoring of patients with active disease must take into consideration the prolonged survival of GEP-NETs, presence of endocrinopathy, and ability to treat progression of disease (please see Table 18.14).

Table 18.14 Surveillance and monitoring in GEP-NETs

		Modality	Frequency	Consideration for more frequent follow-up[a]
Pancreas – resected		CT abdo-pelvis Nonfunctioning: no lab Functioning: measure of relevant hormonal assay	Q 1 year × 3 years Q 2 years thereafter until 10 years Discuss with patient after 10 years	Higher grade (Ki76 > 5%) Positive lymph nodes
Small intestine **Colon – resected**		CT abdo-pelvis No routine lab	Q 1y × 3 years Q 2 years thereafter until 10 years Discuss with patient after 10 years	Higher grade (Ki67 > 10%) Higher ratio of positive lymph nodes
Appendix – resected	**<1 cm** **Appendectomy**	Low clinical risk: minimal or no follow-up.		G2 >2 cm Positive lymph nodes
	G1 **1-2 cm** **Appendectomy or right hemicolectomy**	CT abdo-pelvis No routine lab	Q 1y × 3 years Q 2 years thereafter until 10 years Discuss with patient after 10 years	

Table 18.14 (continued)

		Modality	Frequency	Consideration for more frequent follow-up[a]
Rectum – resected	**T1** **No nodal disease** **R0 resection**	No follow-up		T2 G2 Positive lymph nodes
	T1 **No nodal disease** **R1 resection or margin unknown**	Sigmoidoscopy	Q 1 year Duration undetermined	
	Others	CT abdo-pelvis No routine lab	Q 1y × 3 years Q 2 years thereafter until 10 years Discuss with patient after 10 years	
Metastatic or visible disease – monitoring (with or without resection)		CT abdo-pelvis CT chest if thoracic disease requiring monitoring Lab: relevant hormonal assay if elevated	Q 6 months Duration: while active disease under treatment	

Adapted from Singh S et al. JAMA Oncol. 2018;4(4):583–5 [31]

[a]Increasing frequency of follow-up may be considered in higher risk cases: q6–12 months x 3 years, and q 1 year thereafter until 10 years, discuss with patient after 10 years

Relevant Publications on the Management of GEP NETs

Study	Methods	Results
RADIANT-4 [98]	**Everolimus** vs. placebo Advanced nonfunctional lung and GINET Phase 3 $N = 302$ Primary end point: PFS	Median PFS 11 vs. 3.9 months. Disease control rate 81 vs. 64% OS not different at median f/u 33 months (HR 0.73, 95% CI 0.48–1.11)
NETTER-1 [100]	**Octreotide LAR** 60 mg vs. 117-Lu Dotatate Somatostatin receptor positive midgut GINET with inoperable disease progressing on octreotide LAR 30 mg) Phase 3 $N = 230$ Primary end point: PFS	Median PFS 8.4 months, but not reached at 30 months yet in 117-Lu Dotatate arm Interim analysis suggested improved OS for 117-Lu Dotatate (HR 0.4; $P = 0.0004$) Higher objective response rate with 117-Lu Dotatate (18% vs. 3%)

(continued)

Study	Methods	Results
PROMID [104]	**Octreotide LAR** 30 mg vs. placebo Newly diagnosed, treatment-naïve patients with well-differentiated (G1) midgut NETs (both functional and nonfunctional) Phase 3 Primary end point: TTP	Median TTP 14.3 vs. 6 months ($p < 0.001$) Reduction of disease progression 66%
CLARINET [105]	**Lanreotide** vs. placebo Metastatic or unresectable, G1 or G2, midgut or hindgut NETs Phase 3 $N = 204$ Primary end point: PFS	Median PFS 18.0 vs. median not reached ($p < 0.001$) 24 months PFS 65.1% vs. 33.0% No difference in OS
RADIANT-3 [106]	**Everolimus** (m-TOR inhibitor) vs. placebo Metastatic or unresectable pancreatica NETs with radiologic progression Phase 3 $N = 410$ Primary end point: PFS	Median PFS 11 vs. 4.6 months ($p < 0.001$) Grade 3 or 4 drug-related adverse events 5%
Sutent Trial [95]	**Sunitinib** (tyrosine kinase inhibitor) vs. placebo Well-differentiated metastatic or unresectable pancreatica NETs and no candidates for surgery Phase 3 $N = 171$ Primary end point: PFS	Median PFS 11.4 vs. 5.5 months ($p < 0.001$) Improved OS (HR 0.42; $p = 0.02$) ORR 9.3% ($p = 0.007$)
CAPTEM [107]	**Capecitabine–Temozolomide** as first line in metastatic well to moderately differentiated pancreatica NET Retrospective $N = 30$ Primary end point: ORR	ORR: 70% Median PFS: 18 months

[a]RADIANT-3, Sutent, and CAPTEM results are applicable only for PNETs; *PFS* progression-free survival, *TTP* time to tumor progression, *ORR* objective response rate, *OS* overall survival

Referring to Medical Oncology

1. All NETs, particularly functional, should ideally be managed in conjunction with medical oncology and/or endocrinology as per individual institution [108].
2. Metastatic disease
3. Unresectable pNETs
4. Any poorly differentiated or high grade (G3) NETs
5. Patients with elevated 5-HIAA or carcinoid syndrome preoperatively
6. Patients with carcinoid syndrome requiring somatostatin analogs for symptom control
7. Candidates for clinical trials

Referring to Radiation Oncology/Interventional Radiology

1. Unresectable and metastatic tumors should be referred for discussion of new radioablative and ablative therapies.

Referring to Multidisciplinary Cancer Conference (MCC)

1. All NETs would benefit from discussion and collaboration with MCC, and ideally, due to their unique needs, would be best managed in a conjoint multidisciplinary clinic [108].

Toronto Pearls

- *Pathology*:
  - Pathology interpretation is crucial to the proper identification of neuroendocrine tumors. Review of pathology by a specialized pathologist can alter the grading and therefore management of patients.
  - IHC can help identify suspected primary NET site in case of metastatic presentations.
  - NETs profile can change over the course of disease, or from one site to another. Repeat biopsies can be considered to better tailor treatment [109].
- *Multidisciplinary clinics* can facilitate access to care and multimodal therapy for NETs. Such team include: surgical oncology, medical oncology, radiation oncology, endocrinology, with supportive services from interventional radiology, radiology, cardiology, psychiatric oncology, clinical nutrition, and nursing [108].
- *Surgery*:
  - Surgery has a role in the management of locoregional and metastatic NETs, even with large burden of metastatic disease, but 60% never see a surgeon [110]. All patients with NETs should be assessed by a surgeon with expertise in management of those patients.
  - Treatment of primary neuroendocrine tumors does require some experience in order to ensure that maximum but not over-aggressive LND is done, particularly to intestinal NETs. Mesentery-sparing resections are favored over resection of large extent of intestine, in order to minimize functional impact while ensuring resection of the disease.
  - Surgical therapy of neuroendocrine liver metastases is very different from the strategies used for other cancers, and parenchymal preservation is a very important principle of treatment. Anatomical liver resections should be avoided [111].
  - Cytoreductive surgery for metastatic NETs plays an important therapy-sparing role in the sequencing of therapies. By reducing tumor burden and symptoms, cytoreduction can delay the need to escalate medical therapy,

thereby maintaining treatment options for a longer period of time. This is crucial when managing a chronic malignancy.

- *Multimodal therapy* is key in NETs. Surgical, medical, and ablative therapies can be combined and sequenced for maximal effect for patients.
  - Sequencing of therapies will take place over several years [108].
  - When discussing treatment options and sequencing, it is important to consider tumor grade, primary tumor site, endocrine symptoms, and tumor burden, as well as sparing therapies for the future and not compromising eligibility for future therapies.
  - Treatment options should be re-evaluated at each visit.
- *Patient support*: Serotonin secretion in NETs can be associated with neuropsychological symptoms, including subclinical cognitive and depressive disorders, even when 24 h-u5HIAA is below detectable levels. Patient support should include screening for those symptomatic involvement of psychology or psychiatric oncology services [112, 113].
- *Protocol for liver embolization:*
  - Give 100 μg octreotide iv bolus prior to procedure in angiography holding area (100 μg in 50 ml NS over 10 min).
  - Start continuous infusion of octreotide at 50 μg/h (500 μg in 100 ml NS, i.e., 10 ml/h) for duration of procedure.
  - After 6 h from the start of octreotide infusion, decrease rate to 5 ml/h.
  - Stop infusion after the bag is finished unless patient is clinically symptomatic (e.g., flushing, palpitations, alteration of mental status, diarrhea, wheezing) or vital signs are abnormal.
- *Radiation therapy:*
  - Delivery of *PRRT* requires the use of up-to-date agents, an experienced team, and careful dosimetry.
  - *Radiation* therapy remains an important component of management of GEP-NETs, including all metastatic neuroendocrine tumors. In patients with good performance status, consider ablative approaches to maximize local control, even in the context of metastatic disease.

References

1. Dasari A, Shen C, Halperin D, et al. Trends in the incidence, prevalence, and survival outcomes in patients with neuroendocrine tumors in the United States. JAMA Oncol. 2017;3:1335.
2. Hallet J, Law CH, Cukier M, et al. Exploring the rising incidence of neuroendocrine tumors: a population-based analysis of epidemiology, metastatic presentation, and outcomes. Cancer. 2015;121:589.
3. National Cancer Institute Surveillance, Epidemiology, End Results Program. Cancer Stat Facts [Internet]. National Institutes Heal [Cited 2017 Nov]. Available from https://doi.org/10.1007/SeerCancerGov/Statfacts.
4. Kunz PL. Understanding neuroendocrine tumors – a NET gain. JAMA Oncol. 2017;3:1343–4.
5. Parren A, Couvelard A, Scoazec J, et al. ENETS consensus guidelines for the standards of care in neuroendocrine tumors: pathology, diagnosis and prognostic stratification. Neuroendocrinology. 2017;105:196–200.

6. Singh S, Asa SL, Dey C, et al. Diagnosis and management of gastrointestinal neuroendocrine tumors: an evidence-based Canadian consensus. Cancer Treat Rev. 2016;47:32–45.
7. Boudreaux JP, Klimstra DS, Hassan MM, et al. The NANETS consensus guideline for the diagnosis and management of neuroendocrine tumors: well-differentiated neuroendocrine tumors of the jejunum, ileum, appendix, and cecum. Pancreas. 2010;39:753–66.
8. Rindi G, Klimstra DS, Abedi-Ardekani B, Asa SL, Bosman FT, Brambilla E, et al. A common classification framework for neuroendocrine neoplasms: an International Agency for Research on Cancer (IARC) and World Health Organization (WHO) expert consensus proposal. Mod Pathol. 2018;31:1770–86.
9. Rindi G, Kloppel G, Ahlmann H, et al. TNM staging of foregut (neuro)endocrine tumors: a consensus proposal including a grading system. Virchows Arch. 2006;449:395.
10. Amin MB, Edge S, Greene F, et al. AJCC cancer staging manual. 8th ed. New York: Springer; 2017.
11. Klimstra DS, Modlin IR, Adsay NV, et al. Pathology reporting of neuroendocrine tumors: application of the Delphic consensus process to the development of a minimum pathology data set. Am J Surg Pathol. 2010;34:300–13.
12. Keck KJ, Maxwell JE, Menda Y, et al. Identification of primary tumors in patients presenting with metastatic gastroenteropancreatic neuroendocrine tumors. Surgery. 2017;161:272–9.
13. Massimino KP, Han E, Pommier SJ, Pommier RF. Laparoscopic surgical exploration is an effective strategy for locating occult primary neuroendocrine tumors. Am J Surg. 2012;203:628–31.
14. Clift AK, Drymousis P, Al-Nahhas A, et al. Incidence of second primary malignancies in patients with neuroendocrine tumours. Neuroendocrinology. 2015;102:26–32.
15. Kamp K, Damhuis RA, Feelders RA, et al. Occurrence of second primary malignancies in patients with neuroendocrine tumors of the digestive tract and pancreas. Endocr Relat Cancer. 2012;19:95–9.
16. Kauffmann RM, Wang L, Phillips S, et al. Incidence of additional primary malignancies in patients with pancreatic and gastrointestinal neuroendocrine tumors. Ann Surg Oncol. 2014;21:3422–8.
17. Hope TA, Bergsland EK, Bozkurt MF, Graham M, Heaney AP, Herrmann K, et al. Appropriate use criteria for somatostatin receptor pet imaging in neuroendocrine tumors. J Nucl Med. 2017;59:66–74.
18. Sundin A, Arnold R, Baudin E, et al. ENETS consensus guidelines for the standards of care in neuroendocrine tumors: radiological, nuclear medicine & hybrid imaging. Neuroendocrinology. 2017;105:212–44.
19. Squires MH 3rd, Volkan Adsay N, Schuster DM, et al. Octreoscan versus FDG-PET for neuroendocrine tumor staging: a biological approach. Ann Surg Oncol. 2015;22:2295.
20. Hicks RJ. Use of molecular targeted agents for the diagnosis, staging and therapy of neuroendocrine malignancy. Cancer Imaging. 2010;10:Spec no A:S83–91.
21. National Comprehensive Cancer Network. NCCN Clinical Practice Guideline in Oncology Gastric Cancer v2.2018. http://www.nccn.org/professionals/physician_gls/pdf/gastric.pdf.
22. Vinayek R, LA Capurso G. Grading of EUS-FNA cytologic specimens from patients with pancreatic neuroendocrine neoplasms: it is time move to tissue core biopsy? Gland Surg. 2014;3:222–5.
23. Kulke M, Anthony L, Bushnell D, et al. NANETS treatment guidelines: well-differentiated neuroendocrine tumors of the stomach and pancreas. Pancreas. 2010;39:735–52.
24. Ramage JK, Ahmed A, Ardill J, Bax N, Breen DJ, Caplin ME, et al. Guidelines for the management of gastroenteropancreatic neuroendocrine (including carcinoid) tumours (NETs). Gut. 2012;61:6–32.
25. Knigge U, Capdevila J, Bartsch DK, et al. ENETS consensus recommendations for the standards of care in neuroendocrine neoplasms: follow-up and documentation. Neuroendocrinology. 2017;105:310–9.
26. Soga J. Carcinoids and their variant endocrinomas. An analysis of 11,842 reported cases. J Exp Clin Cancer Res. 2003;22:517–30.
27. Kaltsas G, Caplin M, Davies P, et al. ENETS consensus guidelines for the standards of care in neuroendocrine tumors: pre- and perioperative therapy in patients with neuroendocrine tumors. Neuroendocrinology. 2017;105:245–54.

28. Laskaratos FM, Rombouts K, Caplin M, et al. Neuroendocrine tumors and fibrosis: an unsolved mystery? Cancer. 2017;123:4770–90.
29. Oberg K, Couvelard A, Delle Fave G, et al. ENETS consensus guidelines for standard of care in neuroendocrine tumours: biochemical markers. Neuroendorinology. 2017;105:201–11.
30. Fossmark R, Jianu CS, Martinsen TC, et al. Serum gastrin and chromogranin a levels in patients with fundic gland polyps caused by long-term proton-pump inhibition. Scand J Gastroenterol. 2008;43(1):20–4.
31. Singh S, Moody L, Chan DL, Metz DC, Strosberg J, Asmis T, et al. Follow-up recommendations for completely resected gastroenteropancreatic neuroendocrine tumors. JAMA Oncol. 2018;4:1597.
32. Elias D, Lefevre JH, Duvillard P, et al. Hepatic metastases from neuroendocrine tumors with a "thin slice" pathological examination. Ann Surg. 2010;251:307–10.
33. Ozao-Choy J, Buch K, Strauchen JA, et al. Laparoscopic antrectomy for the treatment of type I gastric carcinoid tumors. J Surg Res. 2010;162:22.
34. Dakin GF, Warner RR, Pomp A, et al. Presentation, treatment, and outcome of type 1 gastric carcinoid tumors. J Surg Oncol. 2006;93:368.
35. Fave GD, O'Toole D, Sundin A, et al. ENETS consensus guidelines update for gastroduodenal neuroendocrine neoplasms. Neuroendocrinology. 2016;103:119–24.
36. Delle Fave G, Kwekkeboom DJ, Van Cutsem E, et al. ENETS consensus guidelines for the management of patients with gastroduodenal neoplasms. Neuroendocrinology. 2012;95:74–87.
37. Kim GH, Kim J II, Jeon SW, et al. Endoscopic resection for duodenal carcinoid tumors: a multicenter, retrospective study. J Gastroenterol Hepatol. 2014;29:318–24.
38. Poultsides GAFW. Carcinoid of the ampulla of Vater: morphologic features and clinical implications. World J Gastroenterol. 2006;12:7058.
39. Carter JT, Grenert JP, Rubenstein L, et al. Neuroendocrine tumors of the ampulla of Vater: biological behavior and surgical managemen. Arch Surg. 2009;144:527.
40. Howe JR, Cardona K, Fraker DL, et al. The surgical management of small bowel neuroendocrine tumors: consensus guidelines of the north American neuroendocrine tumor society. Pancreas. 2017;46:715.
41. Sharpe SM, In H, Winchester DJ, et al. Surgical resection provides an overall survival benefit for patients with small pancreatic neuroendocrine tumors. J Gastrointest Surg. 2015;19:117.
42. Partelli S, Bartsch DK, Capdevila J, et al. ENETS consensus guidelines for standard of care in neuroendocrine tumours: surgery for small intestinal and pancreatic neuroendocrine tumours. Neuroendocrinology. 2017;105:255–65.
43. Keck KJ, Maxwell JE, Utria AF, et al. The distal predilection of small bowel neuroendocrine tumors. Ann Surg Oncol. 2018;25:3207–13.
44. Öhrvall U, Eriksson B, Juhlin C, et al. Method for dissection of mesenteric metastases in mid-gut carcinoid tumors. World J Surg. 2000;24:1402–8.
45. Caplin M, Sundin A, Nilson O, et al. ENETS consensus guidelines for the management of patients with digestive neuroendocrineneoplasms: colorectal neuroendocrine neoplasms. Neuroendocrinology. 2012;95:88–97.
46. Pape UF, Niederle B, Costa F, et al. ENETS consensus guidelines for neuroendocrine neoplasms of the appendix (excluding goblet cell carcinomas). Neuroendocrinology. 2016;103:144–52.
47. Kleiman DA, Finnerty B, Beninato T, et al. Features associated with metastasis among well-differentiated neuroendocrine (carcinoid) tumors of the appendix: significance of small vessel invasion in addition to size. Dis Colon Rectum. 2015;58:1137.
48. Lamberti G, Brighi N, Campana D, et al. Current management and predictive factors of lymph node metastasis of appendix neuroendocrine tumors. A national study from the French Group of Endocrine Tumors (GTE). Ann Surg. 2018;270:165.
49. Brighi N, La Rosa S, Rossi G, et al. Morphological factors related to nodal metastases in neuroendocrine tumors of the appendix: a multicentric retrospective study. Ann Surg. 2018;271:527.

50. Weinstock B, Ward SC, Harpaz N, Warner RRP, Itzkowitz S, Kim MK. Clinical and prognostic features of rectal neuroendocrine tumors. Neuroendocrinology. 2013;98:180–7.
51. McConnell YJ. Surgical management of rectal carcinoids: trends and outcomes from the surveillance, epidemiology, and end results database (1988 to 2012). Am J Surg. 2016;211:877–85.
52. Chan D, Law C, Hallet J, et al. Trans-anal minimally invasive surgery for completion excision of well-differentiated rectal neuroendocrine tumours. Pancreas. 2018;47:334.
53. Kwak MS, Chung SJ, Yang JI, et al. Long-term outcome of small, incidentally detected rectal neuroendocrine tumors removed by simple excisional biopsy compared with the advanced endoscopic resection during screening colonoscopy. Dis Colon Rectum. 2018;61(3):338–46.
54. Kim GU, Kim KJ, Hong SM, et al. Clinical outcomes of rectal neuroendocrine tumors ≤ 10 mm following endoscopic resection. Endoscopy. 2013;45(12):1018–23.
55. Falconi M, Bartsch DK, Eriksson B, et al. ENETS consensus guidelines for the management of patients with digestive neuroendocrine neoplasms of the digestive system: well-differentiated pancreatic non-functioning tumors. Neuroendocrinology. 2012;95:120–34.
56. Partelli S, Gaujoux S, Boninsegna L, et al. Pattern and clinical predictors of lymph node involvement in nonfunctioning pancreatic neuroendocrine tumors (NF-PanNETs). JAMA Surg. 2013;148:932–9.
57. de Herder W, Niederle B, Scoazec J, et al. Well-differentiated pancreatic tumor/carcinoma: insulinoma. Neuroendocrinology. 2006;84(3):183–8.
58. Jensen R, Niederle B, Mitry E, et al. Gastrinoma (duodenal and pancreatic). Neuroendocrinology. 2006;84(3):173–82.
59. Noone TC, Hosey J, Zeynep F, Semelka RC. Imaging and localization of islet-cell tumours of the pancreas on CT and MRI. Best Pract Res Clin Endocrinol Metab. 2005;19:195–211.
60. Singh S, Dey C, Kennecke H, et al. Consensus recommendations for the diagnosis and management of pancreatic neuroendocrine tumors: guidelines from a Canadian National Expert Group. Ann Surg Onco. 2015;22:2685–99.
61. Sadot E, Reidy-Lagunes DL, Tang LH, et al. Observation versus resection for small asymptomatic pancreatic neuroendocrine tumors: a matched case-control study. Ann Surg Oncol. 2016;23(4):1361–70.
62. Gaujoux S, Partelli S, Maire F, et al. Observational study of natural history of small sporadic nonfunctioning pancreatic neuroendocrine tumors. J Clin Endocrinol Metab. 2013;98(12):4784–9.
63. Yohanathan L, Dossa F, St Germain AT, et al. Management and surveillance of non-functional pancreatic neuroendocrine tumours: retrospective review. Pancreatology. 2019;19(2):360–6.
64. Falconi M, Eriksson B, Kaltsas G, et al. ENETS consensus guidelines update for the management of patients with functional pancreatic neuroendocrine tumors and non-functional pancreatic neuroendocrine tumors. Neuroendocrinology. 2016;103:153–71.
65. Cherif R, Gaujoux S, Couvelard A, et al. Parenchyma-sparing resections for pancreatic neuroendocrine tumors. J Gastrointest Surg. 2012;16:2045–55.
66. Conrad C, Kutlu OC, Dasari A, et al. Prognostic value of lymph node status and extent of lymphadenectomy in pancreatic neuroendocrine tumors confined to and extending beyond the pancreas. J Gastrointest Surg. 2016;20:1966–74.
67. Mehrabi A, Fischer L, Hafezi M, et al. A systematic review of localization, surgical treatment options, and outcome of insulinoma. Pancreas. 2014;43:675–86.
68. Chiruvella A, Kooby DA. Surgical management of pancreatic neuroendocrine tumors. Surg Oncol Clin N Am. 2016;25(2):401–21.
69. Service FJ, McMahon MM, O'Brien PC, et al. Functioning insulinoma–incidence, recurrence, and long-term survival of patients: a 60-year study. Mayo Clin Proc. 1991;66(7):711–9.
70. Norton JA, Fraker DL, Alexander HR, et al. Surgery increases survival in patients with gastrinoma. Ann Surg. 2006;244(3):410–9.
71. Bartsch DK, Waldmann J, Fendrich, et al. Impact of lymphadenectomy on survival after surgery for sporadic gastrinoma. Br J Surg. 2012;99(9):1234–40.
72. Norton JA, Fraker DL, Alexander HR, et al. Value of surgery in patients with negative imaging and sporadic Zollinger-Ellison syndrome. Ann Surg. 2012;256(3):509–17.

73. Norton JA, Alexander HR, Fraker DL, et al. Does the use of routine duodenotomy (DUODX) affect rate of cure, development of liver metastases, or survival in patients with Zollinger-Ellison syndrome? Ann Surg. 2004;239(5):617–25.
74. Yu F, Venzon DJ, Serrano J, et al. Prospective study of the clinical course, prognostic factors, causes of death, and survival in patients with long-standing Zollinger-Ellison syndrome. J Clin Oncol. 1999;17(2):615–30.
75. Ito T, Igarashi H, Jensen RT. Pancreatic neuroendocrine tumors: clinical features, diagnosis and medical treatment: advances. Best Pr Res Clin Gastroenterol. 2012;26(6):737–53.
76. Knigge U, Hansen CP. Surgery for GEP-NETs. Best Pr Res Clin Gastroenterol. 2012;26(6):819–31.
77. Falconi M, Plockinger U, Kwekkeboom D, et al. Well-differentiated pancreatic non-functioning tumors/carcinoma: ENETS guidelines. Neuroendocrinology. 2006;84:196–211.
78. Jürgensen C, Schuppan D, Neser F, et al. EUS-guided alcohol ablation of an insulinoma. Gastrointest Endosc. 2006;63(7):1059–62.
79. Limmer S, Huppert PE, Juette V, et al. Radiofrequency ablation of solitary pancreatic insulinoma in a patient with episodes of severe hypoglycemia. Eur J Gastroenterol Hepatol. 2009;21(9):1097–101.
80. Keutgen XM, Hammel P, Choyke PL, et al. Evaluation and management of pancreatic lesions in patients with von Hippel-Lindau disease. Nat Rev Clin Oncol. 2016;13(9):537–49.
81. Frilling A, Li J, Malamutmann E, et al. Treatment of liver metastases from neuroendocrine tumours in relation to the extent of hepatic disease. Br J Surg. 2009;96(2):175–84.
82. Sarmiento JM, Heywood G, Rubin J, et al. Surgical treatment of neuroendocrine metastases to the liver: a plea for resection to increase survival. J Am Coll Surg. 2003;197:29–37.
83. Mayo SC, de Jong MC, Pulitano C, et al. Surgical management of hepatic neuroendocrine tumor metastasis: results from an international multi-institutional analysis. Ann Surg Oncol. 2010;17(12):3129–36.
84. Maxwell JE, Sherman SK, O'Dorisio TM, et al. Liver-directed surgery of neuroendocrine metastases: what is the optimal strategy? Surgery. 2016;159:320–33.
85. Graff-Baker AN, Sauer DA, Pommier SJ, et al. Expanded criteria for carcinoid liver debulking: maintaining survival and increasing the number of eligible patients. Surgery. 2014;156(6):1369–76; discussion 1376–7
86. Morgan RE, Pommier SJ, Pommier RF. Expanded criteria for debulking of liver metastasis also apply to pancreatic neuroendocrine tumors. Surgery. 2018;163(1):218–25.
87. Chan DL, Dixon M, Law CHL, et al. Outcomes of cytoreductive surgery for metastatic low-grade neuroendocrine tumors in the setting of extrahepatic metastases. Ann Surg Oncol. 2018;25(6):1768–74.
88. Bertani E, Fazio N, Radice D, et al. Assessing the role of primary tumour resection in patients with synchronous unresectable liver metastases from pancreatic neuroendocrine tumour of the body and tail. A propensity score survival evaluation. Eur J Surg Oncol. 2017;43(2):372–9.
89. Hüttner FJ, Schneider L, Tarantino I, et al. Palliative resection of the primary tumor in 442 metastasized neuroendocrine tumors of the pancreas: a population-based, propensity score-matched survival analysis. Langenbeck's Arch Surg. 2015;400(6):715–23.
90. Garcia-Carbonero R, Rinke A, Valle JW, et al. ENETS consensus guidelines for the standards of care in neuroendocrine neoplasms. Systemic therapy 2: chemotherapy. Neuroendocrinology. 2017;105:281–94.
91. Kunz PL, Catalano PJ, Nimeiri H, et al. A randomized study of temozolomide or temozolomide and capecitabine in patients with advanced pancreatic neuroendocrine tumors: a trial of the ECOG-ACRIN Cancer Research Group (E2211). J Clin Oncol. 2018;36 no. 15_suppl:4004.
92. Fine RL, Gulati AP, Krantz BA, et al. Capecitabine and temozolomide (CAPTEM) for metastatic, well-differentiated neuroendocrine cancers: the pancreas Center at Columbia University experience. Cancer Chemother Pharmacol. 2013;71(3):663–70.
93. Kunz PL, Balise RR, Fehrenbacher L, et al. Oxaliplatin-fluoropyrimidine chemotherapy plus bevacizumab in advanced neuroendocrine tumors: an analysis of 2 phase II trials. Pancrea. 2016;45:1394.

94. Moertel CG, Lefkopoulo M, Lipsity S, et al. Streptozocin-doxorubicin, streptozocin-fluorouracil or chlorozotocin in the treatment of advanced islet-cell carcinoma. N Engl J Med. 1992;326:519–23.
95. Raymond E, Dahan L, Raoul JL, et al. Sunitinib malate for the treatment of pancreatic neuroendocrine tumors. N Engl J Med. 2011;364:501.
96. Faivre S, Niccoli P, Castellano D, et al. Sunitinib in pancreatic neuroendocrine tumors: updated progression-free survival and final overall survival from a phase III randomized study. 2017;28(2):339–43.
97. Yao JC, Shah MH, Ito T, et al. Everolimus for advanced pancreatic neuroendocrine tumors. N Engl J Med. 2011;364:514.
98. Yao J, Fazio N, Singh S, et al. Everolimus (EVE) in advanced, nonfunctional, well-differentiated neuroendocrine tumors (NET) of gastrointestinal (GI) or lung origin: second interim overall survival (OS) results from the RADIANT-4 study. J Clin Oncol. 2016;34 no. 15_suppl:4090.
99. Pavel ME, Singh S, Strosberg JR, et al. Health-related quality of life for everolimus versus placebo in patients with advanced, non-functional, well-differentiated gastrointestinal or lung neuroendocrine tumours (RADIANT-4): a multicentre, randomised, double-blind, placebo-controlled, phase 3 trial. Lancet Oncol. 2017;18:1411–22.
100. Strosberg J, El-Haddad G, Wolin E, et al. Phase 3 trial of (177)Lu-dotatate for midgut neuroendocrine tumors. N Engl J Med. 2017;376:125.
101. Brabander T, Van der Zwan WA, Teunissen JJ, et al. Long-term efficacy, survival and safety of [177Lu-DOTA0,Tyr3]octreotate in patients with gastroenteropancreatic and bronchial neuroendocrine tumors. Clin Cancer Res. 2017;23(16):4617–24.
102. Condron ME, Jameson NE, Limbach KE, et al. A prospective study of the pathophysiology of carcinoid crisis. Surgery. 2019;165(1):158–65.
103. Massimino K, Harrskog O, Pommier S, et al. Octreotide LAR and bolus octreotide are insufficient for preventing intraoperative complications in carcinoid patients. J Surg Oncol. 2013;107(8):842–6.
104. Rinke A, Müller HH, Schade-Brittinger C, et al. Placebo-controlled, double-blind, prospective, randomized study on the effect of octreotide LAR in the control of tumor growth in patients with metastatic neuroendocrine midgut tumors: a report from the promid study group. J Clin Oncol. 2009;27:4656–63.
105. Caplin ME, Pavel M, Cwikla JB, et al. Lanreotide in metastatic enteropancreatic neuroendocrine tumors. N Engl J Med. 2014;371:224–33.
106. Yao JC, Shah MH, Ito T, et al. RAD001 in advanced neuroendocrine tumors, third trial (RADIANT-3) study group. Everolimus for advanced pancreatic neuroendocrine tumors. N Engl J Med. 2011;364:514–23.
107. Strosberg JR, Fine RL, Choi J, et al. First-line chemotherapy with capecitabine and temozolomide in patients with metastatic pancreatic endocrine carcinomas. Cancer. 2011;117:268–75.
108. Singh S, Law C. Multidisciplinary reference centers: the care of neuroendocrine tumors. J Oncol Pr. 2010;6:e11–6.
109. Singh S, Hallet J, Rowsell C, Law C, et al. Variability of Ki67 labeling index in multiple neuroendocrine tumors specimens over the course of the disease. Eur J Surg Oncol. 2014;40:1517–22.
110. Hallet J, Singh S, Law C. Healthcare utilization in the pre-diagnostic period for neuroendocrine tumors. Ann Surg Oncol. 2014;21:S97.
111. Nadler A, Cukier M, Milot L, et al. Hepatic parenchymal preserving technique in the management of diffuse bilateral neuroendocrine tumour liver metastases: a feasible approach. Can J Surg Can J Surg. 2014;57:e2–8.
112. Hallet J, Davis L, Mahar AL, et al. Symptom burden at the end of life for neuroendocrine tumors: a population-based analysis of patient-reported outcomes. The Oncologist. 2019;24:1384–94.
113. Hallet J, Isenberg-Grzeda E, Kazdan J, et al. Integrating patient reported outcomes (PROs) in Neuroendocrine Tumors (NETs) care: an assessment of cognitive and psychological screening tools during follow-up. J Psychosom Res. 2018;109:106–7.

Non-melanoma Skin Cancer

19

David W. Lim, Lu Yin, Jennifer M. Racz, Anthony Michael Joshua, Wadid W. K. Abadir, Marcus O. Butler, Joan E. Lipa, Alexander Sun, and Frances C. Wright

D. W. Lim
Breast Surgical Oncology, University of Toronto, Toronto, ON, Canada
e-mail: davidw.lim@mail.utoronto.ca

L. Yin
Breast Surgical Oncology, Sunnybrook & University Health Network, University of Toronto, Toronto, ON, Canada

J. M. Racz
Department of Surgery, Mayo Clinic, Rochester, MN, USA
e-mail: Racz.Jennifer@mayo.edu

A. M. Joshua
Kinghorn Cancer Centre, St Vincents Hospital, Sydney, NSW, Australia
e-mail: Anthony.joshua@svha.org.au

W. W. K. Abadir
Department of Dermatology, University of Toronto, Toronto, ON, Canada
e-mail: Wadid.Abadir@sunnybrook.ca

M. O. Butler
Department of Medicine, University of Toronto, Toronto, ON, Canada
e-mail: Marcus.Butler@uhn.ca

J. E. Lipa
Department of Surgery, Division of Plastics and Reconstructive Surgery, University of Toronto, Toronto, ON, Canada
e-mail: Joan.Lipa@sunnybrook.ca

A. Sun
Department of Radiation Oncology, University of Toronto, Toronto, ON, Canada
e-mail: Alex.Sun@rmp.uhn.on.ca

F. C. Wright (✉)
Department of Surgery, Division of Surgical Oncology, University of Toronto, Toronto, ON, Canada
e-mail: frances.wright@sunnybrook.ca

F. C. Wright et al. (eds.), *Surgical Oncology Manual*,
https://doi.org/10.1007/978-3-030-48363-0_19

Introduction

Non-melanoma skin cancers (NMSCs) are the most commonly diagnosed cancers in Canadians, accounting for 28% of all new cancer cases in Canada. In 2014, the Canadian Cancer Society estimated that there will be approximately 76,100 new cases and 440 deaths from squamous cell carcinoma (SCC) and basal cell carcinoma (BCC) combined [1]. The incidence of both tumor types continues to rise despite growing awareness of the risk factors (see Table 19.1) [2, 3]. The American Joint Committee on Cancer (AJCC) eighth edition is the current recommended cutaneous squamous cell carcinoma and other cutaneous carcinoma staging system [4].

Skin lesions in high-risk populations may be challenging to clinically assess. A low threshold for performing skin biopsies is prudent.

Table 19.1 Risk factors [3, 5–10]

Risk factor	BCC	SCC
Exposure to ultraviolet light	Intense, intermittent exposure; burns	Cumulative exposure
Increasing age	++	++
Fair complexion	++	++
Recreational tanning/tanning beds	++ (OR 1.5)	++ (OR 2.5)
Immunosuppression (including transplant patients)	++ (ten-fold)	++++ (40–250-fold)
HPV (especially serotypes 16 and 18) HIV/AIDS and non-Hodgkin lymphoma	+ ++	+++ +++
Exposure to ionizing radiation	++	++
Chemical exposure		
Arsenic, coal tar Tobacco Soot, asphalt, mineral oil	++ +	++ ++ ++
Chronic inflammation and healing scars, burn sites, or ulcers		++ (Marjolin ulcer)
Personal history of skin cancer	++	++
Family history of skin cancer	++ (OR 2.2)	++
Genetic syndromes Xeroderma pigmentosum Albinism Muir–Torre syndrome Fanconi anemia *CSTT1* or *CYP2D6* polymorphisms	++	++
Nevoid basal cell (Gorlin) syndrome	++	
Benign sun-related skin disorders (i.e., actinic keratoses and		++
solar lentigines)		
Psoralen/PUVA therapy for psoriasis	+	++

BCC basal cell carcinoma, *SCC* squamous cell carcinoma, *OR* odds ratio, *PUVA* psoralen and ultraviolet A

Clinical Presentation [3, 5]

Both BCC and SCC characteristically develop on body areas previously exposed to sun.

Early BCCs are small, translucent or pearly, with raised telangiectatic edges; 80% of BCCs occur on the head and neck, followed by trunk (15%) and extremities. Clinical subtypes of BCCs include the following: (1) classic rodent ulcer (indurated edge and ulcerated center), (2) nodular or cystic, (3) superficial, (4) morphoeic (ill-defined borders), and (5) pigmented. Up to 40% of BCCs contain a mixed pattern of two or more histologic subtypes. Nodulocystic BCC is the most common subtype, usually on the head and neck, while superficial BCCs mainly present on the trunk and limbs. BCC is characterized by local and sometimes disfiguring invasiveness if left untreated; however, metastasis is rare, occurring in less than 0.05% of cases [11]. BCC most commonly metastasizes to regional lymph nodes, followed by bone, lung, and liver [7].

SCCs can arise de novo or from premalignant lesions such as actinic keratoses, SCC in situ (Bowen's disease), keratoacanthoma, and cutaneous horns. Individual actinic keratoses are estimated to progress to invasive SCC at 1–10% over 10 years, but the risk is increased with greater than 5 actinic keratoses. Bowen's disease presents as slow-developing erythematous scaly or crusted plaques, with a 3–5% risk of progression to SCC. Keratoacanthomas have a rapid onset, progression, and regression within months, with similar clinicopathologic features to well-differentiated SCC. Cutaneous horns are growths that present as a dense cone of epithelium; up to 15% demonstrate invasive SCC at the base. Given the associated risk of progressing to invasive SCC, these precursor lesions are generally excised or consider cryotherapy, topical 5-fluorouracil, topical imiquimod, photodynamic therapy, or curettage and electrodessication.

All SCCs demonstrate induration, which is usually the first sign of malignancy, and typically have an adherent crust with ill-defined margins. In contrast to BCCs, SCCs are responsible for the majority of deaths from NMSCs as they have a higher metastatic potential (~5% at 5 years) [12]. The most common metastatic site for SCC are regional lymph nodes; distant sites include bone, brain, and lung (parotid gland for head and neck SCCs).

Tables 19.2 and 19.3 describe the low- and high-risk factors for local recurrence or metastasis for BCC and SCC.

Management: Primary Localized Basal and Squamous Cell Carcinoma (No Evidence of Regional or Metastatic Disease) [13, 14, 25, 26]

Management of Low-Risk Basal Cell Carcinoma and Squamous Cell Carcinoma (See Table 19.4)

For patients unable or unwilling to undergo surgical treatment of primary lesions or when clear margins cannot be obtained by Mohs or more extensive surgery,

Table 19.2 Definition: low- and high-risk factors for local recurrence of BCC and metastasis [7, 13–24]

Risk factor	Low risk	High risk
Location and transverse size (i.e., diameter)	Site L— < 20 mm Site M— < 10 mm	Site L— ≥ 20 mm Site M— ≥ 10 mm Any H
Borders	Well defined	Poorly defined
Primary vs. recurrent	Primary	Recurrent
Immunosuppression	Negative	Positive
Site of prior radiation therapy	Negative	Positive
Subtype[a]	Nodular, superficial	Aggressive growth pattern[b]
Perineural or perivascular involvement Residual margins	Negative Negative	Positive Positive

Site L = trunk or extremity location
Site M = cheek, forehead, scalp, neck, or pretibial location
Site H = mask area of face, genitalia, hand, or foot location
[a]Low-risk subtypes include nodular, superficial, and other nonaggressive growth patterns such as keratotic, infundibulocystic, and fibroepithelioma of Pinkus
[b]Having morpheaform, basosquamous (metatypical), sclerosing, mixed infiltrative, micronodular, or carcinosarcomatous features in any portion of the tumor

Table 19.3 Definition: low- and high-risk factors for local recurrence or metastases for SCC [3, 14–24]

Risk factor	Low risk	High risk
Location and transverse size (must include peripheral rim of erythema)	Site L— < 20 mm Site M— < 10 mm	Site L— ≥ 20 mm Site M— ≥ 10 mm Any H
Borders	Well defined	Poorly defined
Primary vs. recurrent	Primary	Recurrent
Immunosuppression	Negative	Positive
Site of prior radiation therapy, scar, or chronic inflammation	Negative	Positive
Rapid growth rate	Negative	Positive
Neurologic symptoms	Negative	Positive
Degree of differentiation	Well or moderate	Poor
Adenoid, adenosquamous (mucin), desmoplastic, or metaplastic (carcinosarcomatous) subtypes	Negative	Positive
Depth (thickness or level of invasion)[a]	≤6 mm and no invasion beyond subcutaneous fat	>6 mm or invasion beyond subcutaneous fat
Perineural, lymphatic, or vascular involvement Excision	Negative Complete	Positive Incomplete

Site L = trunk or extremity location
Site M = cheek, forehead, scalp, neck, or pretibial location
Site H = mask area of face, genitalia, hand, or foot location
[a]Deep invasion = invasion beyond the subcutaneous fat or > 6 mm measured from the granular layer of adjacent normal epidermis to the base of the tumor

radiation therapy should be pursued. Radiation should also be considered for primary treatment (instead of surgery) to sites that cause significant morbidity or require extensive reconstruction. Radiation is not recommended for patients younger than 60 years of age due to inferior long-term cosmesis and potential for carcinogenesis.

Management of High-Risk Basal Cell Carcinoma and Squamous Cell Carcinoma (See Table 19.5)

For patients unable or unwilling to undergo surgical treatment of primary lesions or when clear margins cannot be obtained, radiation therapy should be pursued if over the age of 60 years old. Consider multidisciplinary tumor board consultation to discuss chemoradiation or enrolment into a clinical trial. Radiation should also be considered as primary treatment (instead of surgery) to sites where surgery may be disfiguring, cause significant morbidity, or require extensive reconstruction (i.e., nose, ears, eyelids, lips). Radiotherapy should also be considered in the adjuvant setting if there is extensive perineural or large nerve involvement ($\geq$ 0.1 mm for cutaneous SCC of the head and neck).

Mohs Micrographic Surgery

- Removes malignant skin tumors with rapid, in-office analysis of horizontal frozen-section specimens processed to include 100% of the peripheral and deep surgical margins. If any part of the specimen demonstrates tumor infiltration of a margin, serial margins can be limited to the affected areas, allowing the narrowest possible margin excised.
- Lowest 5-year recurrence rate of any treatment (1% for primary tumors, 5.6% for recurrent tumors), followed by surgical excision, cryosurgery, and curettage and electrodesiccation.
- For most NMSCs, Cancer Care Ontario recommends surgery (with postoperative and intraoperative margin assessment), or radiation for those ineligible for surgery, as standard of care. Their indications for Mohs micrographic surgery are limited to histologically confirmed recurrent BCC of the face, and primary BCCs of the face that are >1 cm in size, have aggressive histology, or are located in the H zone [32]. The consideration of Mohs micrographic surgery for high-risk SCC should be made by a multidisciplinary team.

Role for Sentinel Lymph Node Biopsy

- Although sentinel lymph node biopsy has been used in the management of select patients with high-risk SCC, data remain insufficient to determine whether early detection of microscopic metastatic disease has a beneficial effect on patient

Table 19.4 Management of low-risk BCC and SCC

Work-up	Surgical techniques	Destructive techniques	Nonsurgical options	Follow-up
History and physical examination Complete skin examination Assessment of regional nodal basins (*SCC only*) No labs No imaging studies[a] Biopsy[b]	Wide local excision with postoperative margin assessment (POMA) (*4 mm* margins for BCC and *4–6 mm* margins for SCC)[c] CCPDMA[d]	Curettage + electrodesiccation[e] Cryotherapy[f]	Radiation therapy Topical 5% fluorouracil Imiquimod (Aldara®)[g] Photodynamic therapy (PDT)[h] Intralesional therapies[i]	History and physical with skin examination every 3–12 months for 2 years, then every 6–12 months for 3 years, then annually (SCC) History and physical with skin examination every 6–12 months for 5 years, then at least annually for life (BCC) Sun protection and self-examination education

[a]Unless there is suspicion of deep structural involvement (i.e., CT with contrast for suspected bone or deep soft tissue involvement; MRI with contrast for suspected perineural disease)

[b]Punch or excisional biopsy techniques are preferred as the full thickness of the dermis (including reticular dermis) can be evaluated; incisional biopsy is an option for large lesions, lesions in difficult locations or if an excisional biopsy would be cosmetically disfiguring

[c]Preferred treatment if adipose tissue has been reached vertically; associated with 5-year disease-free survival of >98% for BCC and 92% for SCC [27–29]; may close with linear repair, skin graft, or secondary intention healing

[d]Consider if positive margins following wide local excision (may also re-attempt resection with complete circumferential peripheral and deep margin assessment (CCPDMA) with permanent section or intraoperative frozen-section analysis)

[e]Not appropriate for terminal hair-bearing areas (scalp, pubic, axillary, beard)

[f]Reserved for treatment of patients with low-risk, shallow NMSCs such as *superficial BCC or SCC* in situ (Bowen's disease)

[g]Imiquimod is approved for biopsy-proven, small (<2.0 cm diameter), primary, *superficial* lesions of the trunk, neck, or extremities of adults with normal immune systems; it is not indicated for nodular, recurrent, or aggressive histologic subtypes of BCC or for lesions on the head. Imiquimod 5% is applied daily 5 times per week for 16 weeks

[h]PDT is effective for superficial and nodular BCC (80–100% success) but is associated with high recurrence rates

[i]Intralesional agents for low-risk BCC and SCC have some support in the literature but are not widely used. They can be used when surgical intervention is inappropriate or when the tumor is in cosmetically sensitive areas. Intralesional agents provide deeper penetration of the medication as opposed to topical treatment. As such, intralesional 5-fluorouracil, bleomycin, or interferon-α can be used to treat BCC, and intralesional 5-fluorouracil, bleomycin, interferon-α, or methotrexate can be used to treat SCC [30]. The best results have been reported with keratoacanthoma, a variant of SCC, with a cure rate of 91–100% [31]

Table 19.5 Management of high-risk BCC and SCC

Work-up	Surgical techniques	Nonsurgical options	Follow-up
History and physical examination Complete skin examination Assessment of regional nodal basins (*SCC only*) No labs No imaging studies[a] Biopsy Multidisciplinary consultation (for complicated cases)	Wide local excision with postoperative margin assessment with linear or delayed repair[b] ***Mohs micrographic surgery*** (negative margins)[c] Resection with complete circumferential peripheral and deep margin assessment with frozen or permanent section (CCPDMA)[d] +/− SLNB (SCC only)—See next section	Radiation therapy +/− systemic therapy[e]	History and physical with skin examination every 1–3 months for 1 year, then every 2–4 months for 1 year, then every 4–6 months for 3 years, then every 6–12 months for life (SCC) History and physical with skin examination every 6–12 months for 5 years, then at least annually for life (BCC) Sun protection education and self-examination of skin and lymph nodes

SLNB sentinel lymph node biopsy

[a]Unless there is suspicion of deep structural involvement—fixed lesion/large lesion (i.e., CT with contrast for suspected bone involvement; MRI with contrast for suspected perineural disease or deep soft tissue involvement)

[b]There is no longer a defined margin of standard excision for high-risk BCC and SCC due to wide variation in clinical features that define a high-risk tumor. Complete margin assessment is recommended. Previous NCCN guidelines recommended 6–10 mm for BCC and 10 mm for SCC, but these margins should now be modified based on tumor- and patient-specific factors, with an awareness for subclinical extension

[c]Indications for Mohs procedure are histologically confirmed recurrent BCC of the face and primary BCCs of the face that are >1 cm in size, have aggressive histology, or are located on the H zone of the face. Mohs may be considered in smaller tumors <1 cm in areas of functional or cosmetic significance, complex tumors needing margin control and immunosuppressed patients. Consideration of Mohs surgery for SCC should be evaluated by a multidisciplinary team [32]

[d]Superficial parotidectomy is indicated if parotid fascia is involved

[e]Radiation therapy may be combined with chemotherapy for select patients, or systemic therapy alone if surgery and radiotherapy are both contraindicated. Consider multidisciplinary tumor board consultation after persistent positive margins

outcome. Nevertheless, consider sentinel lymph node biopsy in certain high-risk lesions such as locally advanced SCC and discuss at a multidisciplinary skin cancer tumor board [33–36].

Regional Metastatic Non-melanoma Skin Cancer

Management of Regional and Metastatic BCC [13]

For nodal or distant metastases, consider surgery and/or radiation therapy, and multidisciplinary tumor board consultation for consideration for a hedgehog pathway inhibitor (i.e., vismodegib, sonidegib) or clinical trial.

Management of Regionally Metastatic SCC [9] (See Table 19.6)

Referring to Radiation Oncology

- Patients should be referred to radiation oncology for consideration of radiation as primary therapy if:
  - They have histologically confirmed NMSCs and are unable or unwilling to undergo surgical treatment of their primary lesion.
  - Clear margins cannot be obtained by Mohs or more extensive surgery.
  - Surgery may be disfiguring, cause significant morbidity, or require extensive reconstruction (i.e., nose, ears, eyelids, lips).
- All patients with positive margins, regional or metastatic disease should also be referred to radiation oncology for consideration of adjuvant radiation therapy.
- Data on the value of adjuvant radiation after surgical excision with negative margins (particularly after Mohs micrography surgery) remain conflicting [13, 14].

Referring to Medical Oncology

- All patients with distant metastases or locally advanced disease should be referred to medical oncology for consideration of systemic therapy or clinical trial enrollment.
- Systemic therapy is usually indicated once surgical and radiation options have been exhausted.

Options

- Targeted therapy.
  - Hedgehog pathway inhibitors (i.e., vismodegib, sonidegib) (BCC).
- Immunotherapy.
  - PD-1 inhibitor (i.e., pembrolizumab, cemiplimab).
- Systemic chemotherapy.
  - Cisplatin alone or with paclitaxel (BCC) [25].
  - Cetuximab, cisplatin/5-fluorouracil or α-interferon, retinoic acid, and cisplatin (SCC) [26].
  - There is no standard chemotherapy treatment plan for NMSCs.

BCC: Vismodegib is now standard of care (and paid for by the Provinces) for BCC not amenable to surgery or radiation. Patients with borderline resectable BCC may also be considered for neoadjuvant vismodegib. Pembrolizumab has shown some efficacy in case reports for patients who are refractory to targeted therapy but regulatory approvals have not yet occurred [37, 38].

Table 19.6 Management of regionally metastatic SCC

Work-up	Operable disease	Nonoperable disease	Adjuvant treatment	Follow-up
History and physical examination Complete skin examination and assessment of regional nodal basins Biopsy (FNA or core) of lymph node CT with contrast of nodal basin CT chest, abdomen, and pelvis or PET/CT If locally advanced then use MRI to assess extent of muscle/bone/tendon involvement Multidisciplinary consultation	Wide local excision of primary lesion + regional lymph node dissection[a]	Radiation[b] Multidisciplinary tumor board to discuss systemic therapy with or without radiation or immunotherapy[c]	Radiation therapy to regional lymph node basin[d]	History and physical with complete skin and regional lymph node examination every 4–6 months for 3 years, then every 6–12 months up to 5 years Sun protection education

[a]Regional lymph node dissection is preferred unless the patient is not a surgical candidate. For trunk and extremity cutaneous SCC, perform regional lymphadenectomy and if multiple nodes involved or extracapsular extension is present, consider adjuvant radiation. For head and neck cutaneous SCC: (1) if solitary node ≤3 cm, perform ipsilateral selective neck dissection; (2) if solitary node >3 cm or multiple ipsilateral nodes, perform ipsilateral comprehensive neck dissection; (3) if bilateral nodes, perform comprehensive bilateral neck dissection; (4) if parotid nodes involved, perform superficial parotidectomy and ipsilateral neck dissection

[b]Reassess candidacy for post-radiation lymph node dissection; contrast CT may help evaluate burden of residual disease

[c]Immunotherapy with cemiplimab, an immune checkpoint inhibitor, is recommended for locally advanced or metastatic cutaneous SCC who are not candidates for either curative surgery or curative radiotherapy. This is not an option for solid organ transplant recipients, as immune checkpoint inhibitors can lead to organ rejection. Other options include palliative radiation/surgery if symptomatic and stereotactic body radiotherapy in select patients. Multidisciplinary tumor board consultation is highly recommended

[d]Consider RT for most head and neck primary lesions and lesions of the head and neck, trunk, or extremity that have lymph node basin involvement, especially with multiple nodes or the presence of extracapsular extension. May omit adjuvant radiation for head and neck cutaneous SCC with lymph node involvement if only one positive node ≤3 cm with no extracapsular extension. May consider concurrent systemic therapy with radiation (multidisciplinary consultation) for any node with extracapsular extension or incompletely resected nodal disease

SCC: Phase I and II studies demonstrated a 50% response to cemiplimab in locally advanced or metastatic SCC, with adverse effects in at least 15% of patients limited to diarrhea, fatigue, nausea, and rash [39]. Cemiplimab has since received both FDA and Health Canada approval and is now standard of care for metastatic or locally advanced cutaneous SCCs that are not curable with surgery or radiation.

Referring to Multidisciplinary Cancer Conference

- Patients with positive deep margins following resection with graft/flap reconstruction.
- All patients with regionally metastatic NMSCs.
- All patients with distant metastatic NMSCs.

Toronto Pearls

- Patients with high-risk BCCs or SCCs on the face should be prepared for graft or local flap reconstruction given the cosmetically sensitive nature of this region; high-risk SCCs in other locations may also require graft/flap reconstruction given the potential size of resection.
- If deep margins are positive following resection and reconstruction, consideration should be given to re-resection.
- Level 3 axillary dissection for SCC should be considered for palpable disease in the axilla.

References

1. Canadian Cancer Society: Non-melanoma skin cancer statistics. Available at http://www.cancer.ca/en/cancer-information/cancer-type/skin-non-melanoma/statistics/?region=on.
2. Guenther LC, Barber K, Searles GE, Lynde CW, et al. Non-melanoma skin cancer in Canada chapter 1: introduction to the guidelines. J Cutan Med Surg. 2015;19(3):205–15.
3. Mortenson MM, Herne K, Hymes SR, Cormier JN. Chapter 4 nonmelanoma skin cancer. In: Feig BW, Ching CD, editors. The MD Anderson surgical oncology handbook. 5th ed. Philadelphia: Lippincott Williams and Wilkins; 2012. p. 117–26.
4. Keohane SG, Proby CM, Newlands C, Motley RJ. The new 8th edition of TNM staging and its implications for skin cancer: a review by the British Association of Dermatologists and the Royal College of Pathologists, U.K. Br J Dermatol. 2018;179(4):824–8.
5. Madan V, Lear JT, Szeimies RM. Non-melanoma skin cancer. Lancet. 2010;375(9715):673–85.
6. Wong CSM, Strange RC, Lear JT. Basal cell carcinoma. BMJ. 2003;327:794–8.
7. Rubin AI, Chen EH, Ratner D. Basal-cell carcinoma. N Engl J Med. 2005;353:2262–9.
8. Perkins JL, Liu Y, Mitby PA, et al. Nonmelanoma skin cancer in survivors of childhood and adolescent cancer: a report from the childhood cancer survivor study. J Clin Oncol. 2005;23:3733–41.
9. Karagas MR, Nelson HH, Zens MS, et al. Squamous cell and basal cell carcinoma of the skin in relation to radiation therapy and potential modification of risk by sun exposure. Epidemiology. 2007;18:776–84.
10. Barber K, Searles GE, Vender R, et al. Non-melanoma skin cancer in Canada chapter 2: primary prevention of non-melanoma skin cancer. J Cutan Med Surg. 2015;19(3):216–26.
11. Verkouteren JAC, Ramdas KHR, Wakkee M, Nijsten T. Epidemiology of basal cell carcinoma: scholarly review. Br J Dermatol. 2017;177(2):359–72.
12. Alam M, Ratner D. Cutaneous squamous-cell carcinoma. N Engl J Med. 2001;344(13):975–83.
13. NCCN Clinical Practice Guidelines in Oncology: Basal Cell Skin Cancer. Version 1.2019, August 31, 2018 [online]. Available from URL: http://www.nccn.org/professionals/physician_gls/pdf/nmsc.pdf.
14. NCCN Clinical Practice Guidelines in Oncology: Squamous Cell Skin Cancer. Version 2.2019, October 31, 2018 [online]. Available from URL: http://www.nccn.org/professionals/physician_gls/pdf/squamous.pdf.

15. Boeta-Angeles L, Bennett RG. Features associated with recurrence (basal cell carcinoma). In: Miller SJ, Maloney ME, editors. Cutaneous oncology pathophysiology, diagnosis, and management. Malden: Blackwell Science; 1998. p. 646–56.
16. Haas AF. Features associated with metastasis (squamous cell carcinoma). In: Miller SJ, Maloney ME, editors. Cutaneous oncology, pathophysiology, diagnosis, and management. Malden: Blackwell Science; 1998. p. 500–5.
17. Clayman GL, Lee JJ, Holsinger FC, et al. Mortality risk from squamous cell skin cancer. J Clin Oncol. 2005;23:759–65.
18. Rowe DE, Carroll RJ, Day CL Jr. Prognostic factors for local recurrence, metastasis, and survival rates in squamous cell carcinoma of the skin, ear, and lip. Implications for treatment modality selection. J Am Acad Dermatol. 1992;26:976–90.
19. Thompson AK, Kelley BF, Prokop LJ, et al. Risk factors for cutaneous squamous cell carcinoma recurrence, metastasis, and disease-specific death: a systematic review and meta-analysis. JAMA Dermatol. 2016;152(4):419–28.
20. Randle HW. Basal cell carcinoma. Identification and treatment of the high-risk patient. Dermatol Surg. 1996;22:255–61.
21. Rieger KE, Linos E, Egbert BM, Swetter SM. Recurrence rates associated with incompletely excised low-risk nonmelanoma skin cancer. J Cutan Pathol. 2010;37:59–67.
22. Rowe DE, Carroll RJ, Day CL Jr. Long-term recurrence rates in previously untreated (primary) basal cell carcinoma: implications for patient follow-up. J Dermatol Surg Oncol. 1989;15:315–28.
23. Ulrich C, Kanitakis J, Stockfleth E, Euvrard S. Skin cancer in organ transplant recipients-where do we stand today? Am J Transplant. 2008;8:2192–8.
24. Brantsch KD, Meisner C, Schonfisch B, et al. Analysis of risk factors determining prognosis of cutaneous squamous-cell carcinoma: a prospective study. Lancet Oncol. 2008;9:713–20.
25. Zioty D, Guenther LC, Sapijaszko M, et al. Non-melanoma skin cancer in Canada chapter 4: management of basal cell carcinoma. J Cutan Med Surg. 2015;19(3):239–48.
26. Sapijaszko M, Zioty D, Bourcier M, et al. Non-melanoma skin cancer in Canada chapter 5: management of squamous cell carcinoma. J Cutan Med Surg. 2015;19(3):249–59.
27. Samarasinghe V, Madan V. Nonmelanoma skin cancer. J Cutan Aesthet Surg. 2012;5:3–10.
28. Brodland DG, Zitelli JA. Surgical margins for excision of primary cutaneous squamous cell carcinoma. J Am Acad Dermatol. 1992;27:241–8.
29. Wolf DJ, Zitelli JA. Surgical margins for basal cell carcinoma. Arch Dermatol. 1987;123:340–4.
30. Good LM, Miller MD, High WA. Intralesional agents in the management of cutaneous malignancy: a review. J Am Acad Dermatol. 2011;64(2):413–22.
31. Kirby JS, Miller CJ. Intralesional chemotherapy for nonmelanoma skin cancer: a practical review. J Am Acad Dermatol. 2010;63(4):689–702.
32. Murray C, Sivajohanathan D, Hanna T, et al. Patient indications for Mohs micrographic surgery. Toronto: Cancer Care Ontario; 2018. Program in Evidence-Based Care Guideline No.:8–11.
33. Ross AS, Schmults CD. Sentinel lymph node biopsy in cutaneous squamous cell carcinoma: a systematic review of the English literature. Dermatol Surg. 2006;32:1309.
34. Renzi C, Caggiati A, Mannooranparampil TJ, et al. Sentinel lymph node biopsy for high risk cutaneous squamous cell carcinoma: case series and review of the literature. Eur J Surg Oncol. 2007;33:364.
35. Fahradyan A, Howell AC, Wolfswinkel EM, et al. Updates on the management of non-melanoma skin cancer (NMSC). Healthcare (Basel). 2017;5(4):E82. https://doi.org/10.3390/healthcare5040082.
36. Matthey-Giè ML, Boubaker A, Letovanec I, et al. Sentinel lymph node biopsy in nonmelanoma skin cancer patients. J Skin Cancer. 2013;2013:267474. https://doi.org/10.1155/2013/267474.
37. Lipson EJ, Lilo MT, Ogurtsova A, et al. Basal cell carcinoma: PD-L1/PD-1 checkpoint expression and tumor regression after PD-1 blockade. J Immunother Cancer. 2017 Mar 21;5:23.
38. Cannon JGD, Russell JS, Kim J, et al. A case of metastatic basal cell carcinoma treated with continuous PD-1 inhibitor exposure even after subsequent initiation of radiotherapy and surgery. JAAD Case Rep. 2018;4(3):248–50.
39. Migden MR, Rischin D, Schmults CD, et al. PD-1 blockade with cemiplimab in advanced cutaneous squamous-cell carcinoma. N Engl J Med. 2018;379(4):341–51.

Palliative Surgical Care

20

Erin M. Sadler, Anand Govindarajan, Lucy K. Helyer, and Alexandra M. Easson

Introduction

The most recent statistics generated by the Canadian Cancer Society suggest that despite the fact that one in four Canadians will die from cancer, the incidence of Canadians surviving beyond 5 years of a cancer diagnosis is increasing [1]. These encouraging statistics do not only highlight the improvements that have been made in the provision of modern cancer care, but also emphasize the important role that palliative care will play in the lives of patients both dying from, or, more importantly, living *with* cancer.

There is strong clinical evidence to support the introduction of palliative care early in the treatment of cancer patients. Temel and colleagues showed that early referral to palliative care plus standard oncology care resulted in improved mood, metrics of quality of life, and a survival benefit compared with standard oncology care alone; benefits echoed in multiple studies [2–5]. Despite the evidence and the years of good work by our palliative care colleagues, there remains a strong stigma attached to palliative care, which impairs the effective integration of palliative care into modern surgical oncology [6]. This challenge is deepened by the ever-changing face of cancer treatment and disease trajectories that creates difficulty in accurate

E. M. Sadler
General Surgery, University of Toronto, Toronto, ON, Canada

Department of Surgery, University of Toronto, Toronto, ON, Canada
e-mail: erin.sadler@mail.utoronto.ca

A. Govindarajan · A. M. Easson (✉)
Department of Surgery, University of Toronto, Toronto, ON, Canada
e-mail: Anand.Govindarajan@sinaihealth.ca; Alexandra.Easson@uhn.ca

L. K. Helyer
Department of Surgery, Dalhousie University, Halifax, NS, Canada
e-mail: Lucy.helyer@nshealth.ca

F. C. Wright et al. (eds.), *Surgical Oncology Manual*,
https://doi.org/10.1007/978-3-030-48363-0_20

prognoses of certain diseases and increased uncertainty in a patient's treatment course [7]. Indeed, physicians are accurate in predicting survival only about 50% of the time for patients with advanced cancer [8]. This accuracy is likely to become even more inaccurate as more novel therapeutic options become available.

Palliative care and surgical oncology are two disciplines that are transitioning into a synergistic relationship rather than being perceived historically as mutually exclusive pursuits [9]. Despite a growing body of evidence that this synergy is possible, necessary, and of great benefit to patients across the oncology spectrum, there continue to be challenges in bringing palliative care to the consciousness of surgical oncologists, to the forefront of comprehensive surgical cancer care, and its integration into surgical oncology education. This synergistic relationship is ever more important when one considers that up to 22% of patients undergo a surgical procedure in the last year of their life [10], and 10–20% of all surgical procedures are done with palliative intent [11]. The American College of Surgeons has integrated this philosophy, whereby the College now emphasizes the need for palliative care to be incorporated alongside curative and life-prolonging surgical interventions [12].

Alongside palliative care is the concept of palliative surgery, which is generally defined as a surgical pursuit designed to improve quality of life and relieve or prevent symptoms caused by an advanced disease [13]. *Palliative surgery* must be distinguished from *non-curative surgery*, where the latter's primary intent is not the improvement of quality of life. Together, these complementary concepts fall under the overarching entity of surgical palliative care, defined as the treatment of suffering, and the promotion of quality life for seriously or terminally ill patients under surgical care [14].

Evidence for Palliative Care in Surgical Oncology

In January 2017, the American Society of Clinical Oncology created a new set of guidelines with regard to integration of palliative care into standard oncology care after careful review of the current evidence as derived from the sentinel studies in this area [2, 3, 5, 15–18]. The specific recommendations from this evidence-based document include [19]:

1. Patients with advanced cancer (defined as patients with distant metastases, late-stage disease, cancer that is life limiting, and/or prognosis of 6–24 months) should be referred to interdisciplinary palliative care teams that provide inpatient and outpatient care early in the course of disease, alongside active disease management of their cancer.
2. Palliative care for patients with advanced cancer should be delivered through interdisciplinary palliative care teams with consultation available in both outpatient and inpatient environments.
3. Essential components of palliative care include:
   - Rapport and relationship building with patients and family caregivers
   - Symptom and functional status management

  - Exploration and education of understanding illness and prognosis
  - Clarification of treatment goals
  - Assessment and support of coping needs
  - Assistance with medical decision-making
  - Coordination with other care providers
  - Provision of referrals to other healthcare providers as needed
4. Early palliative care involvement within 8 weeks of diagnosis of advanced cancer
5. Patients with high symptom burden should be provided with outpatient cancer care programs with dedicated resources to deliver palliative care services to complement existing program tools.

Palliative Surgery

Goals of Palliative Surgery

- Primary outcome: Improvement in quality of life through the relief of symptoms caused by an advanced disease [20].
- Secondary outcome (but not primary goal of treatment): Improvement in survival.
- Successful outcome defined by patient and surgeon preoperatively.
  - Relief from distressing symptoms, easing of pain, and improvement in quality of life.
  - May increase response to chemotherapy or radiotherapy in certain circumstances [21].
- The decision to intervene is based on the treatment's ability to meet these goals, rather than its effect on the underlying disease.
- See Table 20.1 for details regarding important aspects of surgical decision-making in patients with advanced cancer
- See Table 20.2 for examples of indications for palliative procedures and surgery

The first step for consideration of palliative surgery is proper patient selection. Patients with at least a 3-month expected survival may be considered adequate candidates [21]. However, acceptable timelines may be variable on an individual patient basis.

Patients' choices are greatly influenced by a physician's recommendations. It has been estimated that physician recommendation is the predominant reason for treatment selection in up to 40% of cases [22]. Therefore, the situation should be managed carefully, ensuring the patient has clear and honest information in order to make the best decision for themselves. When discussing treatment options and a possible surgical approach, the attending physician should choose words wisely, making sure to explain the current status of the patient and disease process, the goals of treatment, its possible benefits, likely outcomes, and also the risks involved. Qualitative research has shown that patients often choose surgical intervention as they feel there are "no other options," and thus it is the physician's role to ensure the patient understands the options and alternatives to surgical intervention [23].

Table 20.1 Surgical decision-making in the advanced cancer patient

Identify	Assess	Discuss and Recommend
Acuity of presentation: Emergent Urgent Elective Symptoms: Nausea/vomiting Anorexia Abdominal distension Pain Bleeding Shortness of breath Weakness/fatigue Potential surgical causes: Mechanical bowel obstruction Bleeding/eroding tumor Tumor bulk Ascites Pleural effusion	Patient factors: Prognosis Goals of care Active/future oncologic treatment Age—biologic, physiologic Concurrent illness and comorbidities Malnutrition and/or cachexia Performance status Technical factors: Degree of invasiveness of the intervention: Interventional radiology < endoscopy < laparoscopy < laparotomy Anesthetic requirements Tumor factors affecting technical success Risk of complications Expected outcome Anticipated length of stay Impact on future treatments	Discuss with patient and family: What do they understand about their disease and where are they on their disease trajectory? Does surgical intervention fit with the patient's goals of care? What are the perceived and/or expected benefits of the surgical intervention from both the patient's and surgeon's perspective? What are the potential risks, and likely outcomes, and are they worth the potential benefit to the patient? Provide a commitment to continue to care for the patient regardless of the outcome of the discussion Formulate recommendation(s) Consider all options and alternatives What is feasible? What is futile? No ethical or legal obligation to offer futile treatment
When decision is to operate: Thorough preoperative evaluation to avoid intraoperative surprises Prevention of emergency situations Clear and honest communication with the patient and family about the goals of care and likelihood of success Discuss all potential outcomes of the procedure A commitment to ongoing care with a clear care plan, whatever the outcome of surgery		

Table 20.2 Examples of indications for palliative surgical procedures

Drainage of fluid Ascites Pleural effusion
Relief of obstruction Gastrointestinal tract from mouth to anus Genitourinary tract from kidney to bladder neck Hepatobiliary system
Treatment/prevention of bleeding From tumor or feeding vessels
Palliative tumor resection Space occupying lesions in the cranium Debulking tumors for symptoms: Pain, distension, biochemically functional tumors Prevent/palliate bleeding, obstruction, fungation, neuropathic pain
Fixation for bony metastases and impending fracture

Postoperative care and recovery should also be discussed with patients and families. Routine postoperative care, the risks of developing complications, the need for additional actions (e.g., ICU, mechanical ventilation), the aggressiveness of treatments in the event of any postoperative complication, the anticipated length of stay, and the risk of spending an important part of their remaining lifespan in the hospital must be addressed [24, 25].

Prognostication

Prognostication is not limited to predicting survival, but rather includes prognoses of response to treatment, ability to cure, attainment of functional goals, relief of symptoms, and risk of recurrence, among others [26]. Awareness of one's prognoses has been associated with improved end of life planning, decreased levels of psychological distress, and more positive bereavement experiences [27–29]. In surgical oncology this is a complex process that must integrate patient factors (surgical fitness, functional status, etc.) and disease factors (tumor type, stage, previous treatments, etc.). For this reason, various tools exist that can aid in the prognostication of patients with advanced cancer (Table 20.3).

Beyond prognostication tools for the physician to determine patient suitability for intervention, another important aspect of prognostication is for the patient to understand the expected benefit and potential for risk and complications. A useful tool for this application is the American College of Surgeons Surgical Risk Calculator [30]. This National Surgical Quality Improvement Program (NSQIP) databased derived instrument can be accessed online, and provides an estimation of risk for complications and expected outcomes provided 20 individualized patient factors. Although this tool is not specific to the palliative context, it is a useful tool to supplement communication with patient and families.

Table 20.3 Examples of tools for prognostication

Tool	Predicts survival	Externally validated	Special notes
Palliative Performance Scale (PPS)	x	x	Studied in largest group of patients Based on Karnofsky Performance Scale but more specific to palliative patient population Survival decreases by ~50% with each performance level Depends largely on functional status
Palliative Prognostic Score (PaP)	x	x	Depends largely on functional status Heavily reliant on physician's expertise in prognostication
Palliative Prognostic Index (PPI)	x	x	Depends largely on functional status Incorporates PPS in its score
Glasgow Prognostic Score (GPS)	x	x	Only two objective parameters (CRP and albumin) Robust evidence for accuracy Quick and easy to use

Evaluation of Outcomes

Currently, there are no validated instruments to measure Quality of Life (QOL) after palliative procedures. In the absence of a good measurement tool, the absence of a postoperative complication has been used as an indicator of QOL [31]. In the absence of a validated instrument, the Palliative Surgery Outcome Score (PSOS) has been used as a measure of symptom resolution after a palliative procedure.

$$\text{Palliative Surgery Outcome Score}\left(\text{PSOS}\right) = \text{SFD}/\text{POD}$$

SFD = Number of days a patient is without symptoms and not in the hospital. The symptoms refer to those that were meant to be treated by the intervention, and include complications related to the surgical procedure.
POD = Number of total days of life after the operation (up to 180 days).

The PSOS score is an estimated measure of the impact of a palliative surgical procedure on patient well-being. A PSOS score > 0.7 is considered to be an acceptable outcome score.

Specific Clinical Scenarios

Malignant Bowel Obstruction

Malignant bowel obstruction (MBO) is estimated to occur in 15% of all palliative care patients and encompasses a heterogeneous clinical syndrome, defined as obstructive symptoms due to the presence of intra-abdominal neoplastic disease. The small bowel is more commonly involved than large bowel, and the most common causes are ovarian and colon cancer [31–34].

MBO can be due to extraluminal compression, intraluminal obstruction, or functional obstruction due to tumor infiltration of the mesentery, nerve involvement, or paraneoplastic neuropathy [33]. Often, obstruction involving the small bowel is multifocal (carcinomatosis), in contrast to large bowel obstruction, which is usually endoluminal and unifocal (solitary tumor). The site and degree of involvement of the bowel determine the treatment path.

High-quality imaging is crucial to rule out signs of a surgical emergency and to properly characterize the obstruction (location, degree, multifocality, and cause). In addition, imaging can rule out other non-neoplastic causes of obstruction, which can be found in up to 15–30% of patients with previously known peritoneal carcinomatosis [33].

Special Notes

- Criteria for MBO:
  - Clinical evidence of bowel obstruction
  - Obstruction beyond the ligament of Treitz

  - Caused by incurable intra-abdominal cancer or extra-abdominal cancer with peritoneal disease
- Clinical variables associated with decreased survival in patients with MBO [25, 35]:
  - ECOG status 2–4
  - Elevated BUN
  - Low albumin
  - Ascites
  - Palpable mass
  - Peritoneal carcinomatosis
  - Progression of symptoms despite active or recent treatment with chemotherapy (within 6 months)
  - Continued postoperative obstruction
- Careful patient selection is important, as operative morbidity and mortality are high.
- Most important prognosticator for survival in these patients is functional status.
- MBOs related to peritoneal carcinomatosis from neuroendocrine tumor may have more favorable outcomes after surgery [35].
- Patients should also be aware of the risk of failure of the intent of surgery.
- Table 20.4 outlines general principles for management of MBO.

Gastric Outlet Obstruction (GOO)

Most common causes are cancers of the stomach, pancreas, and periampullary/biliary tract, as well as lymphoma and metastases [36]. Treatment is necessary, as patients quickly develop vomiting, dehydration, and malnutrition [37]. The goal of therapy is to restore the ability to tolerate diet orally. Table 20.5 outlines treatment options for GOO.

Patient selection for the appropriate therapy is important, because the outcome depends on the clinical condition of the patient and their anticipated lifespan. A WHO performance status >2 or short expected lifespan should prompt consideration for stent therapy, given the poor prognosis of this group of patients.

In patients with periampullary cancer who underwent a surgical exploration and were deemed unresectable, a prophylactic gastrojejunostomy should be considered (up to 20% of these patients will develop GOO). A Cochrane review demonstrated no increased morbidity, and compared to patients with no gastrojejunostomy, their risk of developing GOO in the future was lower (2.5% vs. 28%) [40].

Large Bowel Obstruction (LBO)

About 80% of all LBO are malignant in nature and up to 10–30% of patients with colorectal cancer present with acute obstructive symptoms. Usually, it is associated with fluid and electrolyte disturbances [32].

Table 20.4 Malignant bowel obstruction (MBO) management steps

1. Fluid Resuscitation		
2. Nasogastric Decompression	Should be reserved for the period of initial evaluation, for temporary relief, until more durable measures are initiated or resolution of the episode has occurred or as an adjunct to perioperative care.	
3. Radiologic Investigations	To determine: Single site vs. multiple sites Anatomic site, e.g., gastric outlet, small bowel, large bowel Partial vs. complete obstruction Burden of disease Ascites	
4. Symptom Management	*Anti-secretory*	Octreotide Buscopan
	Antiemetic	Haloperidol Stemetil Gravol Dexamethasone
	Antispasmodic (colicky pain)	Loperamide Buscopan
	Analgesic	Morphine/hydromorphone Fentanyl patch
	Intravenous Hydration	If no reversible cause found for MBO or if no appreciable change with steroids and octreotide Can be maintained via SC boluses if required Controversial when to stop
5. Indications for Surgery	Ischemic complications are rare, allowing for careful patient selection for operative therapy Risk of major surgical complications after surgery is 7–44%. 30 day mortality ranges between 6% and 32% [25, 34] Obstructive symptoms resolution may vary between 32% and 100%, re-obstruction occurs in 6–47% [25] Symptom relief may be short lived, with only 32–71% being symptom free at 60 days postoperatively [25] Surgery as a bridge to palliative chemotherapy is associated with prolonged survival over surgery alone	

MBO malignant bowel obstruction

Table 20.5 Treatment options for gastric outlet obstruction [36, 38]

Gastrojejunostomy (GJ)	Open vs. laparoscopic More medical complications in early postoperative period Consider for patients with longer anticipated survival Better functional outcomes in the long term [39]
Endoscopic Stent	Improved time to PO intake Shorter hospital stay Higher re-obstruction rate and late complications (20–44%) Consider for patients with shorter anticipated survival
Gastrostomy with Tube Decompression	May provide relief from intractable nausea Placement via endoscopy, interventional radiology, or surgically Ideally should be placed into the posterior wall of the stomach

Table 20.6 Treatment options for large bowel obstruction [32, 41]

Surgical Resection and Anastomosis	Option in patients with less advanced disease May involve multistage resection with temporary stoma Considered the ideal management for lesions proximal to the splenic flexure. Patient selection is advised. Anastomotic leak rates of 2.8–16.4% [32] Resolution of obstruction 98%
Surgical Resection and Hartmann's	Less complex procedure in the acute setting Avoids the morbidity of an anastomosis. Reconstruction of the Hartmann's is only attempted in 60% of the patients. Morbidity 5–57% [32]
Surgical Diversion with Stoma	High morbidity and mortality Option in patients with mid or distal rectal tumors: There is no strong evidence for stents in proximal colon or rectal tumors as definitive palliative management [42]. Some patients derive benefit from neoadjuvant therapy. Initially unresectable liver metastasis may become resectable after chemotherapy in 12–26% of the cases [43, 44].
Colonic Stenting	Effective with minimal morbidity Definitive Therapy [42, 45]: Technical success in 88%. Clinical success (evidence of intestinal transit) up to 95% Median patency ranges between 55 and 343 days. Less success in tumors close to anal verge (<5 cm) Compared to surgery, stents had a shorter length of hospital stay, lower rates of ICU admission, lower 30-day mortality rates, lower rates of early complications (<30 days), and a shorter time to initiation of chemotherapy. The overall survival was the same, but there was a lower clinical success rate and higher rate of late (>30 days) complications [45]. Complications: Perforation 10%, migration 9%, and stent obstruction 18% Not recommended if angiogenesis inhibitor (e.g., Bevacizumab) chemotherapy is going to be administered, because of the increased risk of perforation. Bridging therapy to surgery: Technical success in 70%. Clinical success 52.5–78% Increases the possibility of a primary anastomosis and avoiding a stoma [32, 41, 46] No difference in permanent stoma rates, 30-day mortality, surgical site infection, or anastomotic leakage [32, 41, 42, 46]

Obstructive lesions are more commonly found in the left colon, and in the acute obstructive setting they are associated with worse oncological outcomes and a higher incidence of local spread and metastatic disease [41]. See Table 20.6 for treatment option for LBO.

Biliary Duct Obstruction

Malignant bile duct obstruction can be due to intraluminal tumor presence, local invasion of primary disease, extraluminal compression, or metastatic cancers [47]. See Table 20.7 for treatment options.

Table 20.7 Treatment options for biliary duct obstruction [48]

Surgical diversion	Options: Hepaticojejunostomy, Segment III cholangiojejunostomy, right sectoral duct bypass or transtumoral tube placement. Considered in patients deemed unresectable during surgical exploration, or when endoscopic and/or percutaneous stenting has failed.
Endoscopic stenting	Option for patients with obstruction distal to the hilum. Plastic stents (PS) have a patency time of 1.4–3 months. Self-expandable metal stents (SEMS) are patent for 6–10 months [48, 49]. If life expectancy is greater than 4 months, SEMS are recommended [50]
Percutaneous stenting [47]	Option for patients with advanced disease and proximal (common hepatic duct or higher) obstruction. Success in 77–98% of interventions Stent occlusion 5–25%

Malignant Ascites

The pathogenesis of malignant ascites (MA) is multifactorial. Increased production of peritoneal fluid due to high permeability of the tumor-generated neovascularization and diminished reabsorption (secondary in most cases to obstruction of fluid drainage through peritoneal "stomata") are the main causes [51, 52].

Malignant ascites is a sign of poor prognosis; median survivals range from 10 weeks in foregut tumors to 20 weeks in gynecological tumors. See Table 20.8 for treatment options.

Symptoms

Pain

Even though it has been recognized as the fifth vital sign and a lot of research has been done to improve its management, we have not risen to the challenge yet. Currently it is estimated that up to 60% of patients with cancer have pain issues, and up to 75% of the patients who are under treatment for cancer pain are undertreated [59, 60].

Pain Assessment [60–62]

- Routinely screen all patients for pain, at all encounters
- Characterize its dimensions
  - Location, duration, radiation, temporal pattern, provocative or relieving factors
- Formulate an understanding of the nature of the pain
  - Etiology (Cancer related, treatment related, or not related to cancer)
  - Pain mechanism
- Quality:
  - Somatic (dull/aching, well localized)

  - Visceral (dull/sharp/colicky, referred)
  - Neuropathic (burning, stabbing, itching, radicular)
- Impact of pain in activities of daily living
  - Emotional component: *What does it represent to the patient?*
- Severity:
  - 0 (no pain)-10(most severe possible)
- Clarify the extent of the neoplastic disease
- Elucidate comorbidities
  - Screen for alcohol and smoking dependencies
- Treatment:
  - What has been used to relieve the pain
  - Determine the need for other palliative care interventions
  - Identify barriers to treatment (patients' beliefs, physicians' misconceptions, fear of addiction to opioids)

A useful mnemonic is LMNOPQRST (location, medical treatments, number of episodes, onset, position, quality, radiation, severity, and triggers [61]).

There are multiple ways to treat cancer-related pain, and a clinician should always recognize that pharmacological management is only one of them (Table 20.9).

Pharmacological Pain Management

- Degree of pain (mild/moderate/severe) determines selection of analgesic
- Oral route preferred, avoid IM route, IV route for quick onset (severe pain).
  - Subcutaneous route is reserved for advanced disease and management of dehydration.
- At appropriate doses, respiratory depression is uncommon with opioid use in palliative cancer patients
- Addiction is rare when pain is present
- See Table 20.10 for examples of pharmacologic agents for pain treatment

Special Notes

- If there is a decline or fluctuation in renal function, the use of an opioid without active metabolites, such as fentanyl, or with a lower concentration of renally cleared metabolites, such as hydromorphone, is recommended [60].
- Opioid rotation: A change from one opioid to another in patients who are poorly responsive to an initial medication is accompanied by a better therapeutic outcome. Response is evident in approximately 2/3 of the patients who are switched [60].

Adjuvant Analgesics

Adjuvant analgesics are especially useful in cancer-related neuropathic pain [63]. The number needed to treat (NNT) to prevent one episode of pain for many adjuvant drugs is 3–5 [64], and drug toxicity is limiting. The overall clinical picture of the

Table 20.8 Treatment options for malignant ascites [51, 53]

Diuretic Therapy [53]	Successful in approximately 40% of cases. More useful in patients with liver metastasis and portal hypertension Better results when combined with other therapies
Paracentesis	Symptom resolution in 90%. Need for repeated treatments. Especially indicated in patients who need rapid resolution of symptoms. Up to 5 L of fluid can be removed, without requiring IV fluid replacement. No evidence of benefit from albumin replacement. Studies in MA have used D5W [53]
Permanent Catheters (Tunneled) [51, 54]	Ideal for patients requiring frequent paracentesis (<7 days of interval) Risk of peritonitis (1–4.4%). Complications 7%
Intraperitoneal Chemotherapy	Range of success depends on tumor type. Ranges between 33% and 65%
Cytoreductive Surgery (CRS) and Heated Intraperitoneal Chemotherapy (HIPEC) [55]	Resolution of ascites in 93% Resolution of ascites not related to R0–R1 or R2 resection. Magnitude of preoperative ascites did not correlate with the probability of resolution. However there was an inverse correlation between quantity of ascites and R0–R1 resection. Survival advantage with R0–R1 resections Not considered an ideal "palliative option"
Laparoscopic HIPEC [56, 57]	Valuable option for patients not eligible for CRS + HIPEC. Considered a viable "Palliative therapy" Resolution of ascites in 95% of patients. Mean Hospital Stay 2.3 days. No Cytoreductive Surgery required
Surgical Peritoneovenous Shunts [58]	High rates of complications (up to 38%). Occlusion 24% Shunt revision in 12% Use in extremely selected patients with life expectancy greater than 3 months Contraindicated in patients with heart or renal failure, portal hypertension, loculated effusions, and hemorrhagic ascites Prevents protein and fluid loses [53]. Better outcomes in patients with non-gastrointestinal cancer Median patency of peritoneovenous shunt (Denver®) is 3 months

patient and possible secondary benefits (e.g., treatment of concomitant depression) should guide agent selection. Table 20.11 outlines examples of some adjuvant therapies for pain management.

Nausea

About 20–30% of people with advanced cancer suffer from nausea, and the impact nausea can have on their quality of life can be devastating [65]. There are different mechanisms that can cause nausea in palliative cancer patients (Table 20.12). It is

Table 20.9 Categories of treatment for pain-related to cancer

Pharmacologic	Opioids/Non-opioids/Adjuvant Analgesics
Intervention	Implant/Injection Therapies Neural Blockades
Radiation therapy	Treatment of bone pain, malignant spinal cord compression, or brain metastasis [63]
Rehabilitative	Therapeutic Exercise Occupational Therapy Therapies for specific disorders (e.g., Lymphedema)
Psychological	Psychoeducational interventions Cognitive-behavioral therapy
Neurostimulation	Transcutaneous Transcranial
Integrative or Complementary	Acupuncture Massage

Adapted from Portenoy et al. [60] and and Auret et al. [63]

Table 20.10 Pharmacological pain therapies

Mild pain	Moderate pain	Severe pain
Acetaminophen or NSAID (aspirin or ibuprofen)	Single agents: Codeine 5–10% of patients may be slow CYP2D6 metabolizers and experience no benefit from codeine. Oxycodone Combination: Acetaminophen with codeine	First line drug is morphine—Use hydromorphone in elderly or renal impairment Start with routine q4h doses of immediate release until pain control achieved. Do not start sustained release until pain control is stable for a few days Breakthrough (PRN) doses should also be prescribed Monitor and titrate frequently, change q4h dose when you know how much was needed in 24 h, watch for over-sedation and respiratory depression Always prescribe a laxative and antiemetic with opiates 30 mg oral morphine = 20–30 mg oral oxycodone = 7.5 mg oral hydromorphone = 10 mg IV/SC morphine = 2 mg IV/SC hydromorphone Conversion is an estimate, so use 50–75% of new dose to avoid overdosing FENTANYL patch (mcg) = 24 h oral morphine dose/2. Round down to avoid overdosing.

important to try to determine the cause so the treatment can be tailored to it. Nondrug and pharmacologic approaches can be helpful in the management of nausea (Table 20.13).

Nondrug Therapy for Nausea and Vomiting [66]

- Cool cloth, fan
- Bland, room temperature foods; limit fluids with foods
- Decrease: stimuli
- Acupuncture or acupressure

Table 20.11 Adjuvant therapies for pain management

Class	Notes	Examples
Antidepressants	Start low dose Escalate slowly (2–3 days) Discontinue if no effect in 1 week	Amitriptyline Venlafaxine Duloxetine
Anticonvulsants		Gabapentin Pregabalin Carbamazepine
Corticosteroids	Limited for long-term use	Dexamethasone Prednisone
Bisphosphonates	Bone pain from metastases in normocalcemic patients 14–28 days for effect	Pamidronate Zolendronate Denosumab

Adapted from: Dunn et al. 2009 [31] and Auret et al. [65]

Table 20.12 Causes of nausea in the cancer patient [31, 65]

Pharmacologic	Opioids/Nonopioids/Adjuvant Analgesics In patients with reversible causes for nausea, it may be the culprit in up to 50% If related to opioids, a dose reduction or opioid rotation may reduce the severity [65]
Elevated Intracranial Pressure	Metastatic/primary brain lesions Blockage of cerebrospinal fluid collecting system Leptomeningeal disease
Vestibular	Stimulation of vestibular system
Emotional/Psychological	Anticipatory nausea prior to chemotherapy or procedures Anxiety
Gastrointestinal	Impaired gastric motility Constipation Obstruction
Metabolic Causes	Electrolyte disorders

Dyspnea

Dyspnea is the subjective sensation of uncomfortable breathing that may not relate to measured oxygen saturation or blood gases. It is strongly associated with anxiety (feedback loop). There are nondrug and drug therapies that are helpful in the management of dyspnea (Table 20.14).

Nondrug Therapy

- Positioning
- Supplemental oxygen (preferably nasal cannula) titrated to symptom relief not pulse oximetry
- Increase air movement (fans)
- Humidified air
- Behavioral treatment

Table 20.13 Pharmacologic management for nausea and vomiting [66]

Class	Indications	Examples
Serotonin agonist	Stimulation of chemoreceptor trigger zone (CTZ): e.g. morphine, hypercalcemia, uremia	Ondansetron
Dopamine agonist	Stimulation of CTZ	Haloperidol
Promotility	Gastric stasis (should be avoided in patients with query obstruction)	Metoclopramide
Glucocorticoids	Consider in patients with elevated ICP	Dexamethasone
Antihistamine	Vestibular nausea (movement related, tumor, infections, morphine)	Diphenhydramine
Benzodiazepines	Helps prevent anticipatory nausea and vomiting (limbic system)	Lorazepam

ICP intracranial pressure

Table 20.14 Drug therapy for dyspnea [31]

Symptoms	Class	Examples
Cough	Opioid Inhaled local anesthetics may be used for cough, though impairs gag reflex and limits ability to taste	Dextromethorphan, codeine Inhaled lidocaine
Patients with air hunger	Opioids	Morphine
Patients experiencing anxiety, panic, or sense of suffocation	Anxiolytics	Lorazepam Diazepam
Bronchospasm Superior vena cava syndrome Parenchymal metastases	Corticosteroids	Dexamethasone Prednisone
Excessive watery secretions	Anticholinergic	Glycopyrrolate
Excessive thick secretions	Sedatives Avoid anticholinergics (causes increased thickening of secretions) Avoid suctioning if possible (causes patient distress [66])	Chlorpromazine

Constipation

Constipation is a very common symptom in patients with cancer. Its prevalence can be between 70% and 100% [67]. Every patient with new onset constipation or a change from their regular bowel habits should have other processes ruled out to explain the change in presentation, especially obstruction [31, 67].

- Prevention is more effective than cure.
- Considerations include addition of stool softeners or laxatives when ordering opioids (constipation is the most frequent and persistent side effect of opioid therapy) [67]

Table 20.15 Treatment options for constipation [67]

First line	Senna glycoside ± milk of magnesia
Second line	Bisacodyl
Third line	Fleet enema GoLYTELY enema Lactulose Methylnaltrexone IV or SC
Fourth line	Magnesium citrate, repeat enema, manual disimpaction

- Stool softeners or bulking agents alone may not be adequate
  - (See Table 20.15 for treatment options for constipation)

References

1. Canadian Cancer Statistics Advisory Committee. Canadian cancer statistics 2018. Toronto: Canadian Cancer Society; 2018. Available at: cancer.ca/Canadian-Cancer-Statistics-2018-EN (accessed 5 May 2019).
2. Temel JS, Greer JA, Muzikansky A, et al. Early palliative care for patients with metastatic non-small-cell lung cancer. N Engl J Med. 2010;363:733–42.
3. Bakitas MA, Tosteson TD, Li Z, et al. Early versus delayed initiation of concurrent palliative oncology care: patient outcomes in the ENABLE III randomized controlled trial. J Clin Oncol. 2013;33(13):1438–48.
4. Pirl WF, Greer JA, Traeger L, et al. Depression and survival in metastatic non–small-cell lung cancer: effects of early palliative care. J Clin Oncol. 2012;30:1310–5.
5. Zimmerman C, Swami N, Krzyzanowska M, et al. Early palliative care for patients with advanced cancer: a cluster-randomised controlled trial. Lancet. 2014;383:1721–30.
6. Zimmerman C, Swami N, Krzyzanowska M, et al. Perceptions of palliative care among patients with advanced cancer and their caregivers. CMAJ. 2016;188(10):e217–27.
7. Hawley P. The bow tie model of 21st century palliative care. J Pain Symptom Manag. 2014;47(1):e2–5.
8. Gwilliam B, Keeley V, Todd C, et al. Prognosticating in patients with advanced cancer—observational study comparing the accuracy of clinicians' and patients' estimates of survival. Ann Oncol. 2013;24:482–8.
9. Sadler EM, Hawley PH, Easson AM. Palliative care and active disease management are synergistic in modern surgical oncology. Surgery. 2018;163(4):950–3.
10. Olmsted CL, Johnson AM, Kaboli P, et al. Use of palliative care and hospice among surgical and medical specialties in the Veterans Health Administration. JAMA Surg. 2014;149(11):1169–75.
11. Dunn GP, Martensen R, Weissman D. Surgical palliative care: a resident's guide. Essex: American College of Surgeons; 2009.
12. Lilley EJ, Cooper Z, Schwarze ML, et al. Palliative care in surgery: defining the research priorities. Ann Surg. 2017;267:66. https://doi.org/10.1097/SLA.0000000000002253.
13. Wagman LD. Progress in palliative surgery-is it a subspecialty? J Surg Oncol. 2007;96(6):449–50.
14. Cameron JL, Cameron AM, editors. Current surgical therapy. 9th ed. Philadelphia: Mosby Inc.; 2007.
15. Bakitas M, Lyons KD, Hegel MT, et al. Effects of palliative care intervention on clinical outcomes in patients with advanced cancer: the project ENABLE II randomized controlled trial. JAMA. 2009;302:741–9.

16. Scibetta C, Kerr K, McGuire J, et al. The costs of waiting: implications of the timing of palliative care consultation among a cohort of decedents at a comprehensive cancer center. J Palliat Med. 2016;19(1):69–75.
17. Hui D, Kim SH, Roquemore J, et al. Impact of timing and setting of palliative care referral on quality of end-of-life care in cancer patients. Cancer. 2014;120(11):1743–9.
18. Ferrell B, Sun V, Hurria A, et al. Interdisciplinary palliative care for patients with lung cancer. J Pain Symptom Manag. 2015;50(6):758–67.
19. Ferrell B, Temel J, Temin S, et al. Integration of palliative care into standard oncology care: American Society of Clinical Oncology practice guideline update. J Clin Oncol. 2017;35(1):96–112.
20. Ng A, Easson AM. Selection and preparation of patients for surgical palliation. In: Surgical palliative care. New York: Oxford University Press; 2004. p. 16–32.
21. Hanna NN, Bellavance E, Keay T. Palliative surgical oncology. Surg Clin North Am. 2011;91(2):343–53; viii.
22. Collins LK, Goodwin JA, Spencer HJ, Guevara C, Ferrell B, McSweeney J, et al. Patient reasoning in palliative surgical oncology. J Surg Oncol. 2013;107(4):372–5.
23. Hamilton T, Selby S, Tsang M, Kim A, Wright F. Patients' perceptions of palliative surgical procedures: a qualitative analysis. Ann Palliat Med. 2017;6(Suppl 1):S77–84.
24. Kostakou E, Rovina N, Kyriakopoulou M, Koulouris NG, Koutsoukou A. Critically ill cancer patient in intensive care unit: issues that arise. J Crit Care. 2014;29(5):817–22.
25. Paul Olson TJ, Pinkerton C, Brasel KJ, Schwarze ML. Palliative surgery for malignant bowel obstruction from carcinomatosis: a systematic review. JAMA Surg. 2014;149(4):383–92.
26. Lamont EB, Christakis NA. Some elements of prognosis in terminal cancer. Oncology (Williston Park, N.Y.). 1999;13:1165–70; Discussion 1172–1174, 1179–1180.
27. Chochinov HM, Tataryn DJ, Wilson KG, Enns M, Lander S. Prognostic awareness and the terminally ill. Psychosomatics. 2000;41:500–4.
28. Bradley EH, Hallemeier AG, Fried TR, et al. Documentation of discussions about prognosis with terminally ill patients. Am J Med. 2001;111:218–23.
29. Hebert RS, Schulz R, Copeland VC, Arnold RM. Preparing family caregivers for death and bereavement. Insights from caregivers of terminally ill patients. J Pain Symptom Manag. 2009;37:3–12.
30. Bilimoria KY, Liu Y, Paruch JL, et al. Development and evaluation of the universal ACS NSQIP surgical risk calculator: a decision aid and informed consent tool for patients and surgeons. J Am Coll Surg. 2013;217:833–42.
31. Dunn G, Martensen R, Weissman D. Surgical palliative care: a residents guide. Essex: American College of Surgeons/Cunniff-Dixon Foundation; 2009.
32. Frago R, Ramirez E, Millan M, Kreisler E, del Valle E, Biondo S. Current management of acute malignant large bowel obstruction: a systematic review. Am J Surg. 2014;207(1):127–38.
33. Laval G, Marcelin-Benazech B, Guirimand F, Chauvenet L, Copel L, Durand A, et al. Recommendations for bowel obstruction with peritoneal carcinomatosis. J Pain Symptom Manag. 2014;48(1):75–91.
34. Shariat-Madar B, Jayakrishnan TT, Gamblin TC, Turaga KK. Surgical management of bowel obstruction in patients with peritoneal carcinomatosis. J Surg Oncol. 2014;110(6):666–9.
35. De Boer N, Hagemans J, Schultze B, et al. Acute malignant obstruction in patients with peritoneal carcinomatosis. Eur J Surg Oncol. 2019;45:389–93.
36. Ly J, O'Grady G, Mittal A, Plank L, Windsor JA. A systematic review of methods to palliate malignant gastric outlet obstruction. Surg Endosc. 2010;24(2):290–7.
37. Jeurnink SM, Steyerberg EW, Vleggaar FP, van Eijck CH, van Hooft JE, Schwartz MP, et al. Predictors of survival in patients with malignant gastric outlet obstruction: a patient-oriented decision approach for palliative treatment. Dig Liver Dis. 2011;43(7):548–52.
38. Fiori E, Lamazza A, Demasi E, Decesare A, Schillaci A, Sterpetti AV. Endoscopic stenting for gastric outlet obstruction in patients with unresectable antro pyloric cancer. Systematic review of the literature and final results of a prospective study. The point of view of a surgical group. Am J Surg. 2013;206(2):210–7.

39. Jeurnink SM, Steyerberg EW, van Hooft JE, van Eijck CH, Schwartz MP, Vleggaar FP, et al. Surgical gastrojejunostomy or endoscopic stent placement for the palliation of malignant gastric outlet obstruction (SUSTENT study): a multicenter randomized trial. Gastrointest Endosc. 2010;71(3):490–9.
40. Gurusamy KS, Kumar S, Davidson BR. Prophylactic gastrojejunostomy for unresectable periampullary carcinoma. Cochrane Database Syst Rev. 2013;2:CD008533.
41. Tan CJ, Dasari BV, Gardiner K. Systematic review and meta-analysis of randomized clinical trials of self-expanding metallic stents as a bridge to surgery versus emergency surgery for malignant left-sided large bowel obstruction. Br J Surg. 2012;99(4):469–76.
42. van Hooft JE, van Halsema EE, Vanbiervliet G, Beets-Tan RG, DeWitt JM, Donnellan F, et al. Self-expandable metal stents for obstructing colonic and extracolonic cancer: European Society of Gastrointestinal Endoscopy (ESGE) Clinical Guideline. Endoscopy. 2014;46(11):990–1053.
43. Masi G, Cupini S, Marcucci L, Cerri E, Loupakis F, Allegrini G, et al. Treatment with 5-fluorouracil/folinic acid, oxaliplatin, and irinotecan enables surgical resection of metastases in patients with initially unresectable metastatic colorectal cancer. Ann Surg Oncol. 2006;13(1):58–65.
44. Loupakis F, Cremolini C, Masi G, Lonardi S, Zagonel V, Salvatore L, et al. Initial therapy with FOLFOXIRI and bevacizumab for metastatic colorectal cancer. N Engl J Med. 2014;371(17):1609–18.
45. Zhao XD, Cai BB, Cao RS, Shi RH. Palliative treatment for incurable malignant colorectal obstructions: a meta-analysis. World J Gastroenterol. 2013;19(33):5565–74.
46. Cirocchi R, Farinella E, Trastulli S, Desiderio J, Listorti C, Boselli C, et al. Safety and efficacy of endoscopic colonic stenting as a bridge to surgery in the management of intestinal obstruction due to left colon and rectal cancer: a systematic review and meta-analysis. Surg Oncol. 2013;22(1):14–21.
47. Bosscher MR, van Leeuwen BL, Hoekstra HJ. Surgical emergencies in oncology. Cancer Treat Rev. 2014;40(8):1028–36.
48. Rerknimitr R, Angsuwatcharakon P, Ratanachu-ek T, Khor CJ, Ponnudurai R, Moon JH, et al. Asia-Pacific consensus recommendations for endoscopic and interventional management of hilar cholangiocarcinoma. J Gastroenterol Hepatol. 2013;28(4):593–607.
49. Webb K, Saunders M. Endoscopic management of malignant bile duct strictures. Gastrointest Endosc Clin N Am. 2013;23(2):313–31.
50. Razumilava N, Gores GJ. Cholangiocarcinoma. Lancet. 2014;383(9935):2168–79.
51. Cavazzoni E, Bugiantella W, Graziosi L, Franceschini MS, Donini A. Malignant ascites: pathophysiology and treatment. Int J Clin Oncol. 2013;18(1):1–9.
52. Sangisetty SL, Miner TJ. Malignant ascites: a review of prognostic factors, pathophysiology and therapeutic measures. World J Gastrointest Surg. 2012;4(4):87–95.
53. Becker G, Galandi D, Blum HE. Malignant ascites: systematic review and guideline for treatment. Eur J Cancer. 2006;42(5):589–97.
54. Lungren MP, Kim CY, Stewart JK, Smith TP, Miller MJ. Tunneled peritoneal drainage catheter placement for refractory ascites: single-center experience in 188 patients. J Vasc Interv Radiol. 2013;24(9):1303–8.
55. Randle RW, Swett KR, Swords DS, Shen P, Stewart JH, Levine EA, et al. Efficacy of cytoreductive surgery with hyperthermic intraperitoneal chemotherapy in the management of malignant ascites. Ann Surg Oncol. 2014;21(5):1474–9.
56. Facchiano E, Risio D, Kianmanesh R, Msika S. Laparoscopic hyperthermic intraperitoneal chemotherapy: indications, aims, and results: a systematic review of the literature. Ann Surg Oncol. 2012;19(9):2946–50.
57. Valle M, Van der Speeten K, Garofalo A. Laparoscopic hyperthermic intraperitoneal peroperative chemotherapy (HIPEC) in the management of refractory malignant ascites: a multi-institutional retrospective analysis in 52 patients. J Surg Oncol. 2009;100(4):331–4.
58. White MA, Agle SC, Padia RK, Zervos EE. Denver peritoneovenous shunts for the management of malignant ascites: a review of the literature in the post LeVeen era. Am Surg. 2011;77(8):1070–5.

59. Paice JA, Von Roenn JH. Under- or overtreatment of pain in the patient with cancer: how to achieve proper balance. J Clin Oncol. 2014;32(16):1721–6.
60. Portenoy RK, Ahmed E. Principles of opioid use in cancer pain. J Clin Oncol. 2014;32(16):1662–70.
61. Hui D, Bruera E. A personalized approach to assessing and managing pain in patients with cancer. J Clin Oncol. 2014;32(16):1640–6.
62. Gough N, Miah AB, Linch M. Nonsurgical oncological management of cancer pain. Curr Opin Support Palliat Care. 2014;8(2):102–11.
63. Auret K, Schug SA. Pain management for the cancer patient—current practice and future developments. Best Pract Res Clin Anaesthesiol. 2013;27(4):545–61.
64. Ripamonti CI, Santini D, Maranzano E, Berti M, Roila F, ESMO Guidelines Working Group. Management of cancer pain: ESMO Clinical Practice Guidelines. Ann Oncol. 2012;23(Suppl 7):vii139–54.
65. Gordon P, LeGrand SB, Walsh D. Nausea and vomiting in advanced cancer. Eur J Pharmacol. 2014;722:187–91.
66. Old JL, Swagerty D. A practical guide to palliative care. Philadelphia: Wolters Kluwer Health; 2007. p. xii, 348.
67. Clemens KE, Faust M, Jaspers B, Mikus G. Pharmacological treatment of constipation in palliative care. Curr Opin Support Palliat Care. 2013;7(2):183–91.

Adenocarcinoma of the Pancreas

21

Christopher R. Shubert, Carol-anne E. Moulton, Ali Hosni, Grainne M. O'Kane, and Steven Gallinger

Introduction

Pancreatic cancer is the 12th most common cancer and the 10th most common solid organ malignancy with approximately 5500 new diagnosis per year in Canada. It has one of the lowest relative survival rates, making it the fourth most common cause of cancer death. In Canada, the lifetime probability of developing pancreatic cancer is 1 in 72 and the 5-year overall survival for pancreatic cancer is 8% [1]. Incidence rates of pancreatic cancer have remained relatively unchanged since 1992 [2]. However, if current trends continue, pancreatic cancer will surpass breast cancer to become the third leading cause of cancer-related death after lung and colorectal cancers [2]. The stage at diagnosis is the most important prognostic factor. Most patients are diagnosed with metastatic disease, where survival is limited (Table 21.1).

With regard to incidence, there is great variability among ethnic groups with Northern, Central, and Eastern Europeans and African Americans having high incidence rates of 10–15/100,000 whereas Asians and native Africans have low rates of <1/100,000.

C. R. Shubert
Hepatopancreatobiliary Surgery, University of Toronto, Toronto, ON, Canada
e-mail: christopher.shubert@uhn.ca

C.-a. E. Moulton · S. Gallinger (✉)
Department of Surgery, University of Toronto, Toronto, ON, Canada
e-mail: Carol-anne.Moulton@uhn.ca; steven.gallinger@uhn.ca

A. Hosni
Department of Radiation Oncology, University of Toronto, Toronto, ON, Canada
e-mail: Ali.Hosni@rmp.uhn.on.ca

G. M. O'Kane
Department of Medical Oncology, University of Toronto, Toronto, ON, Canada
e-mail: Grainne.O'kane@uhn.ca

F. C. Wright et al. (eds.), *Surgical Oncology Manual*,
https://doi.org/10.1007/978-3-030-48363-0_21

Table 21.1 Prognosis by stage at presentation

Presentation	Prognosis 5-year overall survival (OS)
Resectable disease (10–20%)	15–34%
Borderline resectable disease (5–10%)	15–20%
Unresectable disease—locally advanced (20–40%)	<5%
Metastatic disease (40–60%)	0%

Table 21.2 Most common genetic disorders associated with pancreatic cancer

Genetic disorder	Gene implicated	Approximate relative risk
Hereditary pancreatitis	SPINK1/PRSS1	50–70
Peutz–Jeghers syndrome	LKB1/STK11	>100
Cystic fibrosis	CFTR	2, 6–60
Familial atypical, multiple-mole melanoma	CDKN2A	13–39
Hereditary breast ovarian cancer syndrome	BRCA1/2/PALB2	2, 3–10
Lynch syndrome	MSH2/MLH1/MSH6/PMS2	4–5
Familial adenomatous polyposis	APC	4–5
Li–Fraumeni	p53	Unknown
Familial pancreatic cancer	Multiple, unidentified	4–32

The most significant risk factor for the development of pancreatic cancer is age, with a rapid rise in incidence after the age of 50. Smoking has been clearly causally related to an increased risk of pancreatic cancer in epidemiological studies, and risk increases with extent of exposure. Pancreatic cancer is more common in people with diabetes. Interestingly, many patients present with new onset or worsening diabetes around the time of diagnosis although the association between pancreatic cancer and diabetes are not fully understood. Obesity and chronic pancreatitis are more controversial; while statistical associations exist, the relative risk is low (1.2–1.5) and it is difficult to confirm causality [3–7].

A few uncommon genetic disorders contribute to 10–15% of cases [7, 8]. The recognition of the presence of an underlying genetic disorder may have significant implications for the treatment of pancreatic cancer (Table 21.2). For example, some patients with a BRCA or PALB2 mutation who develop pancreatic cancer have exceptional response to platinum-based chemotherapy, some demonstrating significant tumor regression, even with metastatic disease [9].

There is no level I evidence to support screening of pancreas cancer in the general population. Investigational screening protocols are underway for high-risk individuals with Peutz–Jeghers syndrome, known BRCA mutation, FAMM, familial pancreatic cancer, and hereditary pancreatitis. The diagnostic yield of screening in these groups varies from 1% to 50% [3, 8, 10]. Subjects from high-risk families should be enrolled in investigational surveillance protocols.

Diagnosis and Staging

Work-Up

- History and physical exam
- Performance status assessment
  - A careful examination of performance status is essential, as it may greatly affect the sequencing and choice of treatment. Performance status is one of the primary indicators of long-term survival in patients with metastatic disease.
- Labs:
  - Liver function tests: Including albumin and coagulation profile (specifically INR)
  - Serum CA 19-9 (also consider CEA)
    - Tumor marker CA 19-9 should be performed. Elevated CA 19-9 has been shown to be a biological indicator of advanced disease and poor prognosis [11, 12]. Some evidence has shown that even among early-stage resectable pancreatic cancer, CA 19-9 elevation is associated with worse prognosis and may warrant chemotherapy as first approach to treatment [11]. Results should be interpreted with caution, however, as strict cutoff levels have not been established and jaundice artificially elevates serum levels [12].
  - Consider IgG4 in selected cases to exclude autoimmune pancreatitis.
- Imaging:
  - Pancreas protocol CT scan
  - Chest imaging (ideally CT chest but X-ray could also be accepted)
  - Consider EUS, MRI, and/or staging laparoscopy in selected cases

Classification and Staging

The most well established, CT-based classification of resectability was developed at the MD Anderson Cancer Center (MDACC) and uses key parameters based on preoperative, multi-detector CT imaging. This classification is accepted by AHPBA, SSO, and SAT since 2009 and was incorporated into the NCCN guidelines since [13] (Table 21.3).

The American Joint Committee on Cancer/Union for International Cancer Control (AJCC/UICC) TNM 8th edition staging system is the most current recommended staging system for pathology reporting. The TNM staging system provides a unified and standard staging language for communication of the extent of cancer. This information conveys useful and objective information for prognosis and is the basis of treatment decisions for individual patients. As well, TNM staging aids in the evaluation of treatment response, facilitates exchange of information among centers and oncology professionals, is critical to cancer registries, and policy development and implementation.

Table 21.3 CT-based classification of resectability

	Metastatic disease	Nodal disease	Relationship to SMV-PV	Relationship to arteries
Resectable disease (RES) (all criteria must be met)	None	Allowed within regional nodes	No evidence of PV or SMV distortion	Normal tissue planes
Borderline Resectable (BOR) (any criteria fulfilled)	None	Allowed within regional nodes	Venous involvement of PV or SMV with distortion, narrowing or occlusion of the vein Must be suitable for reconstruction Contact with IVC	Tumor contact with CHA or variant of arterial anatomy Tumor contact with SMA 0–180 ° Body-tail tumor with tumor contact with CA 0–180 °
Unresectable—Locally Advanced (LA) (any criteria fulfilled)	None	Allowed within regional nodes	Unreconstructible PV and/or SMV occlusion	SMA > 180 ° CA > 180 ° Aortic invasion
Metastatic disease	Yes (e.g., peritoneum, liver, lung, bones)	Non-regional lymph node metastasis (e.g., celiac, peri-aortic)	Any	Any

Based on NCCN criteria defining resectability status (Version 1.2019) [13, 14]
CA celiac axis, *CHA* common hepatic artery, *PV* portal vein, *SMA* superior mesenteric artery, *SMV* superior mesenteric vein

Imaging Studies

- CT scan of the abdomen:
  - Thin slice pancreatic protocol CT including arterial and pancreatic phases via a high-quality scanner is mandatory for accurate preoperative staging of pancreatic cancer and represents the single best test for determining resectability [15–18].
  - CT review by an experienced HPB radiologist and standardized, structured, synoptic reporting is recommended [19]
  - CT should be evaluated with detailed comments on the following [15–19]:
    - Presence or suspicion of metastatic disease (e.g., liver, peritoneum, omentum)
    - Presence or suspicion of nodal disease outside the resected field (aortocaval nodes)
    - Presence of a hypodense mass and/or pancreatic duct dilatation and/or biliary duct dilatation

    - Presence of SMV-PV involvement and/or arterial involvement including name of the vessel with degree of involvement
    - Presence of aberrant vascular anatomy and if involved by tumor
  - CT should be performed prior to any interventional endoscopic procedure, as both biliary decompression and lesion biopsy can result in pancreatitis that can preclude the necessary detailed anatomical evaluation of the lesion. Furthermore, high-quality CT may prove these interventions unnecessary.
  - The addition of the borderline resectable and locally advanced categories identify groups of patients at higher risk for positive resection margins and worse outcomes who may benefit from neoadjuvant therapy [20].
- Magnetic Resonance Imaging (MRI) [21]
  - Magnetic resonance cholangio-pancreatography (MRCP) may have a role in diagnosis for patients with a differential diagnosis of distal common bile duct tumors (CBD), cystic pancreatic lesions.
  - MRI can be useful when CT is contraindicated.
  - MRI is less sensitive for detecting pancreatic lesions than CT and is equivalent for determining resectability.
  - Equivocal hepatic lesions may be better defined with MRI or transabdominal US.
- Endoscopic Ultrasound (EUS):
  - Diagnostic EUS may be useful when:
    - A lesion is not clearly visible, despite associated pancreatic duct/common bile duct dilatation
    - To allow fine needle aspiration of the primary lesion for tissue diagnosis if needed
  - It is also useful when highly suspicious nodes in the peri-aortic and celiac area are identified on CT that, if confirmed metastatic, would preclude surgical resection.
  - Due to the increasing use and investigation of neoadjuvant treatments, there is a growing role for EUS to obtain preoperative tissue diagnosis.
- PET/CT Scan:
  - The role of PET/CT in the diagnosis and staging of pancreatic cancer is controversial.
  - PET/CT does not appear to have sensitivity advantage over CT alone in identifying small-volume metastatic hepatic or peritoneal disease.

Tissue Diagnosis

Biopsy should not be performed in patients whose presentation and imaging findings are classic for pancreas cancer and are planned to undergo a surgery-first approach.

Tissue diagnosis is necessary for patients with unresectable and metastatic disease prior to definitive chemotherapy, as well for neoadjuvant therapy for those with borderline resectable and locally advanced lesions. Brushings can be obtained at the time of ERCP. When the pancreas lesion is targeted, endoscopic ultrasound-fine needle aspiration (EUS-FNA) has the best overall operating characteristics and is most cost-effective [22]. EUS-FNA should be favored when ERCP is not indicated and/or brushings are negative. Additionally, CT or US-guided percutaneous biopsy is also acceptable.

Biopsy of a potential metastatic lesion is often preferred over biopsy of the primary, as confirmation of the metastatic lesion in question would change staging and subsequent treatment.

Biopsy for Molecular Analysis

Molecular profiling studies, primarily in patients with resectable PDAC, have described genomic and gene expression profiles [23–27]. To date, these have not informed clinical practices. Furthermore, in the clinical setting, physicians choose between modified FOLFIRINOX and gemcitabine/nab-paclitaxel as a chemotherapy backbone; however, biomarkers to aid the choice of treatment are lacking. As a result, the Comprehensive Molecular Characterization of Advanced PDAC for Better Treatment Selection: A Prospective Study (COMPASS, NCT02750657) was established at Princess Margaret Cancer Centre. Patients with advanced PDAC (locally advanced and metastatic), suitable for combination chemotherapy, enroll in the COMPASS study and have a fresh biopsy for whole genome sequencing (WGS) and RNAseq prior to treatment.

As part of this high content trial, a poor prognostic group of patients has been reported (modified Moffitt basal-like RNA signature) which encompasses 25% of patients with metastatic PDAC [28]. In addition, it has been shown that GATA6 expression can dichotomize the 'classical' and basal-like (modified Moffitt) subgroups. GATA6 can be reliably determined by RNA in situ hybridization (ISH).

The COMPASS trial represents an ongoing real-world analysis linking outcomes to molecular profiles, and early data suggest tumors scored as GATA6 low using RNA ISH are particularly resistant to modified FOLFIRINOX therefore representing a potential predictive biomarker [29]. Similar to other groups [30–32], WGS has also identified potentially actionable variants in advanced cases, primarily in patients with KRAS wild-type tumors (~8–10%) and the small cohort of patients (~5–8%) with tumors deficient in homologous recombination repair.

A cross-Canada multisite neoadjuvant FOLFIRINOX trial evaluating the GATA6 biomarker in patients with resectable PDAC is planned and opening Summer 2020.

Staging Laparoscopy

Staging laparoscopy should be reserved for selected cases where the yield is likely to justify the additional procedural risks and costs [33]. The literature suggests that 10–36% of patients can be spared an unnecessary laparotomy [34]. As a guide, patients with tumors >3 cm, tumors in the neck, body, or tail, or with equivocal CT findings for metastatic disease may benefit from laparoscopy [35]. Additionally, prior to neoadjuvant therapy, staging laparoscopy should be considered. Patients selected for neoadjuvant therapy typically have locally advanced lesions with higher risk of distant spread of disease which if found would change treatment intent and sequence. Also, knowledge of metastatic disease prior to therapy would allow more accurate patient counseling and informed consent.

Biliary Decompression

Preoperative biliary decompression should be used selectively, as routine biliary drainage increases the rate of perioperative infectious complications, in addition to the risks of the procedure itself [36–39]. Biliary decompression with metal stent should be performed prior to neoadjuvant therapy. When biliary decompression is indicated, it is typically achieved via ERCP. One possible exception is biliary obstruction in the setting of simultaneous gastric outlet obstruction, whereby an operative double bypass should be considered if a Whipple is not indicated, assuming sufficient performance status and expected survival to warrant operative intervention (Table 21.4).

One special consideration when metal common bile duct stents are placed, attention must be paid to the location of the cystic duct (if the gallbladder is in-situ) as coverage of the cystic duct by the stent can cause cystic duct obstruction and precipitate acute cholecystitis.

Table 21.4 Biliary decompression considerations

Presentation	Recommendation	Procedure
Cholangitis	Urgent Biliary Decompression	ERCP + 10Fr plastic stent or SEMS
Preoperative elective	Routine biliary drainage is not recommended in mild/moderate jaundice due to higher overall risks Selective approach is recommended with consideration for stent if severe jaundice AND expected delay to surgery (>7–10 days)	±ERCP + 10Fr plastic stent or short metal stent
Consideration for neo-adjuvant therapy	Self-expanding metal stents should be considered	ERCP + short metal stent
Unresectable or metastatic	Consider stent if symptomatic or elevated bilirubin The choice of metallic or plastic stent depends on life expectancy. The significantly higher price of SEMS suggests their use in selected cases (life expectancy > 3 months) [40]	ERCP + SEMS or 10Fr plastic stent

ERCP endoscopic retrograde cholangio-pancreatography, *SEMS* self-expanding metal stent

Oncologic Management

Referring to Multidisciplinary Cancer Conference (MCC)

1. All patients should be presented early for multidisciplinary review to enable appropriate and efficient sequencing of investigations and treatments.
2. All patients should be offered to participate in clinical trials when available and appropriate for their stage and situation.

Systemic Chemotherapy

Neoadjuvant Therapy

Surgery alone, even for resectable PDAC, often leads to poor outcomes. Due to the relatively high morbidity of the procedure, only 59–95% of the patients have adequately recovered to receive adjuvant chemotherapy within 3 months of resection [41–44]. In addition, the aggressive nature of PDAC and its propensity to metastasize are arguments in favor of earlier systemic treatments.

There is some concern regarding the potential for "loss of the surgical window" due to local (or distant) progression during neoadjuvant therapy that could ultimately preclude surgery. However, proponents argue that neoadjuvant therapy allows for a more appropriate selection of patients for surgery by assessing tumor biology via response/stability of the tumor to chemotherapy prior to surgical resection. Studies suggest that 16–27% of patients progress during neoadjuvant therapy and do not proceed to surgical resection [45–47]. Most patients who progressed developed metastases during induction therapy and therefore were not offered surgery. This is a subgroup of patients with very poor cancer biology who may be spared a futile operation. In this setting, neoadjuvant therapy may increase the ability to identify patients who are most likely to not benefit from surgery.

The role of neoadjuvant therapy for PDAC continues to be defined. There is tremendous variability of its use worldwide. Patients with resectable or borderline disease should be offered the opportunity to participate in clinical trials examining this question where available.

In general, the goal of neoadjuvant therapy is to improve DFS and OS. Additionally, neoadjuvant therapy objectives are to expand operative eligibility and increase the rate of margin-negative resections (R0) in patients with locally advanced and borderline resectable disease.

Currently available data largely comes from small and heterogeneous retrospective studies and Phase 1–2 studies. In general, neoadjuvant regimens with CT restaging have shown partial response (PR) in 0–31%, stable disease (SD) in 60%, and progression (PD) in 17–32%. Interestingly, in the previously resectable group, 0–17% of the specimens have shown complete histological responses [48, 49]. One recent meta-analysis from the Dutch Pancreatic Cancer Group compared upfront surgery to neoadjuvant therapy with resectable and borderline resectable pancreatic cancer. They reported intention to treat improvement in overall survival despite lower resection rates [50].

To date, there has been only one published randomized controlled study comparing neoadjuvant therapy (chemoradiotherapy) and up-front surgery in the setting of resectable or borderline disease; however, there are many studies currently open and accruing and others starting to report. In the aforementioned multicenter study, 66 patients with resectable disease were randomized to surgery vs. neoadjuvant chemoradiotherapy (gemcitabine and cisplatin plus radiotherapy 50.4 Gy) plus surgery and both groups received adjuvant gemcitabine. Unfortunately, the trial was terminated early due to slow accrual. Median OS was 14.4 vs. 17.4 months with an intention-to-treat analysis and 18.9 vs. 25.0 months after resection [51].

Another study recently reported that patients with proven borderline resectable disease were randomized to preoperative chemoradiotherapy (36 Gray with gemcitabine) or immediate surgery, both followed by adjuvant chemotherapy. This study observed a significant improvement in overall survival (13.5 vs. 17.1 months, HR 0.71; $p = 0.047$) as well as an improvement in R0 resection rate (31% vs. 65%, $p < 0.001$) [52]. Another recently reported abstract of a randomized phase II/III trial of neoadjuvant gemcitabine and S-1 versus up front surgery for resectable disease showed a significant improvement in median overall survival (36.7 versus 26.6 months; HR 0.72, $p = 0.015$) [53].

FOLFIRINOX-based regimens have been studied in selected patients with borderline resectable or LAPC and have shown PR in 28–44% with resection made possible in 22–67% and an overall R0 rate of 28–67% [48, 54–56]. Noteworthy, in locally advanced cases despite post-neoadjuvant therapy imaging continuing to show locally advanced/unresectable disease, a margin negative (R0) resection is possible in >90% of cases after FOLFIRINOX. This same study showed that patients who received neoadjuvant therapy had decreased rates of lymph node involvement, lymphovascular invasion, perineural invasion, and resulted in a smaller tumors compared to those who had no neoadjuvant therapy [57]. One recent phase 2 study studying a combination of neoadjuvant FOLFIRINOX followed by radiotherapy for borderline resectable disease resulted in 66% of patients proceeding to surgery, 97% RO resection rate, median OS for all patients being 37.7 months, and 2-year OS for all patients being 56%; and among surgically resected patients, median OS had not been reached with a 2-year OS of 72% [58] (Table 21.5).

FOLFIRINOX, gemcitabine–paclitaxel, and chemoradiation protocols have been introduced into novel multimodality treatment, but further study is required to clarify the optimal sequence and strategy of treatment.

Adjuvant Therapy

Adjuvant therapy is generally recommended for all resected patients who are able to tolerate therapy regardless of final pathology stage. Adjuvant therapy is well established following surgical resection and improves long-term survival (5 years OS increases from 11% to 22% with gemcitabine vs. observation) [59].

The current standard of care in Ontario has been for postoperative chemotherapy with gemcitabine for 6 months post resection and should be started within 3 months of surgery. While there has been no evidence demonstrating superiority of Gemcitabine over 5-FU-based chemotherapy, Gemcitabine has a lower toxicity

Table 21.5 Landmark trials of systemic therapy for PDAC

Study comparison	Publication	Year	Main findings
Adjuvant chemoradiotherapy	EORTC-GITG [63]	1985 Ann Surg	NS improvement in OS—discouraged use of adjuvant chemoradiotherapy
Adjuvant chemoradiotherapy vs. chemotherapy alone	ESPAC-1 [64]	2001 Lancet	5 years OS: chemotherapy (20%) vs. chemoradiotherapy (10%)
Adjuvant gemcitabine vs. observation	CONKO-001 [59]	2007 JAMA	Median DFS: 13.4 vs. 6.9 months 5 years OS: 22.5% vs. 11.5%
Adjuvant 5-FU vs. gemcitabine	ESPAC-3 [60]	2010 JAMA	No difference in median overall survival (23 months), fewer adverse events with gemcitabine
FOLFIRINOX vs. gemcitabine (metastatic)	PRODIGE 4 (Accord 11) Trial [65]	2011 NEJM	Median survival 11.1 months vs. 6.8 months Increased toxicity with FOLFIRINOX, reserved for ECOG performance status 0 and 1 patients
Gemcitabine–paclitaxel vs. gemcitabine (metastatic) [66]		2013 (NEJM)	Median survival 8.5 months vs. 6.7 months Slightly increased toxicity with gemcitabine–paclitaxel
Adjuvant Gemcitabine vs. Gemcitabine-Capecitabine	ESPAC-4 [62]	2017 Lancet	Median survival 28.0 vs. 25.5 months
FOLFIRINOX or Gemcitabine as adjuvant therapy for pancreatic cancer	PRODIGE 24 [61]	2018 NEJM	Adjuvant therapy with a modified FOLFIRINOX regimen led to significantly longer survival than gemcitabine among patients with resected pancreatic cancer, at the expense of a higher incidence of toxic effects.

NS nonsignificant, *OS* overall survival, *DFS* disease-free survival, *ECOG* Eastern Cooperative Oncology Group

profile [60]. However, recently the PRODIGE trial comparing FOLFIRINOX to Gemcitabine as adjuvant therapy found significantly improved survival with FOLFIRINOX at the expense of higher incidence of toxicity [61]. Additionally, the ESPAC-4 trial compared adjuvant Gemcitabine to combination Gemcitabine and Capecitabine found and improvement in median overall survival for combination Gemcitabine and Capecitabine [62] (Table 21.5).

Referring to Medical Oncology

1. All patients who underwent resection *should* be referred for adjuvant chemotherapy.
2. Patients with unresectable or metastatic disease *should* be referred for consideration of systemic treatment.

3. Patients with borderline disease *could* be referred preoperatively for consideration of neoadjuvant treatment in the setting of a clinical trial.
4. Patients with unresectable/locally advanced disease *could* be considered for neoadjuvant therapy in the setting of a clinical trial.

Radiation Therapy

Neoadjuvant therapy:
Patients with borderline resectable pancreatic cancer likely receive systemic chemotherapy followed by chemoradiation aiming to achieve higher R0 resection rates. Patients who complete this multimodality regimen without evidence of disease progression undergo curative-intent surgery. This approach leverages theoretical benefits associated with *"systemic"* chemotherapy and *"targeted"* radiation.

Definitive therapy:
The addition of chemoradiation to chemotherapy showed better overall survival in ECOG 4201 randomized controlled trial and GERCOR Phase II and III studies [67, 68]. However, it showed inferior overall survival in phase III 2000–01 FFCD-SFRO study [69]. In phase III GERCOR LAP07 trial, chemoradiation was associated with decreased local progression (32% vs. 46%, $p = 0.03$) with no overall survival benefit [70].

Results of SBRT in patients with locally advanced pancreatic cancer are encouraging. Phase I/II studies showed excellent local control at 1 year (>90% for single fraction 25 Gy, and 78% following 33 Gy in 5 fractions), with less reported toxicity for fractionated (i.e., 5 fraction) SBRT regimen [71]. A multi-center phase III randomized study (NCT01926197) is currently recruiting locally advanced unresectable pancreatic cancer to evaluate the addition of SBRT to systemic chemotherapy, by which patients who show stable disease or response following 4 cycles of mFOLFIRINOX will be randomized to receive sequential SBRT then mFOLFIRINOX or continue with mFOLFIRINOX only [72].

Referring to Radiation Oncology

1. Patients with unresectable disease *could be* referred for consideration of radiotherapy as an adjunct to chemotherapy.
2. The routine use of radiotherapy in the adjuvant setting remains controversial. Patients who underwent resection and had positive margins *could be* referred for consideration of adjuvant radiotherapy adjunct to chemotherapy.
3. Some neoadjuvant protocols utilize pre-operative chemoradiotherapy for locally advanced lesions where there is high risk of positive margin.

Surgery

The tumor is located in the head of the pancreas or the uncinate process in approximately 45% of cases. Among resectable cases, 80% of tumors are located in the head/uncinate. For lesions of the pancreatic head and uncinate, patients should be offered a pancreatoduodenectomy (PD—Whipple procedure). When the tumor is located in the body-tail and judged resectable, distal pancreatectomy with splenectomy is the procedure of choice.

Outcomes following pancreatoduodenectomy (PD) vary widely with the volume of cases performed. This is reflected in recent series from high-volume centers, which reported peri-operative mortality between 1% and 2%, median LOS of 6–9 days, and median OS of 22–27 months after PD for pancreas cancer. About 20–25% of the surgeries included a PV-SMV resection and reconstruction. Positive surgical margins occur in 13–50% of patients undergoing resection. Positive surgical margin may negate the benefits of surgical resection, although pathological reporting of margins is inconsistent.

Arterial resection for borderline resectable and locally advanced pancreas cancer is now being performed in some high-volume centers with tailored neoadjuvant treatment protocols. Arterial resections are typically only entertained after extensive neoadjuvant chemotherapy often followed by chemo-radiotherapy, with proven stability/non-progression of disease on treatment. Postoperative morbidity is significantly increased for arterial resection compared to non-arterial resections. However, survival appears to be comparable to pancreatectomy without arterial resection [73, 74] (Table 21.6).

Table 21.6 Technical aspects of surgery. Multiple controversies exist regarding various technical aspects of pancreatic resection and reconstruction. These are summarized here

	Evidence	Recommendation
Extended lymphadenectomy vs. regular [77–79]	No survival advantage with extended lymphadenectomy, increased early morbidity	Standard lymphadenectomy
Venous resection [80–82]	Need for venous resection does not impact survival if R0 resection obtained	Venous resection is standard of care if reconstruction is possible and R0 resection is obtainable
PPPD vs. standard [83]	No difference in clinically relevant outcome between the two techniques	PPPD and standard Whipple are acceptable
PJ vs. PG [84]	Meta-analysis shows no difference in overall morbidity, DGE, bleeding, reoperation, or mortality. Possible decreased incidence of POPF and intra-abdominal collection with PG	PJ and PG are acceptable Even among high-risk anastomoses, PJ is most commonly performed
Pancreatic duct stent [85, 86]	No evidence to support decrease in POPF rate with trans-anastomotic pancreatic duct stenting. Possible increase in morbidity with stenting	No evidence to support internal stenting decreased morbidity

Table 21.6 (continued)

	Evidence	Recommendation
Somatostatin analogues [87–89]	Conflicting data from European and US trials Meta-analysis suggests reduction in POPF rate RCT suggests a decreased rate of clinically significant POPF from 21% to 9% No difference in mortality	Consider administration of peri-op somatostatin analogues for those at higher risk of POPF
Intra-abdominal drain [90–94]	Conflicting data among RCTs One trial failed to show a reduction in the number of deaths or complications with the addition of surgical intraperitoneal closed suction drainage after pancreatic resection [90] Another trial was stopped early due to increase in mortality and morbidity among PD patients without drain [91] Amylase value >5000 on POD#1 can predict POPF [94] Drain amylase analysis identifies which moderate/ high risk patients benefit from early drain removal [93].	Selective use of drain Early drain removal (on POD 3) [57, 92]
Open vs. laparoscopic distal pancreatectomy (DP)	Systematic review and meta-analysis: lap DP could decrease EBL, transfusion rate, LOS, and infections [95] Small retrospective series of 23 Lap DP for pancreas cancer: similar short- and long-term oncologic outcomes compared with open technique, with potentially shorter hospital stay [96]	Laparoscopic DP for pancreas cancer is feasible and safe in experienced hands.
Open vs. laparoscopic pancreatoduodenectomy (PD) [44]	Large retrospective series of 108 totally laparoscopic PD for pancreatic ductal adenocarcinoma (PDAC) Decreased EBL, transfusion rate, LOS, DGE grade B/C, and time to adjuvant chemotherapy. No difference in R0 rate, OS. Improved PFS	Laparoscopic PD for pancreas cancer is feasible and safe in experienced hands at select centers
Arterial Resection [73, 74]	After extensive neoadjuvant therapy, survival is comparable to non-arterial resections Increased postoperative complications compared to non-arterial resections	Arterial resections should only be considered at select high volume centers with particular expertise in arterial resection with arterial resection protocols.

DGE delayed gastric emptying, *PJ* pancreatojejunostomy, *PG* pancreatogastrostomy, *POPF* post-operative pancreatic fistula, *PPPD* pylorus preserving pancreatoduodenectomy, *EBL* estimated blood loss, *LOS* length of stay, *DGE* delayed gastric emptying

[a]Soft gland or small pancreatic duct

Special Notes

Clinical pathways to standardize recovery and mitigate risks of post-surgical complications after PD have been shown to decrease morbidity, decrease resource utilization including decreased LOS and decreased postoperative interventional radiology procedures while not increasing mortality or readmission rate [75].

- Laparoscopic PD for pancreas cancer is feasible and safe in select centers with experienced surgeons. It may decrease LOS and time to adjuvant chemotherapy and prolong PFS [44].
- In the setting of good imaging techniques, exploratory laparotomy for the purpose of determining resectability should be avoided.
- Patients with large lesions of the neck or body or those with associated main duct intraductal papillary mucinous neoplasm (IPMN) may require total pancreatectomy and splenectomy.
- Palliative surgical biliary ± gastric bypass may be considered at the time of exploration if the disease is deemed unresectable or metastatic and patient has an expected survival greater than 12 months (good performance status, absence of risk factors of poor survival) and with poor access to interventional/radiologic stenting [76].

Toronto Pearls

- High-quality CT imaging with biphasic pancreas protocol is essential for accurate staging and operative planning.
- All patients should be presented early for multidisciplinary review at a high-volume HPB center to enable appropriate and efficient sequencing of investigations and treatments.
- The sequencing of treatment should be individualized.
- Patients should routinely be given an opportunity to participate in clinical trials.
- Reconstructable venous involvement requires PV and/or SMV resection and reconstruction. The procedure is considered technically safe; therefore, this subgroup of borderline disease is treated like resectable disease.
- Arterial involvement does not absolutely preclude resection. Whether these tumors are classified as "borderline-artery" or "locally advanced-unresectable," the cases should be reviewed at a tertiary center. These patients should be given an opportunity to participate in trials or clinical protocols and considered for neoadjuvant chemotherapy [26] (Table 21.7).

Table 21.7 Summary of treatment by resectability classification

Classification	Neoadjuvant therapy	Surgery	Adjuvant treatment	Follow-up (F/U)
Resectable disease (RES)	Under investigation	R0 Resection	Chemotherapy × 6 months should be initiated within 12 weeks Gemcitabine × 6 months Level 1 evidence to supporting FOLFIRINOX in adjuvant setting Consider radiation for positive margins	Initial follow-up 2–4 weeks H&P q 3–6 months × 2 years, then annually Include assessment for pancreatic insufficiency Consider CT and CA 19-9 q 3–6 months × 2 year (level 5) There is no data to support that aggressive postoperative surveillance alters outcome in this disease.
Borderline resectable (BOR)	*Very controversial: resection* vs. *neoadjuvant therapy.* Patients should be included in clinical trials if possible Consider neoadjuvant therapy Decision to proceed to surgery is usually based on "non-progression"	*Borderline – Vein*: Consider up-front surgery. Will likely require a PV-SMV resection and reconstruction. *Borderline – Artery*: Consider neoadjuvant systemic chemotherapy ± chemoradiotherapy. Resectability status should be based on the ability to obtain negative margin	Chemotherapy × 6 months (same as resectable) Patients who have received neoadjuvant therapy may be candidates for additional adjuvant chemotherapy Consider radiation for positive margins	Same as RES
Unresectable—locally advanced (LA)	Select patients with arterial involvement should be considered for neoadjuvant treatment followed by pancreatectomy with vascular resection Those who progress on neoadjuvant therapy or who are not surgical candidates should receive chemotherapy with palliative intent (same as metastatic) Biliary decompression with stent where indicated When found during surgical exploration; consider surgical biliary ± gastric bypass			
Metastatic disease	Chemotherapy with palliative intent FOLFIRINOX (preferred) or Gemcitabine–paclitaxel (preferred) or Gemcitabine (for patients with poor performance status) Biliary decompression with stent where indicated When found during surgical exploration; consider surgical biliary ± gastric bypass			

References

1. Canadian Cancer Society. Canadian Cancer Statistics Advisory Committee. Canadian cancer statistics 2018. 2018.
2. Canadian Cancer Society. Canadian cancer statistics 2017 special topic: pancreatic cancer [Internet]. [cited 2019 Jan 15]. Available from: http://www.cancer.ca/~/media/cancer.ca/CW/cancerinformation/cancer101/Canadian-Cancer-Statistics-2017-EN.pdf.
3. Brand RE, Lerch MM, Rubinstein WS, Neoptolemos JP, Whitcomb DC, Hruban RH, et al. Advances in counselling and surveillance of patients at risk for pancreatic cancer. Gut. 2007;56:1640.
4. Iodice S, Gandini S, Maisonneuve P, Lowenfels AB. Tobacco and the risk of pancreatic cancer: a review and meta-analysis. Langenbeck's Arch Surg. 2008;393:535.
5. Stoita A, Penman ID, Williams DB. Review of screening for pancreatic cancer in high risk individuals. World J Gastroenterol. 2011;17:2365.
6. Lowenfels AB, Maisonneuve P, Whitcomb DC. Risk factors for cancer in hereditary pancreatitis. International Hereditary Pancreatitis Study Group. Med Clin North Am. 2000;84:565.
7. Maisonneuve P, Lowenfels A. Epidemiology and prospects for prevention of pancreatic cancer. In: Pancreatic cancer [Internet]. 2nd ed. New York: Springer New York; 2016. p. 1–16; [cited 15 Jan 2019]. Available from: http://link.springer.com/10.1007/978-1-4939-6631-8_73-1.
8. Del Chiaro M, Segersvärd R, Löhr M, Verbeke C. Early detection and prevention of pancreatic cancer: is it really possible today? World J Gastroenterol. 2014;20:12118.
9. Sonnenblick A, Kadouri L, Appelbaum L, Peretz T, Sagi M, Goldberg Y, et al. Complete remission, in BRCA2 mutation carrier with metastatic pancreatic adenocarcinoma, treated with cisplatin based therapy. Cancer Biol Ther. 2011;12:165.
10. Greer JB, Brand RE. Screening for pancreatic cancer: current evidence and future directions. Gastroenterol Hepatol. 2007;3:929.
11. Bergquist JR, Puig CA, Shubert CR, Groeschl RT, Habermann EB, Kendrick ML, et al. Carbohydrate antigen 19-9 elevation in anatomically resectable, early stage pancreatic cancer is independently associated with decreased overall survival and an indication for neoadjuvant therapy: a National Cancer Database Study [Internet]. J Am Coll Surg. 2016;223(1):52–65; available from: https://linkinghub.elsevier.com/retrieve/pii/S1072751516001642.
12. Boeck S, Stieber P, Holdenrieder S, Wilkowski R, Heinemann V. Prognostic and therapeutic significance of carbohydrate antigen 19-9 as tumor marker in patients with pancreatic cancer. Oncology. 2006;70:255.
13. Callery MP, Chang KJ, Fishman EK, Talamonti MS, William Traverso L, Linehan DC. Pretreatment assessment of resectable and borderline resectable pancreatic cancer: expert consensus statement [Internet]. Ann Surg Oncol. 2009;16(7):1727–33; [cited 7 Jan 2019]. Available from: http://www.springerlink.com/index/10.1245/s10434-009-0408-6.
14. National Comprehensive Cancer Network. Pancreatic adenocarcinoma: NCCN clinical practice guidelines in oncology version 1. 2019 [Internet]. 2018 [cited 15 Jan 2019]. Available from: www.nccn.org/patients.
15. Tamm E, Charnsangavej C, Szklaruk J. Advanced 3-D imaging for the evaluation of pancreatic cancer with multidetector CT. Int J Gastrointest Cancer. 2001;30:65.
16. Tamm EP. Imaging of pancreatic ductal adenocarcinoma: state of the art. World J Radiol. 2013;5:98.
17. Tummala P, Junaidi O, Agarwal B. Imaging of pancreatic cancer: an overview. J Gastrointest Oncol. 2011;2:168.
18. Prokesch RW, Schima W, Chow LC, Jeffrey RB. Multidetector CT of pancreatic adenocarcinoma: diagnostic advances and therapeutic relevance. Eur Radiol. 2003;13:2147.
19. Al-Hawary MM, Francis IR, Chari ST, Fishman EK, Hough DM, Lu DS, et al. Pancreatic ductal adenocarcinoma radiology reporting template: consensus statement of the Society of Abdominal Radiology and the American Pancreatic Association. Gastroenterology. 2014;146:291.

20. Varadhachary GR, Tamm EP, Abbruzzese JL, Xiong HQ, Crane CH, Wang H, et al. Borderline resectable pancreatic cancer: definitions, management, and role of preoperative therapy. Ann Surg Oncol. 2006;13:1035.
21. Turowska A, Łebkowska U, Kubas B, Janica JR, Ładny RJ, Kordecki K. The role of magnetic resonance imaging (MRI) with magnetic resonance cholangiopancreatography (MRCP) in the diagnosis and assessment of resectability of pancreatic tumors [Internet]. Med Sci Monit. 2007;13(Suppl 1):90–7; [cited 16 Jan 2019];. Available from: http://www.ncbi.nlm.nih.gov/pubmed/17507892.
22. Harewood GC, Wiersema MJ. Endosonography-guided fine needle aspiration biopsy in the evaluation of pancreatic masses. Am J Gastroenterol. 2002;97:1386.
23. Connor AA, Denroche RE, Jang GH, Timms L, Kalimuthu SN, Selander I, et al. Association of distinct mutational signatures with correlates of increased immune activity in pancreatic ductal adenocarcinoma. JAMA Oncol. 2017;3:774.
24. Bailey P, Chang DK, Nones K, Johns AL, Patch AM, Gingras MC, et al. Genomic analyses identify molecular subtypes of pancreatic cancer. Nature. 2016;531:47.
25. Moffitt RA, Marayati R, Flate EL, Volmar KE, SGH L, Hoadley KA, et al. Virtual microdissection identifies distinct tumor- and stroma-specific subtypes of pancreatic ductal adenocarcinoma. Nat Genet. 2015;47:1168.
26. Waddell N, Pajic M, Patch AM, Chang DK, Kassahn KS, Bailey P, et al. Whole genomes redefine the mutational landscape of pancreatic cancer. Nature. 2015;518:495.
27. Collisson EA, Sadanandam A, Olson P, Gibb WJ, Truitt M, Gu S, et al. Subtypes of pancreatic ductal adenocarcinoma and their differing responses to therapy. Nat Med. 2011;17:500.
28. Aung KL, Fischer SE, Denroche RE, Jang GH, Dodd A, Creighton S, et al. Genomics-driven precision medicine for advanced pancreatic cancer: early results from the COMPASS trial. Clin Cancer Res. 2018;24:1344.
29. O'Kane GMFS, Denroche R, Jang GH, Zhang A, Dodd A, Grant RCGB, Masoomian MM, Moura S, Elimova E, Prince RM, Zogopoulos G, Notta F, Wilson J, Gallinger S, Knox J. Integrative molecular profiling and response to chemotherapy on the COMPASS trial. J Clin Oncol. 2019;37(4 Suppl):188.
30. Lowery MA, Jordan EJ, Basturk O, Ptashkin RN, Zehir A, Berger MF, et al. Real-time genomic profiling of pancreatic ductal adenocarcinoma: potential actionability and correlation with clinical phenotype. Clin Cancer Res. 2017;23:6094.
31. Aguirre AJ, Nowak JA, Camarda ND, Moffitt RA, Ghazani AA, Hazar-Rethinam M, et al. Real-time genomic characterization of advanced pancreatic cancer to enable precision medicine. Cancer Discov. 2018;8:1096.
32. Pishvaian MJ, Bender RJ, Halverson D, Rahib L, Hendifar AE, Mikhail S, et al. Molecular profiling of patients with pancreatic cancer: initial results from the know your tumor initiative. Clin Cancer Res. 2018;24:5018.
33. Friess H, Kleeff J, Silva JC, Sadowski C, Baer HU, Büchler MW. The role of diagnostic laparoscopy in pancreatic and periampullary malignancies. J Am Coll Surg. 1998;186:675.
34. Stefanidis D, Grove KD, Schwesinger WH, Thomas CR. The current role of staging laparoscopy for adenocarcinoma of the pancreas: a review. Ann Oncol. 2006;17:189.
35. Brooks AD, Mallis MJ, Brennan MF, KCP C, Pitt HA, Matthews J, et al. The value of laparoscopy in the management of ampullary, duodenal, and distal bile duct tumors. J Gastrointest Surg. 2002;6:139.
36. Saleh MM, Norregaard P, Jorgensen HL, Andersen PK, Matzen P. Preoperative endoscopic stent placement before pancreaticoduodenectomy: a meta-analysis of the effect on morbidity and mortality [Internet]. Gastrointest Endosc. 2002;56(4):529–34; [cited 26 Sept 2002]. Available from: http://www.ncbi.nlm.nih.gov/pubmed/12297769.
37. van der Gaag NA, Rauws EA, van Eijck CH, Bruno MJ, van der Harst E, Kubben FJ, et al. Preoperative biliary drainage for cancer of the head of the pancreas. N Engl J Med. 2010;362(2):129–37.
38. Temudom T, Sarr MG, Douglas MG, Farnell MB. An argument against routine percutaneous biopsy, ERCP, or biliary stent placement in patients with clinically resectable periampullary

masses: a surgical perspective [Internet]. Pancreas. 1995;11(3):283–8; available from: http://www.ncbi.nlm.nih.gov/pubmed/8577683.
39. Howard TJ, Yu J, Greene RB, George V, Wairiuko GM, Moore SA, et al. Influence of Bactibilia after preoperative biliary stenting on postoperative infectious complications. J Gastrointest Surg. 2006;10:523–31.
40. Boulay BR, Parepally M. Managing malignant biliary obstruction in pancreas cancer: choosing the appropriate strategy. World J Gastroenterol. 2014;20:9348.
41. Bilimoria KY, Bentrem DJ, Ko CY, Stewart AK, Winchester DP, Talamonti MS. National failure to operate on early stage pancreatic cancer. Ann Surg. 2007;246(2):173–80.
42. Bergquist JR, Ivanics T, Shubert CR, Habermann EB, Smoot RL, Kendrick ML, et al. Type of resection (whipple vs. distal) does not affect the national failure to provide post-resection adjuvant chemotherapy in localized pancreatic cancer. Ann Surg Oncol. 2017;24(6):1731.
43. Serrano PE, Cleary SP, Dhani N, Kim PTW, Greig PD, Leung K, et al. Improved long-term outcomes after resection of pancreatic adenocarcinoma: a comparison between two time periods. Ann Surg Oncol. 2015;22:1160.
44. Croome KP, Farnell MB, Que FG, ReidLombardo K, Truty MJ, Nagorney DM, et al. Total laparoscopic pancreaticoduodenectomy for pancreatic ductal adenocarcinoma oncologic advantages over open approaches? Ann Surg. 2014;260(4):633.
45. Shubert CR, Bergquist JR, Groeschl RT, Habermann EB, Wilson PM, Truty MJ, et al. Overall survival is increased among stage III pancreatic adenocarcinoma patients receiving neoadjuvant chemotherapy compared to surgery first and adjuvant chemotherapy: an intention to treat analysis of the National Cancer Database. Surgery (United States). 2016;160(4):1080.
46. Andriulli A, Festa V, Botteri E, Valvano MR, Koch M, Bassi C, et al. Neoadjuvant/preoperative gemcitabine for patients with localized pancreatic cancer: a meta-analysis of prospective studies. Ann Surg Oncol. 2012;19:1644.
47. Gillen S, Schuster T, Meyer Zum Buschenfelde C, Friess H, Kleeff J. Preoperative/neoadjuvant therapy in pancreatic cancer: a systematic review and meta-analysis of response and resection percentages [Internet]. PLoS Med. 2010;7(4):e1000267; [cited 28 Apr 2010]. Available from: http://www.ncbi.nlm.nih.gov/pubmed/20422030.
48. Bittoni A, Santoni M, Lanese A, Pellei C, Andrikou K, Stefano C. Neoadjuvant therapy in pancreatic cancer: an emerging strategy. Gastroenterol Res Pract. 2014;2014:183852.
49. Heinemann V, Haas M, Boeck S. Neoadjuvant treatment of borderline resectable and non-resectable pancreatic cancer. Ann Oncol. 2013;24(10):2484–92; 16 Jul 2013.
50. Versteijne E, Vogel JA, Besselink MG, ORC B, Wilmink JW, Daams JG, et al. Meta-analysis comparing upfront surgery with neoadjuvant treatment in patients with resectable or borderline resectable pancreatic cancer. Br J Surg. 2018;105:946.
51. Golcher H, Brunner TB, Witzigmann H, Marti L, Bechstein W-O, Bruns C, et al. Neoadjuvant chemoradiation therapy with gemcitabine/cisplatin and surgery versus immediate surgery in resectable pancreatic cancer. Strahlenther Onkol. 2015;191:7.
52. Van Tienhoven G, Versteijne E, Suker M, Groothuis KBC, Busch OR, Bonsing BA, et al. Preoperative chemoradiotherapy versus immediate surgery for resectable and borderline resectable pancreatic cancer (PREOPANC-1): a randomized, controlled, multicenter phase III trial [Internet]. J Clin Oncol. 2018;36(18_suppl):LBA4002; [cited 2 Apr 2019]. Available from: http://ascopubs.org/doi/10.1200/JCO.2018.36.18_suppl.LBA4002.
53. Unno M, Motoi F, Matsuyama Y, Satoi S, Matsumoto I, Aosasa S, et al. Randomized phase II/III trial of neoadjuvant chemotherapy with gemcitabine and S-1 versus upfront surgery for resectable pancreatic cancer (Prep-02/JSAP-05) [Internet]. J Clin Oncol. 2019;37(4_suppl):189; [cited 2019 Apr 2]. Available from: http://ascopubs.org/doi/10.1200/JCO.2019.37.4_suppl.189.
54. Hosein PJ, Macintyre J, Kawamura C, Maldonado JC, Ernani V, Loaiza-Bonilla A, et al. A retrospective study of neoadjuvant FOLFIRINOX in unresectable or borderline-resectable locally advanced pancreatic adenocarcinoma. BMC Cancer. 2012;12:199.
55. Christians KK, Tsai S, Mahmoud A, Ritch P, Thomas JP, Wiebe L, et al. Neoadjuvant FOLFIRINOX for borderline resectable pancreas cancer: a new treatment paradigm? [Internet]. Oncologist. 2014;19:266–74; available from: http://www.ncbi.nlm.nih.gov/pubmed/24569947

56. Faris JE, Blaszkowsky LS, McDermott S, Guimaraes AR, Szymonifka J, Huynh MA, et al. FOLFIRINOX in locally advanced pancreatic cancer: the Massachusetts General Hospital Cancer Center experience. Oncologist. 2013;18:543.
57. Ferrone CR, Warshaw AL, Rattner DW, Berger D, Zheng H, Rawal B, et al. Pancreatic fistula rates after 462 distal pancreatectomies: staplers do not decrease fistula rates. J Gastrointest Surg. 2008;12:1691–7.
58. Murphy JE, Wo JY, Ryan DP, Jiang W, Yeap BY, Drapek LC, et al. Total neoadjuvant therapy with FOLFIRINOX followed by individualized chemoradiotherapy for borderline resectable pancreatic adenocarcinoma [Internet]. JAMA Oncol. 2018;4(7):963; [cited 10 Jan 2019]. Available from: http://www.ncbi.nlm.nih.gov/pubmed/29800971.
59. Oettle H, Post S, Neuhaus P, Gellert K, Langrehr J, Ridwelski K, et al. Adjuvant chemotherapy with gemcitabine vs observation in patients undergoing curative-intent resection of pancreatic cancer: a randomized controlled trial. J Am Med Assoc. 2007;297:267.
60. Neoptolemos JP, Stocken DD, Bassi C, Ghaneh P, Cunningham D, Goldstein D, et al. Adjuvant chemotherapy with fluorouracil plus folinic acid vs gemcitabine following pancreatic cancer resection: a randomized controlled trial. JAMA. 2010;304:1073.
61. Conroy T, Hammel P, Hebbar M, Ben Abdelghani M, Wei AC, Raoul J-L, et al. FOLFIRINOX or gemcitabine as adjuvant therapy for pancreatic cancer [Internet]. N Engl J Med. 2018;379(25):2395–406; [cited 7 Jan 2019]. Available from: http://www.nejm.org/doi/10.1056/NEJMoa1809775.
62. Neoptolemos JP, Palmer DH, Ghaneh P, Psarelli EE, Valle JW, Halloran CM, et al. Comparison of adjuvant gemcitabine and capecitabine with gemcitabine monotherapy in patients with resected pancreatic cancer (ESPAC-4): a multicentre, open-label, randomised, phase 3 trial [Internet]. Lancet (London, England). 2017;389(10073):1011–24; [cited 2 Apr 2019]. Available from: http://www.ncbi.nlm.nih.gov/pubmed/28129987.
63. Klinkenbijl JH, Jeekel J, Sahmoud T, Van Pel R, Couvreur ML, Veenhof CH, et al. Adjuvant radiotherapy and 5-fluorouracil after curative resection of cancer of the pancreas and periampullary region: phase III trial of the EORTC Gastrointestinal Tract Cancer Cooperative Group. Ann Surg. 1999;230:776.
64. Neoptolemos JP, Stocken DD, Friess H, Bassi C, Dunn JA, Hickey H, et al. A randomized trial of chemoradiotherapy and chemotherapy after resection of pancreatic cancer. N Engl J Med. 2004;350:1200.
65. Conroy T, Desseigne F, Ychou M, Bouché O, Guimbaud R, Bécouarn Y, et al. FOLFIRINOX versus gemcitabine for metastatic pancreatic cancer. N Engl J Med. 2011;364(19):1817–25.
66. Von Hoff DD, Ervin T, Arena FP, Chiorean EG, Infante J, Moore M, et al. Increased survival in pancreatic cancer with nab-paclitaxel plus gemcitabine. N Engl J Med. 2013;369:1691.
67. Loehrer PJ, Feng Y, Cardenes H, Wagner L, Brell JM, Cella D, et al. Gemcitabine alone versus gemcitabine plus radiotherapy in patients with locally advanced pancreatic cancer: an Eastern Cooperative Oncology Group trial. J Clin Oncol. 2011;29:4105.
68. Huguet F, André T, Hammel P, Artru P, Balosso J, Selle F, et al. Impact of chemoradiotherapy after disease control with chemotherapy in locally advanced pancreatic adenocarcinoma in GERCOR phase II and III studies. J Clin Oncol. 2007;25:326.
69. Chauffert B, Mornex F, Bonnetain F, Rougier P, Mariette C, Bouché O, et al. Phase III trial comparing intensive induction chemoradiotherapy (60 Gy, infusional 5-FU and intermittent cisplatin) followed by maintenance gemcitabine with gemcitabine alone for locally advanced unresectable pancreatic cancer. Definitive results of the 2000-01 FFCD/SFRO study. Ann Oncol. 2008;19:1592.
70. Hammel P, Huguet F, Van Laethem JL, Goldstein D, Glimelius B, Artru P, et al. Effect of chemoradiotherapy vs chemotherapy on survival in patients with locally advanced pancreatic cancer controlled after 4 months of gemcitabine with or without erlotinib the LAP07 randomized clinical trial. JAMA. 2016;315:1844.
71. Schellenberg D, Kim J, Christman-Skieller C, Chun CL, Columbo LA, Ford JM, et al. Single-fraction stereotactic body radiation therapy and sequential gemcitabine for the treatment of locally advanced pancreatic cancer. Int J Radiat Oncol Biol Phys. 2011;81:181.

72. Herman JM, Chang DT, Goodman KA, Dholakia AS, Raman SP, Hacker-Prietz A, et al. Phase 2 multi-institutional trial evaluating gemcitabine and stereotactic body radiotherapy for patients with locally advanced unresectable pancreatic adenocarcinoma. Cancer. 2015;121:1128.
73. Tee MC, Krajewski AC, Groeschl RT, Farnell MB, Nagorney DM, Kendrick ML, et al. Indications and perioperative outcomes for pancreatectomy with arterial resection [Internet]. J Am Coll Surg. 2018;227(2):255–69; [cited 7 Jan 2019]. Available from: http://www.ncbi.nlm.nih.gov/pubmed/29752997.
74. Loveday BPT, Zilbert N, Serrano PE, Tomiyama K, Tremblay A, Fox AM, et al. Neoadjuvant therapy and major arterial resection for potentially reconstructable arterial involvement by stage 3 adenocarcinoma of the pancreas [Internet]. HPB. 2018;21:643; [cited 7 Jan 2019]. Available from: https://www.sciencedirect.com/science/article/abs/pii/S1365182X18344770.
75. Shubert CR, Kendrick ML, Habermann EB, Glasgow AE, Borah BJ, Moriarty JP, et al. Implementation of prospective, surgeon-driven, risk-based pathway for pancreatoduodenectomy results in improved clinical outcomes and first year cost savings of $1 million. Surgery (United States). 2017;163:495.
76. Müller MW, Friess H, Köninger J, Martin D, Wente MN, Hinz U, et al. Factors influencing survival after bypass procedures in patients with advanced pancreatic adenocarcinomas. Am J Surg. 2008;195:221.
77. Farnell MB, Aranha GV, Nimura Y, Michelassi F. The role of extended lymphadenectomy for adenocarcinoma of the head of the pancreas: strength of the evidence [Internet]. J Gastrointest Surg. 2008;12(4):651–6; [cited 19 Dec 2007]. Available from: http://www.ncbi.nlm.nih.gov/pubmed/18085343.
78. Yeo CJ, Cameron JL, Lillemoe KD, Sohn TA, Campbell KA, Sauter PK, et al. Pancreaticoduodenectomy with or without distal gastrectomy and extended retroperitoneal lymphadenectomy for periampullary adenocarcinoma, part 2: randomized controlled trial evaluating survival, morbidity, and mortality. Ann Surg. 2002;236(3):355–8; 23 Aug 2002.
79. Tol JA, Gouma DJ, Bassi C, Dervenis C, Montorsi M, Adham M, et al. Definition of a standard lymphadenectomy in surgery for pancreatic ductal adenocarcinoma: a consensus statement by the International Study Group on Pancreatic Surgery (ISGPS). Surgery (United States). 2014;156:591.
80. Tseng JF, Raut CP, Lee JE, Pisters PWT, Vauthey JN, Abdalla EK, et al. Pancreaticoduodenectomy with vascular resection: margin status and survival duration. J Gastrointest Surg. 2004;8:935.
81. Bockhorn M, Uzunoglu FG, Adham M, Imrie C, Milicevic M, Sandberg AA, et al. Borderline resectable pancreatic cancer: a consensus statement by the International Study Group of Pancreatic Surgery (ISGPS). Surgery (United States). 2014;155:977.
82. Kim PTW, Wei AC, Atenafu EG, Cavallucci D, Cleary SP, Moulton CA, et al. Planned versus unplanned portal vein resections during pancreaticoduodenectomy for adenocarcinoma. Br J Surg. 2013;100:1349.
83. Diener MK, Fitzmaurice C, Schwarzer G, Seiler CM, Hüttner FJ, Antes G, et al. Pylorus-preserving pancreaticoduodenectomy (pp Whipple) versus pancreaticoduodenectomy (classic Whipple) for surgical treatment of periampullary and pancreatic carcinoma. Cochrane Database Syst Rev. 2014;2:CD006053.
84. Hallet J, Zih FSW, Deobald RG, Scheer AS, Law CHL, Coburn NG, et al. The impact of pancreaticojejunostomy versus pancreaticogastrostomy reconstruction on pancreatic fistula after pancreaticoduodenectomy: meta-analysis of randomized controlled trials. HPB. 2015;17:113.
85. Winter JM, Cameron JL, Campbell KA, Chang DC, Riall TS, Schulick RD, et al. Does pancreatic duct stenting decrease the rate of pancreatic fistula following pancreaticoduodenectomy? Results of a prospective randomized trial [Internet]. J Gastrointest Surg. 2006;10(9):1280–90; 23 Nov 2006; discussion 1290. Available from: http://www.ncbi.nlm.nih.gov/pubmed/17114014.
86. Moriya T, Clark CJ, Kirihara Y, Kendrick ML, Reid Lombardo KM, Que FG, et al. Stenting and the rate of pancreatic fistula following pancreaticoduodenectomy. Arch Surg. 2012;147:35–40.

87. Connor S, Alexakis N, Garden OJ, Leandros E, Bramis J, Wigmore SJ. Meta-analysis of the value of somatostatin and its analogues in reducing complications associated with pancreatic surgery [Internet]. Br J Surg. 2005;92(9):1059–67; 27 Jul 2005. Available from: http://www.ncbi.nlm.nih.gov/pubmed/16044410.
88. Alghamdi AA, Jawas AM, Hart RS. Use of octreotide for the prevention of pancreatic fistula after elective pancreatic surgery: a systematic review and meta-analysis [Internet]. Can J Surg. 2007;50(6):459–66; 7 Dec 2007. Available from: http://www.ncbi.nlm.nih.gov/pubmed/18053374.
89. Allen PJ, Gönen M, Brennan MF, Bucknor AA, Robinson LM, Pappas MM, et al. Pasireotide for postoperative pancreatic fistula [Internet]. N Engl J Med. 2014;370(21):2014–22. Available from: http://www.ncbi.nlm.nih.gov/pubmed/24849084.
90. Conlon KC, Labow D, Leung D, Smith A, Jarnagin W, Coit DG, et al. Prospective randomized clinical trial of the value of intraperitoneal drainage after pancreatic resection. Ann Surg. 2001;234:487.
91. Van Buren G, Bloomston M, Hughes SJ, Winter J, Behrman SW, Zyromski NJ, et al. A randomized prospective multicenter trial of pancreaticoduodenectomy with and without routine intraperitoneal drainage. Ann Surg. 2014;259:605.
92. Bassi C, Molinari E, Malleo G, Crippa S, Butturini G, Salvia R, et al. Early versus late drain removal after standard pancreatic resections: results of a prospective randomized trial. Ann Surg. 2010;252(2):207–14; 14 Jul 2010.
93. McMillan MT, Malleo G, Bassi C, Allegrini V, Casetti L, Drebin JA, et al. Multicenter, prospective trial of selective drain management for pancreatoduodenectomy using risk stratification. Ann Surg. 2016;265:1209.
94. Molinari E, Bassi C, Salvia R, Butturini G, Crippa S, Talamini G, et al. Amylase value in drains after pancreatic resection as predictive factor of postoperative pancreatic fistula: results of a prospective study in 137 patients [Internet]. Ann Surg. 2007;246(2):281–7; 2 Aug 2007. Available from: http://www.ncbi.nlm.nih.gov/pubmed/17667507.
95. Jin T, Altaf K, Xiong JJ, Huang W, Javed MA, Mai G, et al. A systematic review and meta-analysis of studies comparing laparoscopic and open distal pancreatectomy. HPB. 2012;14:711.
96. Kooby DA, Hawkins WG, Schmidt CM, Weber SM, Bentrem DJ, Gillespie TW, et al. A multicenter analysis of distal pancreatectomy for adenocarcinoma: is laparoscopic resection appropriate? J Am Coll Surg. 2010;210:779.

Peritoneal Surface Malignancies 22

Jessica Bogach, Andrea McCart, Danielle Bischof, and Anand Govindarajan

Introduction

Peritoneal surface malignancy can be defined as any cancer that has either originated from the peritoneum itself (primary peritoneal malignancy) or has metastasized to the peritoneum from a different primary site (secondary peritoneal malignancy).

Although peritoneal spread is described from many malignancies, peritoneal surface malignancies can be subdivided into three main categories based on common sites of origin: peritoneal, gastrointestinal, and ovarian (Table 22.1).

This chapter focuses on peritoneal mesothelioma and peritoneal carcinomatosis arising from the appendix, colon, and rectum.

J. Bogach
General Surgical Oncology, University of Toronto, Toronto, ON, Canada
e-mail: Jessica.Bogach@one-mail.on.ca

A. McCart · A. Govindarajan (✉)
Department of Surgery, University of Toronto, Toronto, ON, Canada
e-mail: andrea.mccart@sinaihealth.ca; anand.govindarajan@sinaihealth.ca

D. Bischof
Department of Surgery, Sinai Health System, Toronto, ON, Canada
e-mail: Danielle.Bischof@sinaihealth.ca

F. C. Wright et al. (eds.), *Surgical Oncology Manual*,
https://doi.org/10.1007/978-3-030-48363-0_22

Table 22.1 Common sites and histologies that have peritoneal involvement

Site of origin	Common histologies
Peritoneum	Mesothelioma Primary peritoneal carcinoma
Gastrointestinal tract (stomach, appendix, colon, rectum, pancreas)	Low Grade Appendiceal Mucinous Neoplasm (LAMN) Intestinal/colonic-type adenocarcinoma Signet ring cell adenocarcinoma Goblet cell adenocarcinoma/Adenocarcinoma ex-goblet cell
Ovary	Epithelial carcinoma (often low- or high-grade serous carcinoma)

Table 22.2 PSOGI classification of appendiceal tumors

Lesion	Terminology
Mucinous neoplasm with low-grade cytologic atypia[a]	Low-grade appendiceal mucinous neoplasm (LAMN)
Mucinous neoplasm with architectural features of LAMN, no invasion, with high-grade cytologic atypia	High-grade appendiceal mucinous neoplasm (HAMN)
Mucinous neoplasm with infiltrative invasion	Mucinous adenocarcinoma (moderately, or poorly differentiated)
Neoplasm with signet ring cells (<50%)	Poorly differentiated (mucinous) adenocarcinoma with signet ring cells
Neoplasm with signet ring cells (>50%)	Mucinous signet ring cell carcinoma
Non-mucinous adenocarcinoma resembling traditional colorectal type	Adenocarcinoma (well, moderately, or poorly differentiated)

Table adapted from Carr et al. [6]

[a]May include loss of muscularis mucosa, submucosal fibrosis, acellular mucin dissecting the wall, appendix rupture, mucin outside of the appendix, flattened epithelial growth

Peritoneal Carcinomatosis Arising from the Appendix

Neoplasms of the appendix have an incidence rate of 0.12–2 cases per 1 million people, with female predominance, and are most commonly epithelial tumors [1]. Peritoneal carcinomatosis from mucinous tumors has a better prognosis than carcinomatosis from non-mucinous tumors [2].

Mucinous Appendiceal Neoplasms

Approximately 50% of appendiceal adenocarcinomas will have mucinous histology [3]. There are several classification systems for mucinous tumors arising in the appendix. The WHO and the Ronnett histologic classification are two commonly used systems [4, 5]. A consensus paper was published from the Peritoneal Surface Oncology Group International (PSOGI) that classifies both the tumor in the appendix and the peritoneal disease (Table 22.2).

Table 22.3 Classification systems for appendiceal mucinous tumors

Ronnett	WHO	AJCC 8th edition	PSOGI
DPAM	LAMN	Well Differentiated or LAMN (G1)	LAMN
Intermediate/ Discordant		Moderately Differentiated (G2)	HAMN[a] Moderately differentiated mucinous adenocarcinoma
PMCA	MACA	Poorly differentiated (G3)	Poorly differentiated mucinous adenocarcinoma (with or without signet ring cells) Signet ring cell carcinoma

[a]The metastatic potential of HAMN is not well known. Although there should be no invasion, it is not classified with LAMN

The WHO uses the term Mucinous Adenocarcinoma (MACA) to reflect infiltrative tumors from the appendix [3, 5, 7]. The Ronnett histologic classification uses Disseminated Peritoneal Adenomucinosis (DPAM) and Peritoneal Mucinous Carcinomatosis (PMCA) to represent low- and high-grade mucinous tumors, respectively, arising from appendiceal or colorectal origin (see Table 22.3) [4, 8]. These descriptors have generally been replaced by the PSOGI terminology. Terms such as mucinous cystadenoma or cystadenocarcinoma should be avoided as a pathologic descriptor [6].

The 8th edition of the American Joint Council on Cancer (AJCC) staging manual has recommended a three-tier grading scheme with well, moderately, and poorly differentiated mucinous tumors [3].

- *Well differentiated (G1)* tumors typically push, rather than infiltrate; have low cellularity; and mucin is often acellular. These are classified as LAMNs and are considered low grade (G1) despite extensive peritoneal mucinous disease.
- *Moderately differentiated (G2)* tumors often show features of invasion and higher cellularity.
  - Rarely, there are High-Grade Appendiceal Mucinous Neoplasms (HAMN), which have moderate or high-grade (G2) cytologic features without signs of invasion. This is a rare diagnosis and the entire appendix specimen needs to be evaluated to confirm this diagnosis [7, 9].
- *Poorly differentiated (G3)* tumors are high grade, invasive, and often have a signet ring component [3].

At the University of Toronto, the PSOGI classification is accepted and the distinction in management is made when a tumor is low grade (G1 or LAMN) compared to higher grade because of the prognostic significance of grade [10].

Pseudomyxoma peritonei (PMP) is defined as the accumulation of mucin in the peritoneal cavity, secondary to mucinous epithelial tumors. The term encompasses mucinous ascites, peritoneal implants, ovarian metastases, and omental caking [6]. Ninety percent of cases originate from appendiceal tumors, but can also arise from the ovary, colon, and infrequently from pancreas, gallbladder, and urachus [7]. Although the term PMP is often used to describe mucinous disease in the peritoneum secondary to a low-grade appendiceal

Table 22.4 Pathologic description and terminology as per PSOGI

Lesion	Terminology
Mucin with no epithelial cells present	Acellular mucin
PMP with low-grade histology	Low-grade mucinous carcinoma peritonei (synonymous with DPAM)
PMP with high-grade histology	High-grade mucinous carcinoma peritonei (synonymous with PMCA)
PMP with signet ring cells	High-grade mucinous carcinoma peritonei with signet ring cells

Adapted from Carr et al. [6]

Table 22.5 Cancer-specific survival for Stage IV appendiceal tumors according to grade [13]

	5-year cancer specific survival	
Tumor grade	Mucinous (%)	Non-mucinous (%)
Well differentiated (G1)	71	48
Moderately differentiated (G2)	51	9
Poorly differentiated (G3)	0	5

primary, the term is best used only as a clinical description rather than a pathologic one [3]. The PSOGI consensus paper classifies peritoneal spread into four categories (see Tables 22.4 and 22.5).

This is supported by the AJCC classification where acellular mucin is considered M1a disease, cellular mucin is M1b, and peritoneal disease with other metastatic sites as M1c [3].

Non-mucinous Appendiceal Neoplasms

- Adenocarcinoma
- Signet ring cell carcinoma (>50% signet ring cells)
  - This is associated with a poor prognosis with rapid dissemination in the peritoneal cavity.
- Goblet cell carcinoids (GCC)
  - These demonstrate both endocrine and exocrine differentiation. They behave more like adenocarcinomas and are therefore staged as appendiceal carcinoma unlike low-grade neuroendocrine tumors, which should be classified as gastrointestinal neuroendocrine tumors.
  - The WHO classification distinguishes "goblet cell carcinoids" from "mixed goblet cell carcinoid/adenocarcinoma (adenocarcinoma ex-goblet cell)". The latter suggests a more aggressive subtype [11]
  - Tang et al. have classified GCC into three prognostic groups: typical GCC (Group A), signet ring cell adenocarcinoma ex-GCC (Group B), and poorly differentiated adenocarcinoma ex-GCC (Group C) [12]

All non-mucinous neoplasms are approached as high-grade tumors.

Peritoneal Carcinomatosis Arising from the Colon And Rectum

Peritoneal carcinomatosis will affect 30% of patients with colorectal cancer, and 5–10% of these patients will have synchronous disease [14]. In 25% of these cases, the peritoneal cavity seems to be the only site of metastatic disease [15]. Patients with peritoneal metastases from colorectal cancer are more likely to be female, have colon primaries, have BRAF mutant tumors, and have worse performance status [16]. Having peritoneal involvement is associated with worse overall survival [16]. It is important to recognize this because surgical treatment for peritoneal disease is often compared to systemic treatment for Stage IV colorectal cancer, and it is essential to understand the prognostic implications of peritoneal disease.

This is reflected in the 8th edition of the AJCC staging. For colorectal origin, M1a disease represents metastasis confined to one organ or site (e.g., liver, lung, ovary, non-regional node) without peritoneal metastasis, M1b disease represents metastasis in more than one organ/site without peritoneal metastasis. M1c disease represents peritoneal metastasis with or without other organs involved. Peritoneal carcinomatosis is classified as stage IV C disease [3].

Peritoneal Mesothelioma

Mesothelioma is a rare condition with approximately 500 cases a year in Canada, 10–30% present as peritoneal mesothelioma, which is the second most common site after the pleura [17]. Asbestos is associated with peritoneal mesothelioma in 33% of cases, opposed to >80% seen in pleural mesothelioma [17]. Other associated exposures include talc, mica, erionite, thorotrast, Hodgkin's disease, chronic peritonitis, and therapeutic radiation [18]. There is no uniformly accepted staging system for mesothelioma. A TNM staging system has been proposed by the Peritoneal Surface Oncology Group which uses Peritoneal Cancer Index (PCI) for T stage (Table 22.6) [19]. Prognostic factors for survival include histologic subtype, completeness of cytoreduction and stage according to this system (Table 22.7) [18–20]. Epithelioid subtypes, which are most common, are associated with a better prognosis, while sarcomatoid and biphasic histology are associated with worse prognosis [17–21]. Mortality of peritoneal mesothelioma is often secondary to disease progression in peritoneum and not due to distant metastases.

Table 22.6 Prognostic factors for survival in peritoneal mesothelioma

Histologic subtype [21]	Tumor	Nodal status	Metastases
Epithelioid subtypes: Tubulopapillary Micropapillary Solid Sarcomatoid (rare) Biphasic (combination of epithelioid and sarcomatoid)	T1: PCI 1-10 T2: PCI 11-20 T3: PCI 21-30 T4: PCI >30	N0: No nodal disease N1: Nodal disease	M0: No distant metastases M1: Presence of distant metastases

Table 22.7 Survival based on stage for peritoneal mesothelioma

Stage	5-year overall survival[a]
Stage I (T1 N0 M0)	87%
Stage II (T2-3 N0 M0)	53%
Stage III (T4 or N1 or M1)	29%

[a]Prognosis is with cytoreductive surgery and heated intra-peritoneal chemotherapy

Management of Peritoneal Surface Malignancies

Management of peritoneal malignancies can include cytoreductive surgery (CRS) and heated intra-peritoneal chemotherapy (HIPEC), chemotherapy, surgery alone, or palliative treatment only. This chapter will focus on CRS and HIPEC.

In candidates for CRS, the best results are achieved when a patient is able to undergo a complete cytoreduction [22]. CRS is scored based on completeness of cytoreduction (CC). Patient selection to determine those who might benefit from CRS and HIPEC is critical.

Assessment of Extent of Disease

The peritoneal cancer index (PCI) is a score calculated intraoperatively indicating the extent of peritoneal disease (Fig. 22.1). PCI represents one of the most significant prognostic factors, along with the completeness of cytoreduction [23–25]. The PCI score is also used to estimate the likelihood of proceeding with cytoreduction, and to determine if the procedure is beneficial to the patient. The score is a summation of cancer lesions size (scored 0–3) present in the 13 abdominopelvic regions, with a maximum score of 39.

CT is the most commonly used imaging modality to characterize peritoneal carcinomatosis, although, recently, some groups are incorporating MRI. Sugarbaker has defined criteria on cross-sectional imaging as predictors of unresectability: implant >5 cm in epigastrium, loss of normal architecture of small bowel, matted adjacent small bowel loops, segmental obstruction, distorted or thickened bowel, and inability to identify mesenteric vessels [26, 27]. However, conventional cross-sectional imaging can incorrectly estimate the degree of peritoneal disease by 20–30%, making laparoscopy a useful tool for those patients [28]. Although specificity of detecting small bowel peritoneal disease is over 90%, the sensitivity is limited. The use of MRI may have benefit in identifying small bowel and mesenteric disease, but this is not routinely used [29].

Diagnostic laparoscopy has been shown to be beneficial to evaluate the extent of disease and resectability [28, 30, 31]. Laparotomy may be superior to laparoscopy for visualizing the right hemidiaphragm, omental bursa, and pelvis, and remains the most accurate way to evaluate the extent of PCI. Laparoscopy serves to determine PCI score more as a threshold to assess resectability than for accuracy and reduces the number of non-therapeutic laparotomies for patients found with extensive

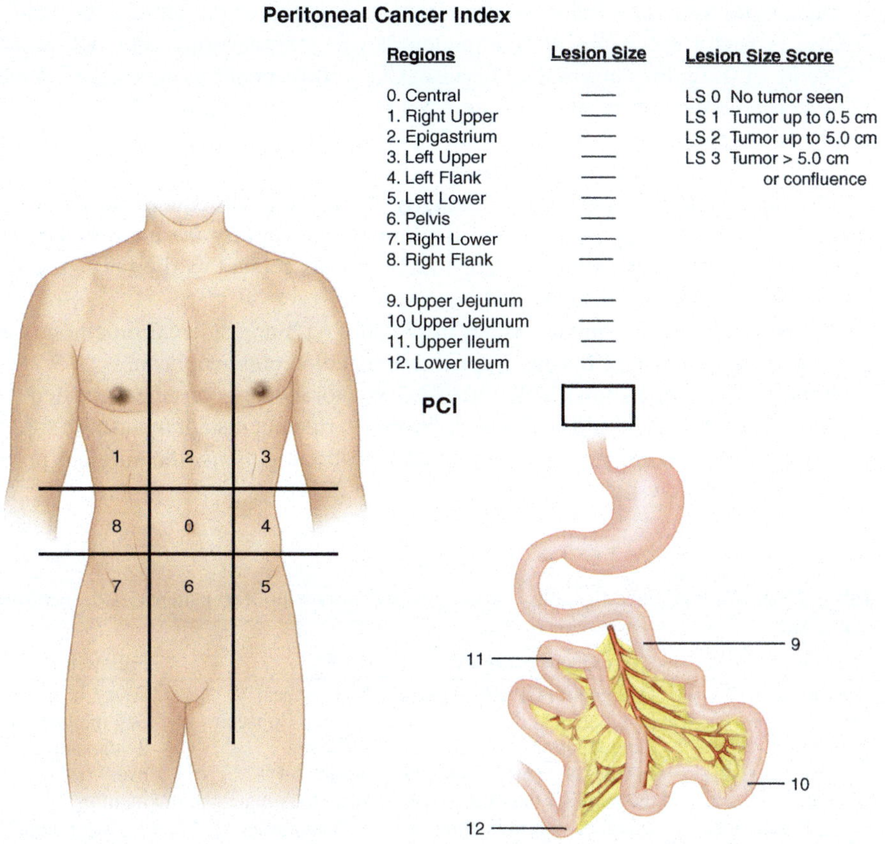

Fig. 22.1 Peritoneal cancer index scoring system based on location and amount of carcinomatosis in each region

disease or without peritoneal carcinomatosis. Laparoscopy may also allow one to obtain tissue for diagnostic confirmation.

A low PCI indicates a better probability of achieving complete cytoreduction, and is associated with better survival than patients with a high PCI. With regard to mucinous adenocarcinoma of the appendix, Sugarbaker reported that PCI ≤10 is associated with a 50% 5-year survival, PCI of 11–20 with a 20% 5-year survival, and a PCI >20 with a 0% 5-year survival [32]. Thus, a PCI <20 is recommended to perform CRS + HIPEC in these cases. For peritoneal carcinomatosis from colorectal origin, a similar threshold of PCI <20 is used to determine candidacy for CRS + HIPEC; moreover, some suggest that optimal outcomes are achieved in patients with PCI ≤17 [33]. For patients with PMP from LAMN, high PCI (>20) does not necessarily preclude CRS + HIPEC. CRS can thus be performed in one or two separate procedures, proceeding with the infra-mesocolic part first and the supra-mesocolic part done subsequently [34]. For mesothelioma, PCI is considered in some staging systems and is considered prognostic but is not necessarily used to select patients for surgery.

Once cytoreductive surgery is completed, evaluation of the amount of residual disease is performed using the completeness of cytoreduction score (CC-score). CC-score of 0 signifies no residual disease; CC-1 corresponds to deposits < 2.5 mm; CC-2 corresponds to deposits between 2.5 mm and 2.5 cm. Finally, CC-3 score corresponds to deposits > 2.5 cm. This number represents the largest deposit remaining and not a sum of the residual disease.

The Peritoneal Surface Disease Severity Score of colon cancer developed by Esquivel et al. may also be useful to determine resectability in carcinomatosis of colorectal origin, as it includes preoperative factors related to the patient, tumor histology, and extent of disease [35].

Colonoscopy should be performed in patients with appendiceal mucinous neoplasms, as there is risk of finding a synchronous colorectal neoplasm.

If thoracic imaging shows a pleural effusion, thoracentesis or video-assisted thoracic surgery (VATS) should be done for biopsy to rule out distant metastatic spread.

The next table summarizes the preoperative investigations, the surgical procedures, and the follow-up of these patients (Table 22.8).

Table 22.8 Workup, investigations, procedure and follow-up for patients with peritoneal malignancy

Workup	Cytoreductive surgery	HIPEC	Follow-up
History and physical exam Labs[a]: Tumor markers Imaging: CT abdomen/pelvis CT chest Colonoscopy (appendix and colorectal) ±Diagnostic laparoscopy (evaluate extent of disease and resectability) Pathology review MCC review of case Consider referral to medical oncology	Document PCI and estimate completeness of cytoreduction In LAMN or mesothelioma the inability to obtain CC-0 is not a contraindication to proceeding with CRS Remove all visible disease CC-0/CC-1 resection Selective peritonectomy Omentectomy Multivisceral resections if necessary Resect previous port sites and scars or biopsy site if involved with disease	Approaches: Open Coliseum Closed Agents for mesothelioma: Oxaliplatin[b] MMC Doxorubicin Cisplatin Agent for appendix: MMC Oxaliplatin Agents for colorectal: Oxaliplatin (concurrently used with IV 5FU-leucovorin) MMC	Every 3–6 months for 2 years, then every 6–12 months[d]: History and clinical exam CT of abdomen–pelvis CT of chest for colorectal primary Consider tumor markers if elevated pre-operatively[c]

MCC Multidisciplinary Cancer Conference, *MMC* mitomycin-C

[a]Tumor markers (CA-125, Mesothelin, CA-19.9, CEA) are not routinely done, but can be followed for post-treatment surveillance and elevation may represent more advanced disease [36–38]

[b]Used at the University of Toronto

[c]Based on an international consensus statement

[d]Due to late recurrences associated with LAMN, the duration of follow up period is extended long term

Cytoreductive Surgery (CRS) and Hyperthermic Intraperitoneal Chemotherapy (HIPEC)

Cytoreductive surgery is the first step of the procedure, and the extent of disease is assessed using the peritoneal cancer index (PCI) score. CRS generally includes resection of organs affected by peritoneal disease, followed by peritoneal stripping of involved surfaces of the abdomen, diaphragm, and pelvis. Electro-evaporation of small implants on serosa of small bowel, liver capsule, and other solid viscera is then undertaken, using fulguration by electrocautery or argon beam coagulation.

An incomplete resection of peritoneal carcinomatosis from colorectal cancer is not usually recommended, as median survival with incomplete resection equates to that with systemic chemotherapy alone. However, in LAMN or mesothelioma, small volume residual disease may have acceptable duration of survival and symptomatic benefit.

The administration of HIPEC follows the cytoreductive phase of the operation. HIPEC consists of intraoperative perfusion of the abdominal cavity with heated chemotherapy solution for a specific length of time. Common intraperitoneal agents used are oxaliplatin, cisplatin, and mitomycin-C (MMC). Chemotherapy agents are heated between 40 °C and 43 °C, for 30–90 min. Intravenous infusion of 5-FU and leucovorin are given preceding intraperitoneal oxaliplatin treatment in colorectal carcinomatosis. There is however no international consensus on the standard agent or dosing for HIPEC treatment [34]. Several retrospective studies have reviewed the use of oxaliplatin and MMC in the setting of colorectal carcinoma. Some have shown longer median survival with oxaliplatin, while others have not identified a difference in complications or efficacy [39, 40]. A comparative prospective study between intraperitoneal administration of MMC vs. oxaliplatin for peritoneal carcinomatosis arising from appendiceal tumors demonstrated different toxicity profiles but was not powered to show a survival difference [41, 42].

Intraperitoneal chemotherapy cannot penetrate more than 2–3 mm depth and, thus, it is generally administered only after a CC-0 or CC-1 resection. However, there may be a therapeutic benefit with the addition of HIPEC in CC2-3 resection in the setting of LAMN and mesothelioma. HIPEC can be performed in a closed or open technique, with no documented differences in outcomes between the two methods. It has been shown that heating the chemotherapy allows for better penetration into tissues and potentiates the cytotoxicity of the chemotherapeutic agent [35, 43, 44]. The hyperthermia itself is also thought to have an independent cytotoxic effect [45].

The addition of HIPEC to CRS has been shown to be associated with improved outcomes in non-randomized studies only. Prodige 7 is a phase III French multicenter randomized controlled trial comparing complete CRS + HIPEC vs. CRS alone for peritoneal metastases arising from colorectal cancer with PCI <25. Although not yet published at the time this chapter was written, the presented abstract suggests there is no overall survival advantage to the addition of HIPEC with oxaliplatin to CRS [46]. The final publication will be informative to understand the findings and determine their applicability.

Table 22.9 Inclusion and exclusion criteria for CRS and HIPEC at the University of Toronto [30, 34, 48, 49]

Inclusion	Exclusion
Diagnosis of carcinomatosis from colorectal origin (resectable), appendiceal neoplasms or mesothelioma Medically fit for surgery Completely cytoreducible disease Generally <70 years old (relative)	Other primaries (e.g., gastric, breast, cholangiocarcinoma, pancreas) Malignant small bowel obstruction (relative) Ureteric obstruction (relative) Biliary obstruction Extraperitoneal metastases (relative) Retroperitoneal lymphadenopathy Progression on chemotherapy

A systematic review on CRS + HIPEC for peritoneal carcinomatosis arising from colorectal cancer reported an overall morbidity from 22% to 76% (mean 49%), and mortality of 3.6% related to the procedure [47].

Patient Selection for Surgery

Patient selection is essential for successful surgery. Patient factors, tumor biology, and extent of disease constitute the main factors to consider for the selection of patients (Table 22.9).

Special Note

Tumor biology and histology play an important role in evaluation of candidates for CRS + HIPEC. Patients harboring poorly differentiated carcinoma from the appendix or colorectal have a lower median survival than those who have moderately differentiated tumor histology (17.7 vs. 41.3 months, respectively). For signet ring cell carcinomas, median survival is 7.2 vs. 29.4 months for those without signet ring cell features [50]. Although, high-grade and signet ring cell histology are not contraindications to CRS + HIPEC, these features must be considered in the decision to pursue CRS + HIPEC.

Histology-Based Considerations in Managing Peritoneal Surface Malignancy

Appendix

Role for Right Hemicolectomy

The presence of a malignancy of the appendix requires consideration of performing a right hemicolectomy to complete staging and assess for residual disease in the bowel wall and the regional lymph nodes. The decision about performing a right hemicolectomy does depend on the histology and pathologic features of the appendiceal tumors.

Patients with high-grade tumors of the appendix (G2/3, mucinous adenocarcinoma, adenocarcinoma ex goblet cell, etc.) should undergo right hemicolectomy as part of their treatment plan in order to assess the regional nodes. The role for right hemicolectomy in HAMN is unknown as the rate of lymph node metastases is not known due to the new use and rarity of this diagnosis. However, patients with low-grade histology (LAMN) do not require a right hemicolectomy. The risk of lymph node metastases is low and right hemicolectomy should generally be performed only if required to remove the primary appendiceal tumor.

Additionally, if a patient is being considered for CRS + HIPEC, timing of right hemicolectomy is an important consideration. The mobilization involved in a right hemicolectomy exposes the retroperitoneum and can make CRS more technically challenging and possibly even result in non-resectability due to retroperitoneal disease at the time of CRS. If necessary and if possible, right hemicolectomy should be performed at the time of CRS.

Colon

In recent case series and multi-institutional studies, the 5-year overall survival of patients treated for colorectal peritoneal carcinomatosis with CRS + HIPEC ranges from 20% to 51% [15, 33, 51–53]. Compared to patients undergoing CRS + HIPEC, patients with colorectal cancer and peritoneal carcinomatosis treated non-surgically with systemic chemotherapy have 5-year overall survival of 13% [51]. In these trials, chemotherapy was used prior to or after HIPEC and therefore many consider the results of this trial applicable only in combination with the use of systemic chemotherapy.

The main prognostic factors are completeness of cytoreduction, extent of disease (PCI), lymph node status, disease-free interval and histologic features (high-grade, signet ring).

Mesothelioma

Well-differentiated papillary mesothelioma and multicystic subtypes have a high rate of cure with complete surgical resection. Often observation alone is considered for these subtypes, and usually CRS + HIPEC are reserved for mesothelioma progression recurrence or presence of extensive disease [36].

CRS + HIPEC are generally not offered in peritoneal mesothelioma presenting with sarcomatoid and biphasic subtypes. Similarly, patients presenting with nodal involvement are not offered CRS + HIPEC. Presence of these features correlates with poor prognosis and no significant oncologic benefit from surgery. Compared to patients undergoing CRS + HIPEC, median survival for untreated mesothelioma is 6 months, and patients treated with chemotherapy alone (pemetrexed and cisplatin based regimen) can expect a median overall survival between 10 and 26.8 months [54].

Of note, some groups recommend complete (rather than selective) parietal peritonectomy as part of CRS for mesothelioma [55].

Extraperitoneal Disease and Extensive Peritoneal Carcinomatosis

The presence of disease beyond the peritoneum is a *relative* contraindication to performing CRS + HIPEC. In patients with synchronous peritoneal disease and liver metastases, overall survival is lower after CRS + HIPEC and liver resection than in patients without liver metastases (27% vs. 66%) [56]. However, selected patients with synchronous peritoneal disease and liver metastases may have improved overall survival after CRS + HIPEC and liver resection compared to treatment with systemic chemotherapy alone [57]. In a study by Maggiori et al., patients with a PCI <12 and three or fewer liver metastases achieved a median survival of 40 months [58]. Retroperitoneal lymphadenopathy and extra-abdominal metastases are generally viewed as absolute contraindications to CRS + HIPEC.

The Canadian HIPEC Collaborative Group recommends different strategies for patients with extensive carcinomatosis. Closure of the abdomen followed by systemic chemotherapy and reassessment for response to treatment can be undertaken. If there is significant tumor response, CRS + HIPEC can then be considered. For patients who are not candidates for CRS and HIPEC for tumor or patient-related reasons, a referral to medical oncology for systemic palliative chemotherapy should be discussed. Patients not candidate for chemotherapy should be referred for best supportive care [34].

Second Look Laparotomy and Prophylactic HIPEC

Second look laparotomy may be useful to diagnose early peritoneal metastases that could not be diagnosed by imaging and clinical evaluation. Since PCI is the strongest predictor of outcome, this strategy has the potential advantage of identifying peritoneal carcinomatosis at a low burden with concomitantly improved survival.

The population at highest risk of developing peritoneal carcinomatosis is patients with perforated tumors, patients who underwent resection of limited peritoneal implants simultaneously with primary tumor, and patients with ovarian metastases [59]. In a study by Elias et al., routine second look laparotomy was performed if metastatic work up was negative 1 year after diagnosis of cancer and 6 months after the end of systemic chemotherapy [56]. When macroscopic peritoneal carcinomatosis was found, Elias et al. performed CRS + HIPEC, and HIPEC alone was performed in those without recurrence resulting in a 5-year disease-free survival of 44%.

If no peritoneal carcinomatosis is found, prophylactic HIPEC may be undertaken. One French study reported a 17% recurrence rate for patients with prophylactic HIPEC from colorectal cancer vs. 43% for those without prophylactic HIPEC [60]. The Prodige 15 (ProphyloChip) study is a multicenter randomized trial comparing second look laparotomy followed by prophylactic HIPEC vs. observation alone for colorectal patients at high-risk of developing peritoneal carcinomatosis, with negative metastatic workup. The study randomized 150 patients to surveillance versus second look laparotomy and HIPEC. Disease-free survival, 3-year overall survival, and rate of peritoneal relapse were the same between the two arms [61].

The COLOPEC trial [62] failed to show a difference in 18 month peritoneal metastasis recurrence in patients who had adjuvant HIPEC along with systemic chemotherapy in patients with high-risk (T4 or perforated) colorectal cancer compared to systemic therapy alone [63]. Early results were presented but the final publication is awaited.

Recurrent Disease and Palliation

There is very little data on how to treat patients with recurrence of peritoneal surface malignancy. In selected patients with a low PCI and good performance status, a repeat CRS + HIPEC may be performed. This was investigated by Brouquet et al. for a variety of histologies. With a mean PCI of 7.6 and a recurrence-free interval time of at least 12 months, 5 and 10 years actuarial survival rates were 72.5% and 58%, respectively [64]. Prolonged survival of 12 months with a second complete CRS + HIPEC have been reported in other studies. However, the majority of those patients develop recurrence [65].

For patients with symptomatic peritoneal disease that are not candidates for curative-intent surgery, repeated surgical debulking may offer palliation. Surgery can palliate obstructive symptoms due to peritoneal carcinomatosis in 32–100% of cases. However, surgical treatment may also lead to prolonged time of hospitalization and significant complications (7–44%), and recurrence of obstruction is reported to be as high as 47% [66]. Patients and family must be fully informed of the potential benefits and risks of palliative surgery for obstructive disease related to peritoneal carcinomatosis. HIPEC can also be beneficial for the treatment of high-volume malignant ascites in mesothelioma, even in the absence of complete cytoreduction [67].

Other Histologies Where CRS and HIPEC May Be Considered for Peritoneal Involvement

Gastric Adenocarcinoma

The high rates of peritoneal spread in advanced gastric cancer has led to investigation of the use of CRS + HIPEC as treatment and prophylaxis for peritoneal carcinomatosis. In several retrospective series, CRS + HIPEC survival outcomes for gastric cancer are poor compared to colorectal, appendiceal, and ovarian histologies, with median overall survival of 9–13 months and 14% 5-year survival [68, 69]. Attempts have been made to identify which patients would benefit most from aggressive surgical treatment of carcinomatosis arising from gastric cancer. Glehen et al. identified that the best prognostic factor for long-term survival was the ability to achieve complete cytoreduction (CC-0), which led to 23% 5-year survival. The best results were seen in patients with very low (0-6) PCI. This suggests that there may be a select group of patients who can have long-term survival with CRS and HIPEC, but careful patient selection is essential.

The role of CRS and HIPEC in these low PCI patients is being investigated in the PERISCOPE trial, and results are awaited [70]. There is some survival advantage seen in retrospective studies for prophylactic HIPEC in high-risk resected patients [71], but this needs prospective study to confirm this.

Desmoplastic Small Round Cell Tumor

Desmoplastic Small Round Cell Tumor (DSRCT) is an abdominal sarcoma that arises most commonly in children and young adults. It often presents with metastatic disease limited to the peritoneum. Traditional treatment consists of surgical resection, systemic therapies, and whole abdomen radiation. The role of CRS + HIPEC has been investigated given that this disease is often limited to the peritoneum. In a retrospective series of 48 patients who underwent CRS for DSRCT, survival was prolonged in patients who had post-operative whole-abdomen radiation but there was no survival advantage with the use of HIPEC [72].

Another series of patients undergoing CRS + HIPEC showed that CC-0 or CC-1 resection was associated with significantly longer median survival than patients with CC-2 resection (63.4 vs 26.7 months) [73]. Although studies have shown the benefit of complete cytoreduction when possible, the role of HIPEC needs to be studied prospectively.

Epithelial Ovarian Cancer

A recently published phase 3 randomized trial from van Driel et al. identified that patients with stage III epithelial ovarian cancer have significantly longer median recurrence free and overall survival (HR 0.67, $p = 0.02$) with the addition of cisplatin HIPEC to cytoreductive surgery [74].

Landmark Studies

Appendix

Study	Methods	Results
Sugarbaker et al. 1999 [32]	Retrospective $N = 385$ DPAM + Intermediate PMCA CRS + HIPEC (MMC) ± 5-FU postoperative intraperitoneal for 5 days for PMCA	DPAM/PMP 5-year OS: 86% Intermediate PMCA 5-year OS: 50% Incomplete CRS 5-year OS: 20%
Chua et al. 2012 [75]	Multi-Institutional Retrospective $N = 2298$ PMP originating from appendiceal mucinous neoplasm	Median survival: 196 mos (16.3 year) Median PFS: 96 mos (8.2 year) 10-year OS: 63% 15-year OS: 59% Predictors of poorer OS: older age, PMCA subtype, CCR-2 or 3, prior chemotherapy, major post-operative complications

Study	Methods	Results
Levine et al. 2018 [42]	RCT $N = 121$ Appendiceal carcinoma (low and high grade) undergoing CRS and HIPEC Randomized to MMC vs. Oxaliplatin for HIPEC	Hematologic outcomes: MMC associated with more neutropenia and oxaliplatin had more thrombocytopenia PFS: 66.8% (MMC) vs. 64.8% (oxali) 3-year OS: 83.7% (MMC) vs. 86.9% (oxali)

OS overall survival, *PFS* progression-free survival, *CRS* cytoreductive surgery, *MMC* Mitomycin-C, *HIPEC* hyperthermic intraperitoneal chemotherapy, *DPAM* disseminated peritoneal adenomucinosis, *PMCA* peritoneal mucinous carcinomatosis, *PMP* pseudomyxoma peritonei

Colorectal

Study	Methods	Results
Verwaal et al. 2003, 2008 [15, 76]	RCT $N = 105$ Colorectal and Appendiceal Adenocarcinomatosis (PMCA) CRS + HIPEC (MMC) + systemic post-op 5-FU/LV vs. 5-FU/LV systemic chemo ± palliative surgery	DSS: Improved with CRS + HIPEC (43 vs. 23 mos) Median FU of 8 year: 45% of patients in experimental arm who had CC-0 resection were still alive
Glehen et al. 2004 [52]	Multi-institutional Retrospective $N = 506$Colorectal CRS + HIPEC or EPIC (various agents)	1-year OS: 72% 3-year OS: 39% 5-year OS: 19%
Elias et al. 2009 [51]	Retrospective $N = 96$ Colorectal CRS + HIPEC (Oxaliplatin) vs. Systemic (various regimens including Folfox, Folfiri, 5-FU etc.)	Improved OS with CRS + HIPEC 2-year OS: 81% vs. 65% 5-year OS: 51% vs. 13% However, age and tumor differentiation were not comparable in both groups
Elias et al. 2010 [33]	Multi-institutional Retrospective $N = 523$ Colorectal CRS + perioperative intraperitoneal chemotherapy HIPEC or EPIC (MMC or Oxaliplatin)	Median OS: 30.1 mos 5-year OS: 27% 5-year DFS: 10%

EPIC early postoperative intraperitoneal chemotherapy, *RCT* randomized controlled trial, *CRS* cytoreductive surgery, *MMC* Mitomycin-C, *PMCA* peritoneal mucinous carcinomatosis, *HIPEC* hyperthermic intraperitoneal chemotherapy, *DSS* disease-specific survival, *OS* overall survival, *DFS* disease-free survival

Mesothelioma

There are no randomized controlled trials in peritoneal mesothelioma. The following are the most significant studies:

Study	Methods	Results
Yan et al. 2009 [77]	Multi-institutional series *N* = 405 CRS ±HIPEC Cisplatin + Doxorubicin; Cisplatin, Mitomycin C or both	46% of patients had CC-0/CC-1 3 year-OS: 60% 5 year-OS: 47%
Deraco et al. 2003 [78]	Phase II multi-institutional series *N* = 61 CRS +HIPEC (C + D or C + MMC)	74% of patients had CC-0/CC-1 5 year-OS: 54%
Deraco et al. 2006 [75]	Phase II trial *N* = 49 CRS +HIPEC (C + D or C + MMC)	88% of patients had CC-0/CC-1 3 year-OS: 65% 5 year-OS: 57%
Feldman et al. 2003 [49]	Phase II trial *N* = 49 CRS HIPEC-Cisplatin ±a single postoperative intraperitoneal dose of fluorouracil and paclitaxel between day 7–10	88% of patients had CC-0/CC-1 1 year-OS: 86% 3 year-OS: 59%

CRS cytoreductive surgery, *HIPEC* hyperthermic intraperitoneal chemotherapy, *C* cisplatin, *D* doxorubicin, *MMC* Mitomycin C, *OS* overall survival

Referring to Medical Oncology

1. All patients with high-grade gastrointestinal peritoneal surface malignancy should be referred to medical oncology. Systemic chemotherapy can be used to:
   - Ensure disease stability pre-operatively
   - Downstage disease in patients with unresectable disease or very high PCI
   - Treat patients that are not surgical candidates
   - Treat micrometastatic disease
   - See in vivo tumor response
2. The most common systemic chemotherapy used for peritoneal mesothelioma patients are pemetrexed ±cisplatin, carboplatin or gemcitabine [79, 80]. Another regimen used is cisplatin + irinotecan [81].
3. Multiple regimens have been used for carcinomatosis of appendiceal origin including 5-FU alone or in combination with oxaliplatin, irinotecan, ±bevacizumab or cetuximab [82]. A phase II trial with MMC and capecitabine showed a 38% benefit in the form of stabilization or reduction of peritoneal disease [83]. A neoadjuvant prospective trial of 34 patients using FOLFOX showed partial or complete responses in 29% of patients [84].

4. Many trials have been performed to evaluate the best systemic treatment for metastatic colorectal cancer. These trials have included patients with carcinomatosis. A detailed discussion is beyond the scope of this chapter. Most regimens used included FOLFOX or FOLFIRI ± bevacizumab, cetuximab, or panitumumab. The Combatac study evaluated perioperative chemotherapy with oxaliplatin or irinotecan based regimen + cetuximab combined with CRS + HIPEC for wild-type KRAS peritoneal carcinomatosis from colorectal or appendiceal adenocarcinoma and showed that this is a safe and feasible regimen [85].
5. Neoadjuvant chemotherapy for higher grade appendiceal malignancies and all peritoneal carcinomatosis from colorectal cancer prior to CRS + HIPEC should be considered.

Referring to Radiation Oncology

1. Radiation therapy is not indicated for peritoneal surface malignancies outside of clinical trials.

Referring to Multidisciplinary Cancer Conference (MCC)

1. All patients should be discussed in multidisciplinary cancer conference.

Toronto Pearls

- When faced with an unexpected finding of peritoneal implants during elective or emergency surgery, we recommend aborting the procedure following tissue confirmation of peritoneal carcinomatosis when the primary lesion is asymptomatic. For symptomatic primary lesions, we recommend doing the minimum possible (i.e. diversion is preferable to resection when obstructed) to address the symptoms with an effort to preserve, as much as possible, the integrity of the peritoneal barrier and not hinder cytoreduction in the future. In selected cases, minimal, localized, and completely resectable implants may be removed if included in the resection. For appendiceal tumors, the appendectomy should be performed if it is safe to do so for diagnostic purposes. Carefully document the PCI. Do a full investigation post-operatively with imaging, and refer the patient to a tertiary care center specialized in the treatment of peritoneal surface malignancies.
- Biopsies are ideally done under either image-guidance or diagnostic laparoscopy, targeting high-grade or suspicious-looking lesion. Fine needle aspiration (FNA) and aspiration of intraperitoneal mucin for cytology are usually inadequate for diagnosis.

- Careful pathologic review by expert pathologist is essential to accurately diagnose peritoneal surface malignancies and their subtypes, especially for uncommon tumors such as appendiceal neoplasms and mesothelioma.
- For selected patients with colorectal and high-grade appendiceal carcinomatosis, we recommend pre-operative systemic chemotherapy for 6 months, for the reasons listed above. Additionally, some patients may not be fit for adjuvant chemotherapy post-operatively due to complications or slow recovery. Delivery of chemotherapy in the neoadjuvant setting mitigates this.
- Diagnostic laparoscopy is performed to evaluate the extent of disease in high-grade adenocarcinoma of the appendix and peritoneal carcinomatosis from colorectal origin.
  - This is often performed after completion of pre-operative chemotherapy
  - After chemotherapy, if patients have an acceptable PCI on laparoscopy and have completely resectable disease, we proceed to CRS + HIPEC
- In patients that are not surgical candidates, chemotherapy alone may be the treatment of choice. We have seen some excellent clinical responses to systemic chemotherapy, including some patients who later became candidates for CRS + HIPEC.

References

1. McCusker ME, Coté TR, Clegg LX, Sobin LH. Primary malignant neoplasms of the appendix: a population-based study from the surveillance, epidemiology and end-results program, 1973-1998. Cancer. 2002;94(12):3307–12.
2. Rouzbahman M, Chetty R. Republished: mucinous tumours of appendix and ovary: an overview and evaluation of current practice. Postgrad Med J. 2015;91(1071):41–5.
3. AJCC. In: Amin MB, editor. AJCC cancer staging manual. 8th ed. Chicago: Springer; 2017.
4. Ronnett BM, Zahn CM, Kurman RJ, Kass ME, Sugarbaker PH, Shmookler BM. Disseminated peritoneal adenomucinosis and peritoneal mucinous carcinomatosis. A clinicopathologic analysis of 109 cases with emphasis on distinguishing pathologic features, site of origin, prognosis, and relationship to "pseudomyxoma peritonei". Am J Surg Pathol. 1995;19(12):1390–408.
5. Bosman F, Carneiro F, Hruban R, Theise ND. WHO classification of tumors of the digestive system. 4th ed. Lyon: IARC; 2010.
6. Carr NJ, Cecil TD, Mohamed F, Sobin LH, Sugarbaker PH, González-Moreno S, et al. A consensus for classification and pathologic reporting of pseudomyxoma peritonei and associated appendiceal neoplasia: the results of the peritoneal surface oncology group international (PSOGI) modified Delphi process. Am J Surg Pathol. 2016;40(1):14–26.
7. Misdraji J, Yantiss RK, Graeme-Cook FM, Balis UJ, Young RH. Appendiceal mucinous neoplasms: a clinicopathologic analysis of 107 cases. Am J Surg Pathol. 2003;27(8):1089–103.
8. Ronnett BM, Yan H, Kurman RJ, Shmookler BM, Wu L, Sugarbaker PH. Patients with pseudomyxoma peritonei associated with disseminated peritoneal adenomucinosis have a significantly more favorable prognosis than patients with peritoneal mucinous carcinomatosis. Cancer. 2001;92(1):85–91.
9. Pai RK, Beck AH, Norton JA, Longacre TA. Appendiceal mucinous neoplasms: clinicopathologic study of 116 cases with analysis of factors predicting recurrence. Am J Surg Pathol. 2009;33(10):1425–39.

10. Miner TJ, Shia J, Jaques DP, Klimstra DS, Brennan MF, Coit DG. Long-term survival following treatment of pseudomyxoma peritonei: an analysis of surgical therapy. Ann Surg. 2005;241(2):300–8.
11. Reid MD, Basturk O, Shaib WL, Xue Y, Balci S, Choi HJ, et al. Adenocarcinoma ex-goblet cell carcinoid (appendiceal-type crypt cell adenocarcinoma) is a morphologically distinct entity with highly aggressive behavior and frequent association with peritoneal/intra-abdominal dissemination: an analysis of 77 cases. Mod Pathol. 2016;29(10):1243–53.
12. Tang LH, Shia J, Soslow RA, Dhall D, Wong WD, O'Reilly E, et al. Pathologic classification and clinical behavior of the spectrum of goblet cell carcinoid tumors of the appendix. Am J Surg Pathol. 2008;32(10):1429–43.
13. Overman MJ, Fournier K, Hu CY, Eng C, Taggart M, Royal R, et al. Improving the AJCC/TNM staging for adenocarcinomas of the appendix: the prognostic impact of histological grade. Ann Surg. 2013;257(6):1072–8.
14. Cao C, Yan TD, Black D, Morris DL. A systematic review and meta-analysis of cytoreductive surgery with perioperative intraperitoneal chemotherapy for peritoneal carcinomatosis of colorectal origin. Ann Surg Oncol. 2009;16(8):2152–65.
15. Verwaal VJ, van Ruth S, de Bree E, van Slothen GW, van Tinteren H, Boot H, et al. Randomized trial of cytoreduction and hyperthermic intraperitoneal chemotherapy versus systemic chemotherapy and palliative surgery in patients with peritoneal carcinomatosis of colorectal cancer. J Clin Oncol. 2003;21(20):3737–43.
16. Franko J, Shi Q, Meyers JP, Maughan TS, Adams RA, Seymour MT, et al. Prognosis of patients with peritoneal metastatic colorectal cancer given systemic therapy: an analysis of individual patient data from prospective randomised trials from the Analysis and Research in Cancers of the Digestive System (ARCAD) database. Lancet Oncol. 2016;17(12):1709–19.
17. Broeckx G, Pauwels P. Malignant peritoneal mesothelioma: a review. Transl Lung Cancer Res. 2018;7(5):537–42.
18. Boussios S, Moschetta M, Karathanasi A, Tsiouris AK, Kanellos FS, Tatsi K, et al. Malignant peritoneal mesothelioma: clinical aspects, and therapeutic perspectives. Ann Gastroenterol. 2018;31(6):659–69.
19. Yan TD, Deraco M, Elias D, Glehen O, Levine EA, Moran BJ, et al. A novel tumor-node-metastasis (TNM) staging system of diffuse malignant peritoneal mesothelioma using outcome analysis of a multi-institutional database*. Cancer. 2011;117(9):1855–63.
20. Krasinskas AM, Borczuk AC, Hartman DJ, Chabot JA, Taub RN, Mogal A, et al. Prognostic significance of morphological growth patterns and mitotic index of epithelioid malignant peritoneal mesothelioma. Histopathology. 2016;68(5):729–37.
21. Kim J, Bhagwandin S, Labow DM. Malignant peritoneal mesothelioma: a review. Ann Transl Med. 2017;5(11):236.
22. Sugarbaker PH. Surgical management of carcinomatosis from colorectal cancer. Clin Colon Rectal Surg. 2005;18(3):190–203.
23. Glehen O, Cotte E, Schreiber V, Sayag-Beaujard AC, Vignal J, Gilly FN. Intraperitoneal chemohyperthermia and attempted cytoreductive surgery in patients with peritoneal carcinomatosis of colorectal origin. Br J Surg. 2004;91(6):747–54.
24. Koppe MJ, Boerman OC, Oyen WJ, Bleichrodt RP. Peritoneal carcinomatosis of colorectal origin: incidence and current treatment strategies. Ann Surg. 2006;243(2):212–22.
25. Pestieau SR, Sugarbaker PH. Treatment of primary colon cancer with peritoneal carcinomatosis: comparison of concomitant vs. delayed management. Dis Colon Rectum. 2000;43(10):1341–6; discussion 7–8
26. Yan TD, Haveric N, Carmignani CP, Chang D, Sugarbaker PH. Abdominal computed tomography scans in the selection of patients with malignant peritoneal mesothelioma for comprehensive treatment with cytoreductive surgery and perioperative intraperitoneal chemotherapy. Cancer. 2005;103(4):839–49.
27. Low RN, Barone RM, Gurney JM, Muller WD. Mucinous appendiceal neoplasms: preoperative MR staging and classification compared with surgical and histopathologic findings. AJR Am J Roentgenol. 2008;190(3):656–65.

28. Jayakrishnan TT, Zacharias AJ, Sharma A, Pappas SG, Gamblin TC, Turaga KK. Role of laparoscopy in patients with peritoneal metastases considered for cytoreductive surgery and hyperthermic intraperitoneal chemotherapy (HIPEC). World J Surg Oncol. 2014;12:270.
29. Menassel B, Duclos A, Passot G, Dohan A, Payet C, Isaac S, et al. Preoperative CT and MRI prediction of non-resectability in patients treated for pseudomyxoma peritonei from mucinous appendiceal neoplasms. Eur J Surg Oncol. 2016;42(4):558–66.
30. Baratti D, Kusamura S, Nonaka D, Langer M, Andreola S, Favaro M, et al. Pseudomyxoma peritonei: clinical pathological and biological prognostic factors in patients treated with cytoreductive surgery and hyperthermic intraperitoneal chemotherapy (HIPEC). Ann Surg Oncol. 2008;15(2):526–34.
31. Laterza B, Kusamura S, Baratti D, Oliva GD, Deraco M. Role of explorative laparoscopy to evaluate optimal candidates for cytoreductive surgery and hyperthermic intraperitoneal chemotherapy (HIPEC) in patients with peritoneal mesothelioma. In Vivo. 2009;23(1):187–90.
32. Sugarbaker PH, Chang D. Results of treatment of 385 patients with peritoneal surface spread of appendiceal malignancy. Ann Surg Oncol. 1999;6(8):727–31.
33. Elias D, Gilly F, Boutitie F, Quenet F, Bereder JM, Mansvelt B, et al. Peritoneal colorectal carcinomatosis treated with surgery and perioperative intraperitoneal chemotherapy: retrospective analysis of 523 patients from a multicentric French study. J Clin Oncol. 2010;28(1):63–8.
34. Dubé P, Sideris L, Law C, Mack L, Haase E, Giacomantonio C, et al. Guidelines on the use of cytoreductive surgery and hyperthermic intraperitoneal chemotherapy in patients with peritoneal surface malignancy arising from colorectal or appendiceal neoplasms. Curr Oncol. 2015;22(2):e100–12.
35. Esquivel J, Farinetti A, Sugarbaker PH. Elective surgery in recurrent colon cancer with peritoneal seeding: when to and when not to proceed. G Chir. 1999;20(3):81–6.
36. Baratti D, Kusamura S, Martinetti A, Seregni E, Oliva DG, Laterza B, et al. Circulating CA125 in patients with peritoneal mesothelioma treated with cytoreductive surgery and intraperitoneal hyperthermic perfusion. Ann Surg Oncol. 2007;14(2):500–8.
37. Wheatley-Price P, Yang B, Patsios D, Patel D, Ma C, Xu W, et al. Soluble mesothelin-related peptide and osteopontin as markers of response in malignant mesothelioma. J Clin Oncol. 2010;28(20):3316–22.
38. van Ruth S, Hart AA, Bonfrer JM, Verwaal VJ, Zoetmulder FA. Prognostic value of baseline and serial carcinoembryonic antigen and carbohydrate antigen 19.9 measurements in patients with pseudomyxoma peritonei treated with cytoreduction and hyperthermic intraperitoneal chemotherapy. Ann Surg Oncol. 2002;9(10):961–7.
39. van Eden WJ, Kok NFM, Woensdregt K, Huitema ADR, Boot H, Aalbers AGJ. Safety of intraperitoneal Mitomycin C versus intraperitoneal oxaliplatin in patients with peritoneal carcinomatosis of colorectal cancer undergoing cytoreductive surgery and HIPEC. Eur J Surg Oncol. 2018;44(2):220–7.
40. Leung V, Huo YR, Liauw W, Morris DL. Oxaliplatin versus Mitomycin C for HIPEC in colorectal cancer peritoneal carcinomatosis. Eur J Surg Oncol. 2017;43(1):144–9.
41. Hompes D, D'Hoore A, Wolthuis A, Fieuws S, Mirck B, Bruin S, et al. The use of Oxaliplatin or Mitomycin C in HIPEC treatment for peritoneal carcinomatosis from colorectal cancer: a comparative study. J Surg Oncol. 2014;109(6):527–32.
42. Levine EA, Votanopoulos KI, Shen P, Russell G, Fenstermaker J, Mansfield P, et al. A multicenter randomized trial to evaluate hematologic toxicities after hyperthermic intraperitoneal chemotherapy with oxaliplatin or mitomycin in patients with appendiceal tumors. J Am Coll Surg. 2018;226(4):434–43.
43. Sugarbaker PH. Managing the peritoneal surface component of gastrointestinal cancer. Part 1. Patterns of dissemination and treatment options. Oncology (Williston Park). 2004;18(1):51–9.
44. Ceelen WP, Påhlman L, Mahteme H. Pharmacodynamic aspects of intraperitoneal cytotoxic therapy. Cancer Treat Res. 2007;134:195–214.
45. Elias D, Bonnay M, Puizillou JM, Antoun S, Demirdjian S, El OA, et al. Heated intra-operative intraperitoneal oxaliplatin after complete resection of peritoneal carcinomatosis: pharmacokinetics and tissue distribution. Ann Oncol. 2002;13(2):267–72.

46. Quenet F, Elias D, Roca L, Goere D, Ghouti L, Pocard M, et al. A UNICANCER phase III trial of hyperthermic intra-peritoneal chemotherapy (HIPEC) for colorectal peritoneal carcinomatosis (PC): PRODIGE 7. J Clin Oncol. 2018;36:LBA3503.
47. Nadler A, McCart JA, Govindarajan A. Peritoneal carcinomatosis from colon cancer: a systematic review of the data for cytoreduction and intraperitoneal chemotherapy. Clin Colon Rectal Surg. 2015;28(4):234–46.
48. Yan TD, Brun EA, Cerruto CA, Haveric N, Chang D, Sugarbaker PH. Prognostic indicators for patients undergoing cytoreductive surgery and perioperative intraperitoneal chemotherapy for diffuse malignant peritoneal mesothelioma. Ann Surg Oncol. 2007;14(1):41–9.
49. Feldman AL, Libutti SK, Pingpank JF, Bartlett DL, Beresnev TH, Mavroukakis SM, et al. Analysis of factors associated with outcome in patients with malignant peritoneal mesothelioma undergoing surgical debulking and intraperitoneal chemotherapy. J Clin Oncol. 2003;21(24):4560–7.
50. Van Sweringen HL, Hanseman DJ, Ahmad SA, Edwards MJ, Sussman JJ. Predictors of survival in patients with high-grade peritoneal metastases undergoing cytoreductive surgery and hyperthermic intraperitoneal chemotherapy. Surgery. 2012;152(4):617–24; discussion 24-5
51. Elias D, Lefevre JH, Chevalier J, Brouquet A, Marchal F, Classe JM, et al. Complete cytoreductive surgery plus intraperitoneal chemohyperthermia with oxaliplatin for peritoneal carcinomatosis of colorectal origin. J Clin Oncol. 2009;27(5):681–5.
52. Glehen O, Kwiatkowski F, Sugarbaker PH, Elias D, Levine EA, De Simone M, et al. Cytoreductive surgery combined with perioperative intraperitoneal chemotherapy for the management of peritoneal carcinomatosis from colorectal cancer: a multi-institutional study. J Clin Oncol. 2004;22(16):3284–92.
53. Gervais MK, Dubé P, McConnell Y, Drolet P, Mitchell A, Sideris L. Cytoreductive surgery plus hyperthermic intraperitoneal chemotherapy with oxaliplatin for peritoneal carcinomatosis arising from colorectal cancer. J Surg Oncol. 2013;108(7):438–43.
54. Helm JH, Miura JT, Glenn JA, Marcus RK, Larrieux G, Jayakrishnan TT, et al. Cytoreductive surgery and hyperthermic intraperitoneal chemotherapy for malignant peritoneal mesothelioma: a systematic review and meta-analysis. Ann Surg Oncol. 2015;22(5):1686–93.
55. Baratti D, Kusamura S, Cabras AD, Deraco M. Cytoreductive surgery with selective versus complete parietal peritonectomy followed by hyperthermic intraperitoneal chemotherapy in patients with diffuse malignant peritoneal mesothelioma: a controlled study. Ann Surg Oncol. 2012;19(5):1416–24.
56. Elias D, Goéré D, Dumont F, Honoré C, Dartigues P, Stoclin A, et al. Role of hyperthermic intraoperative peritoneal chemotherapy in the management of peritoneal metastases. Eur J Cancer. 2014;50(2):332–40.
57. de Cuba EM, Kwakman R, Knol DL, Bonjer HJ, Meijer GA, Te Velde EA. Cytoreductive surgery and HIPEC for peritoneal metastases combined with curative treatment of colorectal liver metastases: systematic review of all literature and meta-analysis of observational studies. Cancer Treat Rev. 2013;39(4):321–7.
58. Maggiori L, Goéré D, Viana B, Tzanis D, Dumont F, Honoré C, et al. Should patients with peritoneal carcinomatosis of colorectal origin with synchronous liver metastases be treated with a curative intent? A case-control study. Ann Surg. 2013;258(1):116–21.
59. Honoré C, Goéré D, Souadka A, Dumont F, Elias D. Definition of patients presenting a high risk of developing peritoneal carcinomatosis after curative surgery for colorectal cancer: a systematic review. Ann Surg Oncol. 2013;20(1):183–92.
60. Elias D, Honoré C, Dumont F, Ducreux M, Boige V, Malka D, et al. Results of systematic second-look surgery plus HIPEC in asymptomatic patients presenting a high risk of developing colorectal peritoneal carcinomatosis. Ann Surg. 2011;254(2):289–93.
61. Goere D, Glehen O, Quenet F, Ducreux M, Guilloit J-M, Texier M, et al. Results of a randomized phase 3 study evaluating the potential benefit of a second-look surgery plus HIPEC in patients at high risk of developing colorectal peritoneal metastases (PROPHYLOCHIP-NTC01226394). J Clin Oncol. 2018;36(15_suppl):3531.

62. Klaver CE, Musters GD, Bemelman WA, Punt CJ, Verwaal VJ, Dijkgraaf MG, et al. Adjuvant hyperthermic intraperitoneal chemotherapy (HIPEC) in patients with colon cancer at high risk of peritoneal carcinomatosis; the COLOPEC randomized multicentre trial. BMC Cancer. 2015;15:428.
63. Klaver C, Tanis P. Adjuvant HIPEC in patients with colon cancer at high risk of peritoneal metastases: primary outcome of the COLOPEC multicentre randomized trial. In: Gastrointestinal Cancers Symposium. San Francisco: ASCO; 2019.
64. Brouquet A, Goéré D, Lefèvre JH, Bonnet S, Dumont F, Raynard B, et al. The second procedure combining complete cytoreductive surgery and intraperitoneal chemotherapy for isolated peritoneal recurrence: postoperative course and long-term outcome. Ann Surg Oncol. 2009;16(10):2744–51.
65. Klaver YL, Chua TC, Verwaal VJ, de Hingh IH, Morris DL. Secondary cytoreductive surgery and peri-operative intraperitoneal chemotherapy for peritoneal recurrence of colorectal and appendiceal peritoneal carcinomatosis following prior primary cytoreduction. J Surg Oncol. 2013;107(6):585–90.
66. Paul Olson TJ, Pinkerton C, Brasel KJ, Schwarze ML. Palliative surgery for malignant bowel obstruction from carcinomatosis: a systematic review. JAMA Surg. 2014;149(4):383–92.
67. Patriti A, Cavazzoni E, Graziosi L, Pisciaroli A, Luzi D, Gullà N, et al. Successful palliation of malignant ascites from peritoneal mesothelioma by laparoscopic intraperitoneal hyperthermic chemotherapy. Surg Laparosc Endosc Percutan Tech. 2008;18(4):426–8.
68. Passot G, Vaudoyer D, Villeneuve L, Kepenekian V, Beaujard AC, Bakrin N, et al. What made hyperthermic intraperitoneal chemotherapy an effective curative treatment for peritoneal surface malignancy: a 25-year experience with 1,125 procedures. J Surg Oncol. 2016;113(7):796–803.
69. Glehen O, Gilly FN, Boutitie F, Bereder JM, Quenet F, Sideris L, et al. Toward curative treatment of peritoneal carcinomatosis from nonovarian origin by cytoreductive surgery combined with perioperative intraperitoneal chemotherapy: a multi-institutional study of 1,290 patients. Cancer. 2010;116(24):5608–18.
70. van der Kaaij RT, Braam HJ, Boot H, Los M, Cats A, Grootscholten C, et al. Treatment of peritoneal dissemination in stomach cancer patients with cytoreductive surgery and Hyperthermic intraperitoneal chemotherapy (HIPEC): rationale and design of the PERISCOPE study. JMIR Res Protoc. 2017;6(7):e136.
71. Desiderio J, Chao J, Melstrom L, Warner S, Tozzi F, Fong Y, et al. The 30-year experience-A meta-analysis of randomised and high-quality non-randomised studies of hyperthermic intraperitoneal chemotherapy in the treatment of gastric cancer. Eur J Cancer. 2017;79:1–14.
72. Honoré C, Atallah V, Mir O, Orbach D, Ferron G, LePéchoux C, et al. Abdominal desmoplastic small round cell tumor without extraperitoneal metastases: is there a benefit for HIPEC after macroscopically complete cytoreductive surgery? PLoS One. 2017;12(2):e0171639.
73. Hayes-Jordan A, Green HL, Lin H, Owusu-Agyemang P, Fitzgerald N, Arunkumar R, et al. Complete cytoreduction and HIPEC improves survival in desmoplastic small round cell tumor. Ann Surg Oncol. 2014;21(1):220–4.
74. van Driel WJ, Koole SN, Sonke GS. Hyperthermic intraperitoneal chemotherapy in ovarian cancer. N Engl J Med. 2018;378(14):1363–4.
75. Chua TC, Moran BJ, Sugarbaker PH, Levine EA, Glehen O, Gilly FN, et al. Early- and long-term outcome data of patients with pseudomyxoma peritonei from appendiceal origin treated by a strategy of cytoreductive surgery and hyperthermic intraperitoneal chemotherapy. J Clin Oncol. 2012;30(20):2449–56.
76. Verwaal VJ, Bruin S, Boot H, van Slooten G, van Tinteren H. 8-year follow-up of randomized trial: cytoreduction and hyperthermic intraperitoneal chemotherapy versus systemic chemotherapy in patients with peritoneal carcinomatosis of colorectal cancer. Ann Surg Oncol. 2008;15(9):2426–32.
77. Yan TD, Deraco M, Baratti D, Kusamura S, Elias D, Glehen O, et al. Cytoreductive surgery and hyperthermic intraperitoneal chemotherapy for malignant peritoneal mesothelioma: multi-institutional experience. J Clin Oncol. 2009;27(36):6237–42.

78. Deraco M, De Simone M, Rossi CR, Cavaliere F, Difilippo F, Scuderi S, et al. An Italian multicentric phase II study on peritonectomy and intra peritoneal hyperthermic perfusion (IPHP) to treat patients with peritoneal mesothelioma. J Exp Clin Cancer Res. 2003;22(4 Suppl):41–5.
79. Simon GR, Verschraegen CF, Jänne PA, Langer CJ, Dowlati A, Gadgeel SM, et al. Pemetrexed plus gemcitabine as first-line chemotherapy for patients with peritoneal mesothelioma: final report of a phase II trial. J Clin Oncol. 2008;26(21):3567–72.
80. Carteni G, Manegold C, Garcia GM, Siena S, Zielinski CC, Amadori D, et al. Malignant peritoneal mesothelioma-results from the international expanded access program using pemetrexed alone or in combination with a platinum agent. Lung Cancer. 2009;64(2):211–8.
81. Le DT, Deavers M, Hunt K, Malpica A, Verschraegen CF. Cisplatin and irinotecan (CPT-11) for peritoneal mesothelioma. Cancer Investig. 2003;21(5):682–9.
82. Shapiro JF, Chase JL, Wolff RA, Lambert LA, Mansfield PF, Overman MJ, et al. Modern systemic chemotherapy in surgically unresectable neoplasms of appendiceal origin: a single-institution experience. Cancer. 2010;116(2):316–22.
83. Farquharson AL, Pranesh N, Witham G, Swindell R, Taylor MB, Renehan AG, et al. A phase II study evaluating the use of concurrent mitomycin C and capecitabine in patients with advanced unresectable pseudomyxoma peritonei. Br J Cancer. 2008;99(4):591–6.
84. Sugarbaker PH, Bijelic L, Chang D, Yoo D. Neoadjuvant FOLFOX chemotherapy in 34 consecutive patients with mucinous peritoneal carcinomatosis of appendiceal origin. J Surg Oncol. 2010;102(6):576–81.
85. Glockzin G, Zeman F, Croner RS, Königsrainer A, Pelz J, Ströhlein MA, et al. Perioperative systemic chemotherapy, cytoreductive surgery, and hyperthermic intraperitoneal chemotherapy in patients with colorectal peritoneal metastasis: results of the prospective multicenter phase 2 COMBATAC trial. Clin Colorectal Cancer. 2018;17(4):285–96.

Rectal Cancer

23

Ricky Jrearz, Shady Ashamalla, Marcus J. Burnstein,
William Chu, Erin Kennedy, and Peter K. Stotland

Introduction

In 2019, an estimated 26,300 Canadians will be diagnosed with colorectal cancer and 9500 will die of the disease. Overall, colorectal cancer is the second leading cause of cancer death in men and the third most common cause of cancer death in women [1]. The death rate is declining in both sexes. Population-based screening has been shown to reduce mortality (see Table 23.1) from colorectal cancer [2].

The American Joint Committee on Cancer 8th edition is the current recommended Colorectal Cancer staging system.

In this chapter, the term rectal cancer refers to adenocarcinoma of the rectum, that is, adenocarcinoma arising at or above the anorectal junction (the pelvic floor) and at or below the rectosigmoid junction (where the taenia coli coalesce to form the confluent longitudinal muscle layer of the rectum).

R. Jrearz
General Surgical Oncology, University of Toronto, Toronto, ON, Canada

S. Ashamalla · M. J. Burnstein · E. Kennedy · P. K. Stotland (✉)
Department of Surgery, University of Toronto, Toronto, ON, Canada
e-mail: shady.ashamalla@sunnybrook.ca; burnsteinm@smh.ca; erin.kennedy@sinaihealthsystem.ca; peter.stotland@nygh.on.ca

W. Chu
Department of Radiation Oncology, University of Toronto, Toronto, ON, Canada
e-mail: william.chu@sunnybrook.ca

F. C. Wright et al. (eds.), *Surgical Oncology Manual*,
https://doi.org/10.1007/978-3-030-48363-0_23

Table 23.1 Prognosis of colorectal cancer

Presentation	Prognosis: 5-year relative survival [3]
Localized disease (stages I and II)	89%
Regional disease (stage III)	70%
Distant metastasis (stage IV)	15%

Definitions/Terminology

- *Localized Rectal Cancer:* rectal adenocarcinoma without distant metastases, which can be divided into early (T1-2N0) and advanced (T3-4 any N) disease.
- *Locally Advanced Rectal Cancer (LARC)*: a non-specific term that encompasses a range of pathology from bulky T3 tumors (+/− lymphadenopathy) to those requiring multivisceral resection.
- *Total Mesorectal Excision (TME)*: excision of the rectum and the mesorectum in the plane between the visceral mesorectal fascia and parietal fascia.
- *Transanal Excision (TAE)*: localized excision of a rectal lesion; in general, a full-thickness, intact, disc of the wall with a 1 cm mucosal margin.
- *Transanal Minimally Invasive Surgery (TAMIS)/Transanal Endoscopic Microsurgery (TEM):* transanal excision of a rectal lesion with the use of a specialized video operating system; these systems include the establishment of a pneumorectum and provide access to the middle and upper rectum.
- *Transanal Total Mesorectal Excision (TaTME):* a novel technique using a TAMIS system to resect low rectal tumors. A low TME resection is achieved under direct visualization for a bottom-up approach.
- *Low Anterior Resection (LAR):* a sphincter-preserving TME with colorectal or coloanal anastomosis.
- *Anterior Resection (AR):* a tumor-specific mesorectal excision, dividing the mesorectum and rectum 5 cm below the distal extent of the lesion, at a right angle to the long axis of the rectum.
- *Abdominoperineal Resection (APR):* TME with en bloc excision of the anus.
- *Extramural venous invasion (EMVI):* Direct invasion of a vascular structure by tumor that can be detected on MRI. EMVI is an independent prognostic factor for rectal cancer.
- *Positive Margin:* tumor cells extending to the cut edge of a specimen. In a TME specimen, a circumferential resection margin (CRM) of ≤1 mm is considered positive. Quirke et al. have identified six modes of margin involvement: [4]
  - *Direct extension*
  - *Discontinuous tumor spread*
  - *Lymph node involvement*
  - *Venous invasion*
  - *Lymphatic invasion*
  - *Perineural spread*

Management

see Table 23.2

Table 23.2 Management of localized rectal cancer

Clinical scenario	Workup	Surgical management	Follow-up[a] [5, 9]
Early rectal cancer (T1-T2, N0)	History and physical: Assessment of preoperative continence, sexual function, neurologic and vascular symptoms Family history (cancer syndromes) DRE Labs: CEA	Upper/middle rectum: LAR Lower rectum: TME or APR *Select T1 cancers with favorable features (confirmed T1 by TRUS) may beconsidered for local excision (TAMIS/TEM)	**CCO** History & physical, CEA q6 months × 5 years CT chest/abdo/pelvis q12 months for 3 years or CXR, U/S abdo/pelvis q6–12 months × 3 years then q12 months for next 2 years
Locally advanced resectable rectal cancer (T3-T4, N0, or N+ disease)	Colonoscopy Imaging: CT chest/abdo/pelvis Pelvic MRI Trans-rectal ultrasound (TRUS) Repeat MRI after nCRT to restage and assess tumor response	Upper rectum LAR (nCRT only in select patients) Middle rectum: nCRT followed by LAR Lower rectum: nCRT followed by TME or APR *Multivisceral resection as required to obtain R0 resection	Colonoscopy 1 year unless not performed preoperatively, then it should be done within 3–6 months Frequency of surveillance colonoscopies to be determined by findings. If normal, repeat in 5 years **NCCN** History and physical q3–6 months for first 2 year then q6 months for next 3 years CT chest/abdo/pelvis q6–12 months × 5 years (stage II/III) or q6 months × 2 years then q12 months for next 3 years (stage IV) CEA q6 months × 2 years then q12 months for next 3 years Colonoscopy 1 year unless not performed preoperatively, then it should be done within 3–6 months. If normal, repeat in 3 years then in 5 years

DRE digital rectal exam, *LAR* low anterior resection, *TAMIS* transanal minimally invasive surgery, *nCRT* neoadjuvant chemoradiation, APR abdominoperineal resection, TRUS transrectal ultrasound, TME total mesorectal excision

[a]Follow-up guidelines vary between institutions. Multiple studies have shown no difference in OS, cancer-specific mortality, recurrence rates, time to recurrence detection, or rates of resection for cancer recurrences in high intensity or low intensity surveillance protocols [73, 74]

Localized Rectal Cancer

Special Notes

- The likelihood of synchronous colon carcinoma is 3–5% and synchronous neoplasia is 10–20%.
- TRUS is the most accurate imaging modality for differentiating T1 from T2 tumors, but MRI is superior for more advanced T stages, N stage, assessment of the circumferential resection margin, and response to neoadjuvant therapy [6, 7].
- PET scan is a useful adjunct in detecting local or distant recurrence in the context of a rising CEA with no disease detected on a CT scan or endoscopy. It can also distinguish local recurrence from postoperative changes [8].
- APR is indicated for cancer invading or very closely encroaching upon the external anal sphincter. Compared to low anterior resection, APR is associated with higher rates of specimen perforation, circumferential margin positivity and local recurrence, and lower overall survival [12–14]. An extra-levator perineal approach, which can be facilitated by the prone jack-knife position, may provide a superior oncologic resection to conventional APR [15, 16].
- nCRT has been shown to significantly decrease lymph node yield after resection for rectal cancer, with some evidence that this mirrors tumor regression in response to treatment [17, 18]. The relevance of the 12 lymph node benchmark in this context has been called into question [19].
- Pathologic tumor regression grade (TRG) (see Table 23.3) is a measure of response to neoadjuvant therapy, based on degree of fibrosis and percentage viable cells. TRG is correlated with outcome, with a greater degree of regression predicting better survival [20]. The College of American Pathologists classifies treatment effect according to the following schema [21]:
- An analogous classification of radiologic TRG based on pre- and post-neoadjuvant MRI has been shown to predict disease-free survival (DFS) and overall survival (OS) [22]. The degree of tumor regression on post-treatment

  MRI was more closely correlated with survival than T stage.

Table 23.3 Tumor regression grade

Description	Tumor regression grade
No viable cancer cells	0 (complete response)
Single cells or small groups of cancer cells	1 (moderate response)
Residual cancer outgrown by fibrosis	2 (minimal response)
Minimal or no tumor kill; extensive residual cancer	3 (poor response)

Special Considerations

Local Excision for Rectal Cancer

Traditional criteria for transanal excision (TAE) have been expanded with the evolution of TAMIS/TEM:

1. *Curative resection of low-risk T1 lesions* [23]
   - T1N0
   - Well differentiated
   - No lymphatic, vascular, or perineural invasion
   - Less than 4 cm in width
   - Less than 50% circumferential
   - Within 15 cm of anal verge
   - Mobile
     - At least 1 cm margin of normal tissue surrounding the tumor is required.
     - Tumor fragmentation is associated with a higher incidence of local recurrence [24].
     - Immediate salvage resection is indicated for adverse pathologic findings. The evidence indicates that the oncologic outcomes of immediate salvage resection are equivalent to primary resection [25, 26]. However, there is concern that local excision renders subsequent salvage more technically challenging, and in some circumstances may preclude sphincter sparing reconstruction [27, 28].
2. *Palliation of T2/T3 lesions*
   - For local control in patients who cannot tolerate radical resection.
3. *Excision of lesions with suspected complete clinical response (cCR) following nCRT*
   - Results are mixed and controversy exists regarding whether organ preservation through local excision alone is appropriate for higher stage tumors that responded well to nCRT [29–31, 46, 47].
   - Multiple smaller studies show a large proportion (>25%) of patients with cCR following nCRT who undergo local excision harbor residual disease [106, 107].
   - A large multicenter observational trial is underway to further elucidate the oncologic safety of this approach [108].

Recommended Margins

- Proximal: minimum 5 cm (gross margins).
- Distal:
  - Upper and middle rectum: minimum 5 cm (gross margins in the rectal wall and in the mesorectum).
  - Lower rectum: ideally 2 cm[a] (gross margins).
- Circumferential radial margin: minimum 1 mm (microscopic margins) [32] [b].

a For low rectal tumors, a distal resection margin of 1 cm can be accepted to allow sphincter preservation. With appropriate technique and neoadjuvant therapy, a 1 cm margin is associated with rates of local recurrence and survival that are equivalent to wider margins [33].

b A positive CRM significantly increases the risk of local recurrence and is associated with decreased survival. In multivariate analyses, it has been identified as the single most important prognostic factor for local recurrence [34].

Chemoradiation in Rectal Cancer

- Neoadjuvant RT or chemoradiation (CRT) is indicated for T3–4 lesions, any N+, or threatened circumferential radial margin.
- Extraperitoneal location of the rectum allows for radiotherapy with minimal toxicity to intra-abdominal structures (e.g., small bowel).
- Radiotherapy reduces the relative risk of local recurrence by 50% [35, 36].

MRI and "Good Prognosis" Tumors [76]

- Quicksilver is a multicenter Canadian study that aimed to identify patients with "good prognosis" rectal tumors amenable to primary surgery without neoadjuvant chemoradiation (nCRT). Good and poor prognostic factors as defined by the study are presented in Table 23.4:
- +CRM rates were 4.9%. LR results are pending
- This studied aimed to validate the results of prior studies such as MERCURY and OCUM which addressed a similar clinical question. +CRM rates in these studies after primary surgery with no nCRT ranged from 2.8% to 3.3%. Five-year LR ranged from 2.7% to 3.3% [38].
- These initial results are promising and may allow clinicians to be more selective in treating patients with nCRT in the near future. However, omitting nCRT for these "good prognosis" tumors is not yet standard of care. Patients with a "good prognostic" tumor should be offered this non-standard treatment pathway only in high-volume centers as part of a trial until further validating studies are completed.

Table 23.4 Quicksilver MRI criteria for good and poor prognosis tumors

MRI criteria [76]	Good prognosis	Poor prognosis
Predicted CRM	>1 mm (non-threatened)	≤1 mm (threatened)
T-category[a] and EMD	Definite T2, T2/early T3, or definite T3 with EMD ≤ 5 mm	Definite T3 with EMD >5 mm or T4
N-category	Any N0, N1, or N2	Any N0, N1, or N2
Extramural venous invasion (EMVI)	Absent or equivocal	Present

EMD extramural depth of invasion
[a]Definite T1 and T1/early T2 tumors excluded from study

Neoadjuvant Versus Adjuvant Chemoradiation [39–41, 70, 71]

- Advantages of neoadjuvant therapy:
  - Significantly lower local recurrence rate, no difference in overall survival.
  - Possibility of tumor downstaging, down-sizing, and possibly increased rate of sphincter preservation.
  - Higher treatment compliance and completion rate.
  - Lower rates of acute and chronic toxicity.
  - Lower rate of anastomotic stricture.
  - Improved functional outcomes.
- Disadvantage of neoadjuvant therapy:
  - Overtreatment of some patients.

Total Neoadjuvant Therapy (TNT)

- TNT is a treatment regimen for LARC that shifts the planned adjuvant chemotherapy to the neoadjuvant setting to be given with nCRT.
- With modern TME techniques and nCRT, recent studies have suggested that adjuvant chemotherapy in rectal cancer has no significant impact on overall survival or disease-free survival [77]. Adjuvant chemotherapy also has generally poor compliance. It is with these limitations in mind that alternate treatment pathways such as TNT were developed.
- Multiple studies have demonstrated a lower toxicity profile and higher compliance rate when chemotherapy is given in a neoadjuvant setting [78, 79].
- Currently, there is no standardized TNT regimen. Neoadjuvant chemotherapy has been given before or after nCRT.
- Many studies show an improved pathologic complete response (pCR) rate with various regimens of TNT [78, 80, 81].
- A clear and consistent survival benefit of TNT has not yet been established. However, no study has shown TNT to have inferior long-term outcomes compared to standard adjuvant chemotherapy regimens [79]. Prospective phase II/III RCTs are underway to better understand long-term outcomes [82].
- A notable downside of TNT is that the additional delay in definitive surgery for non-responders could result in disease progression.
- A potential benefit is early stoma closure after resection of the primary tumor.
- TNT is a viable treatment pathway and can be considered in well-selected patients following a multidisciplinary discussion. Participation in a clinical trial for patients undergoing TNT is encouraged.

Short- Versus Long-Course Radiotherapy [42, 43]

- Short-course RT = 25 Gy in 5 fractions followed by surgery in 1 week.
- Long-course CRT = 50.4 Gy in 28 fractions +5FU followed by surgery in 8–12 weeks.

- No difference in overall survival, disease-free survival, local recurrence, or APR rates.
- Higher rate of pathologic downstaging with long-course CRT, including more complete pathologic responses.
- More acute toxicity with long-course CRT [44, 45].
- Long-course CRT is standard of care in many North American centers, whereas short-course RT is widely practiced in Europe.

Timing to Surgery After Radiation

- There remains debate regarding optimal timing of surgery after nCRT. Some studies suggest a higher downstaging and pCR rate with a longer wait interval (≥8 weeks) [83, 84].
- A recent RCT showed no difference in survival or recurrence outcomes between short-course RT without delay to surgery and regimens of short- and long-course RT with delay. Short-course RT with delay had more radiation induced toxicity, but less postoperative complications [85].
- Another RCT compared surgery at 7 weeks vs. 11 weeks after nCRT. No difference in pCR rates were found. Surgery after 11 weeks was associated with increased morbidity and worse quality of mesorectal excision [86].
- The majority of surgeons at the University of Toronto wait at least 8 weeks and up to 12 weeks (if there is evidence of ongoing clinical response) after nCRT before resection. Short-course RT with delay is used selectively in some patients who would benefit from downstaging, but have comorbidities that prevent use of long-course RT.

"Watch-and-Wait" (W/W)

- Organ preservation and observation after cCR post nCRT ("watch-and-wait") is being studied as a viable treatment pathway for well-selected patients.
- A large meta-analysis [87] reports on oncologic outcomes in W/W patients after cCR:
  - 2-year LR: 16%.
  - Salvage surgery after LR: 95%.
  - DFS is improved in patients with a confirmed pCR after resection compared to those with a cCR after nCRT.
  - No difference in OS, cancer-specific mortality, or non-regrowth recurrence.
- The majority of LR are endoluminal (86–97%) [88–90].
- Watch-and-wait after cCR is not considered standard of care. Although recent observational data shows promising results, prospective data evaluating long-term oncologic outcomes are needed to validate its safety.
- Clinicians who opt to employ watch-and-wait in a carefully selected patient (e.g., poor operative candidate with cCR) should do so after a multidisciplinary

Active Surveillance Schedule														
Month	3	6	9	12	15	18	21	24	30	36	42	48	54	60
DRE	X	X	X	X		X		X		X		X		X
Endoscopy	X	X	X	X		X		X		X		X		X
Pelvic MRI	X	X	X	X		X		X		X		X		X
CEA	X	X	X	X	X	X	X	X	X	X	X	X	X	X
CT CAP		X		X		X		X		X		X		X

Fig. 23.1 Non-validated active surveillance schedule in "watch-and-wait" patients [91]

discussion. Informed consent should be obtained from the patient acknowledging this non-standard approach. An intensive endoscopic, clinical, and radiographic surveillance protocol should be used.
- There is currently no standardized surveillance schedule available.
- Figure 23.1 shows a *non-validated, non-standardized* surveillance schedule currently being used at the University of Toronto for "watch-and wait" patients enrolled in a clinical trial [91].
- All "watch-and-wait" patients should be followed as part of a clinical trial.
- Radical resection remains the standard of care.

Laparoscopic Versus Open Resection

- Two RCTs initially suggested laparoscopic resections to be not non-inferior to open resections based on a non-validated composite measure of surgical resection quality with regard to long-term oncologic outcomes [92, 93].
- Updated long-term oncologic results from both RCTs show no differences between laparoscopic and open surgery in LR, DFS, and OS [94, 95]. This finding is concordant with multiple prior RCTs that also show equivalent oncologic outcomes between both modalities [10, 11, 75].
- There have been no RCTs showing inferior long-term oncologic outcomes of laparoscopic to open surgery.
- A recent, large meta-analysis showed that laparoscopic surgery is non-inferior to open surgery in all individual pathologic outcomes such as circumferential resection margin, completeness of mesorectal excision, and distal resection margin [96].
- Laparoscopic resections from surgeons with minimally invasive expertise are a safe modality from pathologic and long-term oncologic outcome perspectives.

Transanal Total Mesorectal Excision (TaTME)

- TaTME is a novel technique where the rectum and mesorectum are mobilized in a retrograde fashion. A major benefit is better visualization of the distal rectal tumor from an intraluminal perspective. Theoretical advantages include more precise identification and division of the distal margin, more complete dissection of the distal mesorectum, lower rates of +CRM, and increasing the rate of sphincter saving procedures.

- There are currently no standardized indications for TaTME. Recent consensus guidelines strongly suggested TaTME be reserved for low rectal tumors [97].
- Previous consensus statements suggest that TaTME may be useful in patients with a narrow pelvis, obesity (BMI > 30), distorted or inflamed tissue planes (e.g., secondary to nCRT), unclear distal margin, prostatic hypertrophy, or bulky tumor [98].
- T4 tumors and T3 tumors with <1 mm margin to endopelvic fascia are contraindicated for TaTME [99, 100].
- A major complication is damage to the prostatic urethra in males (0.8% risk) [101].
- Reported anastomotic leak rate from a large international registry is 9.8%. Risk factors are presented in Table 23.5 [101]:
- Pathological outcomes from recent studies show low +CRM (~4–8%), + distal resection margin (~0.3–3%), and high complete TME rates (88–96%) [101–103].
- Long-term oncologic data evaluating TaTME is not yet available. A prospective RCT comparing TaTME to conventional laparoscopic TME is underway [99].
- TaTME is an emerging technique with a steep learning curve that is still under investigation. Currently, it should not be performed outside of specialized, high-volume centers. Patients undergoing this procedure should be followed in prospective registries.

Lateral Lymph Node Dissection (LLND)

- There has been a dichotomy in the management of lateral lymph nodes between the East and the West. Western clinicians have primarily used nCRT whereas

Table 23.5 Risk factors in TaTME

Early anastomotic leak (<30 days from resection) risk factors	Anastomotic failure risk factors[a]
Male sex	Male sex
Obesity (BMI >30)	Obesity (BMI >30)
Smoking (borderline significance)	Smoking
Diabetes	Diabetes
Tumor size >2.5 cm	Tumor size >2.5 cm
Tumor height <4 cm from anorectal junction	Manual anastomosis (hand sewn anastomosis)[b]
Estimated blood loss >500 mL	Estimated blood loss >500 mL
	Perianal operative time >1.5 h

Risk factors derived from multivariate analysis.

[a]Anastomotic failure defined as all anastomotic morbidity including early and late leaks, pelvic abscess, fistula, chronic sinus, persistent stricture

[b]Hand-sewn anastomoses increased late structuring rates

Table 23.6 Locally advanced rectal cancer management

Workup	Perioperative treatment	Surgery
History and physical: Focus on urinary, gynecologic, neurologic symptoms, pain, lymphadenopathy Labs: CEA Imaging: CT chest/abdo/pelvis MRI pelvis PET or PET/CT—has been reported to change the management plan in 14% of cases [48]	nCRT in primary disease Evaluate for re-irradiation in previously irradiated pelvis [49] Consider intraoperative radiotherapy if available and applicable [50] Due to the high rate of distant failure, adjuvant systemic therapy is indicated	En bloc resection of all involved structures to achieve an R0 resection margin [51, 52] Early involvement of other surgical subspecialties (e.g., Urology, Orthopedics, Vascular)

many Eastern surgeons include a LLND as part of their surgical management without nCRT [104].

- A recent RCT from Japan showed that adding a LLND to a standard TME decreased local recurrence rates especially in the lateral pelvis. However, TME alone was non-inferior to TME + LLND with regard to survival outcomes [105].
- A large multicenter retrospective review shows a high lateral lymph node recurrence rate if the nodes are greater than 7 mm on pretreatment MRI and do not completely disappear with nCRT. Patients with LLN ≥7 mm who underwent nCRT and LLND had a significantly lower 5-year lateral lymph node recurrence and overall local recurrence rate [104].
- Lateral lymph nodes that grow or remain enlarged after nCRT should be removed and cannot be ignored.
- Convergence of East and West management techniques may help improve recurrence outcomes.

Locally Advanced Rectal Cancer (LARC) (See Table 23.6) **and Locally Recurrent Rectal Cancer (LRRC)** (See Table 23.7)

Distant Metastatic Disease (Stage IV) (See Table 23.8)

In patients with unresectable metastases, the median survival without systemic chemotherapy is 6–9 months. The addition of 5-fluorouracil (5-FU)-based regimens improves survival to 12 months. Adding irinotecan or oxaliplatin to 5-FU extends survival to 20 months. More recently, with the identification of molecular targets and development of biologic agents, median survival has exceeded 30 months [54].

Table 23.7 Locally recurrent rectal cancer

Patterns of recurrence [53]	
Site	Comment
Anastomotic recurrence Inferior/perineal recurrence Central recurrence (involving the rectum or urogenital structures)	Amenable to resection
Posterior recurrence	Amenable to salvage resection when sacral involvement at or below S2
Lateral recurrence	May preclude resection with negative margins due to involvement of bony pelvis, major blood vessels, and other lateral structures
Criteria for unresectability [43]	
Anatomic involvement: Above S2 or sacral ala Acetabular involvement Common or external iliac artery (relative) Sciatic nerve or sciatic notch (relative) Bilateral hydronephrosis (relative) Biologic factors: Unresectable metastatic disease Para-aortic lymph node involvement	Patient factors: Refusal Poor performance status Unacceptable surgical risk Technical factors: Inability to obtain a negative margin

Table 23.8 Metastatic rectal cancer management

Workup	Surgery (referral to appropriate surgical subspecialty)	Follow-up
History and physical Labs: CEA Imaging: CT chest/abdo/pelvis MRI liver as indicated US if ovarian metastases suspected CT head/bone scan for symptoms Consider PET/PET-CT to evaluate limited metastatic disease prior to planned resection [55]	Liver: Complete surgical resection with modern chemotherapy offers a 5-year overall survival up to 58% [56–58] Lung: Complete surgical resection with modern chemotherapy offers a 5-year overall survival up to 55% [59–61] Peritoneum: Cytoreductive surgery and HIPEC for colorectal metastases has a 5-year overall survival of 22–49% [62] Ovary: Prophylactic oophorectomy is not routinely indicated, but bilateral oophorectomy is indicated if one ovary is involved Brain: Palliative resection may be indicated for carefully selected limited metastatic disease [63] Bone: Palliative radiotherapy	Patients with potentially resectable disease undergoing chemotherapy should have imaging every 3 cycles to assess response Monitor for toxicity depending on chemotherapeutic regimen used CEA should be done only if patients do not have measurable disease on imaging Patients undergoing palliation should only have blood tests and/or imaging as dictated by clinical condition

Special Notes

- In synchronous stage IV colorectal cancer, resection of the primary tumor has traditionally been discouraged in the absence of symptoms (e.g., bleeding, obstruction, perforation). This is based on the low proportion of asymptomatic primary tumors that progress to require intervention and the need for urgent systemic therapy in this population [64]. However, recent data question this dogma by demonstrating a survival advantage with resection of the primary in synchronous stage IV disease [65]. A prospective RCT is underway to help clarify the debate [66].

Landmark Trials

See Table 23.9

Referring to Medical Oncology

1. ≥T3
2. ≥N1
3. Recurrent rectal cancer
4. Metastatic disease

Referring to Radiation Oncology

1. ≥T3
2. ≥N1
3. EMVI
4. Recurrent rectal cancer
5. Ambiguous T staging (T2/T3) and suspected close circumferential margin
6. T1/T2 tumors if:
   (a) There is residual tumor or fragmentation after local excision
   (b) There are adverse features on final pathology of local excision

Referring to Multidisciplinary Cancer Conference (MCC)

- All rectal cancer patients should be presented at a MCC [72].

Toronto Pearls

- There is strong evidence, including RCTs, that placing a loop ileostomy at LAR decreases clinical leak rates and re-operation rates [69]. This is advised for anastomoses within 3–4 cm of the pelvic floor.

Table 23.9 Landmark trials for rectal cancer

Study	Methods	Results
Heald et al. [67]	Retrospective review *N* = 113 Examination of local recurrence after TME	LR = 0% at 2 years with TME
Dutch Colorectal Cancer Group Trial Kapiteijn et al. [68]	RCT *N* = 1861 Pre-op RT and TME vs. TME only	LR: 2.4% with pre-op RT and TME vs. 8.2% TME only
Swedish Rectal Cancer Trial Gastrointestinal Tumour Study Group [23] Birgisson et al. [24]	RCT *N* = 1168 Comparing pre-op RT and surgery vs. surgery alone	LR: 5 years: 11% with pre-op RT vs. 27% with surgery alone 13 years: 9% with pre-op RT vs. 26% with surgery alone OS: 5 years: 58% with pre-op RT vs. 48% with surgery alone 13-years: 38% with pre-op RT vs. 30% with surgery alone
German Rectal Cancer Trial Sauer et al. [25]	RCT *N* = 823 Pre-op CRT vs. post-op CRT	LR: 6% pre-op CRT vs. 13% post-op CRT No difference in 5-, 10-year OS Toxicity (Grade 3/4): 27% pre-op vs. 40% post-op
NSABP R-03 Roh et al. [27]	RCT *N* = 267 Pre-op CRT vs. post-op CRT	LR: 11% in both arms
Polish Trial Bujko et al. [28]	RCT *N* = 316 Pre-op CRT vs. short-course RT	No difference in LR, DFS, sphincter preservation Higher rate of pCR with pre-op CRT (16% vs. 1%) Higher acute toxicity with pre-op CRT (18% vs. 3%)
Trans-Tasman Radiation Oncology Group (TROG) Trial Ngan et al. [29]	RCT *N* = 326 Pre-op CRT vs. short-course RT	No difference in LR, DFS, OS, sphincter preservation Higher rate of pCR with pre-op CRT (15% vs. 1%)
COLOR II [10] Bonjer et al.	RCT *N* = 1044 Laparoscopic vs. open rectal surgery	No difference in 3-year LR, DFS, OS

Table 23.9 (continued)

Study	Methods	Results
Dossa et al. [87]	Meta-analysis Watch-and-wait (W/W): cCR after nCRT $N = 867$ W/W vs. pCR after resection W/W vs. resection for cCR	T3: 67%, N+: 52% LR after W/W: 15.7% Salvage therapy after LR: 95.4% W/W vs. pCR after resection No difference in OS, cancer-specific mortality or non-regrowth recurrence, DFS better in pCR group W/W vs. resection for cCR No difference in OS, DFS, cancer-specific mortality, non-growth recurrence
GRECCAR-6 [86] Lefevre et al.	RCT $N = 265$ Surgery 7 weeks post nCRT vs. 11 weeks cT3/4 or Tx/N+, mid to low tumors	No difference in pCR rates Increased morbidity and decreased quality of TME in 11-week group
QUICKSILVER [76] Kennedy et al.	Prospective, non-randomized phase 2 12 Canadian colorectal centers $N = 82$ "good prognosis" rectal cancers Primary surgery for "good prognosis" tumors MRI "good prognosis" definition: CRM >1 mm from primary tumor, discontinuous tumor nodule, +LN T2, T2/early T3, or T3b (less than 5 mm of extramural depth of invasion) Absent/equivocal EMVI Any N	+CRM 4.9% +Distal margin 1.2% Complete/near complete TME—98% Awaiting LR results
MERCURY study Taylor et al. [37, 38]	Prospective observational study $N = 122$ Primary surgery for "good prognosis" tumors MRI "good prognosis" definition: Clear CRM >1 mm to MRF No EMVI T3b or less (less than 5 mm from muscularis propria) N any Not invading sphincters/levators	Overall LR 3.3% 5-year OS 68.2 5-year DFS 84.7% +CRM 3.3%

RCT randomized controlled trial, *TME* total mesorectal excision, *RT* radiotherapy, *LR* local recurrence, *CRM* circumferential radial margin, *OS* overall survival, *nCRT* neoadjuvant chemoradiation, *EMVI* extramural venous invasion, *DFS* disease-free survival, *DRM* distal resection margin, *W/W* watch-and-wait, *cCR* clinical complete response, *pCR* pathologic complete response

- The rate of anastomotic leak after LAR is most consistently associated with the level of the anastomosis. Achieving a tension-free anastomosis to the distal rectum or anus is facilitated by ligation of the IMA at its origin and separate ligation of the IMV at the inferior border of the pancreas
- A 5–6 cm colonic J pouch for patients undergoing LAR ameliorates the functional disturbance known as low anterior resection syndrome.
- In pelvic exenteration, early ligation of the internal iliac vessels facilitates hemostasis.
- When a vertical rectus abdominis myocutaneous (VRAM) flap is needed for reconstruction of the perineum, it is advised to take it ipsilateral to the ileoconduit, rather than the colostomy to avoid colostomy prolapse.
- If a surgeon encounters an unexpected locally advanced rectal cancer in a curable patient and is not prepared to perform appropriate multivisceral resection, the procedure should be aborted, after possible creation of a stoma, and the patient referred for multidisciplinary consultation.
- In the dissection of anterior rectal tumors, or in the event of a threatened CRM, Denonvilliers' fascia should be taken with the rectum. Otherwise, it should be left intact in order to preserve autonomic nerve function.

References

1. Canadian Cancer Society, Statistics Canada. Canadian Cancer Statistics 2017.
2. Baxter NN, Goldwasser MA, Paszat LF, et al. Association of colonoscopy and death from colorectal cancer. Ann Intern Med. 2009;150(1):1–8.
3. Noone AM, Howlader N, Krapcho M, Miller D, Brest A, Yu M, Ruhl J, Tatalovich Z, Mariotto A, Lewis DR, Chen HS, Feuer EJ, Cronin KA, editors. SEER Cancer Statistics Review, 1975–2015, National Cancer Institute. Bethesda, https://seer.cancer.gov/csr/1975_2015/, based on November 2017 SEER data submission, posted to the SEER web site, April 2018.
4. Nagtegaal ID, Quirke P. What is the role for the circumferential margin in the modern treatment of rectal cancer? J Clin Oncol. 2008;26(2):303.
5. Members of the Colorectal Cancer Survivorship Group. Follow-up care, surveillance protocol, and secondary prevention measures for survivors of colorectal cancer. Toronto: Cancer Care Ontario; 2012 Feb 3 [Being Updated 2018 Jun]. Program in Evidence-based Care Evidence-Based Series No.: 26-2 Version 2. Being updated.
6. Bipat S, Glas AS, Slors FJ, et al. Rectal cancer: local staging and assessment of lymph node involvement with endoluminal US, CT, and MR imaging–a meta-analysis. Radiology. 2004;232(3):773.
7. Al-Sukhni E, Milot L, Fruitman M, et al. Diagnostic accuracy of MRI for assessment of T category, lymph node metastases, and circumferential resection margin involvement in patients with rectal cancer: a systematic review and meta-analysis. Ann Surg Oncol. 2012;19(7):2212–23.
8. Mittal BR, Senthil R, Kashyap R, Bhattacharya A, Singh B, Kapoor R, et al. 18F-FDG PET-CT in evaluation of postoperative colorectal cancer patients with rising CEA level. Nucl Med Commun. 2011;32(9):789–93.
9. National Comprehensive Cancer Network. Rectal Cancer (Version 2.2019). https://www.nccn.org/professionals/physician_gls/PDF/rectal.pdf. Accessed 4 June 2019.
10. Bonjer HJ, Deijen CL, Abis GA, Cuesta MA, Pas MHVD, Klerk ESDL-D, et al. A randomized trial of laparoscopic versus open surgery for rectal cancer. N Engl J Med. 2015;372(14):1324–32.

11. Jeong SY, Park JW, Nam BH, et al. Open versus laparoscopic surgery for mid-rectal or low rectal cancer after neoadjuvant chemoradiotherapy (COREAN trial): survival outcomes of an open-label, non-inferiority, randomized controlled trial. Lancet Oncol. 2014;15(7):767–74.
12. Marr R, Birbeck K, Garvican J, et al. The modern abdominoperineal excision: the next challenge after total mesorectal excision. Ann Surg. 2005;242:74–82.
13. Nagtegaal D, van de Velde C, Marijnen CAM, et al. Low rectal cancer: a call for a change of approach in abdominoperineal resection. J Clin Oncol. 2005;23:9257–64.
14. Wibe A, Syse A, Andersen E, et al. Oncological outcomes after total mesorectal excision for cure for cancer of the lower rectum: anterior vs abdominoperineal resection. Dis Colon Rectum. 2004;47:48–58.
15. Han JG, Wang ZJ, Wei GH, et al. Randomized clinical trial of conventional versus cylindrical abdominoperineal resection for locally advanced lower rectal cancer. Am J Surg. 2012;204(3):274–82.
16. West NP, Finan PJ, Anderin C, et al. Evidence of the oncologic superiority of cylindrical abdominoperineal excision for low rectal cancer. J Clin Oncol. 2008;26(21):3517.
17. Persiani R, Biondi A, Gambacorta MA, et al. Prognostic implications of the lymph node count after neoadjuvant treatment for rectal cancer. Br J Surg. 2014;101(2):133–42.
18. Awwad GE, Tou SI, Rieger NA. Prognostic signifi cance of lymph node yield after long-course preoperative radiotherapy in patients with rectal cancer: a systematic review. Color Dis. 2013;15(4):394–403.
19. Miller ED, Robb BW, Cummings OW, et al. The effects of preoperative chemoradiotherapy on lymph node sampling in rectal cancer. Dis Colon Rectum. 2012;55(9):1002–7.
20. Fokas E, Liersch T, Fietkau R, et al. Tumor regression grading after preoperative chemoradiotherapy for locally advanced rectal carcinoma revisited: updated results of the CAO/ARO/AIO-94 trial. J Clin Oncol. 2014;32(15):1554.
21. Protocol for the examination of specimens from patients with primary carcinoma of the colon (Version Colon Rectum 4.0.1.0). https://documents.cap.org/protocols/cp-gilower-colonrectum-17protocol-4010.pdf. Protocol web posting date: June 2017. Accessed 4 June 2019.
22. Patel UBP, Taylor F, Blomqvist L, et al. Magnetic resonance imaging-detected tumor response for locally advanced rectal cancer predicts survival outcomes: MERCURY experience. J Clin Oncol. 2011;29(28):3753–60.
23. Heidary B, Phang TP, Raval MJ, et al. Transanal endoscopic microsurgery: a review. Can J Surg. 2014;57(2):127–38.
24. Bouvet M, Milas M, Giacco GG, et al. Predictors of recurrence after local excision and postoperative chemoradiation therapy of adenocarcinoma of the rectum. Ann Surg Oncol. 1999;6:26–32.
25. Hahnloser D, Wolff BG, Larson DW, et al. Immediate radical resection after local excision of rectal cancer: an oncologic compromise? Dis Colon Rectum. 2005;48:429–37.
26. Levic K, Bulut O, Hesselfeldt P, et al. The outcome of rectal cancer after early salvage TME following TEM compared with primary TME: a case-matched study. Tech Coloproctol. 2013;17(4):397–403.
27. Bujko K, Richter P, Kolodziejczyk M, et al. Preoperative radiotherapy and local excision of rectal cancer with immediate radical re-operation for poor responders. Radiother Oncol. 2009;92(2):195–201.
28. Habr-Gama A, Sao Juliao GP, Perez RO. Pitfalls of transanal endoscopic microsurgery for rectal cancer following neoadjuvant chemoradiation therapy. Minim Invasive Ther. 2014;23(2):63–9.
29. Guerrieri M, Baldarelli M, Rimini M, et al. Transanal endoscopic microsurgery for rectal tumors: an option to radical surgery? Minerva Chir. 2013;68(3):289–98.
30. Perez RO, Habr-Gama A, Lynn PB, et al. Transanal endoscopic microsurgery for residual rectal cancer (ypT0-2) following neoadjuvant chemoradiation therapy: another word of caution. Dis Colon Rectum. 2013;56(1):6–13.
31. Pucciarelli S, De Paoli A, Guerrieri M, et al. Local excision after preoperative chemoradiotherapy for rectal cancer: results of a multicenter phase II clinical trial. Dis Colon Rectum. 2013;56(12):1349–56.

32. Adam IJ, Mohamdee MO, Martin IG, et al. Role of circumferential margin involvement in local recurrence of rectal cancer. Lancet. 1994;344:707–11.
33. Fitzgerald TL, Brinkley J, Zervos EE. Pushing the envelope beyond a centimeter in rectal cancer: oncologic implications of close, but negative margins. J Am Coll Surg. 2011;213(5):589–95.
34. Nagtegaal ID, Gosens MJ, Marijnen CA, et al. Combinations of tumor and treatment parameters are more discriminative for prognosis than the present TNM system in rectal cancer. J Clin Oncol. 2007;25:1647–50.
35. Swedish Rectal Cancer Trial, Cedermark B, Dahlberg M, Glimelius B, Påhlman L, Rutqvist LE, Wilking N. Improved survival with preoperative radiotherapy in resectable rectal cancer. Swedish Rectal Cancer Trial. N Engl J Med. 1997;336(14):980–7.
36. Folkesson J, Birgisson H, Pahlman L, et al. Swedish rectal cancer trial: long lasting benefits from radiotherapy on survival and local recurrence rate. J Clin Oncol. 2005;23(24):5644–50.
37. Taylor FGM, Quirke P, Heald RJ, et al. Preoperative high-resolution magnetic resonance imaging can identify good prognosis stage I, II, and III rectal cancer best managed by surgery alone. Ann Surg. 2011;253(4):711–9.
38. Taylor FGM, Quirke P, Heald RJ, et al. Preoperative magnetic resonance imaging assessment of circumferential resection margin predicts disease-free survival and local recurrence: 5-year follow-up results of the MERCURY study. J Clin Oncol. 2014;32(1):34–43.
39. Sauer R, Becker H, Hohenberger W, et al. Preoperative versus postoperative chemoradiotherapy for rectal cancer. N Engl J Med. 2004;351(17):1731–40.
40. Sauer R, Liersch T, Merkel S, et al. Preoperative versus postoperative chemoradiotherapy for locally advanced rectal cancer: results of the German CAO/ARO/AIO-94 randomized phase III trial after a median follow-up of 11 years. J Clin Oncol. 2012;30(16):1926–33.
41. Roh MS, Colangelo LH, O'Connell MJ. Preoperative multimodality therapy improves disease free survival in patients with carcinoma of the rectum: NSABP R-03. J Clin Oncol. 2009;27(31):5124–30.
42. Bujko K, Nowacki MP, Nasierowska-Guttmejer A, et al. Long-term results of a randomized trial comparing preoperative short-course radiotherapy with preoperative conventionally fractionated chemoradiation for rectal cancer. Br J Surg. 2006;93:1215–23.
43. Ngan S, Fisher R, Goldstein D, et al. A randomized trial comparing local recurrence (LR) rates between short-course (SC) and long-course (LC) preoperative radiotherapy (RT) for clinical T3 rectal cancer: an intergroup trial (TROG, AGITG, CSSANZ, RACS). J Clin Oncol. 2010;28:15s.
44. Bosset JF, Collette L, Calais G, et al. Chemotherapy with preoperative radiotherapy in rectal cancer. EORTC Radiotherapy Group Trial 22921. N Engl J Med. 2006;355(11):1114.
45. McCarthy K, Pearson K, Fulton R, et al. Pre-operative chemoradiation for non-metastatic locally advanced rectal cancer. Cochrane Database Syst Rev. 2012;12:CD008368.
46. Callender GG, Das P, Rodriguez-Bigas MA, et al. Local excision after preoperative chemoradiation results in an equivalent outcome to total mesorectal excision in selected patients with T3 rectal cancer. Ann Surg Oncol. 2010;17(2):441.
47. Borschitz T, Wachtlin D, Möhler M, et al. Neoadjuvant chemoradiation and local excision for T2-3 rectal cancer. Ann Surg Oncol. 2008;15(3):712.
48. Faneyte IF, Dresen RC, Edelbrok MA, et al. Preoperative staging with positron emission tomography in patients with pelvic recurrence of rectal cancer. Dig Surg. 2008;25:202–7.
49. Das P, Delclos ME, Skibber JM, et al. Hyperfractionated accelerated radiotherapy for rectal cancer in patients with prior irradiation. Int J Radiat Oncol Biol Phys. 2010;77:60–5.
50. Hyngstrom JR, Tzeng CW, Beddar S, et al. Intraoperative radiation therapy for locally advanced primary and recurrent colorectal cancer: ten-year institutional experience. J Surg Oncol. 2014;109(7):652–8.
51. Lehnert T, Methner M, Pollok A, et al. Multivisceral resection for locally advanced primary colon and rectal cancer. An analysis of prognostic factors in 201 patients. Anal Surg. 2002;235:217–35.

52. Bhangu A, Ali SM, Darzi A, et al. Meta-analysis of survival based on resection margin status following surgery for recurrent rectal cancer. Color Dis. 2012;14(12):1457–66.
53. Rodriguez-Bigas M, Chang C, Skibber J. Multidisciplinary approach to recurrent/unresectable rectal cancer: how to prepare for the extent of resection. Surg Oncol Clin N Am. 2010;19:847–59.
54. Sridharan M, Hubbard JM, Grothey A. Colorectal cancer: how emerging molecular understanding affects treatment decisions. Oncology. 2014;28(2):110–8.
55. Culverwell AD, Chowdhury FU, Scarsbrook AF. Optimizing the role of FDG PET-CT for potentially operable metastatic colorectal cancer. Abdom Imaging. 2012;37(6):1021–31.
56. Choti MA, Sitzmann JV, Tiburi MF, et al. Trends in long-term survival following liver resection for hepatic colorectal metastases. Ann Surg. 2002;235(6):759–66.
57. Abdalla EK, Vauthey JN, Ellis LM, et al. Recurrence and outcomes following hepatic resection, radiofrequency ablation, and combined resection/ablation for colorectal liver metastases. Ann Surg. 2004;239(6):818–25.
58. Fernandez FG, Drebin JA, Linehan DC, et al. Five-year survival after resection of hepatic metastases from colorectal cancer in patients screened by positron emission tomography with F-18 fl uorodeoxyglucose (FDG-PET). Ann Surg. 2004;240(3):438–47.
59. Kanzaki R, Higashiyama M, Oda K, et al. Outcome of surgical resection for recurrent pulmonary metastasis from colorectal carcinoma. Am J Surg. 2011;202(4):419–26.
60. Blackmon SH, Stephens EH, Correa AM, et al. Predictors of recurrent pulmonary metastases and survival after pulmonary metastasectomy for colorectal cancer. Ann Thorac Surg. 2012;94(6):1802.
61. Iida T, Nomori H, Shiba M, Metastatic Lung Tumor Study Group of Japan, et al. Prognostic factors after pulmonary metastasectomy for colorectal cancer and rationale for determining surgical indications: a retrospective analysis. Ann Surg. 2013;257(6):1059.
62. Yan TD, Black D, Savady R, et al. Systematic review on the efficacy of cytoreductive surgery combined with perioperative intraperitoneal chemotherapy for peritoneal carcinomatosis from colorectal carcinoma. J Clin Oncol. 2006;24(24):4011.
63. Lemke J, Scheele J, Kapapa T, et al. Brain metastases in gastrointestinal cancers: is there a role for surgery? Int J Mol Sci. 2014;15(9):16816–30.
64. Poultsides GA, Servais EL, Saltz LB, et al. Outcome of primary tumor in patients with synchronous stage IV colorectal cancer receiving combination chemotherapy without surgery as initial treatment. J Clin Oncol. 2009;27:3379–84.
65. Tarantino I, Warschkow R, Worni M, et al. Prognostic relevance of palliative primary tumor removal in 37,793 metastatic colorectal cancer patients. Ann Surg. 2015;262(1):112–20.
66. Rahbari NN, Lordick F, Fink C, et al. Resection of the primary tumour versus no resection prior to systemic therapy in patients with colon cancer and synchronous unresectable metastases (UICC stage IV): SYNCHRONOUS – a randomized controlled multicenter trial (ISRCTN30964555). BMC Cancer. 2012;12:142.
67. Heald RJ, Husband EM, Ryall RD. The mesorectum in rectal cancer surgery: the clue to pelvic recurrence? Br J Surg. 1982;69:613–6.
68. Kapiteijn E, Marijen CA, Nagtegaal ID, et al. Preoperative radiotherapy combined with total mesorectal excision for resectable rectal cancer. N Engl J Med. 2001;345:638–46.
69. Tan WS, Tang CL, Shi L, et al. Meta-analysis of defunctioning stomas in low anterior resection for rectal cancer. Br J Surg. 2009;96(5):462–72.
70. Frykholm GJ, Glimelius B, Påhlman L. Preoperative or postoperative irradiation in adenocarcinoma of the rectum. Dis Colon Rectum. 1993;36(6):564–72.
71. Minsky BD, Cohen AM, Kemeny N, Enker WE, Kelsen DP, Reichman B, et al. Combined modality therapy of rectal cancer: decreased acute toxicity with the preoperative approach. J Clin Oncol. 1992;10(8):1218–24.
72. Kennedy E, Vella ET, MacDonald DB, Wong CS, McLeod R. Optimisation of preoperative assessment in patients diagnosed with rectal cancer. Clin Oncol. 2015;27(4):225–45.

73. Snyder RA, Hu C-Y, Cuddy A, Francescatti AB, Schumacher JR, Loon KV, et al. Association between intensity of posttreatment surveillance testing and detection of recurrence in patients with colorectal cancer. JAMA. 2018;319(20):2104.
74. Wille-Jørgensen P, Syk I, Smedh K, Laurberg S, Nielsen DT, Petersen SH, et al. Effect of more vs less frequent follow-up testing on overall and colorectal cancer–specific mortality in patients with stage II or III colorectal cancer. JAMA. 2018;319(20):2095.
75. Clinical Outcomes of Surgical Therapy Study Group, Nelson H, Sargent DJ, Wieand HS, Fleshman J, Anvari M, Stryker SJ, Beart RW Jr, Hellinger M, Richard Flanagan WP Jr, Ota D. A comparison of laparoscopically assisted and open colectomy for colon cancer. N Engl J Med. 2004;350(20):2050–9.
76. Kennedy ED, Simunovic M, Jhaveri K, Kirsch R, Brierley J, Drolet S, et al. Safety and feasibility of using magnetic resonance imaging criteria to identify patients with "good prognosis" rectal cancer eligible for primary surgery. JAMA Oncol. 2019;5(7):961–6.
77. Bosset J-F, Calais G, Mineur L, Maingon P, Stojanovic-Rundic S, Bensadoun R-J, et al. Fluorouracil-based adjuvant chemotherapy after preoperative chemoradiotherapy in rectal cancer: long-term results of the EORTC 22921 randomised study. Lancet Oncol. 2014;15(2):184–90.
78. Cercek A, Roxburgh CS, Strombom P, Smith JJ, Temple LK, Nash GM, et al. Adoption of total neoadjuvant therapy for locally advanced rectal cancer. JAMA Oncol. 2018;4(6):e180071.
79. Fernandez-Martos C, Garcia-Albeniz X, Pericay C, Maurel J, Aparicio J, Montagut C, et al. Chemoradiation, surgery and adjuvant chemotherapy versus induction chemotherapy followed by chemoradiation and surgery: long-term results of the Spanish GCR-3 phase II randomized trial. Ann Oncol. 2015;26(8):1722–8.
80. Deng Y, Chi P, Lan P, Wang L, Chen W, Cui L, et al. Modified FOLFOX6 with or without radiation in neoadjuvant treatment of locally advanced rectal cancer: final results of the Chinese FOWARC multicenter randomized trial. J Clin Oncol. 2018;36(15_suppl):3502.
81. Garcia-Aguilar J, Chow OS, Smith DD, Marcet JE, Cataldo PA, Varma MG, et al. Effect of adding mFOLFOX6 after neoadjuvant chemoradiation in locally advanced rectal cancer: a multicentre, phase 2 trial. Lancet Oncol. 2015;16(8):957–66.
82. Schrag D. Alliance for clinical trials in oncology. 2012 January. PROSPECT: Chemotherapy alone or chemotherapy plus radiation therapy in treating patients with locally advanced rectal cancer undergoing surgery. (ClinicalTrials.gov Identifier NCT0151578). Retrieved from: https://clinicaltrials.gov/ct2/show/NCT01515787#moreinfo.
83. Petrelli F, Sgroi G, Sarti E, Barni S. Increasing the interval between neoadjuvant chemoradiotherapy and surgery in rectal cancer. Ann Surg. 2016;263(3):458–64.
84. Du D, Su Z, Wang D, Liu W, Wei Z. Optimal interval to surgery after neoadjuvant chemoradiotherapy in rectal cancer: a systematic review and meta-analysis. Clin Colorectal Cancer. 2018;17(1):13–24.
85. Erlandsson J, Holm T, Pettersson D, Berglund Å, Cedermark B, Radu C, et al. Optimal fractionation of preoperative radiotherapy and timing to surgery for rectal cancer (Stockholm III): a multicentre, randomised, non-blinded, phase 3, non-inferiority trial. Lancet Oncol. 2017;18(3):336–46.
86. Lefevre JH, Mineur L, Kotti S, Rullier E, Rouanet P, Chaisemartin CD, et al. Effect of interval (7 or 11 weeks) between neoadjuvant radiochemotherapy and surgery on complete pathologic response in rectal cancer: a multicenter, randomized, controlled trial (GRECCAR-6). J Clin Oncol. 2016;34(31):3773–80.
87. Dossa F, Chesney TR, Acuna SA, Baxter NN. A watch-and-wait approach for locally advanced rectal cancer after a clinical complete response following neoadjuvant chemoradiation: a systematic review and meta-analysis. Lancet Gastroenterol Hepatol. 2017;2(7):501–13.
88. Smith JJ, Strombom P, Chow OS, Roxburgh CS, Lynn P, Eaton A, et al. Assessment of a watch-and-wait strategy for rectal cancer in patients with a complete response after neoadjuvant therapy. JAMA Oncol. 2019;5(4):e185896.

89. Renehan AG, Malcomson L, Emsley R, Gollins S, Maw A, Myint AS, et al. Watch-and-wait approach versus surgical resection after chemoradiotherapy for patients with rectal cancer (the OnCoRe project): a propensity-score matched cohort analysis. Lancet Oncol. 2016;17(2):174–83.
90. Van Der Valk MJM, Hilling DE, Bastiaannet E, Kranenbarg EM-K, Beets GL, Figueiredo NL, et al. Long-term outcomes of clinical complete responders after neoadjuvant treatment for rectal cancer in the International Watch & Wait Database (IWWD): an international multicentre registry study. Lancet. 2018;391(10139):2537–45.
91. Kennedy E. Mount Sinai Hospital, Canada. 2017 June. Non-operative management for locally advanced rectal cancer (NOM). (ClinicalTrials.gov Identifier NCT03179540). Retrieved from: https://clinicaltrials.gov/ct2/show/record/NCT03179540?view=record.
92. Stevenson ARL, Solomon MJ, Lumley JW, Hewett P, Clouston AD, Gebski VJ, et al. Effect of laparoscopic-assisted resection vs open resection on pathological outcomes in rectal cancer. JAMA. 2015;314(13):1356.
93. Fleshman J, Branda M, Sargent DJ, Boller AM, George V, Abbas M, et al. Effect of laparoscopic-assisted resection vs open resection of stage II or III rectal cancer on pathologic outcomes. JAMA. 2015;314(13):1346.
94. Stevenson ARL, Solomon MJ, Brown CSB, Lumley JW, Hewett P, Clouston AD, et al. Disease-free survival and local recurrence after laparoscopic-assisted resection or open resection for rectal cancer. Ann Surg. 2019;269(4):596–602.
95. Fleshman J, Branda ME, Sargent DJ, Boller AM, George VV, Abbas MA, et al. Disease-free survival and local recurrence for laparoscopic resection compared with open resection of stage II to III rectal cancer. Ann Surg. 2019;269(4):589–95.
96. Acuna SA, Chesney TR, Ramjist JK, Shah PS, Kennedy ED, Baxter NN. Laparoscopic versus open resection for rectal cancer. Ann Surg. 2019;269(5):849–55.
97. Adamina M, Buchs NC, Penna M, Hompes R. St.Gallen consensus on safe implementation of transanal total mesorectal excision. Surg Endosc. 2017;32(3):1091–103.
98. Motson RW, Whiteford MH, Hompes R, Albert M, Miles WFA. Current status of trans-anal total mesorectal excision (TaTME) following the second international consensus conference. Color Dis. 2016;18(1):13–8.
99. Deijen CL, Velthuis S, Tsai A, Mavroveli S, ESM De Lange-De Klerk, Sietses C, et al. COLOR III: a multicentre randomised clinical trial comparing transanal TME versus laparoscopic TME for mid and low rectal cancer. Surg Endosc. 2015;30(8):3210–3215.
100. Vignali A, Elmore U, Milone M, Rosati R. Transanal total mesorectal excision (TaTME): current status and future perspectives. Updat Surg. 2019;71(1):29–37.
101. Penna M, Hompes R, Arnold S, Wynn G, Austin R, Warusavitarne J, et al. Incidence and risk factors for anastomotic failure in 1594 patients treated by transanal total mesorectal excision. Ann Surg. 2019;269(4):700–11.
102. Simillis C, Hompes R, Penna M, Rasheed S, Tekkis PP. A systematic review of transanal total mesorectal excision: is this the future of rectal cancer surgery? Color Dis. 2016;18(1):19–36.
103. Lacy FBD, Jacqueline J, Van Laarhoven EM, Pena R, Arroyave MC, Bravo R, Cuatrecasas M, et al. Transanal total mesorectal excision: pathological results of 186 patients with mid and low rectal cancer. Surg Endosc. 2017;32(5):2442–7.
104. Ogura A, Konishi T, Cunningham C, Garcia-Aguilar J, Iversen H, Toda S, et al. Neoadjuvant (chemo)radiotherapy with total mesorectal excision only is not sufficient to prevent lateral local recurrence in enlarged nodes: results of the multicenter lateral node study of patients with low cT3/4 rectal cancer. J Clin Oncol. 2019;37(1):33–43.
105. Fujita S, Mizusawa J, Kanemitsu Y, Ito M, Kinugasa Y, Komori K, et al. Mesorectal excision with or without lateral lymph node dissection for clinical stage II/III lower rectal cancer (JCOG0212). Ann Surg. 2017;266(2):201–7.
106. Issa N, Murninkas A, Powsner E, Dreznick Z. Long-term outcome of local excision after complete pathological response to neoadjuvant chemoradiation therapy for rectal cancer. World J Surg. 2012;36(10):2481–7.

107. Debove C, Guedj N, Tribillon E, Maggiori L, Zappa M, Panis Y. Local excision of low rectal cancer treated by chemoradiotherapy: is it safe for all patients with suspicion of complete tumor response? Int J Color Dis. 2016;31(4):853–60.
108. Barina A, Paoli AD, Delrio P, Guerrieri M, Muratore A, Bianco F, et al. Rectal sparing approach after preoperative radio- and/or chemotherapy (RESARCH) in patients with rectal cancer: a multicentre observational study. Tech Coloproctol. 2017;21(8):633–40.

Retroperitoneal and Extremity Soft Tissue Sarcomas

24

Dario Callegaro, Samir Fasih, Charles Catton, Brendan C. Dickson, Peter C. Ferguson, Abha A. Gupta, and Rebecca A. Gladdy

Introduction

Soft tissue sarcomas are rare malignant neoplasms that arise from mesenchymal tissues including fat, muscle, fibrous tissue, nerves, and blood vessels [1]. Although these are mostly sporadic, there are several hereditary cancer syndromes such as Li–Fraumeni syndrome and neurofibromatosis type 1 that are associated with an increased risk of developing soft tissue sarcoma. Rarely, radiation-induced sarcomas can also arise as a late complication, often 10–15 years after treatment [2]. Approximately 1300 cases of soft tissue sarcoma are diagnosed annually in Canada, representing less than 1% of all new cancers [3]. This chapter addresses the workup

D. Callegaro
General Surgical Oncology, University of Toronto, Toronto, ON, Canada
e-mail: dario.callegaro@one-mail.on.ca

S. Fasih
Medical Oncology, University of Toronto, Toronto, ON, Canada
e-mail: samir.fasih@uhn.ca

C. Catton
Department of Radiation Oncology, University of Toronto, Toronto, ON, Canada
e-mail: charles.catton@rmp.uhn.on.ca

B. C. Dickson
Department of Laboratory Medicine and Pathobiology, University of Toronto, Toronto, ON, Canada
e-mail: brendan.dickson@sinaihealthsystem.ca

P. C. Ferguson · R. A. Gladdy (✉)
Department of Surgery, University of Toronto, Toronto, ON, Canada
e-mail: peter.ferguson@sinaihealthsystem.ca; rgladdy@mtsinai.on.ca

A. A. Gupta
Division of Medical Oncology, University of Toronto, Toronto, ON, Canada
e-mail: abha.gupta@sickkids.ca

F. C. Wright et al. (eds.), *Surgical Oncology Manual*,
https://doi.org/10.1007/978-3-030-48363-0_24

and management of retroperitoneal and extremity soft tissue sarcoma. Gastrointestinal stromal tumors, desmoids, and dermatofibrosarcoma protuberans are covered elsewhere.

Special Notes

- Sarcomas grow by direct local extension into adjacent tissues and structures. Muscle fasciae, joint capsules, tendons, epineurium, vascular adventitia, cartilage, periosteum, and mesothelial tissues are less prone to be directly invaded by soft tissue sarcoma and can be considered as relative barriers to tumor spread. Lymph node involvement is uncommon, although there are notable exceptions (e.g., clear cell sarcoma, epithelioid sarcoma; see section Extremity Sarcoma: Localized Disease) [10].
- The most important prognostic factors for distant recurrence are tumor grade, size, and histology.
- The most important prognostic factor for local recurrence (LR) is completeness of surgical resection. Other relevant prognostic factors for LR are tumor size, grade, histology, and site (higher risk of LR for retroperitoneal sarcoma) [11, 12]. In the extremity, use of radiotherapy is associated with a lower risk of local recurrence. In the retroperitoneum, tumor rupture and multifocality are associated with a higher risk of local recurrence [5].
- Main causes of sarcoma-related death are local recurrence in retroperitoneal sarcomas and distant recurrence in extremity soft tissue sarcomas, with histology-specific patterns (see Table 24.1).
- The American Joint Committee on Cancer (AJCC) 8th edition (2017) is the current recommended sarcoma staging system. In this edition, new site-specific staging systems for soft tissue sarcoma of the head and neck, trunk and extremities, abdomen and thoracic visceral organs, and retroperitoneum have been implemented. It incorporates histologic tumor grade as well as TNM status. Node-positive patients with extremity and trunk soft tissue sarcoma are considered Stage 4 [13].
- A nomogram to predict postoperative DSS of patients with STS was developed and externally validated by MSKCC and is available online at https://www.mskcc.org/nomograms/sarcoma [14]. More recently, nomograms specific for patients with retroperitoneal and extremity STS have been developed and validated in order to more accurately predict postoperative survival and the metastatic risk [15–21]. Two free apps are useful for personalized prognosis prediction in patients with extremity and retroperitoneal soft tissue sarcoma:
  - Sarculator: prediction models for primary RPS (OS, DFS: externally validated, incorporated in AJCC VIII edition), recurrent RPS (OS, DFS: not externally validated), primary extremity STS (OS, DM: externally validated) and extremity STS survivors (OS: externally validated) [22].
  - Persarc: prediction models for high-grade primary extremity STS (OS, LR: not externally validated) and high-grade extremity STS survivors (OS: not externally validated) [23].

Table 24.1 Histotypes and prognosis of primary retroperitoneal and extremity STS

Disease site	Most common soft tissue subtypes (relative incidence, %) [4–9]	Prognosis 5-year overall survival (%)	5-year local recurrence (%)	5-year distant metastasis (%)
Retroperitoneum (15% of STS)		66–75	25–37	21
	Dedifferentiated liposarcoma (37%)			
	G1-G2 G3	67 37	43 36	9 31
	Well-differentiated liposarcoma (26%)	90	23	0
	Leiomyosarcoma (19%)	60	10	50
	Solitary fibrous tumor (6%)	81	10	13
	MPNST (3%)	67	20	17
	UPS[a] (2%)	38	42	41
	Other (7%)	54	18	36
Extremity (45% of STS)		68–80	5–15	25
	UPS (21%) Myxoid liposarcoma (14%) Leiomyosarcoma (13%) Myxofibrosarcoma (12%) Synovial sarcoma (8%) MPNST (5%) Dedifferentiated and pleomorphic liposarcoma (5%)[b] Angiosarcoma (2%) Other (20%)			

STS soft tissue sarcoma, *MPNST* malignant peripheral nerve sheath tumor, *UPS* undifferentiated pleomorphic sarcoma

[a]Previously known as malignant fibrous histiocytoma (MFH). Undifferentiated/unclassified sarcomas show no line of differentiation, they are a diagnosis of exclusion and can be subdivided into spindle cell, round cell, pleomorphic, epithelioid, and not otherwise specified variants [1]

[b]Excluding atypical lipomatous tumors (well-differentiated liposarcoma of the extremities)

Management

Table 24.2 Workup and management of primary retroperitoneal sarcoma

Workup	Neoadjuvant treatment	Surgery	Follow-up [24]
History and physical exam Include nodal basins and testicular exam[a] Labs[a]: β-HCG AFP LDH Imaging: CT chest/abdo/pelvis + percutaneous core needle biopsy Differential renal scan in selected cases at high risk for postoperative kidney failure Pathology review Case discussion at MCC	Consider neoadjuvant radiation or clinical trial if available Consider neoadjuvant chemotherapy: For chemosensitive tumors, such as embryonal/alveolar RMS or Ewing's (all very rare in the retroperitoneum) For possible cytoreduction of borderline resectable high-grade tumors which may be chemosensitive, such as high-grade dedifferentiated liposarcoma and leiomyosarcoma	En bloc resection of tumor and closely associated viscera and retroperitoneal musculature/fat with a goal of complete resection	Low grade tumor—every 6 months for the first 2–3 years, then yearly: History and physical exam CT abdo/pelvis
			High-grade tumor—every 4 months for the first 2–3 years, then every 6 months for the next 2 years, then yearly: History and physical exam CT chest/abdo/pelvis

MCC multidisciplinary cancer conference, *RMS* rhabdomyosarcoma
[a]To rule out primary or metastatic germ cell tumor and lymphoma

<table>
<tr><th colspan="2">Radiotherapy</th></tr>
<tr><td colspan="2">In prospective phase II trials and retrospective studies, perioperative radiation therapy has been associated with a lower local recurrence rate and improved survival in patients with primary RPS. However, results are conflicting, patient's selection criteria are not defined, and no level I data exist [5, 25–29].
An EORTC randomized phase III trial of preoperative radiotherapy and surgery vs. surgery alone in primary retroperitoneal sarcoma patients (EORTC 62092–22,092, STRASS trial) showed no difference in abdominal recurrence-free survival (ARFS) between the two groups. In a sensitivity analysis, 3-year ARFS was higher in patients with liposarcoma treated with preoperative radiotherapy (71.6% vs. 60.4%). Full publication is pending.
When radiotherapy is offered, preoperative radiotherapy is the preferred approach at the University of Toronto and other major sarcoma centers.</td></tr>
<tr><td>Advantages of pre-op RT
In situ tumor allows accurate targeting of radiation volume and precise delivery
Tumor displaces the radiosensitive viscera (i.e., small bowel) outside the treatment field, thereby limiting toxicity and allowing delivery of a higher dose
Radiation is theoretically more biologically effective preoperatively
May extend the surgical margin to reduce the risk of local recurrence</td><td>Disadvantages of pre-op RT
Delay of definitive surgery
Possible increased risk of wound healing complications (the evidence is from extremity STS studies)
Possible increased risk of complications if vascular resection and reconstruction are required</td></tr>
<tr><td colspan="2">Relative contraindications to RT
Li–Fraumeni syndrome
History of prior radiation
Tumor crossing midline
Solitary kidney
Patient preference</td></tr>
</table>

Retroperitoneal Sarcoma Localized Disease

Surgery is the only potentially curative option for patient with primary retroperitoneal sarcoma. Chemotherapy and/or radiotherapy should be considered on a case-by-case basis and in a multidisciplinary setting (see Table 24.2).

Special Notes

- Image-guided percutaneous coaxial core needle biopsy is recommended for preoperative diagnosis. Some RPS may be heterogeneous in morphology; thus, it is essential to ensure adequate sampling in the area that harbor the most viable and highest-grade component(s). A minimum of four large gauge cores (14–16 gauge) are generally advised; these should be divided into multiple cassettes in the pathology laboratory to limit the risk of tissue depletion. In most cases this will provide sufficient tissue for histomorphologic assessment, and ancillary immunohistochemical and molecular analysis (e.g., FISH, RT-PCR, CGH, and/or RNA-Seq). All of these studies can be performed using formalin-fixed paraffin-embedded tissues; thus, it is not necessary to divert fresh tissue for freezing, or cell culture media. The risk for needle tract seeding using a coaxial technique is minimal and local recurrence rates are not different between patients who underwent preoperative biopsy or not [30, 31]. Cytologic assessment of soft tissue tumors by fine needle aspiration is not advised [32]. Open or laparoscopic biopsies should be avoided. In case of a non-diagnostic needle core biopsy, the biopsy should be repeated with the same technique but targeting a different area.
- Criteria for local unresectability of RPS are not clearly defined. Involvement of bony structures (vertebrae, iliac wing) or major vessels (aorta, IVC, iliac vessels) are not absolute contraindications for surgery with curative intent. Extensive unreconstructible involvement of the celiac, SMA, SMV, porta hepatis, and central mediastinal structures are generally seen as criteria of unresectability. Decision-making in locally advanced retroperitoneal sarcoma patients is complex and should take into consideration patient-, tumor-, and treatment-related variables in a multidisciplinary fashion and may involve surgical expertise beyond a sarcoma expert (vascular surgery, HPB/transplant) [33].
- The most common organs removed *en bloc* with a retroperitoneal sarcoma are kidney, adrenal, colon, psoas, spleen, diaphragm, abdominal wall muscles, and distal pancreas [5].
- The same principles that guide surgical excision of extra-abdominal STS should apply to the retroperitoneum, taking into consideration the anatomical constraints of this anatomic region. The concept of compartment is not applicable to the retroperitoneal space. Indeed, there are no true boundaries with the pelvis, the mediastinum, the anterior preperitoneal space, and the contralateral retroperitoneum, and there are vital organs lying within the retroperitoneum itself. Nonetheless, tissues that work as natural barriers to tumor spread such as the muscle fasciae posteriorly, the adventitia of major abdominal vessels medially, and the peritoneum anteriorly are also recognizable. Dissection should be carried

out beyond these structures. In consideration of the large dimensions of RPS (especially retroperitoneal liposarcoma) and of the absence of standardized, shared, protocols for tissue sampling, resection of RPS is usually classified as "macroscopically complete" and "macroscopically incomplete." This means that the distinction of R0 vs. R1 resections is not as meaningful as with other cancers. Surgical margins should also be tailored to the histologic subtype. For example, all retroperitoneal fat from the diaphragm to the external iliac vessels should be resected *en bloc* with the tumor in retroperitoneal liposarcoma; a clear margin on the vein or the nerve of origin should be taken in retroperitoneal leiomyosarcoma and MPNST, respectively [32, 34, 35].

- Radical resection of RPS is associated with a 16% morbidity (Clavien–Dindo≥3) and a 2% mortality at 30 days [36]. Long-term sequelae of this surgery are mainly related to sensory disorders of the thigh, groin, or genital area. Lower limbs motor impairment or severe chronic pain are rare [37].
- Medical therapy:
  - No trials of neoadjuvant/adjuvant chemotherapy in patients with retroperitoneal sarcoma have been run so far. As a result, there is much between centers variability in chemotherapy administration. A randomized phase III trial of preoperative anthracycline-based chemotherapy vs. surgery alone in patients with primary high-grade dedifferentiated liposarcoma and high-grade leiomyosarcoma of the retroperitoneum (STRASS2 trial) is being designed by EORTC and should start recruiting in 2020. This randomized trial will be run in the context of the RESAR study (Retroperitoneal Sarcoma Registry, NCT03838718), a prospective observational registry coordinated by the Transatlantic Australasian Retroperitoneal Sarcoma Working Group (TARPSWG, tarpswg.org). Please see the section "Extremity STS" for considerations about the role of chemotherapy in primary STS.
  - Patients with desmoplastic small round cell tumor should always be referred to medical oncologists for perioperative chemotherapy.

Table 24.3 Workup and management of recurrent retroperitoneal sarcoma

Workup	Neoadjuvant treatment	Surgery	Follow-up
History and physical exam Labs: No specific tests Imaging: CT chest/abdo/pelvis ± core biopsy Pathology review Case discussion at MCC	Consider multimodality treatment in recurrent patients	Resect if technically feasible with acceptable morbidity, in the absence of widespread metastases or multifocal/contralateral disease, with favorable tumor biology (consider histology, grade, disease-free interval, growth rate) and favorable patient-related characteristics [33] No role for incomplete resection, except for palliation of symptoms in select circumstances	Low-grade tumor—every 6 months for the first 2–3 years, then yearly: History and physical exam CT abdo/pelvis High-grade tumor—every 4 months for the first 2–3 years, then every 6 months for the next 2 years, then yearly: History and physical exam CT chest/abdo/pelvis

Retroperitoneal Sarcoma: Locally Recurrent Disease

Overall, abdominal recurrence is common in retroperitoneal sarcoma, with different patterns across different histologies. Local recurrence is associated with a worse prognosis than primary RPS, and its treatment is all the more multidisciplinary (see Table 24.3).

Special Notes

- A period of observation to assess tumor behavior and guide therapeutic decisions can be considered [33, 38].
- Median time from surgery of the primary tumor to LR is 23 months. This interval can be much longer in well-differentiated liposarcoma, whose risk of LR is lower than G2 and G3 liposarcoma but does not tend to decrease with time.
- Surgery of recurrent RPS after wide excision of the primary tumor aims to completely excise the recurrent tumor and the directly invaded organs without seeking wide margins [39].
- The role of completion surgery in patients with residual RPS after grossly incomplete resection of the primary tumor is not clear, with some series showing outcome similar to patients who underwent primary adequate surgery and other showing a particularly poor outcome with high complication rate [38, 40].
- After LR, median OS is 33 months, and 5-year OS is 29%, but post-resection outcome is variable, and prolonged survival after resection of recurrent RPS can be achieved in selected patients. Longer disease-free interval from surgery of the primary to LR and surgical resection of recurrent disease are associated with better post-relapse OS. Multifocality (both in primary and recurrent tumors) and organ invasion at primary surgery are associated with worst post-relapse survival. High grade and fast growth rate ($\geq$1 cm/month) of the recurrent tumor are associated with worst post-recurrence disease-specific survival. A nomogram is available to predict OS and DFS after resection of the local recurrence [19, 39, 41–43].
- Re-irradiation is often contraindicated, but this must be discussed in a tumor board with expert radiation oncologists specialized in sarcoma. The decision to whether re-irradiate a patient with local-regional relapse should take into consideration the previous treatment plan (concern for safety), the goals of re-irradiation (symptom relief vs. part of combined salvage therapy), and the specific clinical scenario (patient status and comorbidities, surgical plan, anatomic concern, availability of alternative treatments).
- Second and third recurrences become more challenging to resect, and with each recurrence survival diminishes while morbidity increases.

Table 24.4 Workup and management of metastatic retroperitoneal sarcoma

Workup	Management
History and physical exam Labs: Nutritional status workup Liver workup if consideration for liver metastasectomy Imaging: CT chest/abdo/pelvis ± core biopsy PET scan and/or bone scan in selected cases Pulmonary function tests if consideration for lung local therapies Case discussion at MCC	Criteria for resectability: Patient can medically tolerate the intervention and its physiologic consequences The primary tumor is fully resected or resectable Complete resection of the metastatic disease seems feasible Tumor has favorable biology (slow growing, isolated/low-volume disease, long disease-free interval, response, or prolonged stable disease to medical therapies) For lung: no extra-thoracic disease (not an absolute contraindication), pleural effusion or mediastinal/hilar adenopathy Predictors of good outcome: Complete R0 resection Less than 50-year-old Interval between primary disease and metastasis greater than 12–18 months Isolated/few metastases Lung: tumor less than 2 cm Liver: histology of LMS Procedure: Non-anatomic lung/liver resection with negative margins

MCC multidisciplinary case conference, *R0* negative microscopic margins, *LMS* leiomyosarcoma

Retroperitoneal Sarcoma: Metastatic Disease

The metastatic propensity of retroperitoneal sarcoma is highly histology-dependent (see Table 24.1). Metastatic RPS includes both systemic disease and multifocal intra-abdominal disease ("sarcomatosis") [44]. Principles of recommended practice are summarized in Table 24.4.

Special Notes

- Surgery in patients with diffuse distant metastases or multiple peritoneal implants is not offered since it does not add any survival benefit [45].
- In metastatic RPS, median OS is 16 months. Overall, in patients with metastatic or locally advanced unresectable STS, 5-year survival is 8% [45, 46].
- Lung or liver lesions with typical CT/MRI appearance in the context of a primary histology-proven RPS, or intra-abdominal/retroperitoneal masses in keeping with multifocal recurrence might not need a confirmatory biopsy [44].
- Locoregional treatment of distant metastasis has been associated with longer survival in multiple retrospective series, but there is no level I evidence showing

a causative relationship [44, 47]. Select patients with suitable performance status suffering from metachronous oligometastatic disease to the lung, liver, or soft tissues with favorable disease biology, in whom complete resection can be carried out with acceptable morbidity, should be considered for metastasectomy. Other local therapies (RFA, microwave ablation, stereotactic body radiotherapy) can be considered as alternative or complementary treatments to surgery. Transarterial embolization or chemoembolization may be considered although the available evidence is limited [47–50].

- In patients with intra-abdominal metastasis (peritoneal sarcomatosis, multifocal recurrent disease), surgery should be limited to symptoms palliation. Incomplete resection is not associated with a survival benefit and can lead to significant morbidity. Hypertermic intraperitoneal chemotherapy is not effective in histological subtypes typically seen in the retroperitoneum [44, 51, 52].
- Prognostic factors associated with longer post-metastasectomy survival include longer disease-free interval between surgery of the primary tumor and DM and complete resection of the metastatic disease [44].
- Palliative chemotherapy can slow disease progression, and possibly reduce tumor size to relieve symptoms, but data showing significant improved survival are lacking. An anthracycline-based regimen is considered first line, with further lines to be determined in a histology-driven fashion. Combination therapy (usually doxorubicin+ifosfamide) can be considered if the aim of the medical treatment is tumor shrinkage in a medically fit patient.

Extremity Soft Tissue Sarcoma: Localized Disease

The only potentially curative option of primary extremity STS is surgery. Perioperative chemotherapy and radiotherapy may also play a role and should be discussed in a multidisciplinary setting (see Table 24.5).

Special Notes

- If surgical biopsy is performed, care must be taken not to compromise definitive excision—longitudinal incision in the long axis of the limb, meticulous hemostasis, and avoid mobilizing skin flaps and violating fascial planes.
- Resect outside the tumor pseudocapsule, excising a margin of normal tissue around the tumor. A 1–2 cm margin of uninvolved tissue is ideal, but often not feasible. A closer margin is acceptable if it includes tissues that are more resistant to tumor spread (muscular fascia, vessel adventitia, periosteum, epineurium, paratenon).
- Preoperative and postoperative radiation have similar local control rates. Preoperative radiation is associated with higher rates of acute wound healing

Table 24.5 Workup and management of primary extremity STS

Workup	Adjunctive treatment	Surgery	Follow-up
History and physical exam Labs: No specific tests Imaging: MRI + core biopsy or surgical biopsy CT chest for staging CT abdomen/pelvis or PET scan or whole-body MRI in myxoid liposarcoma US or CT of regional nodes in epithelioid sarcoma, rhabdomyosarcoma, clear cell sarcoma, angiosarcoma Pathology review Case discussion at MCC	Neoadjuvant or adjuvant radiation if high risk of local recurrence or particularly sensitive histotypes (myxoid liposarcoma) Chemotherapy in patients with specific histologic subtypes (alveolar/embryonal RMS, Ewing's sarcoma) is considered mandatory for cytoreduction of primary and also to reduce risk of distant metastases. In other subtypes (synovial sarcoma, angiosarcoma, high-grade myxoid liposarcoma, leiomyosarcoma), chemotherapy may facilitate limb salvage in borderline resectable lesions Isolated limb perfusion with melphalan and TNF may be of help in unresectable tumors	Goal: complete (R0) resection with preservation of maximal function Limb salvage is possible most of the time In superficial or locally advanced STS may require plastic surgery for reconstruction	For low recurrence risk (i.e., stage 1 STS): every 6 months for 2 years, then, then annually for 3 years: History and physical exam Chest X-ray For high recurrence risk: (i.e., stage 2 and 3) every 3 months for 2 years then every 6 months for 3 years than annually for 5 years History and physical exam Chest X-ray MRI primary site every 4–6 months for 2 years, then yearly up to 5 years[a]

[a]Positive margins or difficult area to examine (e.g., pelvis)

complications, whereas postoperative radiation entails higher rates of late, irreversible toxicities [53].

- Radiotherapy can be omitted in small (<5 cm), superficial, low-grade tumors resected with margins >1 cm [54].
- Indication for primary amputation should take into consideration involvement of structures which are essential for the limb (bone, vessels, and nerves), likelihood of obtaining significant tumor shrinkage with neoadjuvant therapies (radiotherapy, chemotherapy, ILP), expected functional outcome with limb salvage, and patient preference. Primary amputation occurs in approximately 1% of cases [55].
- Resection of the primary tumor in the setting of widespread metastatic disease requires multidisciplinary discussion; it may be considered for control of symptoms in patients with anticipated prolonged survival.

- Isolated limb perfusion is used preoperatively in STS that would not be upfront resectable (e.g., multicompartmental, multifocal) to obtain tumor shrinkage and allow a limb-preserving surgery. Response rate is in the 60–90% range in various series. It can be used in different sarcoma subtypes [56].
- Medical therapy in localized STS:
  - Doxorubicin-based chemotherapy is the most commonly used first line.
  - Certain subtypes, including angiosarcoma, synovial sarcoma, and myxoid/round cell liposarcoma, are considered more sensitive than other histologies.
  - Soft tissue Ewing's sarcoma and alveolar/embryonal rhabdomyosarcoma are highly chemosensitive tumors. All patients with these tumors should receive multi-agent chemotherapy by following a published protocol as well as careful local control with surgery and/or radiation [24, 57].
  - An individual-patient data meta-analysis of 1568 patients in 14 trials of doxorubicin-based adjuvant chemotherapy showed better local relapse-free survival (HR 0.71), distant relapse-free interval (HR 0.70), and overall relapse-free survival (0.75) with adjuvant chemotherapy, with an absolute 10-year benefit of 6%, 10%, and 10%, respectively. For OS, the HR of 0.89 was not significant but represent an absolute benefit of 4% at 10 years [58].
  - Another meta-analysis of RCTs of adjuvant chemotherapy in localized resectable STS was published in 2008. This meta-analysis incorporated four new RCTs for a total of 18 trials and 1953 patients. In this study, adjuvant chemotherapy was associated with a lower local (OR 0.73) and distant (HR 0.67) relapse rate. There was a significant OS benefit (HR 0.56) only for the combination doxorubicin-ifosfamide [59].
  - The larger RCT of adjuvant chemotherapy vs. surgery alone in resectable STS did not show a survival benefit for CTx. However, a recent unplanned subgroup analysis on patients with extremity and trunk wall STS who had a predicted 5-year survival calculated with the Sarculator nomogram lower than 60% showed that chemotherapy administration was associated with a significant higher OS (HR 0.50) and DFS (HR 0.49) [60, 61].
  - In 2017 a phase III trial comparing the administration of a short full-dose conventional anthracycline and ifosfamide chemotherapy to histology tailored chemotherapy in patients with resectable high risk (G3, ≥5 cm) STS of the extremity and trunk was closed early due to a significant benefit in favor of the use of conventional chemotherapy. However, the difference in disease-free survival in favor of anthracycline+ifosfamide chemotherapy was not confirmed in the final analysis [62, 63].
  - Currently, neoadjuvant/adjuvant chemotherapy is not standard of care in resectable STS and at the University of Toronto neoadjuvant chemotherapy is offered only for borderline resectable extremity or retroperitoneal STS.
  - The optimal duration of neoadjuvant chemotherapy is not well established. A randomized phase III trial compared three courses of preoperative epirubicin-ifosfamide vs. a total of five courses (three preoperative and two postoperative) of the same regimen in high-risk STS. This study showed no survival difference between the two arms [64]. At University of Toronto, the standard is to assess

Table 24.6 Workup and management of recurrent extremity STS

Workup	Adjunctive treatment	Surgery	Follow-up
History and physical exam Labs: No specific tests Imaging: MRI ± core biopsy/open biopsy CT chest Path review Case discussion at MCC	Neoadjuvant radiation (or chemoradiation) if not previously irradiated Consider high precision techniques (e.g., IMRT) if previously irradiated Consider isolated limb perfusion if expertise in sarcoma center	Limb-sparing re-resection Amputation if limb salvage not feasible (10–25%)	Every 3 months for 2 years, then every 6 months for 3 years, then annually for 5 years: History and physical exam Chest X-ray or CT chest For high recurrence risk[a], MRI primary site every 4–6 months for 2 years, then yearly up to 5 years

[a]Positive margins or difficult area to examine (e.g., pelvis)

tumor response after 2 cycles and, in case of SD or PR (by RECIST) and/or clinical improvement, complete total of 5 cycles in the neoadjuvant setting.

Historically, the treatment of extremity sarcoma was amputation. Limb salvage techniques ± radiation have proven equally effective. In a landmark trial comparing amputation vs. resection with adjuvant radiation, there was no difference in disease-free or overall survival [65]. Function is paramount when considering limb salvage. Major arteries and veins are preserved whenever possible, and preoperative radiation may improve the quality of surgical margins to allow preservation of structures. However, if needed, arteries can be resected and reconstructed, tendon or nerve transfers can restore function if major nerves must be sacrificed, veins can be reconstructed or simply ligated in order to achieve complete resection, and bone can be partially resected or replaced with bone graft or endoprostheses.

Extremity Soft Tissue Sarcoma: Locally Recurrent Disease

Local recurrence in extremity STS is rarely a threat for patient life, unless it occurs in close proximity to the abdomen or the chest. Nevertheless, it can be associated with severe functional sequelae. Workup and management of recurrent extremity STS are summarized in Table 24.6.

Special Notes

- Five to 10% of patients will recur even after complete resection and radiation therapy, usually within the first 2 years [66, 67].
- In Europe, isolated limb perfusion/infusion with TNF and melphalan has been studied with promising preliminary results [68].

Table 24.7 Workup and management of metastatic extremity STS

Workup	Management
History and physical exam Labs: No specific tests Imaging: CT chest +/− abdo/ pelvis to r/o other sites of disease Case discussion at MCC	Criteria for resectability: Patient can medically tolerate the intervention and its physiologic consequences The primary tumor is fully resected or resectable[a] Complete resection seems feasible Tumor has favorable biology (slow growing, isolated/ low-volume disease, long disease-free interval) No extra-thoracic disease (relative contraindication), pleural effusion, or mediastinal/hilar adenopathy Predictors of good outcome: Complete R0 resection Less than 50-year-old Interval between primary disease and metastasis greater than 12–18 months Isolated/few metastases Tumor less than 2 cm Low-intermediate grade Three or fewer metastases/unilateral disease Procedure: Pulmonary wedge resection (open/VATS) Consider chemotherapy for unresectable lesions, in the neoadjuvant setting to facilitate surgical resection in sensitive histologies, or in patients who present with metastatic disease

[a]Patients presenting with synchronous lung metastasis have a poor outcome and are less likely to be treated with lung metastasectomy

- Recurrence rate is higher in myxofibrosarcoma, which shows an infiltrative growth pattern.

Extremity Sarcoma: Lung Metastases

Distant metastases to the lungs are the main cause of sarcoma-related death in patients with extremity STS. The management of patients with lung metastasis is summarized in Table 24.7.

Special Notes

- Five-year overall survival up to 40% has been reported after pulmonary metastasectomy [69–72].
- Patients presenting with synchronous lung metastasis have a poor outcome (5-year OS 8%) despite aggressive surgical management of their primary tumor [73].
- Approximately 1–2% of extremity STS patients have lymph node metastasis at presentation. Histological subtypes that are more prone to giving lymph node metastasis are clear cell sarcoma (11–16%), epithelioid sarcoma (13–20%), angiosarcoma (6–11%), and rhabdomyosarcoma (19%). Routine regional lymphadenectomy is not recommended. Sentinel node biopsy is performed in

very high-risk histologies such as clear cell sarcoma and alveolar RMS if imaging of lymph nodes is unremarkable. In case of enlarged regional lymph nodes at clinical examination or on imaging, confirmatory biopsy is recommended. In the absence of concomitant distant metastasis, resection of the primary and concomitant regional lymphadenectomy should be considered [74–78].

- Medical therapy in advanced STS:
  - In the palliative setting, single-agent doxorubicin is the most commonly used agent in first line. In a phase III trial, the combination of doxorubicin+ifosfamide showed a higher overall response rate compared to doxorubicin alone (26 vs. 14%) with no difference in OS and greater toxicity with the combination. As such, combination of doxorubicin + ifosfamide in the metastatic setting is reserved for situations where the specific goal of treatment is tumor shrinkage [79].
  - In 2016, a phase II trial of doxorubicin alone vs. doxorubicin in combination with olaratumab (a PDGFR-α blocking anti-body) in patients with unresectable/metastatic STS, showed a survival advantage for the combination therapy [80]. Unfortunately, the results were not confirmed in a recently completed phase III trial (NCT02451943, ANNOUNCE trial) testing the same question, and olaratumab is no longer approved for use in metastatic STS [81, 82].
  - After failure of first-line therapy, further lines are administered in a histology-driven fashion considering the particular sensitivity of some histologies to available drugs. Examples of agents that showed to be particularly active in selective histologies include high-dose ifosfamide in synovial sarcoma, trabectedin in liposarcoma and leiomyosarcoma, eribulin in liposarcoma, pazopanib in non-liposarcoma STS, gemcitabine alone or in combination with DTIC for all STS but specially LMS and UPS, tyrosine kinase inhibitors (sunitinib, pazopanib, sorafenib) in SFT, mTOR inhibitors in PEComa, and paclitaxel in angiosarcoma.
  - The opportunity to participate in available clinical trials should be offered to all patients with metastatic disease.
  - The use of checkpoint inhibitors still remains limited in STS [83]. A phase II trial of nivolumab alone vs. nivolumab + ipilimumab (Alliance A091401) in patients with advanced STS showed an overall response rate (ORR) of 5% in the monotherapy arm and 16% in the combination arm. Responses in the combination arm occurred in UPS, LMS, myxofibrosarcoma, and angiosarcoma [84]. A phase II trial (SARC028) of pembrolizumab in advanced sarcoma showed an ORR of 18% and a 12-week PFS of 55%. Responses were observed in patients with UPS (40%), LPS (20%), and synovial sarcomas (10%) [85]. The more promising exploration of adoptive T-cell therapy for patients with NY-ESO-1-positive sarcoma continues [86, 87].

Landmark Publications

In this section are listed significant studies and RCTs regarding retroperitoneal (Table 24.8) and extremity (Table 24.9) soft tissue sarcomas.

Table 24.8 Landmark publications: retroperitoneal sarcoma

Study	Methods	Results
Smith et al. [25]	Prospective *N* = 40 Neoadjuvant EBRT (45–50 Gy), + adjuvant BRT (20–25 Gy) in some patients Median follow-up 106 months	With pre-op EBRT: favorable long-term RFS and OS compared to historical controls. Post-op BRT was not associated with better disease control, resulted in unacceptable toxicity
Gronchi A et al. [5]	Retrospective *N* = 1007 Primary resected RPS	Description of pattern of recurrence by histological subtype
EORTC-62092-22,092 STRASS trial [88]	Phase III randomized trial Neoadjuvant radiotherapy+surgery (RT/S) vs. surgery alone (S) in primary localized retroperitoneal sarcoma Primary endpoint: Abdominal recurrence-free survival (ARFS) *N* = 266	No difference in ARFS In a sensitivity analysis 3-year ARFS in patients with liposarcoma was 71.6% in RT/S group vs. 60.4% in S group (HR = 0.64, $p = 0.049$) Full publication pending

RCT randomized controlled trial, *OS* overall survival, *EBRT* external beam radiation therapy, *BRT* brachytherapy, *RFS* relapse-free survival

Table 24.9 Landmark publications: extremity soft tissue sarcoma

Study	Design	Results
Rosenberg et al. [65]	RCT *N* = 43 Amputation vs. limb-sparing surgery + adjuvant EBRT (50 Gy whole limb + 60–70 Gy boost to tumor bed) Both groups received adjuvant chemo (doxorubicin, cyclophosphamide, high dose methotrexate)	Higher local recurrence rate with limb salvage, but no difference in DFS or OS
Pisters et al. [89]	RCT *N* = 164 Surgery ± adjuvant intraoperative BRT (42–45 Gy) delivered over 4–6 days	With BRT: improved local control for high-grade sarcoma only No difference in survival
Yang et al. [90]	RCT *N* = 141 Limb-sparing surgery ± adjuvant EBRT (45 Gy wide field and 18 Gy boost tumor bed)	With EBRT: decreased local recurrence No difference in OS
O'Sullivan et al. [53]	RCT *N* = 190 Neoadjuvant EBRT (50 Gy) vs. adjuvant EBRT (66 Gy)	No difference in local control, DFS, or OS More grade 2–4 late toxicity with adjuvant EBRT

RCT randomized control trial, *EBRT* external beam radiation therapy, *OS* overall survival, *DFS* disease-free survival, *BRT* brachytherapy

Retroperitoneal Sarcoma

Extremity Soft Tissue Sarcoma

Referring to Medical Oncology

1. For RPS with borderline resectability to use neoadjuvant chemotherapy for the purpose of cytoreduction and facilitating surgical resection.
2. All patients with Ewing's sarcoma, embryonal/alveolar rhabdomyosarcoma.
3. Unresectable and metastatic disease for palliation or for cytoreduction before locoregional therapies.
4. Referral for phase I/II clinical trials for novel agents or drug combinations for (a) metastatic disease or (b) front-line therapy in certain situations of otherwise incurable disease.

Referring to Radiation Oncology

1. All large (>5 cm), deep, G2-G3 extremity sarcomas in a neoadjuvant setting.
2. Extremity STS where surgical margins are expected to be close, in order to preserve critical structures such as major nerves, vessels, or bone.
3. Extremity STS with unexpectedly close margins, for consideration of adjuvant radiation.
4. All primary retroperitoneal STS should be discussed at MCC together with radiation oncologists.
5. Locally recurrent retroperitoneal and extremity STS.
6. Palliation of symptomatic metastatic or locally recurrent unresectable retroperitoneal or extremity sarcoma.

Referring to Multidisciplinary Cancer Conference (MCC)

All sarcoma cases should be discussed with a panel that routinely manages this disease.

Toronto Pearls

- In the event of an unexpected finding of a retroperitoneal mass during emergency surgery or during surgery performed for other reasons, do not attempt to resect or biopsy the retroperitoneal lesion but treat the emergency and close. Investigate the lesion postoperatively with a contrast-enhanced CT scan and refer the patient to a tertiary care center specialized in sarcoma.
- Sample review by a pathologist with subspecialty expertise in sarcoma—and access to the requisite immunohistochemical and molecular diagnostic capabilities—is essential to accurately diagnose and characterize sarcoma.

- For high-risk extremity STS, consider neoadjuvant radiotherapy, as this may result in tumor necrosis and possibly cytoreduction, as well as increase the likelihood of complete R0 resection. Radiation therapy is more accurately delivered to an in situ tumor, with less toxicity.
- For extremity/trunk wall STS consider adjuvant radiotherapy if a complex reconstruction with mesh or alloprosthesis is foreseen, to minimize the risk of postoperative surgical-site infection that might lead to serious complications.
- Myxoid liposarcoma of the retroperitoneum is rare and the presence of a primary myxoid liposarcoma in the extremities (with the retroperitoneal sarcoma being a metastasis) should always be ruled out.
- Pattern of metastasis of myxoid liposarcoma is unpredictable, and whole-body MRI or total-body PET scan should be considered for staging in this histology.
- Patients with Li–Fraumeni syndrome require expert care including involvement of medical genetics team to guide the risk/benefits of cancer treatment including radiation and/or chemotherapy and the need for ongoing comprehensive cancer surveillance that may include whole-body MRI and/or CTs as indicated.

References

1. Fletcher CDM, Bridge JA, Hogendoorn PCW, Mertens F. WHO classification of tumours of soft tissue and bone. Lyon: International Agency for Research on Cancer; 2013.
2. Gladdy RA, Qin LX, Moraco N, Edgar MA, Antonescu CR, Alektiar KM, et al. Do radiation-associated soft tissue sarcomas have the same prognosis as sporadic soft tissue sarcomas? J Clin Oncol. 2010;28(12):2064–9.
3. Canadian Cancer Society. Available at: http://www.cancer.ca/en/cancer-information/cancer-type/soft-tissue-sarcoma/statistics/?region=on.
4. Linehan DC, Lewis JJ, Leung D, Brennan MF. Influence of biologic factors and anatomic site in completely resected liposarcoma. J Clin Oncol. 2000;18(8):1637–43.
5. Gronchi A, Strauss DC, Miceli R, Bonvalot S, Swallow CJ, Hohenberger P, et al. Variability in patterns of recurrence after resection of primary retroperitoneal sarcoma (RPS): a report on 1007 patients from the multi-institutional collaborative RPS working group. Ann Surg. 2015;31
6. Callegaro D, Miceli R, Bonvalot S, Ferguson P, Strauss DC, Levy A, et al. Impact of perioperative chemotherapy and radiotherapy in patients with primary extremity soft tissue sarcoma: retrospective analysis across major histological subtypes and major reference centres. Eur J Cancer. 2018;105:19–27.
7. Heslin MJ, Lewis JJ, Nadler E, Newman E, Woodruff JM, Casper ES, et al. Prognostic factors associated with long-term survival for retroperitoneal sarcoma: implications for management. J Clin Oncol. 1997;15(8):2832–9.
8. Lewis JJ, Leung D, Woodruff JM, Brennan MF. Retroperitoneal soft-tissue sarcoma: analysis of 500 patients treated and followed at a single institution. Ann Surg. 1998;228(3):355–65.
9. Catton CN, O'Sullivan B, Kotwall C, Cummings B, Hao Y, Fornasier V. Outcome and prognosis in retroperitoneal soft tissue sarcoma. Int J Radiat Oncol Biol Phys. 1994;29(5):1005–10.
10. Fong Y, Coit DG, Woodruff JM, Brennan MF. Lymph node metastasis from soft tissue sarcoma in adults. Analysis of data from a prospective database of 1772 sarcoma patients. Ann Surg. 1993;217(1):72–7.
11. Pisters PW, Leung DH, Woodruff J, Shi W, Brennan MF. Analysis of prognostic factors in 1,041 patients with localized soft tissue sarcomas of the extremities. J Clin Oncol. 1996;14(5):1679–89.
12. Singer S, Antonescu CR, Riedel E, Brennan MF. Histologic subtype and margin of resection predict pattern of recurrence and survival for retroperitoneal liposarcoma. Ann Surg. 2003;238(3):358–70.. discussion 370-1

13. American Joint Committee on Cancer 2017. AJCC cancer staging manual. 8th ed. Chicago: Springer; 2017.
14. Kattan MW, Leung DH, Brennan MF. Postoperative nomogram for 12-year sarcoma-specific death. J Clin Oncol. 2002;20(3):791–6.
15. Gronchi A, Miceli R, Shurell E, Eilber FC, Eilber FR, Anaya DA, et al. Outcome prediction in primary resected retroperitoneal soft tissue sarcoma: histology-specific overall survival and disease-free survival nomograms built on major sarcoma center data sets. J Clin Oncol. 2013;31(13):1649–55.
16. Callegaro D, Miceli R, Bonvalot S, Ferguson P, Strauss DC, Levy A, et al. Development and external validation of two nomograms to predict overall survival and occurrence of distant metastases in adults after surgical resection of localised soft-tissue sarcomas of the extremities: a retrospective analysis. Lancet Oncol. 2016;17(5):671–80.
17. Callegaro D, Miceli R, Mariani L, Raut CP, Gronchi A. Soft tissue sarcoma nomograms and their incorporation into practice. Cancer. 2017;123(15):2802–20.
18. van Praag VM, Rueten-Budde AJ, Jeys LM, Laitinen MK, Pollock R, Aston W, et al. A prediction model for treatment decisions in high-grade extremity soft-tissue sarcomas: personalised sarcoma care (PERSARC). Eur J Cancer. 2017;83:313–23.
19. Raut CP, Callegaro D, Miceli R, Barretta F, Rutkowski P, Blay JY, et al. Predicting survival in patients undergoing resection for locally recurrent retroperitoneal sarcoma: a study and novel nomogram from TARPSWG. Clin Cancer Res. 2019;25(8):2664–71.
20. EClinicalMedicine. 2019;17:100215. https://doi.org/10.1016/j.eclinm.2019.11.008. eCollection 2019 Dec. PMID: 31891146
21. Surg Oncol. 2018;27(4):695–701. https://doi.org/10.1016/j.suronc.2018.09.003. Epub 2018 Sep 7. PMID: 30449495
22. DIGITAL FOREST srl. Applestore: https://geo.itunes.apple.com/us/app/sarculator/id1052119173?mt=8 Google Play: https://play.google.com/store/apps/details?id=it.digitalforest.sarculator. Nov, 13th 2015. Accessed 16 Dec 2015.
23. PERSARC. Available at: https://www.lumc.nl/org/oncologie-centrum/patienten/ziektes-en-aandoeningen/wekedelentumor/persarc/.
24. National Comprehensive Cancer Network. Clinical practice guidelines: Soft Tissue Sarcoma (2.2019). Available at: https://www.nccn.org/professionals/physician_gls/pdf/sarcoma.pdf. Accessed 29 Apr 2019.
25. Smith MJ, Ridgway PF, Catton CN, Cannell AJ, O'Sullivan B, Mikula LA, et al. Combined management of retroperitoneal sarcoma with dose intensification radiotherapy and resection: long-term results of a prospective trial. Radiother Oncol. 2014;110(1):165–71.
26. Pawlik TM, Pisters PW, Mikula L, Feig BW, Hunt KK, Cormier JN, et al. Long-term results of two prospective trials of preoperative external beam radiotherapy for localized intermediate- or high-grade retroperitoneal soft tissue sarcoma. Ann Surg Oncol. 2006;13(4):508–17.
27. Leiting JL, Bergquist JR, Hernandez MC, Merrell KW, Folpe AL, Robinson SI, et al. Radiation therapy for retroperitoneal sarcomas: influences of histology, grade, and size. Sarcoma. 2018;2018:7972389.
28. Nussbaum DP, Rushing CN, Lane WO, Cardona DM, Kirsch DG, Peterson BL, et al. Preoperative or postoperative radiotherapy versus surgery alone for retroperitoneal sarcoma: a case-control, propensity score-matched analysis of a nationwide clinical oncology database. Lancet Oncol. 2016;17(7):966–75.
29. Baldini EH, Wang D, Haas RL, Catton CN, Indelicato DJ, Kirsch DG, et al. Treatment guidelines for preoperative radiation therapy for retroperitoneal sarcoma: preliminary consensus of an international expert panel. Int J Radiat Oncol Biol Phys. 2015;92(3):602–12.
30. Berger-Richardson D, Swallow CJ. Needle tract seeding after percutaneous biopsy of sarcoma: risk/benefit considerations. Cancer. 2017;123(4):560–7.
31. Van Houdt WJ, Schrijver AM, Cohen-Hallaleh RB, Memos N, Fotiadis N, Smith MJ, et al. Needle tract seeding following core biopsies in retroperitoneal sarcoma. Eur J Surg Oncol. 2017;43(9):1740–5.

32. Trans-Atlantic RPS Working Group. Management of primary retroperitoneal sarcoma (RPS) in the adult: a consensus approach from the Trans-Atlantic RPS Working Group. Ann Surg Oncol. 2015;22(1):256–63.
33. Ng D, Swallow CJ. Decision-making for palliative versus curative intent treatment of retroperitoneal sarcoma (RPS). Chin Clin Oncol. 2018;7(4):40.
34. Bonvalot S, Raut CP, Pollock RE, Rutkowski P, Strauss DC, Hayes AJ, et al. Technical considerations in surgery for retroperitoneal sarcomas: position paper from E-Surge, a master class in sarcoma surgery, and EORTC-STBSG. Ann Surg Oncol. 2012;19(9):2981–91.
35. Callegaro D, Fiore M, Gronchi A. Personalizing surgical margins in retroperitoneal sarcomas. Expert Rev Anticancer Ther. 2015;15(5):553–67.
36. MacNeill AJ, Gronchi A, Miceli R, Bonvalot S, Swallow CJ, Hohenberger P, et al. Postoperative morbidity after radical resection of primary retroperitoneal sarcoma: a report from the transatlantic RPS working group. Ann Surg. 2018;267(5):959–64.
37. Callegaro D, Miceli R, Brunelli C, Colombo C, Sanfilippo R, Radaelli S, et al. Long-term morbidity after multivisceral resection for retroperitoneal sarcoma. Br J Surg. 2015;102(9):1079–87.
38. Hamilton TD, Cannell AJ, Kim M, Catton CN, Blackstein ME, Dickson BC, et al. Results of resection for recurrent or residual retroperitoneal sarcoma after failed primary treatment. Ann Surg Oncol. 2017;24(1):211–8.
39. MacNeill AJ, Miceli R, Strauss DC, Bonvalot S, Hohenberger P, Van Coevorden F, et al. Post-relapse outcomes after primary extended resection of retroperitoneal sarcoma: a report from the Trans-Atlantic RPS Working Group. Cancer. 2017;123(11):1971–8.
40. Nizri E, Fiore M, Colombo C, Radaelli S, Callegaro D, Sanfilippo R, et al. Completion surgery of residual disease after primary inadequate surgery of retroperitoneal sarcomas can salvage a selected subgroup of patients-A propensity score analysis. J Surg Oncol. 2019;119(3):318–23.
41. Park JO, Qin LX, Prete FP, Antonescu C, Brennan MF, Singer S. Predicting outcome by growth rate of locally recurrent retroperitoneal liposarcoma: the one centimeter per month rule. Ann Surg. 2009;250(6):977–82.
42. Anaya DA, Lahat G, Liu J, Xing Y, Cormier JN, Pisters PW, et al. Multifocality in retroperitoneal sarcoma: a prognostic factor critical to surgical decision-making. Ann Surg. 2009;249(1):137–42.
43. Ikoma N, Roland CL, Torres KE, Chiang YJ, Wang WL, Somaiah N, et al. Salvage surgery for recurrent retroperitoneal well-differentiated liposarcoma: early reoperation may not provide benefit. Ann Surg Oncol. 2018;25(8):2193–200.
44. Trans-Atlantic Retroperitoneal Sarcoma Working Group (TARPSWG). Management of metastatic retroperitoneal sarcoma: a consensus approach from the Trans-Atlantic Retroperitoneal Sarcoma Working Group (TARPSWG). Ann Oncol. 2018;29(4):857–71.
45. Toulmonde M, Bonvalot S, Meeus P, Stoeckle E, Riou O, Isambert N, et al. Retroperitoneal sarcomas: patterns of care at diagnosis, prognostic factors and focus on main histological subtypes: a multicenter analysis of the French Sarcoma Group. Ann Oncol. 2014;25(3):735–42.
46. Blay JY, van Glabbeke M, Verweij J, van Oosterom AT, Le Cesne A, Oosterhuis JW, et al. Advanced soft-tissue sarcoma: a disease that is potentially curable for a subset of patients treated with chemotherapy. Eur J Cancer. 2003;39(1):64–9.
47. Savina M, Le Cesne A, Blay JY, Ray-Coquard I, Mir O, Toulmonde M, et al. Patterns of care and outcomes of patients with METAstatic soft tissue SARComa in a real-life setting: the METASARC observational study. BMC Med. 2017;15(1):78-017-0831-7.
48. Baumann BC, Nagda SN, Kolker JD, Levin WP, Weber KL, Berman AT, et al. Efficacy and safety of stereotactic body radiation therapy for the treatment of pulmonary metastases from sarcoma: a potential alternative to resection. J Surg Oncol. 2016;114(1):65–9.
49. Falk AT, Moureau-Zabotto L, Ouali M, Penel N, Italiano A, Bay JO, et al. Effect on survival of local ablative treatment of metastases from sarcomas: a study of the French sarcoma group. Clin Oncol (R Coll Radiol). 2015;27(1):48–55.
50. Chapiro J, Duran R, Lin M, Mungo B, Schlachter T, Schernthaner R, et al. Transarterial chemoembolization in soft-tissue sarcoma metastases to the liver - the use of imaging biomarkers as predictors of patient survival. Eur J Radiol. 2015;84(3):424–30.

51. Baratti D, Pennacchioli E, Kusamura S, Fiore M, Balestra MR, Colombo C, et al. Peritoneal sarcomatosis: is there a subset of patients who may benefit from cytoreductive surgery and hyperthermic intraperitoneal chemotherapy? Ann Surg Oncol. 2010;17(12):3220–8.
52. Lim SJ, Cormier JN, Feig BW, Mansfield PF, Benjamin RS, Griffin JR, et al. Toxicity and outcomes associated with surgical cytoreduction and hyperthermic intraperitoneal chemotherapy (HIPEC) for patients with sarcomatosis. Ann Surg Oncol. 2007;14(8):2309–18.
53. O'Sullivan B, Davis AM, Turcotte R, Bell R, Catton C, Chabot P, et al. Preoperative versus postoperative radiotherapy in soft-tissue sarcoma of the limbs: a randomised trial. Lancet. 2002;359(9325):2235–41.
54. Al-Refaie WB, Habermann EB, Jensen EH, Tuttle TM, Pisters PW, Virnig BA. Surgery alone is adequate treatment for early stage soft tissue sarcoma of the extremity. Br J Surg. 2010 May;97(5):707–13.
55. Williard WC, Hajdu SI, Casper ES, Brennan MF. Comparison of amputation with limb-sparing operations for adult soft tissue sarcoma of the extremity. Ann Surg. 1992;215(3):269–75.
56. Colombo C, Baratti D, Kusamura S, Deraco M, Gronchi A. The role of hyperthermic intraperitoneal chemotherapy (HIPEC) and isolated perfusion (ILP) interventions in sarcoma. J Surg Oncol. 2015;111(5):570–9.
57. National Comprehensive Cancer Network Clinical Practice Guidelines in Oncology (NCCN guidelines) – Bone Cancer – version 2.2019. Available at: https://www.nccn.org/professionals/physician_gls/pdf/bone.pdf. Accessed 29 Apr 2019.
58. Sarcoma Meta-analysis Collaboration (SMAC). Adjuvant chemotherapy for localised resectable soft tissue sarcoma in adults. Cochrane Database Syst Rev 2000;(4):CD001419.
59. Pervaiz N, Colterjohn N, Farrokhyar F, Tozer R, Figueredo A, Ghert M. A systematic meta-analysis of randomized controlled trials of adjuvant chemotherapy for localized resectable soft-tissue sarcoma. Cancer. 2008;113(3):573–81.
60. Woll PJ, Reichardt P, Le Cesne A, Bonvalot S, Azzarelli A, Hoekstra HJ, et al. Adjuvant chemotherapy with doxorubicin, ifosfamide, and lenograstim for resected soft-tissue sarcoma (EORTC 62931): a multicentre randomised controlled trial. Lancet Oncol. 2012;13(10):1045–54.
61. Pasquali S, Pizzamiglio S, Touati N, Litiere S, Marreaud S, Kasper B, et al. The impact of chemotherapy on survival of patients with extremity and trunk wall soft tissue sarcoma: revisiting the results of the EORTC-STBSG 62931 randomised trial. Eur J Cancer. 2019;109:51–60.
62. Gronchi A, Ferrari S, Quagliuolo V, Broto JM, Pousa AL, Grignani G, et al. Histotype-tailored neoadjuvant chemotherapy versus standard chemotherapy in patients with high-risk soft-tissue sarcomas (ISG-STS 1001): an international, open-label, randomised, controlled, phase 3, multicentre trial. Lancet Oncol. 2017;18(6):812–22.
63. J Clin Oncol. 2020;JCO1903289. https://doi.org/10.1200/JCO.19.03289. Online ahead of print. PMID: 32421444.
64. Gronchi A, Frustaci S, Mercuri M, Martin J, Lopez-Pousa A, Verderio P, et al. Short, full-dose adjuvant chemotherapy in high-risk adult soft tissue sarcomas: a randomized clinical trial from the Italian Sarcoma Group and the Spanish Sarcoma Group. J Clin Oncol. 2012;30(8):850–6.
65. Rosenberg SA, Tepper J, Glatstein E, Costa J, Baker A, Brennan M, et al. The treatment of soft-tissue sarcomas of the extremities: prospective randomized evaluations of (1) limb-sparing surgery plus radiation therapy compared with amputation and (2) the role of adjuvant chemotherapy. Ann Surg. 1982;196(3):305–15.
66. Wilson AN, Davis A, Bell RS, O'Sullivan B, Catton C, Madadi F, et al. Local control of soft tissue sarcoma of the extremity: the experience of a multidisciplinary sarcoma group with definitive surgery and radiotherapy. Eur J Cancer. 1994;30A(6):746–51.
67. McGee L, Indelicato DJ, Dagan R, Morris CG, Knapik JA, Reith JD, et al. Long-term results following postoperative radiotherapy for soft tissue sarcomas of the extremity. Int J Radiat Oncol Biol Phys. 2012;84(4):1003–9.
68. Lans TE, Grunhagen DJ, de Wilt JH, van Geel AN, Eggermont AM. Isolated limb perfusions with tumor necrosis factor and melphalan for locally recurrent soft tissue sarcoma in previously irradiated limbs. Ann Surg Oncol. 2005;12(5):406–11.

69. Billingsley KG, Burt ME, Jara E, Ginsberg RJ, Woodruff JM, Leung DH, et al. Pulmonary metastases from soft tissue sarcoma: analysis of patterns of diseases and postmetastasis survival. Ann Surg. 1999;229(5):602–10; discussion 610–2
70. van Geel AN, Pastorino U, Jauch KW, Judson IR, van Coevorden F, Buesa JM, et al. Surgical treatment of lung metastases: the European Organization for Research and Treatment of Cancer-Soft Tissue and Bone Sarcoma Group study of 255 patients. Cancer. 1996;77(4):675–82.
71. Choong PF, Pritchard DJ, Rock MG, Sim FH, Frassica FJ. Survival after pulmonary metastasectomy in soft tissue sarcoma. Prognostic factors in 214 patients. Acta Orthop Scand. 1995;66(6):561–8.
72. Chudgar NP, Brennan MF, Munhoz RR, Bucciarelli PR, Tan KS, D'Angelo SP, et al. Pulmonary metastasectomy with therapeutic intent for soft-tissue sarcoma. J Thorac Cardiovasc Surg. 2017;154(1):319–330.e1.
73. Ferguson PC, Deheshi BM, Chung P, Catton CN, O'Sullivan B, Gupta A, et al. Soft tissue sarcoma presenting with metastatic disease: outcome with primary surgical resection. Cancer. 2011;117(2):372–9.
74. Sherman KL, Kinnier CV, Farina DA, Wayne JD, Laskin WB, Agulnik M, et al. Examination of national lymph node evaluation practices for adult extremity soft tissue sarcoma. J Surg Oncol. 2014;110(6):682–8.
75. Riad S, Griffin AM, Liberman B, Blackstein ME, Catton CN, Kandel RA, et al. Lymph node metastasis in soft tissue sarcoma in an extremity. Clin Orthop Relat Res. 2004;(426):129–134.
76. Johannesmeyer D, Smith V, Cole DJ, Esnaola NF, Camp ER. The impact of lymph node disease in extremity soft-tissue sarcomas: a population-based analysis. Am J Surg. 2013;206(3):289–95.
77. Keung EZ, Chiang YJ, Voss RK, Cormier JN, Torres KE, Hunt KK, et al. Defining the incidence and clinical significance of lymph node metastasis in soft tissue sarcoma. Eur J Surg Oncol. 2018;44(1):170–7.
78. Jacobs AJ, Morris CD, Levin AS. Synovial sarcoma is not associated with a higher risk of lymph node metastasis compared with other soft tissue sarcomas. Clin Orthop Relat Res. 2018;476(3):589–98.
79. Judson I, Verweij J, Gelderblom H, Hartmann JT, Schoffski P, Blay JY, et al. Doxorubicin alone versus intensified doxorubicin plus ifosfamide for first-line treatment of advanced or metastatic soft-tissue sarcoma: a randomised controlled phase 3 trial. Lancet Oncol. 2014;15(4):415–23.
80. Tap WD, Jones RL, Van Tine BA, Chmielowski B, Elias AD, Adkins D, et al. Olaratumab and doxorubicin versus doxorubicin alone for treatment of soft-tissue sarcoma: an open-label phase 1b and randomised phase 2 trial. Lancet. 2016;388(10043):488–97.
81. Lilly report. Available at: https://investor.lilly.com/news-releases/news-release-details/lilly-reports-results-phase-3-soft-tissue-sarcoma-study. Accessed 29 Apr 2019.
82. JAMA. 2020;323(13):1266–1276. https://doi.org/10.1001/jama.2020.1707. PMID: 32259228.
83. Sebio A, Wilky BA, Keedy VL, Jones RL. The current landscape of early drug development for patients with sarcoma in the immunotherapy era. Future Oncol. 2018;14(12):1197–211.
84. D'Angelo SP, Mahoney MR, Van Tine BA, Atkins J, Milhem MM, Jahagirdar BN, et al. Nivolumab with or without ipilimumab treatment for metastatic sarcoma (Alliance A091401): two open-label, non-comparative, randomised, phase 2 trials. Lancet Oncol. 2018;19(3):416–26.
85. Tawbi HA, Burgess M, Bolejack V, Van Tine BA, Schuetze SM, Hu J, et al. Pembrolizumab in advanced soft-tissue sarcoma and bone sarcoma (SARC028): a multicentre, two-cohort, single-arm, open-label, phase 2 trial. Lancet Oncol. 2017;18(11):1493–501.
86. Robbins PF, Kassim SH, Tran TL, Crystal JS, Morgan RA, Feldman SA, et al. A pilot trial using lymphocytes genetically engineered with an NY-ESO-1-reactive T-cell receptor: long-term follow-up and correlates with response. Clin Cancer Res. 2015;21(5):1019–27.
87. Pollack SM, Lu H, Gnjatic S, Somaiah N, O'Malley RB, Jones RL, et al. First-in-human treatment with a dendritic cell-targeting lentiviral vector-expressing NY-ESO-1, LV305, induces deep, durable response in refractory metastatic synovial sarcoma patient. J Immunother. 2017;40(8):302–6.

88. Bonvalot S, Gronchi A, Le Pechoux C, Swallow CJ, Strauss DC, Meeus P, et al. STRASS (EORTC 62092): A phase III randomized study of preoperative radiotherapy plus surgery versus surgery alone for patients with retroperitoneal sarcoma. J Clin Oncol. 2019;37:15_suppl, 11001.
89. Pisters PW, Harrison LB, Leung DH, Woodruff JM, Casper ES, Brennan MF. Long-term results of a prospective randomized trial of adjuvant brachytherapy in soft tissue sarcoma. J Clin Oncol. 1996;14(3):859–68.
90. Yang JC, Chang AE, Baker AR, Sindelar WF, Danforth DN, Topalian SL, et al. Randomized prospective study of the benefit of adjuvant radiation therapy in the treatment of soft tissue sarcomas of the extremity. J Clin Oncol. 1998;16(1):197–203.

Tumors of the Thyroid Gland

25

Moska Hamidi, Karen Devon, Lorne Rotstein,
and Jesse D. Pasternak

Management of Thyroid Nodules

Background

Recent increased detection of thyroid nodules, and subsequently, thyroid cancer, has been accompanied by scrutiny in the media – suggesting that the rise is due to overdiagnosis and overtreatment of these nodules. Although up to one in seven adults will have thyroid nodules, most are asymptomatic, and fewer than 5% will be malignant [1, 2]. While the incidence of thyroid cancer has risen more than any other type of cancer (6.2% per year in males and 4.3% per year in females) [3], mortality has remained stable. Currently, it is the fifth most common cancer in Canadian women [4].

The morbidity from overtreatment of relatively indolent, or even benign lesions, may result in significant consequences for little, if any, benefit. As a result, these nodules must be appropriately assessed to optimally risk stratify patients who require further investigation and treatment (see Table 25.1).

Staging and Prognostic Scoring Schemes

1. There are several systems which have been proposed to stage and predict oncologic outcomes for differentiated thyroid cancer, including AGES [6], AMES [7], MSKCC [8], MACIS [9], Ohio State [10], EORTC (European Organization for Research on Treatment of Cancer) [11], and NTCTCS (National Thyroid Cancer Treatment Cooperative Study) [12]. We suggest the updated AJCC (American Joint Committee on Cancer) 8th edition [13].

M. Hamidi
General Surgical Oncology, University of Toronto, Toronto, ON, Canada

Department of Surgery, University of Toronto, Toronto, ON, Canada

K. Devon · L. Rotstein · J. D. Pasternak (✉)
Department of Surgery, University of Toronto, Toronto, ON, Canada
e-mail: karen.devon@wchospital.ca; lorne.rotstein@uhn.ca; Jesse.Pasternak@uhn.ca

F. C. Wright et al. (eds.), *Surgical Oncology Manual*,
https://doi.org/10.1007/978-3-030-48363-0_25

Table 25.1 High risk features for thyroid nodules [5]

Thyroid nodule risk stratification			
History	Exposure to ionizing radiation in childhood/ adolescence	Multiple first-degree relatives with thyroid cancer	Familial cancer syndromes (e.g., *MEN2, Cowden)*
Physical	Vocal cord paralysis	Cervical lymphadenopathy	Fixed nodule
US features	Large nodule (>4 cm); taller than wide	Hypoechoic, irregular borders	Contain microcalcifications
Molecular testing	Important for the clinician to understand the pretest probability of malignancy before testing	May help stratify malignancy rate, however, no test has shown cost-effectiveness in Canada	No publically available Canadian test currently

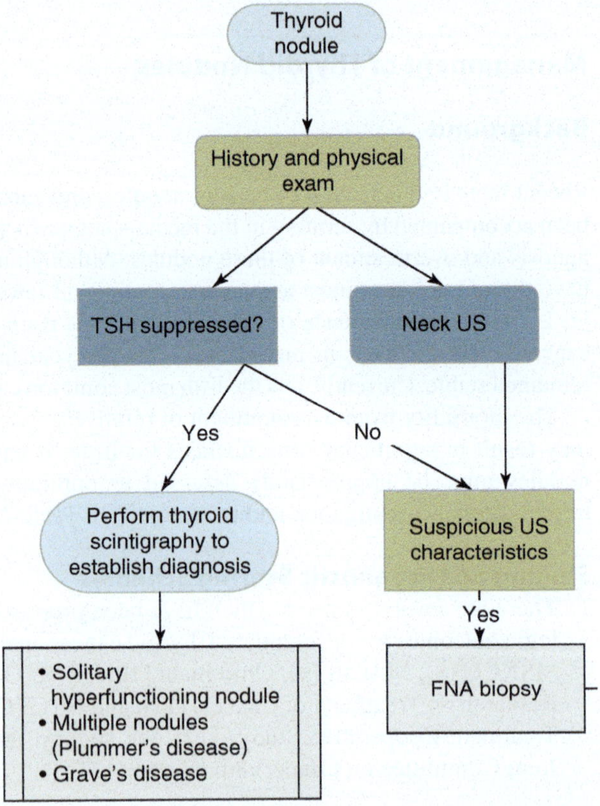

Fig. 25.1 Algorithm for work-up and management of thyroid incidentaloma

Work-Up [5]

- Any thyroid nodule should begin with a clinical evaluation (history, physical) (see Fig. 25.1).
- Routine serum thyroglobulin (Tg) or calcitonin levels for initial evaluation are not standard in Canada and have been shown to be cost-ineffective.
- FNA is the procedure of choice for diagnosis of thyroid nodules.
  - US-guided FNA has lower rates of non-diagnostic and false-negative cytology.

FNA Biopsy [5]
FNA is recommended for the following (ATA):

- Any nodule ≥2 cm
- Nodules ≥1.5 cm with a low suspicion pattern on US
- Nodules ≥1 cm with intermediate or high suspicion pattern on US

FNA Results: Bethesda Classification

- The Bethesda System for Reporting Thyroid Cytopathology was established in 2007 to eliminate the significant variability in reporting of FNA samples [5, 14] (See Fig. 25.2).
- Reports six categories with an estimation of cancer risk.
- It is very important to know the categorical risk of thyroid cancer within your institution. For Bethesda III and V, rates of thyroid cancer can be extremely variable.
- Molecular analysis can help risk stratify indeterminate nodules further*
  - Commercially available tests include Thyroseq V3 and Veracyte's Afirma mRNA gene expression classifier [15].
  - In validation tests, these have a high NPV for AUS/FLUS and FN/SFN categories.
    This reduces the risk of malignancy in these categories allowing the patient to possibly avoid surgery.
  - When pretest risk of malignancy is higher (i.e., if your center's rate of cancer is higher within these categories), this molecular test is less helpful [15].

*These tests are not commercially available in Canada

Management of Thyroid Nodule

Management of Differentiated Thyroid Cancer (DTC)

- DTC arising from epithelial cells accounts for vast majority of thyroid cancer cases.
- Rising incidence of thyroid cancer is largely due to increase in low-risk papillary thyroid cancer (PTC) (>90%) [5].
  - Especially due to increased detection of papillary thyroid microcarcinoma [PTMC] (≤1 cm) using more sensitive diagnostic studies.
  - The disease-specific mortality rates for PMTC following thyroid surgery are <1%.

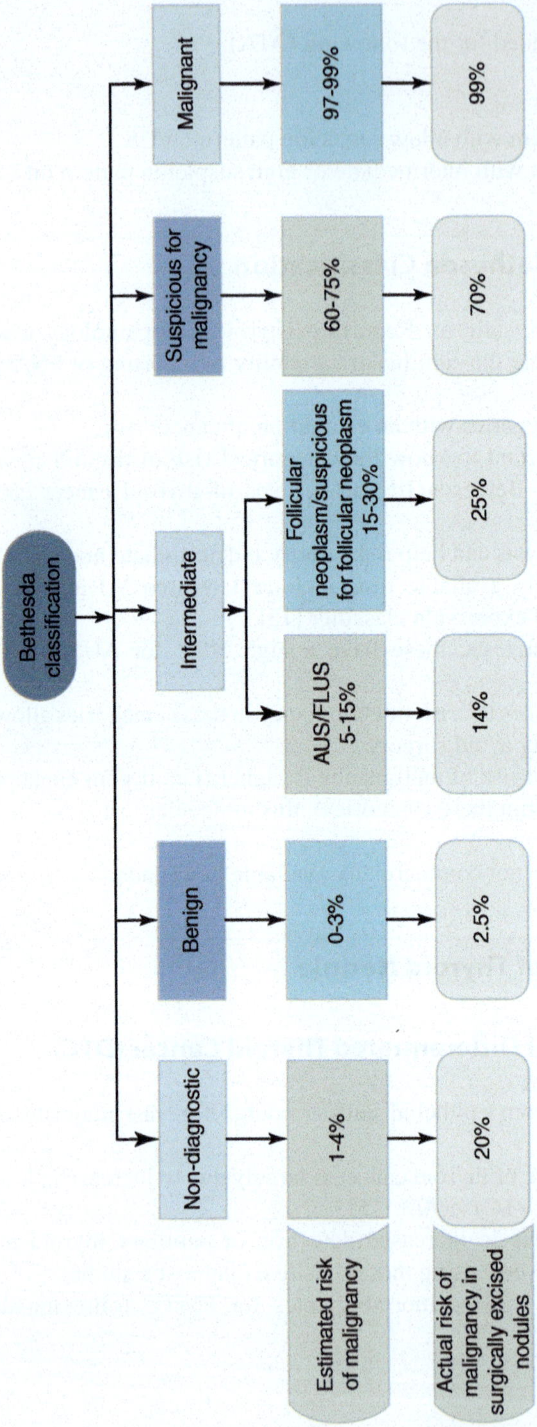

Fig. 25.2 Bethesda classification of thyroid nodule histopathology [14]

- Two prospective studies from Japan followed patients in an active surveillance program for up to 15 years and demonstrated similar clinical outcomes to surgery.
- Currently, active surveillance is offered in a clinical trial setting for patients at UHN with thyroid cancer <2 cm.
- Other rare histologic subtypes include follicular thyroid carcinoma [FTC], medullary thyroid carcinoma [MTC], and anaplastic thyroid carcinoma [ATC]

Surgical Approach [5]

- Considerable de-escalation of intervention over the past years (see Table 25.2).
  - Rarely total ablative surgery (more partial thyroidectomy).
  - Radioactive iodine ablation (RAI) and TSH suppression are adjuncts used only in higher risk patients.
- All patients should have a preoperative neck US and "lymph node mapping" to assess for cervical lymphadenopathy.
  - Cervical lymph node metastases may be present in 2/3 in the central neck and up to 50% in the lateral neck [18]; however, this is often detected in pathologic specimens and not clinically relevant.

Perioperative Considerations

- Preoperative consent should discuss risk of temporary or permanent nerve and parathyroid gland injury.
  - Complication rates for high-volume surgeons are between 7% and 14% [17].
  - Mention clinical sequelae from this, including possible voice/swallowing disability, aspiration risk, need for tracheostomy.

Table 25.2 Management after FNA cytology [5]

Lesion type	Management
Non-diagnostic	Repeat FNA (with US) after 3 months If non-diagnostic again, can observe or proceed to surgery Decision depends on US characteristics and pretest probability of malignancy (based on history and physical exam)
Benign	Consider decrease follow-up depending on ultrasound characteristics and history
AUS/FLUS	Correlate ultrasound findings Repeat FNA as needed Molecular testing can be considered If inconclusive, see above for non-diagnostic pathway
Follicular neoplasm or suspicious for FN	Consider molecular testing if available Surgery for diagnosis and therapeutics
Suspicious for malignancy or malignancy	Surgical resection or active surveillance

  - Hypoparathyroidism and need for calcium/vitamin D supplementation.
- All patients should have a preoperative voice assessment [5].
  - The incidence of preoperative vocal cord abnormalities is 0–3.5% for benign thyroid disease, up to 8% for thyroid cancer.
  - This should be both subjective description by the patient, especially of any vocal changes and objective assessment by laryngoscopy.
- Surgical approach and adjuvant therapy should be individualized to each patient and pathology (see Table 25.3).

Toronto Pearls

- Bilateral superficial cervical plexus blockade for all thyroidectomies using bupivacaine.
- The recurrent laryngeal nerve should be identified and preserved in virtually all instances.
- When the recurrent laryngeal nerve is identified, this is just the onset of the operation, which encompasses a thorough nerve dissection.
- Attempts should be made to preserve the external branch of the superior laryngeal nerve, by ligation of the superior thyroid vessels at the capsule of the thyroid gland, as well as attempted visualization.
- Parathyroid glands should, whenever possible, be identified and preserved. If the vascular supply is deemed to be compromised, the gland should be excised, biopsied, and re-implanted into muscle (i.e., sternocleidomastoid).
- We discourage any intraoperative frozen section analysis on thyroid specimens other than suspicious lymph node diagnosis.

When to Refer to Multidisciplinary Cancer Conference (MCC)

1. All medullary thyroid carcinomas
2. Complex DTC cases
3. Locally advanced DTC
4. All anaplastic thyroid carcinomas

Medullary Thyroid Cancer (MTC)

Overview

- All patients diagnosed with MTC should be screened for pheochromocytoma and referred for genetic counselling (see Table 25.4).

Table 25.3 Work-up and management of DTC [16]

Surgical treatment	Lymph node	Adjuvant treatment			Follow-up	
		Radioactive iodine (RAI)	External beam radiation (EBRT)	TSH	Initial f/u: physical exam, TSH, Tg levels, antithyroglobulin antibodies at 6 & 12 months	
Consider total thyroidectomy if any of the following: Tumor >4 cm Gross extrathyroidal extension (ETE) Regional or distant mets Poorly differentiated (NCCN) Prior radiation exposure (NCCN) High risk cytology *Hemithyroidectomy*: Tumor <4 cm No gross ETE No distant mets Micrometastatic/ low-volume lymph nodal disease	Therapeutic neck dissection of involved compartments for disease that is (NCCN): Clinically apparent Biopsy proven	*Per NCCN*: typically recommended for: Gross extrathyroidal extension Primary tumor >4 cm Postoperative unstimulated Tg >5–10 ng/mL Selectively recommended if: High-risk cytology[a] Cervical LN mets Vascular invasion	Not used routinely; use remains controversial Typically reserved for loco-regionally recurrent disease/in patients who require repeat operations for palliation (ATA)	*From ATA* *High risk*: initial TSH suppression to <0.1 mU/L *Intermediate risk*: initial TSH suppression to 0.1–0.5 mU/L then <2 mU/L *Low risk*: maintain TSH at the lower end of the reference range (0.5–2 mU/L)	*Low risk/disease free:* May extend Tg and antithyroglobulin antibody testing q12–24 months Perform TSH annually for those on hormone replacement Neck US at 6 and 12 months Repeat neck US if suspicion for recurrence	*High risk*: Repeat Neck US q6 months Depends on other factors (Tg, antithyroglobulin antibody levels etc.) Consider CT/MRI with contrast If Tg levels detectable or evidence of distant mets, perform RAI imaging q12–24 months until no response seen to RAI treatment (NCCN)

[a]Poorly differentiated, tall cell, hobnail variants

Table 25.4 Work-up and management of MTC [16]

Work-up	Surgical management of primary tumor	Lymph node management	Adjuvant therapy	Follow-up
History and physical *Laboratory Investigations* Serum calcitonin CEA Pheochromocytoma screening *Genetic/mutational evaluation* Screen for RET proto-oncogene mutations (exons 10–11, 13–16) Referral for genetic counseling *Imaging* Thyroid and neck US Consider contrast-enhanced CT neck Calcitonin levels >200 suggest metastatic disease and CT chest/abdo is indicated	Total thyroidectomy with bilateral prophylactic central neck dissection (level VI)	Consider prophylactic ipsilateral neck dissection if high-volume/gross disease in level VI or higher calcitonin levels without detectable tumor burden elsewhere	EBRT/IMRT if grossly incomplete tumor resection (and further surgical resection attempted or not possible) Use levothyroxine to normalize TSH	2–3 months postoperative Calcitonin CEA If detectable: Neck US [calcitonin] ≥150 pg/mL, cross-sectional contrast-enhanced imaging Consider bone scan when calcitonin very high *Active surveillance* Serum calcitonin, CEA q1 year If MEN2A/2B, annual screening for pheochromocytoma or hyperparathyroidism *Metastatic options* *TKI* (e.g., *Vandetenib) can be used with progressive metastatic disease and no surgical options. Good disease-free survival advantage in responders*

Special Notes

- The high risk of anesthesia and surgery in the presence of a pheochromocytoma dictates that its management takes the highest surgical priority.
- If there is co-existing hyperparathyroidism, surgical management should occur at the time of thyroidectomy.
- FMTC:
  - At least four affected relatives with MTC alone (mild and clinical variant of MEN 2A).

Table 25.5 Work-up and management of ATC [16]

Work-up	Surgical management of primary tumor	Lymph node management	Adjuvant therapy	Follow-up
History and physical *Laboratory investigations* CBC TSH *Imaging* Thyroid and neck US CT head, neck, chest, abdo/pelvis with contrast FDG PET/CT (skull base to mid-thigh) Laryngoscopy (consider bronchoscopy) *Multidisciplinary tumor board*	*Locoregional disease (Stage IVA/B)* Consider total thyroidectomy *if* resectable and not locally advanced *Metastatic disease (Stage IVC)* If aggressive therapy chosen: total thyroidectomy Palliation: radiation, surgery for lesion control	Therapeutic lymph node dissection	Stage IVA/B: R0/R1 resection: EBRT/IMRT +/− systemic therapy If R2 resection: EBRT/IMRT +/− systemic therapy Consider surgery after depending on response Use levothyroxine to normalize TSH Stage IVC: systemic therapy Consider clinical trials Molecular testing	CT/MRI brain/neck/chest/abdo/pelvis as clinically indicated Consider FDG-PET/CT 3–6 months after therapy to assess response

Anaplastic Thyroid Cancer (ATC)

Overview

- Management of anaplastic thyroid carcinoma continues to evolve as novel molecular targeting therapies develop, while surgery remains an important option when possible (see Table 25.5).

References

1. Hoang J. Understanding the risks and harms of management of incidental thyroid nodules: a review. JAMA Otolaryngol Head Neck Surg. 2017;143:718–24.
2. Cabanillas M, Mcadden D, Durante C. Thyroid cancer. Lancet. 2016;388:2783–95.

3. Canadian Cancer Society's Advisory Committee on Cancer. Canadian cancer statistics; 2014. Accessed Dec 2014. Cancer.ca.
4. Topstad D, Dickinson J. Thyroid cancer incidence in Canada: a national cancer registry analysis. CMAJ. 2017;5:612–6.
5. Haugen B, et al. 2015 ATA management guidelines for adult patients with thyroid nodules and differentiated thyroid cancer. Thyroid. 2016;26(1):1–133.
6. Hay ID, Grant CS, Taylor WF, McConahey WM. Ipsilateral lobectomy versus bilateral lobar resection in papillary thyroid carcinoma: a retrospective analysis of surgical outcome using a novel prognostic scoring system. Surgery. 1987;102:1088–95.
7. Cady B, Rossi R. An expanded view of risk-group definition in differentiated thyroid carcinoma. Surgery. 1988;104:947–53.
8. Shah JP, Loree TR, Dharker D, et al. Prognostic factors in differentiated carcinoma of the thyroid gland. Am J Surg. 1992;164:658–61.
9. Hay ID, Bergstralh EJ, Goellner JR, et al. Predicting outcome in papillary thyroid carcinoma: development of a reliable prognostic scoring system in a cohort of 1779 patients surgically treated at one institution during 1940 through 1989. Surgery. 1993;114:1050–7.
10. Mazzaferri EL, Jhiang SM. Long-term impact of initial surgical and medical therapy on papillary and follicular thyroid cancer. Am J Med. 1994;97:418–28.
11. Byar DP, Green SB, Dor P, et al. A prognostic index for thyroid carcinoma. A study of the E.O.R.T.C. Thyroid Cancer Cooperative Group. Eur J Cancer. 1979;15:1033–41.
12. Sherman SI, Brierley JD, Sperling M, et al. Prospective multicenter study of thyroid carcinoma treatment: initial analysis of staging and outcome. National Thyroid Cancer Treatment Cooperative Study Registry Group. Cancer. 1998;83(5):1012–21. https://doi.org/10.1002/(sici)1097-0142(19980901)83:5<1012:aid-cncr28>3.0.co;2-9.
13. Amin M, Edge S, Green F, et al. AJCC cancer staging manual. 8th ed. New York: Springer; 2017.
14. Crippa S, Mazzucchelli L, Cibas ES, Ali SZ. The Bethesda System for reporting thyroid fine-needle aspiration specimens. Am J Clin Pathol. 2010;134:343–4.
15. Nishino M. Molecular cytopathology for thyroid nodules: a review of methodology and test performance. Cancer Cytopathol. 2016;124:14–27.
16. National Comprehensive Cancer Network. Thyroid cancer (version 3.2018). https://www.nccn.org/professionals/physician_gls/pdf/thyroid.pdf. Accessed 20 Jan 2019.
17. Hauch A, Al-Qurayshi Z, Randolph G, Kandil E. Total thyroidectomy is associated with increased risk of complications for low- and high-volume surgeons. Ann Surg Oncol. 2014;21:3844–52.
18. Wada N, Suganuma N, Nakayama H, et al. Microscopic regional lymph node status in papillary thyroid carcinoma with and without lymphadenopathy and its relation to outcomes. Langenbecks Arch Surg. 2007;392:417–22.

Index

F. C. Wright et al. (eds.), *Surgical Oncology Manual*,
https://doi.org/10.1007/978-3-030-48363-0

C

Q

R

The manufacturer's authorised representative in the EU is Springer Nature Customer Service Centre GmbH, Europaplatz 3, 69115 Heidelberg, Germany. If you have any concerns regarding our products, please contact ProductSafety@springernature.com

Printed and bound by CPI Group (UK) Ltd, Croydon, CR0 4YY
30/09/2026
02225587-0011